Sixty-One Years of University of Michigan Pharmacology 1942-2003

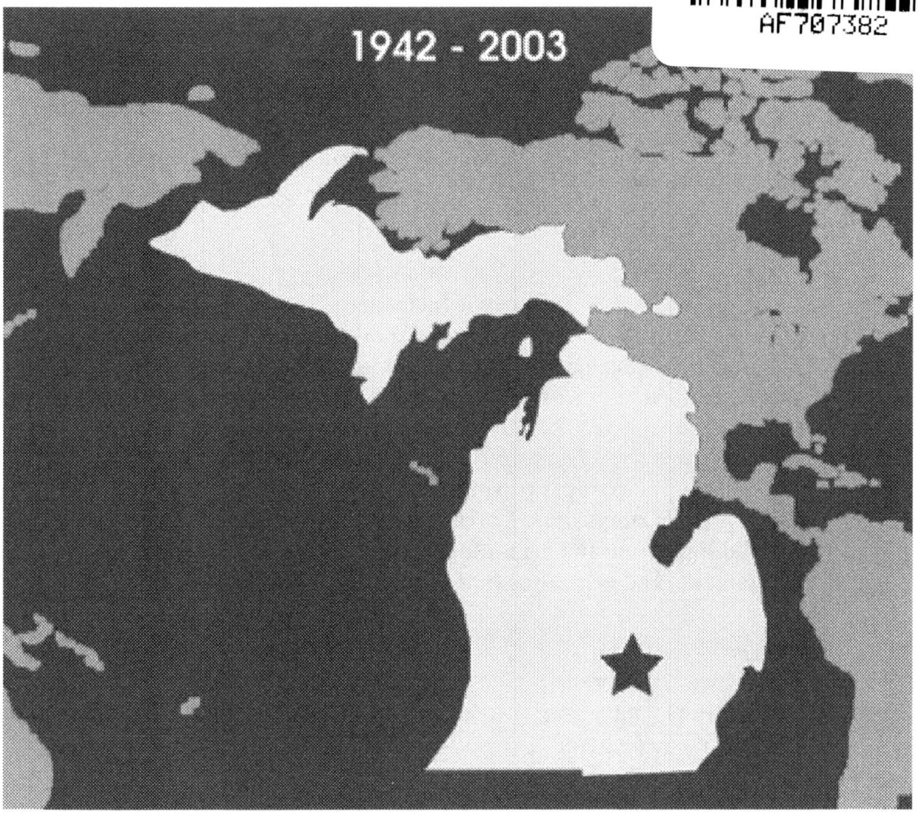

Edward F. Domino, M.D.
Editor

NPP Books
Ann Arbor, Michigan, USA

Publisher:

NPP Books, P.O. Box 1491 Ann Arbor, MI 48106, USA

Printed in the United States of America

International Standard Book Number: 0-916182-13-4
(previously ISBN: 0-916182-12-6)

Library of Congress Control Number: 2003115120

Acknowledgements

This version, prepared in a yearbook format, is the result of the efforts of many people over a seven-year period. The authors of the various contributions are named at the beginning of the written texts and photographs. The initial efforts of Ellen Howard, Linda Ohl, and near the end, Li Ni, Jin Wei (Jane) Ni and Valerie Burnisky allowed this task to proceed to completion.

Wordprocessing by: Kari Fedewa
Compositor: Christopher R. Buchanan
Copy Editing (from the beginning to the very end) by: Jaime Noce
Comments and criticisms (not always heeded by the editor):

Dr. David A. Bloom
Dr. Horace Davenport
Edward B. Goldman Esq.
Dr. Paul F. Hollenberg
Dr. Benedict Lucchesi
Dr. Howard Markel
Dr. Alexandra Stern
Dr. Henry Swain

Dedication

This book is dedicated to the students and staff, academic and nonacademic, past, present, and future, of a remarkable and occasionally a very controversial Department. This is their story, told by those who documented their thoughts and memories.

A special thanks to my wife, Antoinette E Domino, owner and publisher of NPP Books. She provided the impetus, encouragement, and insistence that this project be completed. She was to be the associate editor until she lost her courageous struggle with cancer over two years ago. It was her wish that this volume be the appropriate sequel to Japanese Michigan Fellows in Pharmacology. Toni, I hope you approve of what I have done.

University of Michigan Medical School Center for the History of Medicine Monograph Series No. 8

Preface

As noted above the motto "•artes•scientia•veritas•" is a prominent part of the seal of the University of Michigan. In the center of the seal, on top of a book, is an oil lamp with a flame, symbolizing the presence of light of knowledge where previously there was darkness. The task of combining art, science, and truth is not always easy. Universities, schools, and departments exist primarily to teach. Most of us pay lip service to this task and then concentrate on scientific research in which students are an important, though frequently exploited, resource. In the process of teaching and mentoring, the professor frequently learns far more from the student than he or she gives to the student. Graduate students and fellows need a home with which to identify— a home which a department provides. Administrative, research, and teaching functions all intermingle, requiring the art of communication among department members. Speaking or writing the truth is a virtue that requires great diplomacy in not offending one's colleagues and maintaining some harmony among all. May this volume attempt to come close to describing only some of what has gone on in our Department since the early 1940s while not offending those with totally different recollections.

This book begins with the year 1942, the start of World War II. After the death of Charles W. Edmunds in 1941, Dean Furstenburg of the Medical School appointed a committee to recommend his successor. Maurice H. Seevers was selected. The Department of Materia Medica and Therapeutics became the Department of Pharmacology with the appointment of Seevers as chairman.

Horace W. Davenport's "Fifty Years of Medicine at the University of Michigan 1891-1941," published in 1986 and enlarged and updated in more detail as "Not Just Any Medical School — The Science, Practice, and Teaching of Medicine at the University of Michigan, 1850-1941" published by The University of Michigan Press in 1999 is an excellent source of information. Horace Davenport's Chapter 8 "Materia Medica and Therapeutics, Pharmacology" must be read. On page 89 Davenport summarizes the Search Committee's report that Seevers "was the best of a long list of candidates, but there were problems...[he] had not made a favorable impression on some when he visited Ann Arbor, and there was the possibility that he would display too great aggressiveness... [however] the job was offered to Seevers. He accepted." Although the Committee's concerns were his aggressiveness in who would manage clinical anesthesia, there is no question that the Dean and the Medical School hired a "go-getter."

"The University of Michigan — One Hundred Years of Pharmacology" by Henry H. Swain is another source of departmental history. "The Japanese Michigan Fellows in Pharmacology: 50 Years of Cooperation," edited by myself and Tomoji Yanagita, became available in 1999. The latter describes the Department's connection to post World War II Japanese Pharmacologists in detail. That book was published by my wife's company NPP Books here in Ann Arbor. The book was made available to all members of the Japanese Pharmacological Society.

The present text is a volume, in a yearbook style, with some of the history of the Department since 1942 by many of the people involved.

It is not intended to be a definitive history of all the departmental events in the past 62 years. Rather it is to be a pleasant trip down memory lane. Not all members of our faculty and staff chose to contribute in this style. It is up to others to publish their memories of controversies and departmental failings.

Whenever possible, a chronological then alphabetical organization has been followed. Because I've been a member of our Department for 51 plus years, I thought it important to record the thoughts and memories of those associated with these remarkable events. This effort is a collaboration between all those who wished to tell their more pleasant stories, in few or many words, of their time at Michigan, and how it has affected their lives.

This yearbook took a very long time to prepare even in its present incomplete form. Many were contacted and asked to contribute. Some, due to personal wishes, or because of their time constraints, or unwillingness declined. To those whose recollections are not in this volume, I acknowledge with regret the absence of their comments and memories.

Edward F. Domino, M.D.
May 3, 2004
Ann Arbor, MI

Contents

Section II. Notable Departmental Events

Section III. Reflections of Staff and Students

Section V. The Future of Pharmacology

1

The Years of Maurice H. Seevers, M.D., Ph.D., 1942-1971

Glenn F. Kiplinger, M.D., Ph.D.

Editor's note: Dr. Seevers died on April 20, 1977 and is the only chairman who is unable to provide (in this volume) his thoughts on how he ran the Department and what he accomplished. Fortunately, the following are excerpts written by his students and friends reprinted, with permission, from the University of Michigan Medical Center Journal, 36:(4), Oct.-Dec., 1970.

Maurice Harrison Seevers was born in Topeka, Kansas, October 3, 1901. He received his A. B. degree at Washburn College in 1924 and continued his studies in the graduate school of the University of Chicago where Dr. A. L. Tatum was resident pharmacologist in a combined Department of Pharmacology and Physiological Chemistry. Thus began an association with Dr. Tatum which continued to 1942 when Dr. Seevers accepted the Chair in Pharmacology at the University of Michigan.

Dr. Seevers was granted his Ph.D. degree in 1928 from the University of Chicago. During 1929, while a medical student at Rush Medical School, he served as Instructor in pharmacology at Loyola University in Chicago, filling a need in this department following the death of Dr. Samuel Mathews in 1928. It is of interest to pharmacologists of the University of Michigan that Mathews was a founding member of the American Society for Pharmacology and Experimental Therapeutics (ASPET), and a Michigan graduate in medicine.

After receiving the M.D. degree from Rush Medical School in 1930, Dr. Seevers moved to the University of Wisconsin where he simultaneously assumed the duties of Assistant Professor of Pharmacology and intern. Dr. Tatum had moved to Wisconsin in 1928 and had assumed the chairmanship of that department in 1929 after the death of Dr. A. S. Loevenhardt, another ASPET founder.

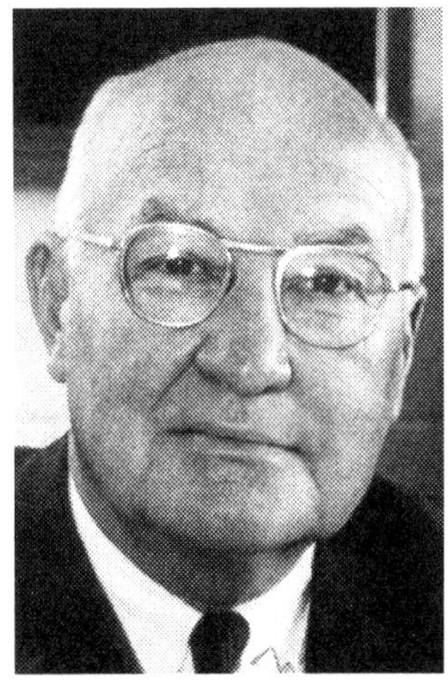

It was at the University of Wisconsin that Dr. M. Seevers came to pharmacological prominence in the fields of anesthesiology and drug dependence. He also married while at Wisconsin in 1936. He and the former Frances Hebl had a daughter (Pamela) and a son (Giles). Mrs. Seevers was well known to former Michigan pharmacologists and visitors to Ann Arbor for her gracious hospitality and her continuing interest in their careers.

In 1930 Dr. Seevers was elected to membership in ASPET at a time when dues were $2 per year and the annual budget of the Society included a $10 contribution to the FASEB Placement Service. His service at the University of Wisconsin included four years as Assistant Professor and a promotion to Associate Professor in 1934. He held this position until 1942 when he became Professor and Chairman of the Department of Pharmacology at the University of Michigan, inheriting the mantle of Abel, Cushny, and Edmunds. He continued to hold this position in 1971, the fourth chairman of the oldest pharmacology department in the United States.

Dr. Seevers' contributions to ASPET are too numerous to detail; however, a few stand out as worthy of mention. In 1937 he was elected councilor. In 1939 Seevers and Tatum jointly approached the Council with suggestions regarding society publications. Tatum suggested a board of trustees for publications and Seevers recommended that more experimental therapeutics be included in the official journal (fully implemented in 1967 when Clinical Pharmacology and Therapeutics became an official organ of the society). It was during his tenure as president of the Society (1946-48) that the Board of Publications Trustees was established, and he served as chairman of that board from 1949-1961.

Dr. Seevers was president of ASPET for two years, presiding at the annual meetings of 1947 and 1948 and serving as chairman of the FASEB Executive Committee in 1948. Dr. Seevers succeeded Dr. Erwin Nelson as president of ASPET; Nelson was a Michigan graduate in medicine who had served as Assistant Professor to C.W. Edmunds while at Michigan. The period of the thirties and forties were times of storm and crisis in pharmacology. Dr. Seevers has written, "It was easy in 1939 for the writer [Seevers] to portray why he contemplated deserting pharmacology for a more promising field. Survival of the subject as an independent discipline was at stake." And Seevers helped to preserve it.

His dedication and service to pharmacology has brought many honors to Dr. Seevers. Dr. K. K. Chen, a former president and official historian of ASPET , writes in ASPET: The First Sixty Years, 1908-1969:

Seevers is an authority on anesthesiology, drug addiction and tolerance, and respiratory physiology. He is a member of APS, SEBM, AMA, and Central Society for Clinical Research. His services to societies and governments range far and wide: Chairman, Section of Experimental Medicine and Therapeutics (1952-53); Council on Pharmacy and Chemistry and the Council on Drugs (1952-62); Committee on Alcoholism and Dependence (1964-70); and Chairman, Committee on Tobacco and Health, AMA (1964-70); Board of Scientific Councilors, National Heart Institute; Surgeon-General's Committee on Smoking and Health, Department of Health, Education and Welfare (1962-63); Chairman, Committee on Behavior Pharmacology, Psychopharmacology Service Center (1964); and American Coordinator, U.S.-Japan Cooperative Science Program on Drug Abuse, National Science Foundation-Japan Science Council (1964-70), Internationally he is a member of the Expert Advisory Panel of Drugs Liable to Produce Addiction, WHO (United Nations) (1951-70); Second Medical Mission to Japan (1951); U.S. National Committee of International Union of Physiological Sciences (IUPS) (1955-59); Chairman, American Team, Conference on Physiological and Pharmacological Basis of Anesthesiology, Japan (1956); Consultant to Minister of Public Health, Thailand (1959); and Consultant to Minister of Health and Welfare, Japan (1963-1970). He was a member of the Editorial Board of Physiological Reviews (1934-1951) and Proceedings of the Society for Experimental Biology and Medicine (1944-59); and was on the Editorial Committee of the Annual Review of Pharmacology (1952-62). He was responsible for the establishment of the Board of Publications Trustees (BPT) of ASPET in 1948 and was its Chairman from 1949 to 1961. He was decorated with the Third Class of the Order of the Rising Sun (1963) and the Second Class of the Order of the Sacred Treasure (1967) in Japan. He received the Distinguished Service Award of the Washburn Alumni Association in 1964, and he was selected Russell Lecturer, University of Michigan in 1967, and Dent Memorial Lecturer, Kings College, University of London, in 1968.

Dr. Seevers' broad vision continues. His students serve in academic institutions, pharmaceutical companies, government agencies and laboratories, and other institutions. Years after leaving the Michigan campus, graduates and former staff members can be heard to say, "I wonder what 'The Boss' thinks about that?"

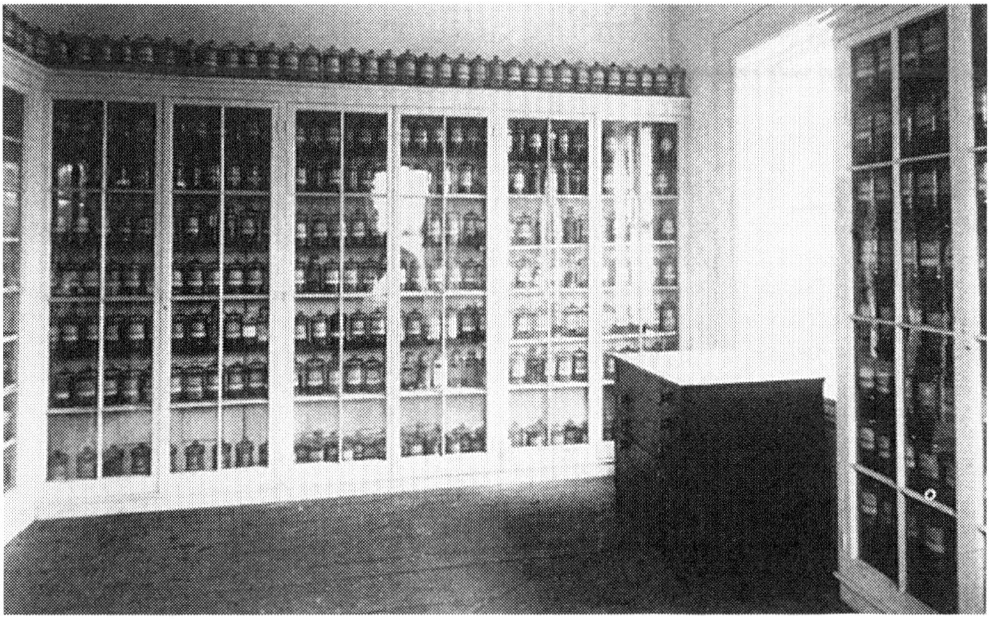

This old materia medica collection from the late 1890s survived via Drs. Abel, Cushny, and Edmunds into the early 1940s. It was then inherited by Dr. Seevers with the challenge to modernize the Department of Pharmacology. The old department title of Materia Medica and Therapeutics was dropped in February, 1942.

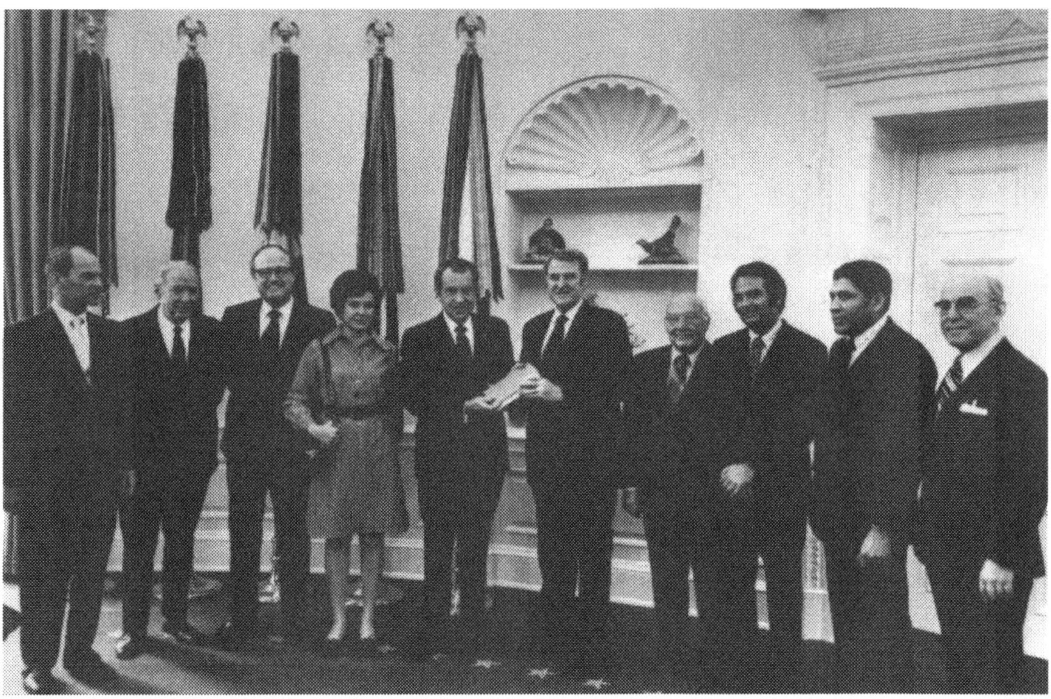

President Nixon officially recognizing members of the Commission on Marijuana and Drug Abuse in 1971. Dr. Seevers was also a member of the Surgeon General's Advisory Committee on Smoking and Health which resulted in the 1964 report that cited chronic tobacco smoking as a cause of lung cancer.

Excerpts from the Seevers Symposium May 28-29, 1970, Ann Arbor, Michigan

After years of service and devotion to pharmacology and to his university, Maurice Harrison Seevers, Professor and Chairman of the Department of Pharmacology, University of Michigan, contemplates retirement. We have prepared this special supplement to The University of Michigan Medical Center Journal [36:(4) Oct.-Dec., 1970 part 2] as an indelible record of appreciation from his students and associates. It contains scientific articles presented at the "Seevers Symposium," held in Ann Arbor, May 28-29, 1970. Reprinted with permission.

the university of michigan

MEDICAL CENTER JOURNAL

SEEVERS SYMPOSIUM
MAY 28-29, 1970
ANN ARBOR, MICHIGAN

Opening Remarks

*Nathan B. Eddy, M.D.**

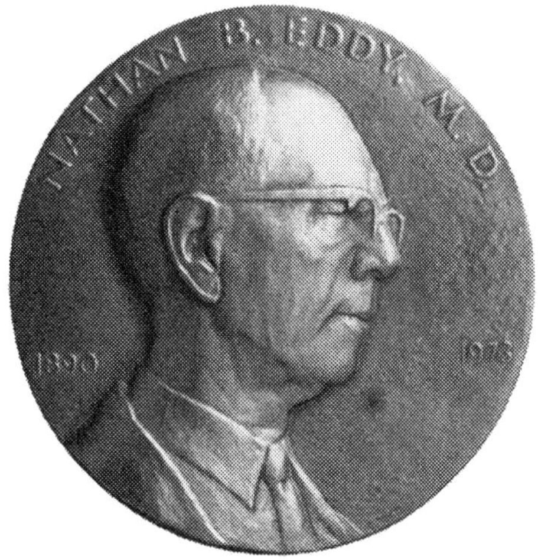

I am indeed honored to be invited to make some comments at the opening of the Maurice H. Seevers Testimonial Symposium. I am undoubtedly among the oldest in years of acquaintance with Dr. Seevers though I cannot remember when we first met. Reminiscing yesterday, Dr. Seevers and I concluded that it might have been in Montreal in 1930. I do know that our association, personal and professional, developed after he came to Ann Arbor and particularly after we both became members of the National Research Council Committee on Drug Addiction and Narcotics in 1948.

Through the years Dr. Seevers has responded most generously to demands upon his knowledge and experience to assist in a wide variety of pharmacological problems, and this has taken him away from Ann Arbor many times. One wondered how he managed to run the department. Perhaps he knew the secret of perpetual motion or had built such a well-oiled, smoothly running machine that it needed little attention. I think he had also learned early that departments are run by the boss' administrative assistant, and, when he has picked the right one, it doesn't matter much if he is there or not.

At home and abroad, Dr. Seevers has given much thought, intensive and constructive, to mechanisms of action and has shared his thinking freely to stimulate research approaches. Dr. Seevers has shared in the formulation of many policy statements and has contributed to innumerable scientific documents; but I think he dislikes to meet a deadline, perhaps partly because he has so many irons in the fire but particularly because of his desire for rightness in the written word.

Dr. Seevers had promised for about ten years, it seems, to get on paper a detailed account of the tolerance and dependence studies which have been going on at the University of Michigan so long. He told Dr. May recently that this is to be the first task in his retirement. However, if his experience of demands on his time in retirement is anything like mine, we will probably wait another ten years, though the invited speakers this morning are going to provide him with a good background and added incentive.

The only time Dr. Seevers and I ever exchanged sharp words had to do with a deadline. We were members of a World Health Organization study group on drug dependence. I happened to be chairman and Dr. Seevers was asked to head a subcommittee to write a description of the concept of dependence. We gave them a free day and I waited a little longer for their statement. Then I chided Dr. Seevers on the delay; we had only a week and we had to approve the statement for our report. In his usual forceful language, Dr. Seevers said that maybe we would get the statement and maybe we wouldn't; it had to be right. He came through in time, as always with a beautiful piece of work.

*Deceased

The interest of Dr. Seevers and myself in the same field covers about the same span of years. Each of us has been intrigued by the multiple elements in the action of morphine and related substances, particularly the phenomena and mechanism of tolerance and dependence and each of us began an experimental approach in the 1920s. I was research professor of pharmacology at Michigan from 1930 to 1939 and was responsible for the pharmacological part of a coordinated attack upon the drug addiction problem under the auspices of the National Research Council. Thus perhaps I had some part in the establishment of the reputation of the Michigan Department of Pharmacology as a research center in the narcotics field.

When Dr. Seevers came to Michigan in 1942 he brought with him, of course, his basic interest, paralleling the activity which had been going on in the department throughout the preceding decade. It was not, however, until the late 1940s that this interest came to the fore, when Dr. Seevers initiated a research program which has occupied a major portion, I would think 60 or 70 percent, of the time and effort of the staff and the department's many graduate students ever since.

Dr. Seevers conceived the idea of using the monkey as the primary research tool and undertook to explore the response of the monkey to morphine and related substances in comparison with the responses of man to the same agents. It is almost incidental that this exploration led to the development of a world-recognized regimen for screening agents for morphine-like physical dependence capacity and that this became a service operated through the Research Council Committee. The department staff have taken advantage of the establishment of his program for intensive research on structure-action relationships of agonist-antagonist agents; on site and mechanism of action; and on tissue distribution, metabolism, and excretion of morphine-like agents. They continue to be willing to furnish this invaluable screening service for the simultaneously available research opportunities. The screening program, too, which is done on a double-blind basis (for both Dr. Seevers and the chemists who provided the drugs), is research oriented since new activities of new compounds require constant alertness and constructive thinking to display and evaluate new profiles of action.

Through 40 years, 30 of which were under the guidance of Dr. Seevers, the Department of Pharmacology of the University of Michigan has built up an enviable reputation in narcotics research along many lines unsurpassed by any other laboratory in the world. The screening program alone is of vital interest to industry, clinical medicine, law enforcement, and public health, and it would be a major calamity if it does not continue.

The passage of time and the scheme of things make retirement inevitable for Dr. Seevers as well as for the rest of us. Our consolation is that he approaches his retirement with such vigor and lively interest across a very broad field. We look forward to having him around for a long time and to continuing to draw upon his counsel and experience.

Editor's note: Charles Edmunds recruited Nathan Browne Eddy to the Pharmacology Department. Eddy was born in 1890 in Glen Falls, New York. In 1911, Eddy received his M.D. from Cornell University. He practiced medicine in New York City for five years and, in 1916, taught physiology at McGill University. Eddy worked in Robert Gesell's laboratory during the summers of 1928 and 1929 here at Michigan.

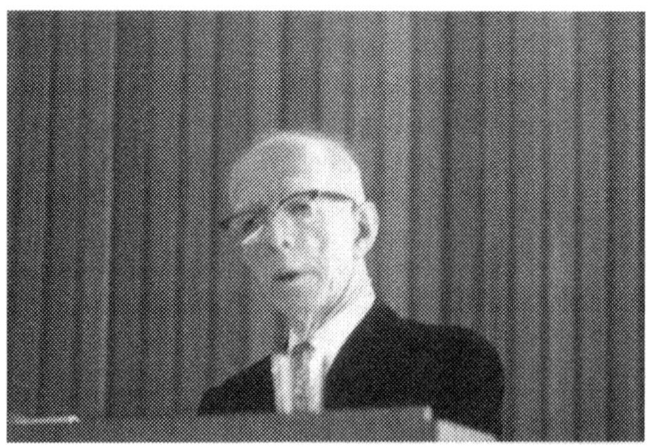

Nathan Eddy speaking at the Seevers' Symposium.

The Monkey Colony in Studies of Tolerance and Dependence

*Gerald A. Deneau, Ph.D.**

The account of the monkey colony in studies of tolerance and dependence begins in the spring of 1925 at the University of Chicago. Young Maurice Seevers had finished his undergraduate work at Washburn College in 1924 and then decided to go to the University of Chicago to study medicine. He found it desirable first of all, however, to take additional courses in physics and organic chemistry, which he did in the fall of 1924. Thus having to wait for several months before the next medical class was admitted, he took an elective course in pharmacology from Dr. A. L. Tatum in the spring of 1925. The class was small—about ten students—and Seevers quickly became fascinated with the subject matter. A mutual respect rapidly developed between teacher and student, with the result that Professor Tatum invited young Seevers to become his laboratory assistant.

Dr. Tatum was then an Associate Professor in the Department of Physiological Chemistry and Pharmacology, which was chaired by Professor F. C. Coke. The department was housed in what was then the Hall Physiological Laboratories. The personnel of the department included Dr. Tatum; Ken Collins, a graduate student; and Maurice Seevers, the laboratory assistant.

In its physical layout, the department where the studies on morphine dependence began, consisted of a combined laboratory and animal room approximately 20 x 30 feet in size. To one end, and adjoining the laboratory, was Professor Tatum's office, a room about 10 x 20 feet. Seevers' assignment was to inject dogs and monkeys with morphine. The dogs were tied to table legs in the laboratory, and the monkey cages were located in Tatum's office. When the professor leaned back in his chair, the monkeys could groom his hair. Besides his personal library, Dr. Tatum had a materia medica collection in his office-until one night when the monkeys got loose; hardly a jar was left unbroken.

In the fall of 1925 a new building was completed, and the Department of Pharmacology occupied the entire fifth floor. Ralph Smith, Ross McIntyre, and W. E. Gower also joined the department at that time. Harry Van Dyke came as a full professor in the fall of 1927.

The first report of the morphine dependence studies was an abstract of a paper given at the fall pharmacology meetings in 1926. Hints of the forthcoming "dual-action" theory are evident in that abstract. Dr. Seevers completed his Ph.D. in 1928. For his thesis work he made a comparative analysis of the use of several laboratory species in the study of morphine dependence and concluded that the monkey was the species of choice. He also found the dog to be the species of choice for studying barbiturate dependence. Many others have since agreed with these conclusions.

In 1928 Dr. Tatum moved to the University of Wisconsin. Dr. Seevers spent the next two years completing his medical studies at Rush Medical School and then moved to Wisconsin at the invitation of Dr. Tatum. At this time Seevers had a four-year medical certificate—the full degree was not to be conferred until a year's internship was completed. In order to be active in the Pharmacology Department during the academic year, he arranged to do his internship in three summer sessions. His work with Dr. Ralph Waters in anesthesiology during these internship sessions led to another fascinating and productive aspect of Dr. Seevers' career.

The first use of the monkey to test the

*Deceased

dependence capacity of an unknown narcotic analgesic occurred in 1933. A morphine derivative that was developed in Germany was tested by Seevers and was found to be morphine-like in its dependence capacity. A year or two later it was suggested that dilaudid, which is more potent than morphine as an analgesic, might be less addicting than morphine. Seevers did a comparative study of dilaudid, morphine, heroin, and codeine in the monkey; this study led to two classic papers on methods for studying opiate addiction in the monkey and the classification of morphine-like abstinence. This research served as the basis for all subsequent studies of narcotic dependence in monkeys.

In the late twenties and early thirties, although quite independently from Tatum and Seevers, Kolb and DuMez also studied opiate dependence in monkeys. Their work naturally varied in minor details from that of Seevers, but their general conclusions were remarkably similar. Dr. Nathan Eddy also used the monkey to study tolerance and dependence to desomorphine while he was a Research Professor here at Michigan during the thirties.

During the latter half of the thirties, Dr. Seevers' interests became directed more toward anesthesiology, with the result that he had little time to continue his studies of narcotic dependence in monkeys. When he came to Michigan as Chairman of the Department of Pharmacology in 1942, his many duties prevented a resumption of these studies for a few more years. He did have a monkey colony, however, for the purpose of studying the toxicity of promising antimalarial drugs. Among the drugs that excited Dr. Gordon K. Moe and Dr. Seevers the most were some 8-aminoquinoline derivatives which produced brain lesions resulting in a central sympathectomy.

From 1929 until 1941, the National Research Council's Committee on Drug Addiction directed a monumental cooperative research program aimed at finding a nonaddicting analgesic drug. Under this program, hundreds of drugs were synthesized by the late Dr. Lyndon Small at the University of Virginia and were evaluated pharmacologically by Dr. Eddy here at Michigan. The more promising drugs were then evaluated for addiction liability in man through the cooperation of the Division of Mental Hygiene of the United States Public Health Service. These studies were conducted at Fort Leavenworth, Kansas, and Lexington, Kentucky. Himmelsbach, Kolb, Isbell, Wikler, and Fraser made important contributions in the development of this area of clinical research.

The National Research Council's efforts were curtailed during World War II, but the Committee on Drug Addiction was revived in 1947. By that time, two new chemical classes of analgesics were available, the meperidine and methadone series. Efforts to separate chemically the desirable properties of these drugs from their undesirable properties resulted in the production of so many derivatives that the available clinical facilities for testing addiction liability at Lexington were swamped. There was a clear need for developing a preclinical technique to evaluate the addictive properties of these new drugs. Because of his classical work with opiate derivatives, Dr. Seevers suggested to the committee that he evaluate the monkey as a subject for preclinical prediction of the physical dependence properties of the new synthetic analgesic drugs. Seevers and his graduate student, Samuel Irwin, began these studies in 1950.

Irwin demonstrated that the monkey did indeed develop physical dependence to such synthetic analgesics as racemorphan, methadone, l-isomethadone and alpha-acetylmethadol, and ketobemidone. He applied a modification of the Himmelsbach point-score system to Seevers' classification of abstinence signs, and his eight-grade scale for determining the abstinence severity is still valid. Cross-tolerance and cross-dependence among the several chemical classes of narcotic analgesics were also clearly demonstrated. One of the most exciting aspects of Irwin's work was his study of the antagonist, N-allylnormorphine (nalorphine). He demonstrated that it would antagonize the depressant effects of all classes of narcotic analgesics and that it would precipitate abstinence signs, which were comparable in severity to those that resulted from abrupt withdrawal of the drug. Thus, with nalorphine it was possible to learn in a few hours what would otherwise require round-the-clock observations for several days.

I was fortunate to be on the scene at the time that Sam Irwin graduated and began to work with the monkeys after most of the housing and care problems had been worked out. We continued to study primary physical dependence to drugs such as codeine and found that the monkey responded to many agents qualitatively the same as man, provided the drugs were administered frequently enough to keep the animals under continuous drug effect. Dr. Eddy helped immensely by providing drugs under code number. He chose a sufficiently wide variety of agents to demonstrate conclusively that the monkey was indeed a suitable subject for the preclinical evaluation of physical dependence capacity of narcotic analgesics.

Duncan McCarthy joined us in 1956 as a graduate student. He demonstrated that the precipitation of morphine abstinence signs by nalorphine was a dose-related response, which indicated a competitive antagonism. Relevant to this was the demonstration that the greater the level of physical dependence to morphine, the greater is the animal's sensitivity to nalorphine. McCarthy also showed that chronic interference with centrally acting sympathetic and parasympathetic agents did not interfere in a major way with the development of physical dependence to morphine. This implies that the mechanisms underlying the development of physical dependence to morphine involve pathways other than those utilizing catecholamines, serotonin, or acetylcholine.

Since the early recognition of the dangers of cocaine, it has been realized that drugs which do not produce physical dependence can have great abuse potential. The common factors in all forms of drug abuse are the development of psychological dependence on an agent and the behavioral or psychotoxicity which results from excessive self-administration of the drug. Spurred by Weeks' success in the development of chronic intravenous catheter systems in the rat, a method for determining psychological dependence in monkeys with chronic indwelling catheters was developed during the early sixties, with the collaboration of Dr. Tomoji Yanagita.

A series of postdoctoral fellows stimulated much thought and contributed much effort in the general areas of tolerance and dependence studies. Among these were Dr. Shuji Takaori, who made a detailed study of electroencephalographic and neuroexcitatory phenomena in the monkey as influenced by a cycle of morphine addiction as well as by several other classes of centrally acting drugs. Dr. Yoshio Ikeda and Dr. Kiro Shimamoto demonstrated the competitive nature of nalorphine antagonism using the Straub tail phenomenon in mice. Dr. Kengo Nakai studied the influence of route of administration of meperidine on its subsequent biotransformation and demonstrated that quantitative differences in metabolic disposition depended upon the route of administration and influenced the nature of the toxic effects of meperidine. Dr. Reizo Inoki demonstrated tolerance development and psychological dependence to nicotine in the monkey. Dr. Shoichi Iida demonstrated the suitability of the monkey as a laboratory subject for studying alcoholism. Dr. Atmakasuma extended the observational technique which is used for grading abstinence syndromes into a system for describing the activity profile of any centrally acting drug in the monkey. Dr. Salamuddin Weiss made further studies of barbiturate dependence in dogs and developed a substitution technique for determining barbiturate-like physical dependence capacity.

None of these studies would have been possible without the strong support and advice of Dr. Seevers and the many contributions of other departmental members in the office, the stockroom, and the shop. It was a great pleasure and privilege for me to have spent 13 years studying tolerance, dependence, and related phenomena in the monkey at the University of Michigan.

Commentary

*Duncan A. McCarthy, Ph.D.**

I wish to express my sincere appreciation to Dr. Seevers and to the Department of Pharmacology at the University of Michigan for providing me with the opportunity for graduate education and research. I consider myself exceptionally fortunate in having worked with Drs. Seevers and Deneau, as well as others on the staff, at the end of the era in the old building and at the beginning of the new one in the new Medical Sciences Building I. I shall not forget the many ways my life was enriched by these years at Michigan, and the friendships and associations established within the department and with Dr. Eddy and others who played their various roles in the Committee on Drug Addiction and Narcotics, as it was then called.

There is little that can be added to the fine resume Dr. Deneau has presented. He has summarized the highlights of the use of the monkey in addiction and physical dependence studies. Out of modesty perhaps, he has understated the importance of his own work in the total endeavor. He did, however, make the point that, for 40 years now, the Department of Pharmacology of the University of Michigan has been a center for animal studies on the intricate inter-relationships that comprise tolerance and physical dependence phenomena. During most of this time, Dr. Seevers, his graduate students, and, from time to time, various associates have sought answers to the riddles of tolerance, habituation, and physical dependence phenomena and how these are interwoven into the psychophysical complex popularly called addiction. Over the years, the succeeding and changing groups focused their attentions on one or more aspects of the overall problem while actively developing appropriate predictive tests for dependence liability of potentially useful analgesic drugs. For the greater part, their endeavors involved the use of the "addiction" colony of rhesus monkeys. I have always viewed this monkey addiction laboratory as one that evolved to meet a basic need for information in a critical area.

Drug abuse has now reached pandemic proportions and is posing a serious threat to our community and our nation as a viable society. As the magnitude of the problem grows arithmetically, the need for quality research to provide preventive and corrective measures increases geometrically. Drs. Seevers, Irwin, Deneau, Yanagita, and Villarreal have developed test procedures that meet the essential requirements for new drug evaluation. The single-dose suppression test, the primary addiction test, self-administration procedures, and tests for agonist-antagonist relationships carried out in monkeys offer a remarkably high level of reliability, reproducibility, and predictive capability for the human response to drugs. Practical use has been made and is being made of these techniques. Over 800 drugs have been tested. The results obtained have assisted drug manufacturers by alerting them to dependence liability and thus saved them from expending unnecessary effort on the development and marketing of analgesics which would offer little or nothing in the way of a medical advance. The nature of psychic dependence presents a more difficult series of problems. Progress has been remarkable.

The laboratory, whose evolution has been so succinctly described by Dr. Deneau, must be continued, if not expanded and enlarged; and the work so well begun must be improved upon and expanded. I call upon all present as part of the "Michigan pharmacology family and tradition" to use such influence and other resources as are available to them to support in one way or another the maintenance of the Michigan Monkey Addiction Laboratory.

*Deceased

Self-Administration Studies on Various Dependence-Producing Agents in Monkeys

Tomoji Yanagita, M.D., Ph.D.

I first joined the Department of Pharmacology of the University of Michigan in 1960, as a postdoctoral fellow. A considerable body of experience and knowledge had already been accumulated in studies on drug dependence. The screening test developed at Michigan for predicting morphine-like physical dependence liability in new compounds was already well established and was meeting national and world demand for such a test. However, the extensive laboratory experience with physical dependence testing in infra-human subjects was making it apparent that recognition of the factor of psychological dependence was just as imperative in these subjects as it was for human subjects, and a means of testing this factor was going to have to be developed. It was fortunate for me that I came to the University just at that juncture, for only here was research so far developed that the recognition of the need for new avenues of investigation could be effectively utilized. Under the guidance and strong support of Drs. Seevers and Deneau, who were already convinced of the necessity for work on the problem, the future of my own research started to take shape as we began to work on new dimensions in the problem of drug dependence through self-administration experiments in monkeys.

Development of Intravenous Self-Administration Techniques

Essential to the development of the new techniques was the equipment to effect the experiments. Two events come to mind when I think of the steps taken in arriving at these new techniques. The first took place on a cold, snowy day early in 1961 when Dr. Deneau and I went to Kalamazoo, Michigan, to see Dr. James Weeks of The Upjohn Company. Dr. Weeks had developed a new technique for chronic catheterization and self-administration of drugs in rats. He briefed us thoroughly on his work, which was very helpful. The second was a long discussion in Dr. Seevers' office on a design that would enable us to chronically restrain a monkey in a cage while yet assuring the animal maximum body freedom. Long after the others had gone home and the sun had set, Dr. Seevers and I stood by the blackboard, chalk in hand.

The product of these technical deliberations was a restraining apparatus developed cooperatively by Drs. Seevers and Deneau and myself, with the aid of the late Mr. Robert Shepherd. Through trial and error with this prototype, we finally arrived at the apparatus presently in use. A monkey is restrained to a front-open cage by a stainless steel restraining arm and harness. He can trigger an automatic injector, which is located outside of the cage, by pressing a lever on the back wall of the cage. The drug solution is delivered to the animal through a catheter which runs inside the arm, enters the animal at the back, and leads into the jugular vein at the cervical region.

Development of a Research Program in Japan

When I returned to Japan in 1965, I took with me a National Institute of Mental Health research grant in the form of a subcontract from the University of Michigan for continuation of my drug dependence studies. This grant encouraged the establishment and future growth of a monkey laboratory called the Medical Research Laboratory of the Central Institute for Experimental Animals (CIEA). The laboratory now has about 100 monkeys and 24 self-administration units.

Commentary

James H. Woods, Ph.D.

It has been said that behavioral pharmacology is an offspring resulting from the marriage of experimental pharmacology and experimental psychology. It is, of course, interesting to observe how this child developed and what it drew from each of its parents' repertoires. The drug self administration techniques, which Dr. Yanagita has been a forerunner in developing, represent a new and, perhaps, important step by the infant.

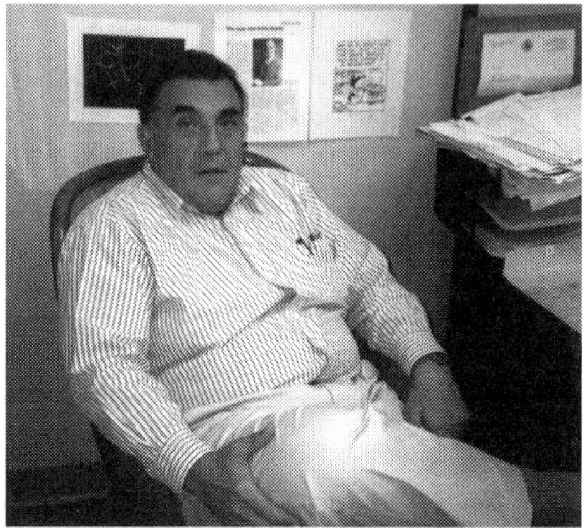

These self-administration techniques weld a drug with behavior in a manner that is novel. A response of the organism, such as a lever press, is required to deliver a drug to the organism by one of the various routes of administration. If no change in behavior occurred when this opportunity was provided, we would have no more than a convenient system for delivering drugs on a chronic basis. However, the frequency of the lever-pressing response changes in many interesting ways. When the frequency of responding increases following the contingent delivery of drug, the drug is said to reinforce the response. Its strength is increased and maintained by this contractual arrangement. When the drug serves as a reinforcer, a number of complex patterns of responding subsequently emerge that depend upon the class of the drug, its dose regimen, its route of administration, and the behavior required. The fact that patterns of self-administration can be altered drastically by these variables is illustrated, for example, by the observed differences among ethanol, cocaine, and morphine self-administration. Both cocaine and ethanol under unlimited-access conditions appear to be self-administered in episodes of severe and prolonged intoxication followed by periods of self-imposed abstinence. Withdrawal is noted with ethanol self-imposed abstinence, but is not observed with cocaine. Morphine, on the other hand, rapidly produces physical dependence under the conditions of Dr. Yanagita's experiments, yet the monkey apparently never stops long enough to become withdrawn significantly as is the case with ethanol.

It should be of no surprise that a considerable effort will have to be applied to the study of these and other patterns of self-administration before they are adequately understood. In an experimental analysis of this kind, the strongest concepts of each parent science about the mechanisms of action of drugs and the mechanisms by which reinforcing effects may be altered and assessed are already showing joint usefulness. The outcome of this and related research should be of interest to both parent sciences and to those urgently concerned with the burden of drug abuse. The sagacious man that we have honored at this Symposium had the foresight not only to recognize the possibilities of the study of drug self-administration but also to urge its realization.

Commentary

Charles R. Schuster, Ph.D.

For as long as recorded history, man has ingested chemical substances in an attempt to bring about an altered state of consciousness. At times, this ingestion of chemicals has become of such frequency and magnitude that the individual becomes physically and/or psychologically dependent upon the drug. For many years infrahuman subjects have been used to study the mechanisms underlying the development of physical dependence. Recently, attempts have been made to understand psychological dependence through self-administration studies in the animal laboratory. The Department of Pharmacology at the University of Michigan under the direction of Dr. Maurice Seevers has for many years been the leading department in the study of drug dependence. The work of Dr. Yanagita on the self-administration of drugs by rhesus monkeys attests to the breadth and depth of the approaches that were developed at the University of Michigan. The concept underlying this approach is based upon the idea that the self-administration of drugs can be viewed as operant behavior in which drugs serve as reinforcers.

One outcome of this research was the discovery that the drugs found reinforcing by man were also found reinforcing by monkeys, while the drugs rejected by man were rejected by monkeys. This discovery lent credence to the belief that findings in animal research could be extrapolated to man. After six years in the animal laboratory at the University of Michigan, I was offered the opportunity to join the Department of Psychiatry at the University of Chicago. This appointment has allowed me to attempt self-administration studies in man similar to those done in monkeys. I would like to briefly report on our pilot studies in this area. This work has been carried out in collaboration with Dr. Jerome Jaffe of the University of Chicago.

The drugs used for the studies were methadone, codeine, and pentazocine and a placebo. Eighty-eight subjects on the waiting list of the State of Illinois Drug Abuse Program were contacted and invited to join the study on an outpatient basis for 10 consecutive days. The subjects were randomly assigned to one of the four medication groups. The study was double-blind. The patients were instructed that eight capsules of medication would be available for them to collect each morning at the clinic for the 10-day period. The series of procedures which had to be completed daily by the subjects to become eligible to receive the medication was submitting a urine specimen, completing a 10-minute pencil and paper test designed to measure opiate withdrawal, and participating in a brief interview to tell about daily drug use, both licit and illicit. The frequency of return to the clinic was used as a measure of the reinforcing efficacy of each drug. Each subject was allowed $2 carfare for the first five days of the study but not the second five days in order to assess the role of monetary reinforcement.

In the second five-day period a significantly greater number of subjects given 400 mg of codeine or 40 mg of methadone continued to report to the clinic than subjects given either 400 mg of pentazocine or the placebo. We may thus conclude that in this subject population methadone and codeine are significantly better reinforcers than pentazocine or a placebo. We feel that this procedure provides an additional means of predicting the dependence liability of new pharmacological compounds.

Biochemical Aspects of Tolerance

*Joseph Cochin, M.D., Ph.D.**

I am most deeply honored by this invitation to speak to you at this symposium. Dr. Seevers, of course, is honored not only by the presentations and activities on this occasion, but even more so by the fact that much of the work which has been and will be described has been done either under the auspices of the department which he has headed so ably or by scientists who have been trained or have taught in that department.

As I mulled over my assigned topic and attempted to put the pieces of my presentation together, I realized that although the topic is rather broad, I could in fact be describing the impact of the Department of Pharmacology at Michigan upon the field of tolerance and dependence. Like the beer that made Milwaukee famous, it is this department that above all else made narcotic research famous. Dr. Seevers is responsible for much of this. This is not to say that the department was not interested in problems of drug dependence before his arrival. Dr. Eddy's cooperative program anticipated Dr. Seevers by some years. But the major thrust came after Maurice Seevers' arrival in Ann Arbor in the forties. Nor does this mean that Dr. Seevers' department was not interested in fields other than narcotic drugs. The program of this symposium certainly tells us otherwise. But it is safe to say that the problems of tolerance to, dependence on, and abuse of certain centrally acting agents is the area of knowledge and research closest to Dr. Seevers' heart.

When Dr. Seevers and Dr. Eddy began their research in the field, it was recognized by all that this was an extraordinarily complex, extremely important, and intensely intriguing problem. In the intervening decades, research techniques, laboratory equipment, and methodological approaches have changed greatly. We know a good deal more and can describe the phenomenon more accurately, but the basic mechanisms underlying tolerance and dependence still elude us.

Many of the early studies in the field that were considered investigations of in vivo drug metabolism could probably be classified as essentially biochemical in nature. I will not restrict myself in any narrow fashion to studies involving NADP, cytochrome P-450, and other currently fashionable terms. Instead, I will present a broad overview of the highlights of work in the field that have to do with the reactions of tissues, either inside or outside the body, to narcotic analgesics under conditions of acute and chronic administration and of cessation of drug administration.

The search for differences tolerant vis-à-vis nontolerant animals goes back a long way. At the turn of the century, Marme hypothesized the conversion of morphine to an oxidized metabolite. This metabolite was a stimulant and counteracted the depressant action of additional morphine doses and whose action was uncovered when the chronic administration of morphine was terminated, thus accounting for both tolerance and dependence. One would hazard a guess that when Tatum, Seevers, and Collins formulated the "dual-action" hypothesis, they were struck by the resemblance of their theoretical formulation of neuronal-receptor combinations, that was neuropharmacological in nature, to the Marme hypothesis that was chemical in nature. By the time Dr. Seevers had taken the chairmanship at Michigan, a number of studies had appeared, purporting to find differences between the way morphine was handled by the tolerant and by the nontolerant animal. The studies of Plant and Pierce, Gross and Thompson, and Oberst are cases in point. Although widely quoted, none of these were convincing, and the need for investigations using newer analytical techniques and improved methods was apparent.

A fortunate series of events (fortunate

*Deceased

for me, that is) brought me to the department at Michigan as a graduate student at a time when Lauren Woods had perfected a novel and fruitful approach to the estimation of amines in body fluids and tissues. Using these methods and some rather ingenious techniques that he devised, we were able to show that there were no really significant differences between tolerant and nontolerant dogs with respect to either plasma levels, tissue distribution, or excretory patterns. What differences that existed, were either too small to be considered relevant or could be explained on the basis of differences in biliary circulation in acutely and chronically treated animals.

Dr. Lauren Woods and a number of his students extended similar studies to other species and to other drugs and have used much more sophisticated techniques and equipment. The results of such studies, including those of Mulé and Mellett, for instance, do not really change the conclusions of our earlier work that altered distribution, altered metabolism, or altered excretory patterns do not account for tolerance.

Avram Goldstein suggested that both tolerance and dependence are completely and rapidly reversible. Tolerance, in part at least, can be explained by an increased rate of conjugation and excretion of the drug (levorphanol in this particular instance). The measure of drug effect was the increase in activity in the mouse after the administration of narcotic drugs. Goldstein described rapid tolerance to this effect. In our laboratory we have never seen the simple effect on activity that he describes nor have we observed tolerance develop at anywhere near the same rate. We do see an initial depression of activity to which tolerance develops in a matter of days and a concomitant increase in activity that seemingly becomes even more marked as time goes on. This increased activity as drug administration continues is, we believe, more indirect than direct, since it apparently is due to the tolerance to the depressant effect of narcotics. In any case, the observations of Goldstein are important if they can be replicated and would be among the few that do not agree with the generally held conclusion mentioned earlier, namely that altered distribution, metabolism, and excretion do not explain tolerance.

There are, of course, a number of explanations of tolerance to mention in passing, such as the receptor-occupation hypothesis first postulated by Schmidt and Livingston was based on their observations of acute tolerance to the vascular effects of morphine. This hypothesis assumed that drug molecules exert their action at the time of occupation of receptor sites. Once attached those drug molecules exert no effect other than preventing the initiation of a new response by receptor combination with additional drug. Although many facets of morphine action are explained by this theory, there are a number of morphine actions that point to much more profound changes. Among these are the persistence of tolerance and the appearance of abstinence symptoms long after the drug has apparently left the body. It is hard to visualize simple occupation of receptor sites for periods of several weeks, let alone the nine months to a year that tolerance has been shown to persist.

The possibility that cellular adaptation based on biochemical changes is one of the mechanisms underlying the development of tolerance has been considered for many years. Enzymatic adaptation is a well-known phenomenon in biology. H^+, SH has been shown by cytochemical studies that the distribution and concentration of H^+, SH groups, and nucleic acids are affected by extrinsic factors such as diet, extremes in temperature, and the physiologic condition of the animal. Such biochemical transformations may take the form of increased or decreased activity of mechanisms normally operating to carry on a function, or the initiation of new mechanisms, or the substitution of alternative pathways. The form that such adaptation can take differs from phenomenon to phenomenon and from preparation to preparation, but the term "adaptation " should be broad enough to cover a wide range of changes, both biochemical and biophysical, that are responses to external stimuli and the external environment. Such changes are intracellular for the most part and include changes in enzyme activity, in the respiration of tissues, in the reaction of offspring of mothers chronically treated with drugs during pregnancy, in the evoking of mechanisms to maintain the status quo (a response that we call homeostasis), and in reactions of the organism to the drugs in patterns that mimic to some extent those seen in immune processes and in the processes involved in memory.

Although many of the theories of tolerance that involve homeostatic adjustments to account for tolerance and dependence could not really be classified as biochemical, many can. The resemblance between those that invoke biochemical adjustments in so many words and those that only infer them indirectly is striking. There is, for instance, much in the "dual-action" theory described by Seevers and Woods that anticipates in a neuropharmacological way the "derepressor" theories of Shuster, Goldstein and Goldstein, and Collier. They all invoke homeostatic adjustments and attempt to explain in a unitary manner both tolerance and dependence, and stimulant and depressant effects existing side by side; but the former are covered by the latter and become "unmasked" during withdrawal.

The dual-action hypothesis of Tatum, Seevers, and Collins, as modified by Seevers and Woods, was a most important contribution. It influenced our thinking about tolerance and dependence for many years and was responsible for the initiation of a great deal of very important work. What is even more interesting from my point of view about the dual-action theory is that its refutation came from the same laboratory in which it was first formulated. Drs. Seevers and Deneau were able to show that the development of physical dependence can be aborted by the concomitant administration of a morphine antagonist such as nalorphine. Their studies demonstrated that the receptors responsible for the depressant action of morphine are also involved in the development of physical dependence, since no dependence develops if the depressant activity of the narcotic analgesic is blocked by the antagonist. In addition, although some of the stimulant actions of morphine are not antagonized by nalorphine, no abstinence signs were seen, so that it appears as if the depressant effect of the narcotic analgesics is the one intimately related with abstinence. Shuster and also Goldstein and Goldstein have shown tolerance to the stimulant effects of dihydromorphinone and levorphanol, respectively; yet we know that physical dependence can be demonstrated after chronic administration of both of these compounds.

In the early 1940s, Drs. Shideman and Seevers undertook a series of investigations on the effects of morphine and its derivatives on intermediary metabolism. Their first paper on the subject, published in 1941, dealt with the inhibitory effects of morphine, codeine, and thebaine on several dehydrogenases prepared from animal tissues and on the oxygen uptake of rat cerebral cortex slices. The results confirmed the earlier work of Quastel and Wheatley and of Gross and Pierce using rat brain minces. Shideman and Seevers questioned the validity of an approach that uses concentrations of morphine far beyond those attained in the intact animal. They then proceeded to study the effects of chronic administration of morphine upon a variety of systems. In a study also published in 1941, they were able to show a significant increase in the oxygen uptake of normal rat skeletal muscle when morphine was added and to show that minced skeletal muscle from chronically morphinized animals utilized oxygen at a considerably greater rate than normal muscle.

Editor's note: Dr. Cochin then extensively reviews the many more recent contributions of former members of our Department, including Sal Mulé, Lauren Woods, Ted Brody, Tai Akera, his own, as well as the research of others, on then current theories and biochemical evidence of opioid mechanisms of tolerance and physical dependence.

I hope that this somewhat discursive and yet cursory overview of some of the work on the biochemical level with respect to tolerance and dependence has been of interest to you. I trust those of you in the audience whose work I haven't mentioned will not take it personally. Inclusion or exclusion does not imply a value judgement but simply choices reflecting my personal interest, not bias. I know that there are dozens of studies going on in the department at present that could have been included had I had sufficient time. I'm also certain that I have not even scratched the surface in outlining the contributions that past and present members of this department have made in the field. All of us are extremely grateful and deeply indebted to the leadership that Dr. Seevers provided that has made much of what I've outlined possible.

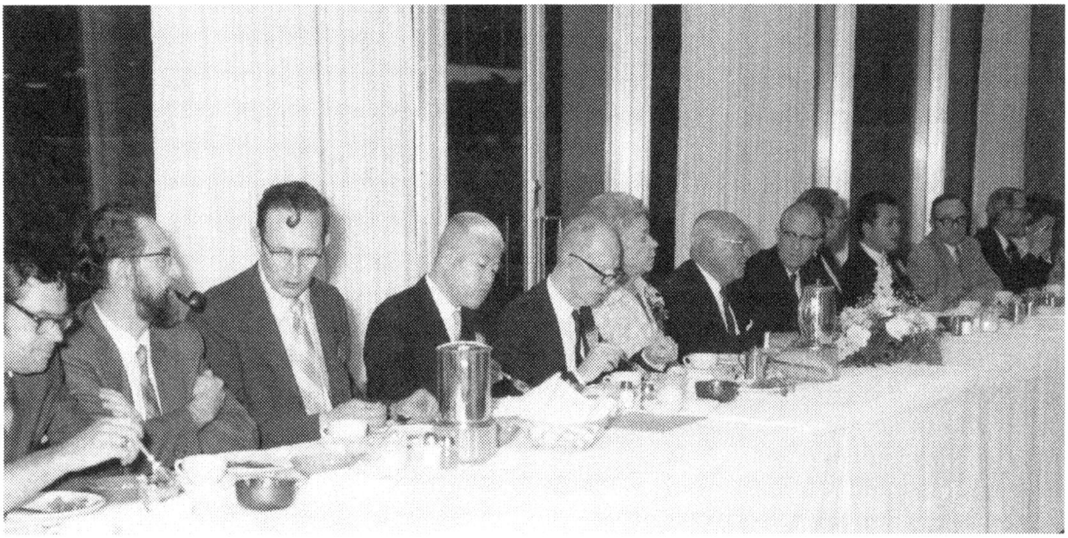

The Seevers Symposium Banquet Head Table pictured from left to right (above) and vice versa (below): Glenn Kiplinger, Maynard Chenoweth, Henry Swain, Eikichi Hosoya, Nathan Eddy, Frankie Seevers, Maurice Seevers, Alan Bass, Lauren Woods, Tomoji Yanagita, Joe Cochin, Frederick Shideman and Dotty Overbeck.

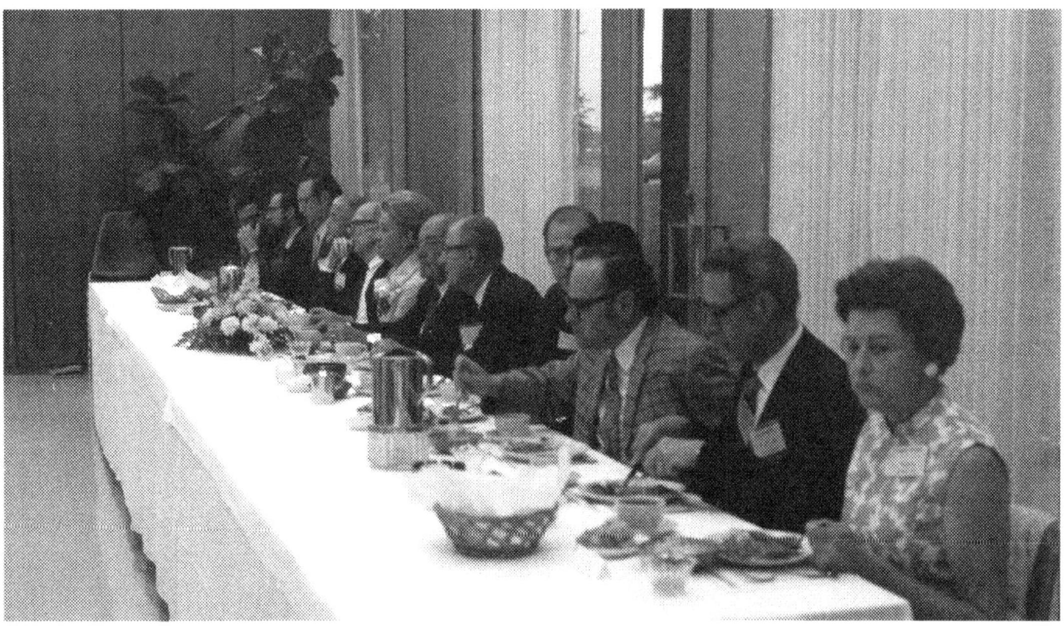

Commentary

*Julian E. Villarreal, M.D., Ph.D.**

I will first express my appreciation for the honor of participating in this testimonial symposium for Dr. Seevers and for the distinction of being called to comment on Dr. Cochin's paper. His presentation has been a comprehensive review of seven decades of biochemical research on the mechanisms of tolerance and physical dependence to narcotic analgesics. In spite of time limitations, Dr. Cochin has managed to cover the results of the most significant lines of investigation in this area. He has been an active contributor to this research since his days as a graduate student in the Department of Pharmacology at the University of Michigan. Not surprisingly, then, I find little that I could add to Dr. Cochin's discussion except for a few elaborations on some isolated points. Because of this and because I am somewhat of a latecomer in this field, I feel it is more appropriate that I take a look at the future, offering some thoughts on what I think are promising areas of productive research on the biochemistry of drug dependence.

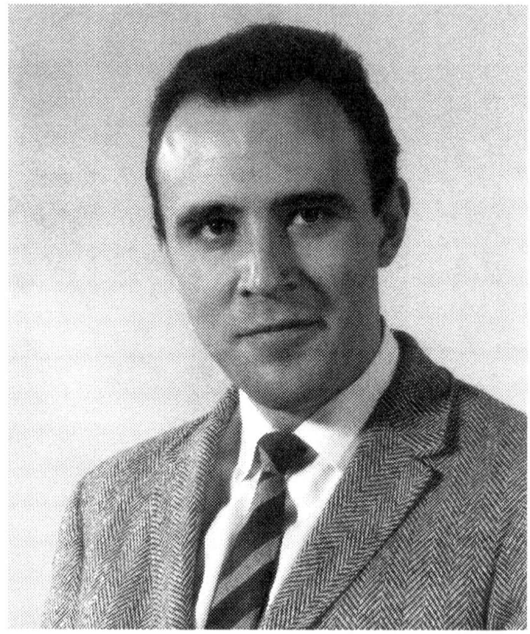

It has been said many times that all drugs which affect the central nervous system are likely to be abused by at least a small number of individuals. However, the drugs that generate compulsive self-administration behavior are members of only a few pharmacological classes. I would like to call attention to the fact that all the drugs which give rise to strong self-administration behavior produce some form of psychomotor stimulation. This is certainly true of cocaine and the amphetamine-like stimulants; but it is also true for morphine, ethanol, and the barbiturate-like sedatives.

In spite of the CNS depressant effects of narcotic analgesics, addicts to these drugs recognize good "dope" by subjective sensations of "drive" and internal energy. Another typical effect of good "dope" is the "soap box" phenomenon (talkativeness), one of the signs which for many years has been employed to help identify new drugs with morphine-like actions.

Narcotic antagonists such as cyclazocine and nalorphine are not liked by former opiate addicts in spite of the fact that these drugs have strong central depressant properties; these two compounds are almost devoid of psychomotor stimulation. Ethanol and the barbiturate-like sedatives are capable of producing gross manifestations of psychomotor stimulation when administered under appropriate circumstances. Schmiedeberg speculated that the stimulant effects of ethanol were due to depression of inhibitory functions. Whatever the mechanism, the fact remains that ethanol as well as the barbiturate-like sedatives and tranquilizers produce central depression mixed with stimulation. In striking contrast, the phenothiazine-like tranquilizers, which are strong depressants and can relieve anxiety, do not have psychomotor stimulant properties and do not produce compulsive self-admin-

*Deceased

istration. It does not seem far-fetched to suggest that the induction of self-administration behavior by the various drugs which produce strong psychological dependence may involve common neurological or biochemical mechanisms.

Studies in physiological psychology are providing other facts which may have a bearing on these mechanisms. A growing body of evidence indicates that another form of "addictive" behavior, intracranial self-stimulation, involves the activation of central aminergic systems in the brain. It may very well be that sympathomimetics such as cocaine and the amphetamine-like stimulants will be found to share common mechanisms with intracranial self-stimulation. With regard to the narcotic analgesics, recent work in our laboratory has shown that a number of morphine-like drugs alter the levels of catecholamines and increase the synthesis of norepinephrine and dopamine in the brain. These effects may play a role in the mechanisms of action of narcotic analgesics because they exhibit the features of the specific effects of the morphine-like drugs: chemical stereospecificity, susceptibility to blockade by low doses of narcotic-antagonists, tolerance, and cross-tolerance.

It is fortunate that we now have powerful techniques for the rigorous study of drug self-administration in animals. The possibilities of combining the tools of biochemistry, physiology, pharmacology, and behavioral analysis are highly promising for the understanding of mechanisms and for the development of methods of control for compulsive drug self-administration.

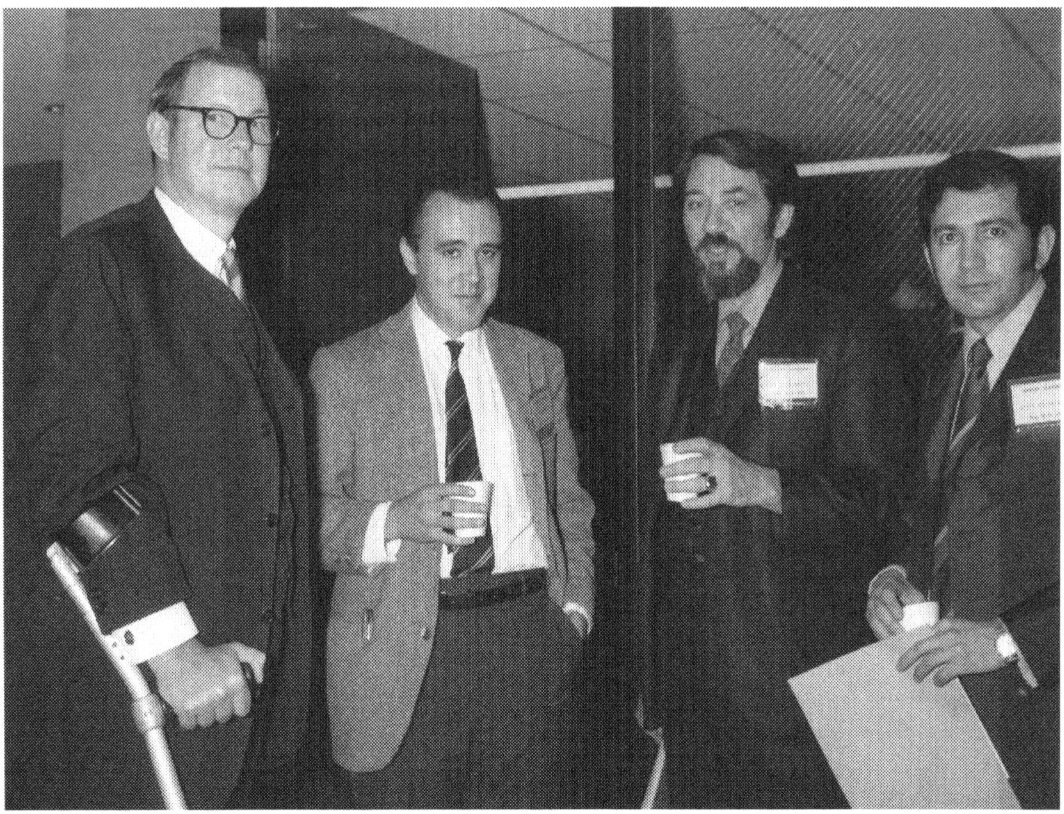

A colleague at the Seevers' Symposium with Julian Villarreal, Charles Schuster and Uriel Estrada from the Department.

Commentary

Carl C. Hug, Jr., M.D., Ph.D.

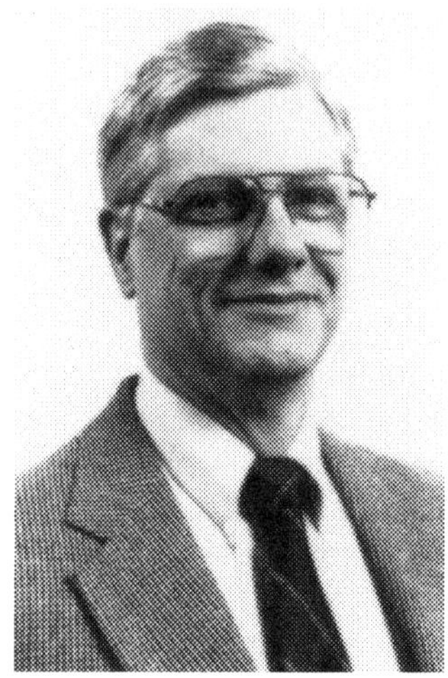

The broad, multidisciplinary nature of the lectures given at this symposium stands in sharp contrast to the assertion of a famous scientist, as related by Dr. Cochin, that investigators in the field of drug dependence and tolerance are narrow in their outlook. Dr. Seevers, as both a teacher and researcher, has set the example by insisting on a broadly based graduate training program in the pharmacology department and by attracting people from different fields to his own area of special research interest. People such as Lauren Woods, a chemist; Bob Schuster and Jim Woods, both psychologists; and many others have been encouraged by Dr. Seevers to help solve some of the riddles of this complex problem of drug dependence. In all of us he has fostered a broad look at the problems we face. He has continued the tradition and advanced the reputation of pharmacology as a science which bridges gaps between disciplines, between basic science and clinical application.

Taking the broad view is especially relevant in listening to Dr. Cochin's summary of the biochemical mechanisms proposed as explanations for drug dependence and tolerance. Allow me to mention two or three examples from Dr. Cochin's presentation.

He cited the work of Smith and of Weinstock on lenticular opacities produced by the administration of narcotic analgesics. The effect is apparently mediated through adrenergic portions of the nervous system. This interesting phenomenon has received a fair amount of attention in the last several years as a model for studies of the role of the adrenergic system in morphine action and in tolerance and dependence. However, the broad view stimulates us to have a healthy skepticism about the appropriateness of this model for study of the mechanism of action of morphine. First of all, what is the relationship of the lenticular opacity to the effects of morphine? Weinstock has reported, at least informally, that if the respiratory depression from morphine is prevented the opacity does not occur. Secondly, one wonders about the stress induced by administration of doses of levorphanol as large as 35 or 100 mg/kg to produce the opacity. There are reports that other forms of stress can result in similar lenticular opacities. Thus, the phenomenon may simply reflect the toxic effects of large doses of narcotic analgesics and really not serve to implicate the adrenergic portion of the nervous system as a specific target site for morphine action.

Another hypothesis of biochemical events underlying the development of tolerance and physical dependence to morphine has been formulated by Eddy Way, our distinguished honorary alumnus, and his associates. Dr. Way has postulated that synthesis of new or increased amounts of protein is linked to the development of tolerance and physical dependence. The hypothesis is based on studies by Way and his colleagues and by at least four other groups of workers, who have reported that administration of inhibitors of protein synthesis prevented the development of tolerance and physical dependence in rodents given morphine chronically. Of course, the inhibitors are highly toxic substances and one wonders about the role of their toxicity and their effect on the animal's ability to respond to the test stimulus under any conditions. As has been pointed out, one has to look beyond the one particular response under study and evaluate the condition of the whole animal. Incidentally, although the various investigators included the usual control group of animals treated with the protein synthesis inhibitor (e.g., cycloheximide) alone, this may not be sufficient, since Loh, Chen, and Way have shown that there is an interaction between cycloheximide and morphine which leads to a greater than additive toxicity when the two drugs are administered in combination.

A final example of the importance of interpreting experimental results in the light of the whole animal can be drawn from a recent article in Science (vol. 167, page 1005, February 13, 1970) by Virginia Davis and Michael Walsh. In their article dealing with alkaloids, amines, and physical dependence to alcohol, they postulated that acetaldehyde, which is formed in the body by metabolism of ethyl alcohol, causes an alteration in the metabolism of dopamine and leads to the synthesis of tetrahydropapaveroline. The latter compound is an intermediate in the synthesis of morphine in the opium poppy. Davis and Walsh postulate that a similar synthesis could occur in the brains of animals given alcohol. Hence, they postulate that physical dependence to alcohol is really physical dependence to morphine.

When you stand back and look at the effects of alcohol and of morphine in the whole animal, it becomes apparent that their hypothesis is untenable. The withdrawal syndromes of alcohol and morphine have very different characteristics, which were evident in the material presented earlier by Dr. Yanagita. For example, convulsions and psychotic behavior do not occur in morphine abstinence but are characteristic of strong physical dependence to alcohol. What about the narcotic antagonists? They produce a sudden, dramatic withdrawal episode in morphine-dependent subjects but not in alcoholics. And what about disulfiram, which stops the metabolism of alcohol at the acetaldehyde stage? Persons ingesting alcohol after the administration of disulfiram do not exhibit the spectrum of signs and symptoms characteristic of morphine action.

There are several other items to be noted in refuting the hypothesis of Davis and Walsh, and Dr. Seevers has done so in a letter to the editors of Science. In closing I would like to quote from that letter written by Dr. Seevers.

"Drug abuse is being recognized increasingly as a major medical and sociologic problem. As a result, research on drug dependence, having been long neglected, is becoming scientifically respectable. Since it is preferentially supported, many investigators from disciplines other than pharmacology are being attracted to the field. Because so little is known of the intimate mechanism of physical dependence this is highly desirable. Sound biochemical and physiological studies are badly needed. However, unless the hypothesis and interpretations based upon such studies are consonant with pharmacologic facts, they have no validity."

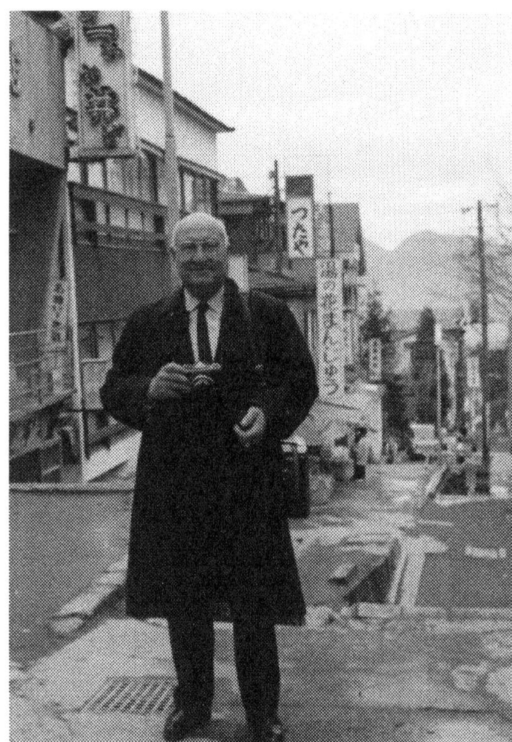

Dr. Seevers on one of his many trips to Japan, ca. 1950s

Albert C. Furstenberg, M.D., Dean 1935-1959*

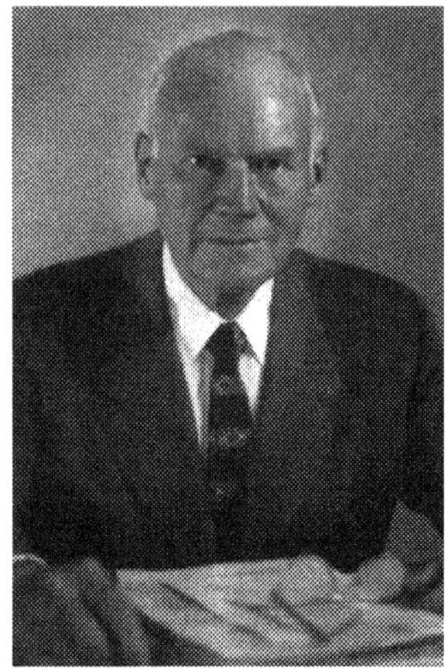

Dr. Albert C. Furstenberg, M.D., was Dean of the University of Michigan Medical School from 1935-1959. He was Michigan-trained both for his undergraduate and graduate work. After an internship at University Hospital in 1915-1916, he began a clinical practice specializing in otolaryngology in Ann Arbor, which he maintained until 1965. In 1918 he was appointed as an instructor in the Department of Otolaryngology and eventually he became chairman of the department in 1932.

After he was appointed dean of the Medical School in 1935, he expanded the teaching, research, and medical facilities of the Medical School with remarkable success. Medical classes increased to 200 students, the largest in the United States. His efforts during World War II included working with the Office of the Surgeon General of the Army and a national accelerated medical program to train more physicians.

Dr. Furstenberg promoted research in the Medical School and selected outstanding persons to head clinical and basic science departments. He appointed chairpersons who had considerable energy, drive, and leadership qualities. He encouraged independence in the affairs of their departments.

In 1942, he appointed Dr. Seevers as head of the Department of Pharmacology, and later as associate dean of the Medical School. This enabled Dr. Seevers to recommend outstanding students for acceptance into the Medical School. Dr. Seevers enthusiastically embraced the concept of dual degrees, and attracted B.S., M.S., and Ph.D. candidates to the Medical School and/or graduate school. He had the full support of Dean Furstenberg to make pharmacology especially attractive. Administratively, Dr. Seevers stressed the fact that the Department of Pharmacology would teach all of the courses in pharmacology in the Nursing, Pharmacy, Dental, and Postgraduate departments as well as in the Medical School. Dean Furstenberg agreed on the condition that its base remain in the Medical School.

In view of Dr. Furstenberg's clinical practice responsibilities, his role as Dean permitted decentralization of authority from the Dean's office to each department. Most departments of the medical school thrived in such an atmosphere. Pharmacology in particular was viewed as a provider of teaching to all units of the University as needed with its base in the Medical School which persists to this day.

Dean Furstenberg's ability to become friends with politicians and philanthropists resulted in Medical Science Building I, the Kresge Research building, the library, the Hearing Institute, the Institute of Industrial Health, and Mott's Children's Hospital. Furstenberg was the last dean to be simultaneously in private practice, head of a department, and dean of the medical school. William Hubbard became full-time dean in 1959.

*Deceased

William N. Hubbard, Jr., M.D., Dean 1959-1970

William N. Hubbard, Jr., was appointed as the first full-time Dean of the Medical School upon the retirement of Dean Furstenberg in 1959. In contrast to the many diverse responsibilities that Dean Furstenberg had, it was decided that Dr. Hubbard should be appointed as a full time dean without departmental administrative responsibilities or private practice privileges. He was only 39 years old at that time. He was also appointed as Professor of Internal Medicine.

In 1942, Dr. Hubbard graduated from Columbia University and in 1944 obtained his M.D. degree from New York University. In 1950, he was chief resident in internal medicine at Bellevue Hospital. Dr. Hubbard then became Assistant Dean at New York University and then full time Dean. At Michigan, he encouraged innovative teaching methods of medical students in the new Medical Science Building I. In addition, Dean Hubbard reorganized medical policy and practices at University Hospital.

In 1969, the Regents of the University of Michigan gave him responsibility of directing the entire Medical Center. In addition, Dean Hubbard directed a major building program to remodel existing facilities as well as construct new buildings in the Medical Center. Dr. Hubbard commented on his career goals, published in the University of Michigan Medical Center Journal 31: 241, 1965, which initially involved general medical practice, subsequently internal medicine, then teaching and research, and finally administration of teaching and research. Dr. Hubbard recruited John A. Gronvall as Associate Dean of the Medical School and Associate Professor of Pathology.

In 1970, Dean Hubbard resigned his position at the University to become Vice President of the Upjohn Pharmaceutical Company in Kalamazoo. Subsequently, he became President of the Upjohn Company. He was very prominent in medically-related issues at the

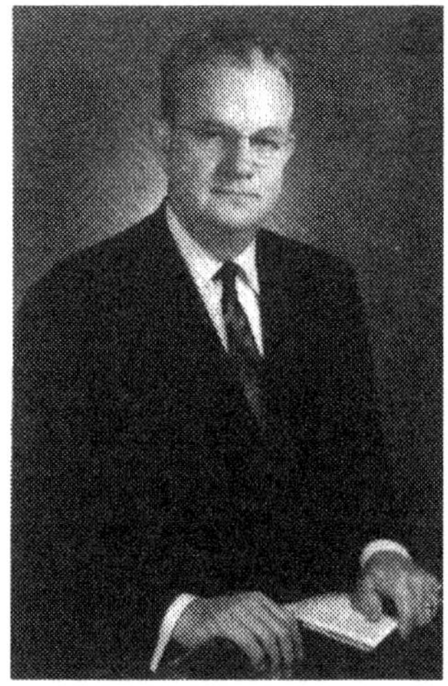

national level, frequently serving as a consultant to the US government, the Association of American Medical Colleges, and the National Library of Medicine.

My Recollections

In 1959 the departments of the basic medical sciences were geographically divided, with Anatomy, Biochemistry, and Pharmacology occupying Med Sci I in new space designed by the departments themselves. Whether by proximity or by intent there was a broad interface with the clinical departments, but most extensively in the Department of Pharmacology. Research with primate models of addiction and habituation in collaboration with human studies conducted in federal institutions in Lexington, Kentucky, were a unique strength of the Department of Pharmacology. Research led by Dr. Domino in the pharmacology of psychoactive drugs was and continues to be a strong programmatic field. Training programs in collaboration with the Department of Medicine were internationally renowned in establishing and defining the discipline of Clinical Pharmacology. Dr. Seevers and other members of the Department were active and influential participants in the evolution of the National Institutes of Health; later Seevers was a member of the Task Force of the Surgeon General that issued the landmark reports on the effects of smoking.

In 1961 Dr. Seevers became a member of the Executive Committee of the Faculty of Medicine and served for three years. It would be difficult to exaggerate the importance of his role during years of what seemed to be radical changes in curriculum, governance of the Medical School, clinical practice arrangements, capital construction programs and clinical faculty titles. He was an ardent and effective spokesman for the preservation of those elements upon which the Medical School had drawn in historically achieving the excellence that characterized it. Most especially did he emphasize the integrity of the department as the locus of responsibility for fostering of development of members of the faculty and for serving as the intellectual "germ plasm" in the evolution of the discipline which it represented; as well as being final arbiter of the content of instruction. At times this advocacy could give the appearance of opposition to change, but this would be inaccurate. In all matters he endorsed and supported change with the condition that it was demonstrably an improvement on what had heretofore been deemed appropriate. He brought vigor, dedication, and discipline to the process of change— a truly invaluable role for the ultimate acceptance by the general faculty.

The Department of Pharmacology was one of the first to change the laboratory component of the instruction of the second year medical students. Using audio-visual demonstrations of experiments before the lab markedly increased the efficiency and the success rate of the students' laboratory exercises. Reducing the set-up requirements increased the opportunity for direct observation. Ultimately much of the "new" student laboratory space was re-assigned as a result of this innovative experience. Among the programs that distinguished the Department was its leadership in developing the field of clinical pharmacology. Based on a long history of collaboration with the clinical departments a post doctoral training program was developed and was among the first to be supported by the National Institutes of Health. The influence was international, but especially strong in Japan where it may reasonably be asserted that in the person of Dr. Seevers the Department established clinical pharmacology as a university discipline in Japan. Years later, when I was with the Upjohn Company, a major research program was started in Japan. The leadership in clinical pharmacology was largely a product of the earlier contacts with the Department.

When a grant from the Upjohn Company was received in the early '80s, for the construction of clinical pharmacology laboratories by the Medical School, it was a tangible recognition of the distinction of existing programs that exemplified collaboration of the clinical departments with the Department of Pharmacology and the administration reflected this joint responsibility. When application was made for a matching grant from N.I.H. that administration was not approved, it being N.I.H. policy at the time that the authority should rest in a department of pharmacology. Changing the administrative structure to comply was discussed. A doubling of the resource was at stake. Without dissent the tradition of collaborative responsibility was maintained. At this writing, the policy has long since been revised.

The close personal friendship of Dr. Harry Towsley, professor of pediatrics and chairperson of postgraduate medicine, and Dr. Seevers contributed to the Department's participation in programs of postgraduate education both within the Medical Center and throughout the state. At a more personal level, their shared interest in horticulture and in hunting or fishing provided many hours of shared recreation. The dedication to fundamental principles along with concern for the broader community and an attitude of personal generosity characterized the leadership of and was reflected in the work of the Department of Pharmacology.

2

Confessions of an Acting Chairman or, Why I Refused to Do the Job a Third Time

Henry H. Swain, M.D.

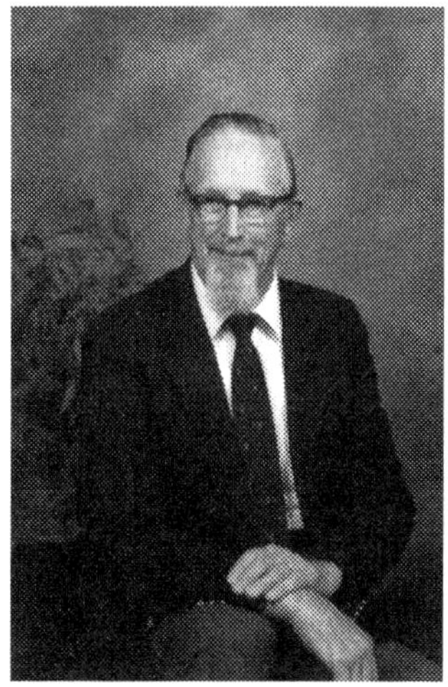

I spent almost the entirety of my professional life in the Department of Pharmacology at the University of Michigan. It is not surprising that I remained for 37 years once I got there, because the department, the University, and the city of Ann Arbor have continued to be attractive through the years. How I got to Ann Arbor in the first place, however, is quite surprising and involved several unlikely events that all meshed together for my ultimate benefit.

When I entered the University of Illinois College of Medicine in 1947, I had no intention of pursuing a career in pharmacology — I was planning to become a psychiatrist. At the end of the first semester of medical school, my biochemistry instructor asked me if I would work in his laboratory during the following summer. I told my fiancee and she asked, "Will you get paid?"

When I relayed her question to my instructor, he replied that he had no funds to support me, and that the biochemistry department would be unable to help. However, upstairs in the pharmacology department was a faculty member who had recently invented a successful antihistamine drug, and since my instructor and I were going to study the actions of histamine injected into the skin, perhaps the pharmacologists could give me a little money.

We were in luck because the head of the Department of Pharmacology, Dr. Carl C. Pfeiffer, was active in recruiting medical students into careers in that science. During the eight years that he was at Illinois, 21 medical students worked during the summers in pharmacology department laboratories and ten of those 21 medical students went on to careers in pharmacology. I was one of the ten. Dr. Pfeiffer paid me a stipend of $125 per month for the three months of the 1948 summer vacation between my freshman and sophomore years in medical school. Further, he enrolled me (as he had enrolled most of the other summer medical students in his department) in graduate school, so that I became a candidate for a master of science degree in pharmacology at the same time that I was a candidate for the M.D. degree. I spent the summers after my sophomore and junior medical school years at the same salary and in the same graduate school enrollment. Then I wrote up the results of my work with my biochemistry instructor as both a journal publication and, in expanded form, as a masters thesis. At the University of Illinois commencement exercises in Chicago in 1951, the speaker was Adlai Stevenson. That day, Stevenson shook my hand twice — once when he presented me my M.D. degree and again when he handed me my master of science diploma.

At the time of graduation, I probably knew less pharmacology than any of the other medical students whom Carl Pfeiffer had lured into the science. While my compatriots were in the laboratories of pharmacology department faculty members and pursuing pharmacological investigations, I was downstairs working for a biochemist who sent me over to the hospital's allergy clinic to inject histamine into the skin of ragweed sufferers. My instructor and I eventually published a paper entitled "Quantative Studies in Skin Testing V. The Whealing Reactions of Histamine and Ragweed Pollen Extract" in the Journal of Allergy. However, my isolation from the rest of the pharmacologists deprived me of the osmotic education that one picks up from the daily association with people who are thinking, talking, reading, and experimenting pharmacology day-in and day-out.

As it turned out, it made very little difference that at the time of my graduation I knew no more pharmacology than a slightly-above-average medical student, even though I had a masters degree in the subject. You see, my timing was excellent. The period around 1950 marked the division between the Old Days, when there was very little research money for the medical sciences, and the New Times, when there was more money available than the existing scientists knew how to spend. In the late 1940s, a woman named Mary Lasker had been successful in lobbying Congress to enormously increase the budgets for the National Institutes of Health. Suddenly, departments of pharmacology across the nation, as well as other medical school departments, could afford to enlarge their faculties. However, there were very few candidates available for these new jobs. There were no large graduate training programs in pharmacology in existence at that time. People like Carl Pfeiffer were recruiting a few medical students into the field, but the pool of candidates was so small that almost anyone who could spell the word pharmacology could probably get a faculty position.

By the fall of my senior year in medical school I still assumed that I was headed for the practice of medicine, despite my impending masters degree in pharmacology. At lunchtime one day that fall I saw Dr. Pfeiffer. Out of the blue he asked, "Henry, why don't I get you a job teaching pharmacology?" Without significant pause, I replied, "OK." In that manner, I chose my life's work.

I discussed my decision with several trusted professors, who all approved of my choice but recommended strongly that I complete an internship and obtain a license to practice medicine before I tried a teaching career. In that way, if the teaching didn't work out, it would be easier to get back into medical training. Therefore, for the year between my graduation and my first faculty appointment I served as an intern at Cook County Hospital in Chicago.

During the year that I was interning I saw Dr. Pfeiffer one day shortly after he had returned from the fall meeting of the American Society for Pharmacology and Experimental Therapeutics, our professional society. He told me that he had just learned of three faculty positions that I should consider. One was at the University of Michigan, one at the University of Iowa, and one at the University of Cincinnati. I wrote letters to each of the three. I received no answer from Michigan, but I was invited to visit both Iowa and Cincinnati. The Iowa job did not materialize, but I received an offer from Cincinnati, which I accepted, effective July 1, 1952.

My Cincinnati career was not entirely successful. My salary the first year was a meager $4,200, which did not support my young family very well. Therefore, I began moonlighting in the emergency rooms of area hospitals to augment my income, which may have suggested to my department chairman that I was not truly dedicated to a career in pharmacology. Whatever his reasons, the chairman notified me after a year and a half there that my appointment would not be renewed after June 30, 1954. Thus I was fired from my first pharmacology faculty position.

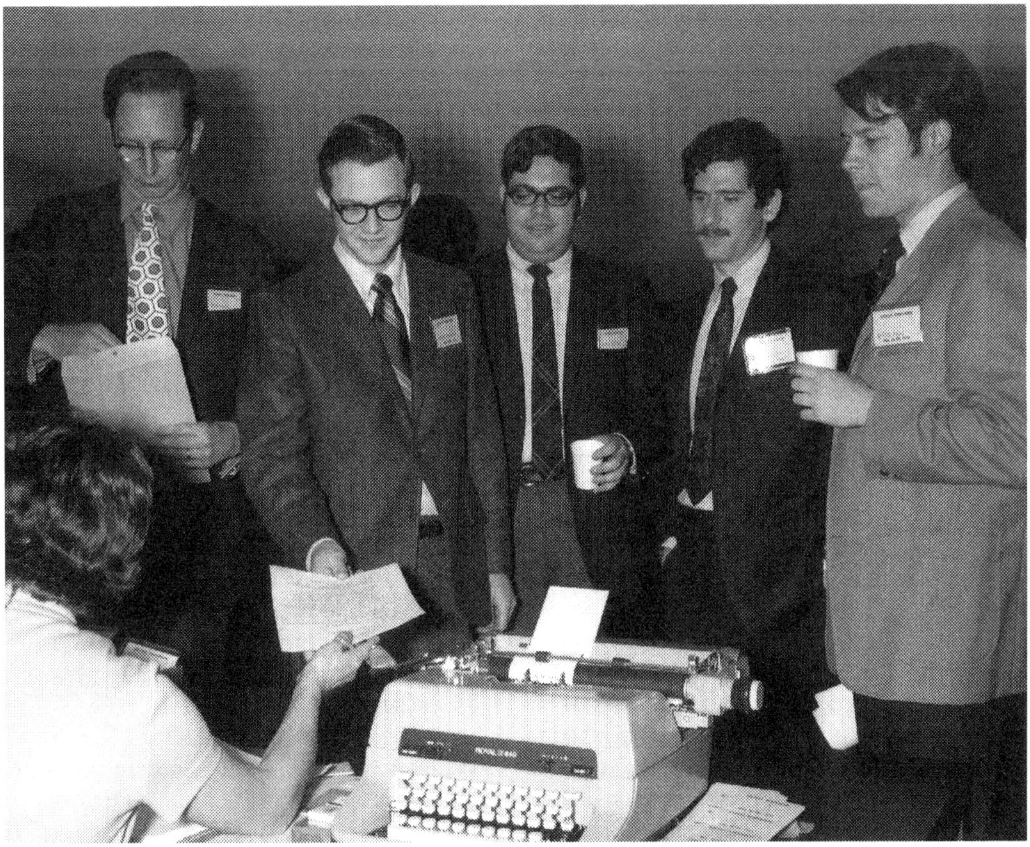

Registering for the Seevers' Symposium 1970— Henry Swain, Ron Chipps, Frank Kniffen, Joe Graedon, and Dennis Dietz.

Remarkable good luck had brought me a piece of information, which served to convert the misfortune of being fired into the happiness of a much better pharmacology position. In those days, a friend of my parents was a dean at the University of Michigan. He had attended a cocktail party in Ann Arbor at which he found himself talking to Dr. M. H. Seevers, Michigan's chairman of pharmacology. Somehow their conversation included a mention of my father, which prompted Dr. Seevers to say, "A couple of years ago I was ready to offer his son a job, but by the time I got around to answering the mail, he had taken a position somewhere else."

The dean told my father what he had learned, and my father told me. Shortly thereafter I was fired. Armed with the information from the dean, I wrote immediately to Dr. Seevers, saying in effect, "I wrote to you two years ago seeking a position in your department. Once again I am looking for such an opportunity." By return mail I received an invitation to go to Ann Arbor to be interviewed. I was offered and accepted a job as an instructor in pharmacology at Michigan, as of September 1, 1954.

The availability of a position in pharmacology at Michigan at that time involved an unrelated element of luck — almost all bad luck. In 1954 Senator McCarthy's anti-communist witch hunt was running rampant throughout the country. In the pharmacology department at that time there was a tenured associate professor named Mark Nickerson who had been a Communist Party member earlier in his life. Under great pressure from the state legislature, the university dismissed Nickerson and one other faculty member because of their communist ties. This action brought great difficulties to the university, to Dr. Seevers, and especially to Dr. Nickerson. As far as I can tell, I am the only person in the United States who profited from this unhappy occurrence. It created a job at the moment when I needed one, it gave me a recently vacated office, and it offered me a block of lectures to give to sophomore medical students.

After eight years in the Michigan Department of Pharmacology, I went crazy. The onset was insidious. In the fall of 1962 I developed a sore mouth. When I opened my mouth and looked in a mirror, I could see a few small reddened areas on my throat. It was not very spectacular, and not even very sore. Mostly it was just annoying. In the department at that time there was a graduate student who had previously been trained as a dentist. I knew that he had seen many throats in his career, and so I showed him mine. He agreed that it looked sore, but he had no useful ideas as to what I should do about it. Eventually he suggested that I go over to the Dental School and see a former professor of his who was a distinguished oral pathologist. The distinguished professor gave me a red medicine and a green medicine to sooth the irritation, but they did not help very much. The sore mouth continued essentially unchanged from September until March.

One day plumbers came to replace a sink in our laboratory. They removed the old sink and dumped the old sink trap into a pan. Out came a handful of mercury. One plumber said to the other, "We got even more mercury out of the other sink." Upon hearing that, I rushed upstairs to the graduate student/ dentist. I asked if my throat irritation could be a sign of mercury poisoning, and he said that it certainly could be. I was fortunate that in the next laboratory was a faculty member who routinely ran urine-mercury-level determinations. (He studied the actions of mercurial diuretics.) Within an hour that colleague had measured the amount of mercury in my urine, and there was quite a bit.

Toxicologists from the School of Public Health then came to our laboratory with their mercury-sniffing machines and found that the place was seriously contaminated. The source was easy to identify. One of our graduate students was using an instrument which measured the concentration of certain gases in blood. The instrument used a drop of mercury to seal the gases into the measuring chamber. Next to the instrument, the student kept a beaker of mercury and an ordinary medicine dropper, which he used to transfer the liquid metal to the instrument. However, mercury is quite heavy and regularly some of it fell out of the dropper and onto the floor.

Organic mercury compounds and many inorganic salts of mercury are quite poisonous, but generally speaking large drops of elemental mercury are harmless. (Countless children have encountered no ill effects when they rubbed metallic mercury on pennies to make them look like dimes.) Older laboratories with wooden floors have tolerated mercury spills without serious consequences. However, the laboratories of the pharmacology department had plastic-tile floors with no cracks in which mercury droplets could hide. Furthermore, every week or two the janitors polished those floors with motor-driven brushes which served to shatter the large mercury droplets into an almost-invisible powder with an enormously increased surface area and a much-increased toxic potential. This poisonous powder settled on flat surfaces throughout the laboratory, including desktops where we rested our luncheon sandwiches between bites. Over time those of us who worked (and ate) in that laboratory ingested a significant amount of mercury, which, because of its finely divided state, was readily absorbed from our guts and produced symptoms of poisoning.

Many of the signs of mercury poisoning are related to the nervous system. The list includes such things as irritability, shyness, and forgetfulness. The intensity of the symptoms depends upon the duration of exposure and the magnitude of the ingestion of mercury, and it can range from nearly imperceptible to catastrophic and even lethal. My laboratory mates and I were lucky to be at the mild end of the spectrum. Though our exposure extended over a period of months, the amount of mercury that we ingested was quite small. At the time I was not aware of anything except the soreness of my mouth, but in retrospect I realized that I had undergone a personality change during that period of my life. That year it was painful for me to stand in front of a class, whereas throughout the rest of my professional life I have thoroughly enjoyed the process of teaching anybody anything.

Once the problem had been identified, the laboratory was cleaned of its mercury content and its inhabitants slowly returned to sanity. I was absolutely delighted to discover that a simple chemical substance was the cause of my encroaching craziness.

After I regained my sanity, I became the acting chairman of the Department of Pharmacology. (A cynical person might suggest that the previous sentence is an oxymoron.) In September, 1971, Dr. Seevers, who had been chairman for 29 years, was rapidly approaching his 70th birthday. In those days there was a general belief in university circles that professors should retire by the time they turned 70 and that they should step down from leadership roles (such as chairman or dean) at age 65. Obviously Seevers had not stepped down as chairman five years before, and so eventually the dean summoned him and explained to him that his years of faithful service to the University of Michigan were now complete. When Seevers returned to the department from the dean's office, he was heard to say, in his usual salty language, something to the general effect that he had been fired.

The same day that Seevers' chairmanship ended, the dean sent word to the department that he wanted to talk to Dr. Swain. However, I was out playing golf with my son that afternoon. (I would prefer to think of myself more as a dedicated dad than as a fastidious pharmacologist.) Thus it was the following day before the dean told me that I should serve as acting chairman of the department until a new permanent chairman could be recruited. We assumed that within a year a new chairman would be in place and that I would return to my regular duties of teaching and research.

It is difficult to be the successor to a legend, and M. H. Seevers was legendary. Perhaps that is why several distinguished and qualified pharmacologists, after being interviewed and approved by the search committee, chose to reject the dean's offer of the chairmanship. In fact, the department was turned down seven times by six nominees. (One person refused the position on two different occasions.) Thus, I served as acting chairman for nearly three years before a new chairman came on board. During that period, in addition to my other adventures, I became involved with the monkeys.

For most of his career at Michigan, Seevers maintained a colony of rhesus monkeys, which he used to test the physical-dependence liability of a variety of pain-killing drugs. For a number of years there had been an interest in developing drugs that had the potent analgesic action of morphine without having morphine's addiction liability. Laboratory animals of several different species show withdrawal signs when their chronic morphine administration is interrupted. The signs in rhesus monkeys are very similar to those in humans and so Seevers had used this species to test new analgesic drugs. Four times every day, each monkey received a maintenance dose of morphine. Approximately every two weeks the morphine administration was interrupted for two doses. At 14 hours after their last dose the monkeys were in "cold turkey," and they were given a test drug. If the drug had morphine-like addiction properties, the "cold turkey" signs disappeared within moments; if the test drug was one which did not produce morphine-like dependence in the monkeys (and, by inference, in man), then the withdrawal signs were unaffected by its administration. When Seevers retired, some of his junior colleagues continued the work with the monkey colony.

I became involved with the monkeys because of then-President Nixon. Mr. Nixon had run successfully for the office of President of the United States on a ticket that emphasized Law and Order. Legend has it that it was only after he was in office that he discovered that most of the serious crimes which concern our society are not the business of the president because such offenses as murder, assault, robbery, and the like are crimes against individual states, not against the United States. There are some crimes which are against the United States, such as treason and income tax evasion, but most of these offenses are not well suited to a new president wishing to bolster his image for Law and Order. Then Mr. Nixon discovered drugs of abuse, against which there are federal statutes. The new president announced a War on Drugs.

Legend further states that the president asked his staff to find out how many heroin addicts there were in the United States, to thus establish a baseline against which to demonstrate the success of his War. Using methods similar to those used in fish-counting studies (where you catch some fish, tag them, throw them back in the lake, catch fish again, and see what percentage of the new catch have tags) or those used in chemical studies (where this is called the "isotope-dilution method"), the federal workers decided that there were 50,000 heroin addicts around. The following year a new count, using somewhat different methods, suggested that the number of addicts was closer to 200,000. The third year's count gave the number 500,000. At that point, apparently, someone had the temerity to say, "Mr. President, I believe that you are losing the War on Drugs."

Regardless of what actually happened in the Oval Office, the fact remains that shortly after I became the acting chairman, the government sent out a letter saying that funds were available to establish Centers of Excellence to study both the basic science and the clinical aspects of substance abuse. Presumably the results of these studies would improve the results of the War on Drugs. My reaction to the government's letter was, "We are already a Center of Excellence in this field of study, so send us some money." As the acting chairman, I was able to persuade several colleagues to join in a grant application that would fund an expansion of our activities. Our proposed Drug Abuse Basic Research Center would include not only the ongoing studies in the monkey colony but also neurophysiological and behavioral studies in whole animals, isolated tissue studies, and the identification of various types of opioid receptors. After the usual study-section review and site visit, we were rewarded with an initial year's budget of approximately $200,000. Because I was (1) the acting chairman, and (2) the typist who wrote most of the grant application, I was allowed to serve as Principal Investigator of the project.

It was my childhood experience as the manager of a baseball team that enabled me to survive as the Principal Investigator when each of my colleagues on the project knew a great deal more about drugs of abuse than I did, when each of them had a much more extensive bibliography than I, and each of them commanded much more research grant money than I commanded. When I was ten years old, I organized, managed, scheduled, and played on a neighborhood baseball team. I was not a good athlete, but I loved the game. (This was many years before the adults had taken over the running of boyhood baseball.) From this managerial baseball experience I learned to sense how far you should try to push people. If you don't push at all, nothing is accomplished; if you push too hard, the other players get angry and go home. There is a middle ground where things actually work pretty well. This principle has aided me in administrative activities throughout my life.

The position of acting chairman is a particularly powerless one because department members know intuitively that time is on their side. They will still be there in their jobs long after the acting chairman has been replaced. The acting chairman cannot fire them or ease them out. He cannot add to their number. They can cooperate with the acting chairman whenever, but only if, they feel like it.

Baseball experience also taught me to recognize a type of activity which might be called an umpire's decision. In baseball, one of the umpire's duties is to declare whether a particular ball was hit fair or foul. If he calls it, "fair ball," the game proceeds; in like manner, if he declares, "foul ball," the game goes on. However, if he says, "I don't know whether it was fair or foul," the game comes to a screeching halt. The point is that under the circumstances of the game, we need an answer, but it does not really matter whether the answer is correct or not. The game can go on, even if the umpire is demonstrably wrong. In life, as in baseball, there are situations in which the making of a decision is more important than being sure that the decision is correct. The acting chairman should recognize such situations when they arise, because they are ideal for exercising the democratic process. The department members can be assembled and given the problem to solve. The acting chairman has already decided that almost any decision is satisfactory, provided only that something is decided. Therefore he can give the members free rein in their activities.

In contrast to umpire's decisions, there are situations in which it is important, at least in the opinion of the acting chairman, that the group follow a particular Plan A instead of some Plan B or Plan C. The wise acting chairman will choose Plan A without discussion and put it into effect. If he is lucky, the members will be so busy debating some previously introduced umpire's decision that Plan A will not be noticed until it is already up and running. Even if the acting chairman's decision is noticed and not particularly popular, it is usually easier to get forgiveness than permission. For a leader who has no real power to enforce his wishes, there is a useful technique that might be called the sequential committee meeting. In this scheme, the chairman visits each member privately, outlines a proposal, listens to the member's response, and incorporates at least a little bit of that response into the final product. This is far more effective (from the chairman's point of view) than having all the staff members sitting around a table, feeding on each other's arguments against the chairman's proposal. The individual member is flattered to think that his opinion is valued, and that he has made a contribution to the decision.

The most interesting moment in my tour of duty as acting chairman did not concern the Michigan pharmacology department at all. It was related to the University of Cincinnati department, from which I had been fired 15 years earlier. The phone rang one day and the caller identified himself as a professor of medicine at Cincinnati. He explained that the school there was in the process of reviewing the chairmanships of their several basic science departments. He wondered if I would be willing to serve as an external reviewer of their pharmacology department chairman. My response was, "I was formerly a member of that department, and so I would be in conflict of interest." He replied that they knew I had been there, and they thought that I would be an apppropriate reviewer. (Notice that I was a little bit short of candor, because I did NOT say, "That guy fired me, so I would be in conflict of interest.") I went to Cincinnati, and with another visiting pharmacologist I listened solemnly to the presentations of the Cincinnati department members as they described their activities and goals. Then, equally solemnly, I recommended that they fire the man who 15 years before had fired me. It was the recommendation that the University of Cincinnati had wanted to hear.

Eventually a new permanent chairman was successfully recruited to Michigan and my acting chairmanship was over, though not for long. The new appointee served his five-year term and then stepped down, thus initiating a new appointment sequence. The same dean who had appointed me in 1971 summoned me again in 1980 to ask me to serve once again as acting chairman. This time around he pointedly explained that I would not be a candidate for the permanent chairmanship. Furthermore, he said that if I would do the job again, he would reward me afterward with a special sabbatical leave, devoid of the expectations of scholarship which normally are a part of sabbatical process. With mixed emotions I accepted the assignment. I served for a little over a year on that occasion, bringing my total acting chairmanship time to approximately four years. When the next chairman was installed, my wife and I climbed into our VW van and spent six months driving happily around the country. We covered 25,000 miles, visiting 35 states and five Canadian provinces. I even did a tiny bit of scholarship in the process of this sabbatical, during which I interviewed Drs. Louis S. Goodman and Alfred Gilman and a number of their colleagues as I prepared a brief history of how it came to pass that Goodman and Gilman wrote "The Pharmacological Basis of Therapeutics."

There might have been a third time around for me as acting chairman. After a number of years, the 1981 appointee left the university, and once again the services of an "acting" chairman were required. Some people suggested that Dr. Swain knew how to do the job, and so why not simply reappoint him. But Dr. Swain said "No! Not again!" By that time I had been serving for several years as the assistant dean for Faculty Affairs of the Medical School, a position to which I had been appointed immediately upon my return from sabbatical.

One of the benefits that I reaped from nearly four years of acting chairmanship was experience, which proved most useful when I was an assistant dean. The faculty-affairs dean is often involved in collisions and abrasions between a professor and his chairman. Having sat on both sides of such encounters, I was often able to lead the contestants to a tolerable win-win situation.

As the assistant dean for faculty affairs, I spent quite a bit of time on cases of plagiarism. In the academic world, ideas are an important commodity. Properly developed ideas can lead to publications, grant support, promotions, and fame. However, it is often difficult to determine which individual had a particular idea first, especially if the dispute is between a pair of people who work in close proximity to one another. I found it useful to make a distinction between that which I labeled felony plagiarism and the far more common misdemeanor plagiarism. The former is out-and-out cheating, and is exemplified by the student who copies an obscure section of the encyclopedia and submits it as his term paper. More serious, but in the same category, is a reviewer for a scientific journal who receives a submitted manuscript and uses it as the basis for his own grant application while delaying the publication of the submitted manuscript.

On the other hand, I used the term misdemeanor plagiarism to describe a situation that arises fairly frequently. If two or more investigators are working together and publishing together, ideas may arise from their interaction in such a manner that neither contributor is clearly the inventor of the concept. If these collaborators subsequently have a falling out, disagreements and bad feelings may result. In cases of felony plagiarism, strong evidence that one document has been copied from another is provided by the demonstration that exactly the same words in exactly the same order appear in the two documents. On the other hand, such evidence is less conclusive in the misdemeanor case. If two investigators have been studying the same phenomena for several years and writing manuscripts together, eventually they begin to use exactly the same words in the same order to describe their observations. An assistant dean trying to sort out an accusation of plagiarism under these circumstances may find complexity and uncertainty instead of a clear-cut bad guy stealing from a noble good guy.

After eight years as assistant dean, I went on retirement furlough, and thereafter retired from the university. Thus there is no possibility that I will ever again be either the acting chairman of the department of pharmacology or the assistant dean for faculty affairs at the University of Michigan Medical School. But it was fun while it lasted.

*John A. Gronvall, M.D., Dean 1970-1983**

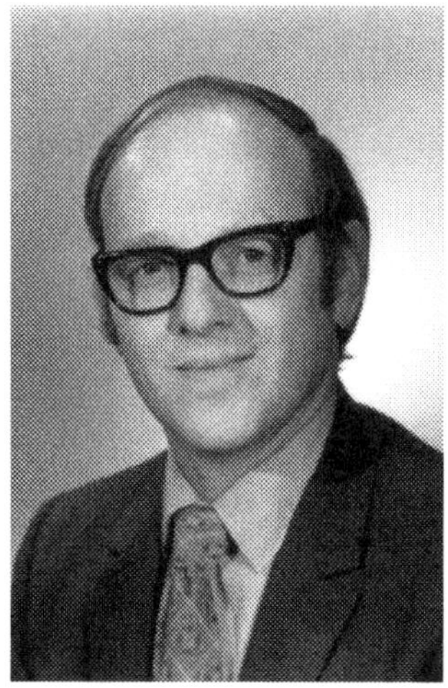

When Dean Hubbard resigned, Dr. Gronvall was first appointed acting Dean in 1970, then Dean of the Medical School and Director of the Medical Center on January 1, 1971. Dr. Gronvall received a B.A. degree in 1953, a B.S. in 1954, and an M.D. degree in 1956, all from the University of Minnesota. He was at Minneapolis General Hospital and subsequently at the University of Mississippi. At the University of Michigan, he was first Associate Professor of Pathology then Associate Dean of the Medical School and Associate Director of the Medical Center. Dr. Gronvall served as Dean of the University of Michigan Medical Center from 1970 to 1982. During this period, with financial support from the federal government, as well as other sources, the Medical School continued to be one of the largest in the nation with a large percentage of women entering its ranks. In addition, the Inteflex program was initiated for rapid facilitation of physician education, integrating undergraduate and medical students in a period of six years. Construction projects at the Medical Center increased enormously, including Medical Science Building II, the A. Alfred Taubman Medical Library, and initiation of plans and construction on the Replacement Hospital Project. Dean Gronvall was especially astute in the early planning years of the new University Hospital. He was asked to appear before a State of Michigan legislative committee, the members of which criticized the enormous outlay of money planned for the replacement hospital. Dean Gronvall pointed out to the legislators that the cost of the replacement hospital was relatively cheap compared to the cost of a single B51 bomber.

When Dr. Seevers retired as Chairman of the Department of Pharmacology, Dean Gronvall appointed Henry Swain as Acting Chairman. This role was one that Dr. Swain was to serve twice during his career at the University of Michigan. In 1974, Dean Gronvall appointed Bert La Du as Chairman of Pharmacology. The Pharmacology Department teaching laboratories on the seventh level of Medical Science Building I were remodeled into research laboratories to accommodate the increasing number of pharmacology staff. Other building projects included construction of Medical Science Research Building I. Five years after Dr. La Du become Chairman of Pharmacology, he stepped down, and again Henry Swain was appointed Acting Chairman. The process of recruiting a new Chairman of Pharmacology continued and resulted in the appointment of Raymond Ruddon in 1981.

After thirteen years of service to the Medical School, Dean Gronvall resigned in 1983 to take a position as Deputy Chief Medical Director at the Veterans Administration in Washington, DC After seven years in this capacity, he died suddenly in 1990.

*Deceased

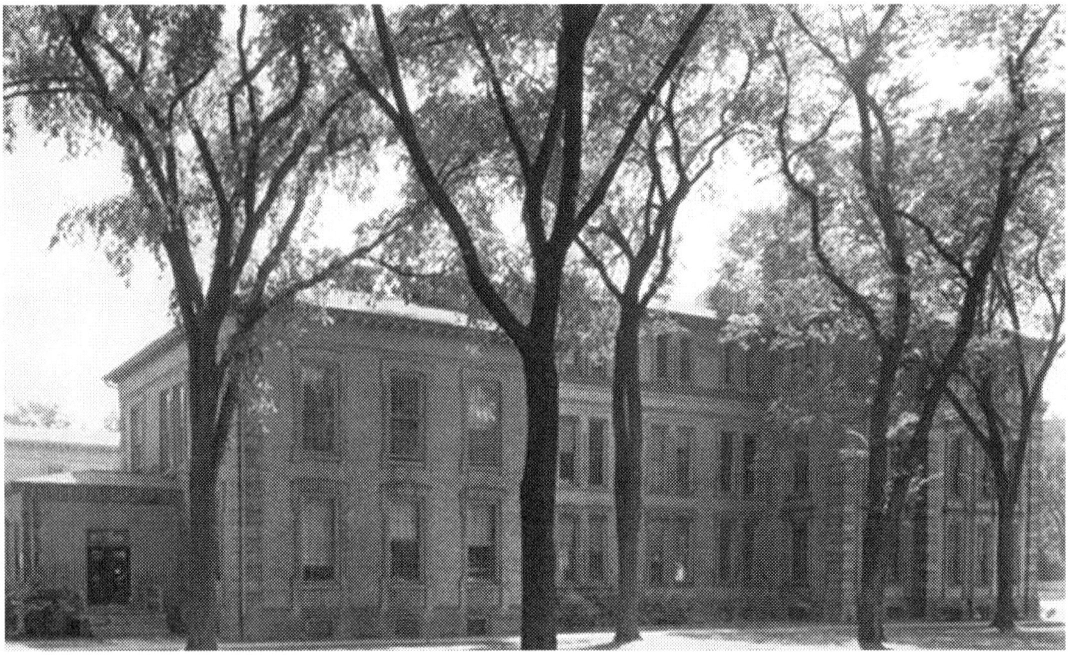

The old Pharmacology Building. Dr. Seevers usually would park his car behind the old loading dock to the left.

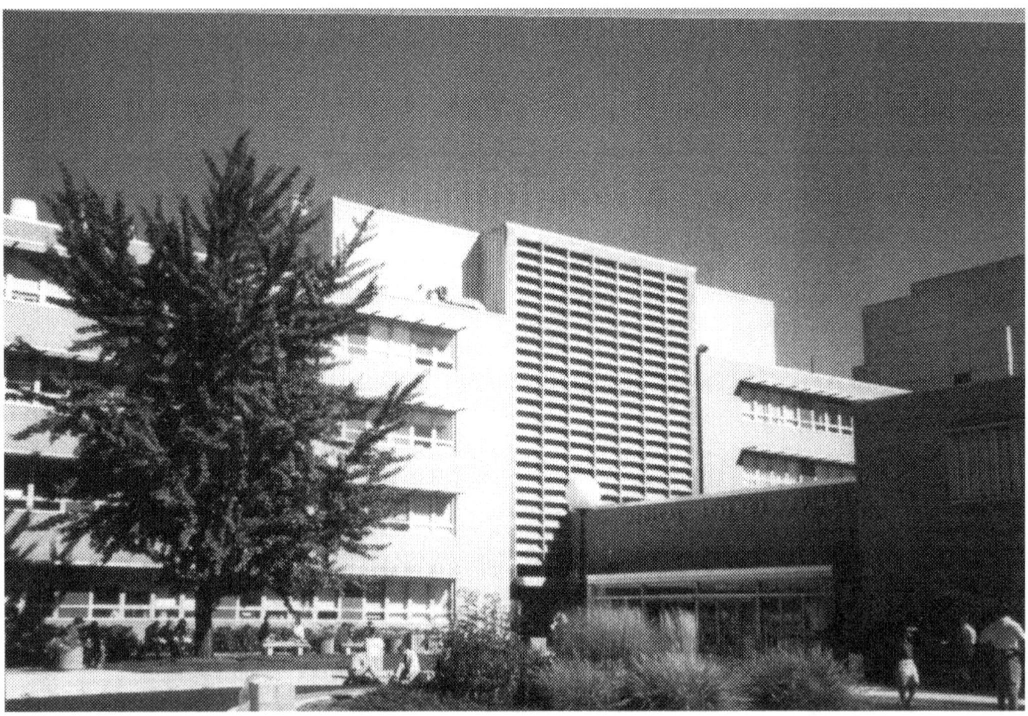

The new home of the Pharmacology Department— Medical Science Building I, 1959.

3

Some Memories of 1974 Through 1980, and Even After That

Bert N. La Du, Jr., M.D., Ph.D.

Arrival in Ann Arbor

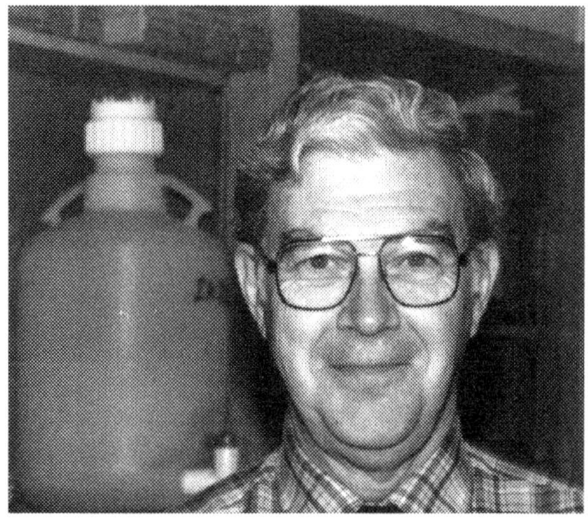

In 1974 I accepted the position of chairman of the Department of Pharmacology at the University of Michigan. A few days before we were to leave New York for Ann Arbor, I was packing papers in my office at New York University Medical School. Suddenly, I noticed my vision had become greatly reduced in my left eye. I had elected to have a cataract operation in New York City a few weeks before our move in order to have that problem all taken care of before starting my new position in Ann Arbor, and everything had been going well, up to that time. The ophthalmologist who did my cataract operation made a quick examination and found an extensive retinal detachment in the operated eye.

He presented me with two choices: either stay on in New York and have another operation at the University Hospital while the rest of my family and two cats moved to Ann Arbor, or fly ASAP out to Ann Arbor and have that operation at the Kellogg Eye Center. I chose the latter to be near my family and start my new job in the Pharmacology Department, even though it would be difficult to undertake many of the things I knew needed to be started as soon as possible, as the new chairman.

Hank Swain had been acting chairman for several years before I came, and he continued to be very helpful with many of the administrative duties. Slowly, I recovered from that second eye operation, unfortunately followed by a third, since the second one under local anesthesia did not completely correct the extensive retinal tear. My first few weeks at Michigan were complicated by my eye problems since I was able to do only a limited amount of reading for several weeks, and many important decisions that had to be made were more difficult to prepare for with my visual handicap. Fortunately, the vision in my left eye gradually improved, and I regained nearly 20/20 vision in that eye over the next few years.

I invited Wendell Weber and Vincent Zannoni to also transfer from NYU to Michigan. Dean John Gronvall and others in his office called us all the "New Yorkers." Zannoni really was a New Yorker; he had grown up in the Yorkville section of New York City. Weber, however, was from Missouri, later Chicago, and came to New York from San Francisco. I was born in Lansing, graduated from Michigan State, the University of Michigan Medical School, and the University of California (Berkeley), so I was coming home.

My medical student memories of the

University of Michigan were a reflection of the unusual time I had been a medical student in Ann Arbor, during World War II. There were relatively few male students on campus at that time, and the medical faculty and we students were trying to adjust to the new Accelerated Medical Teaching Program (four academic years in about three calendar years). I met my future wife, Cathy, at that time in Ann Arbor but we waited to get married until after my year of internship.

Dealing with Dean Gronvall

John Gronvall was an unusual dean, to say the least. I was used to the ways of my previous deans at New York University. The first, Dr. Sam Wortis, was Dean when I came to NYU. He was also chairman of the psychiatry department. He was very astute in sizing up people and very frank in saying exactly what he could and could not do. He came through with all of his promises and was very supportive, as was Dean Lewis Thomas, the next NYU dean. Lewis Thomas was a remarkably gifted man; he was a great scientist, educator, writer and scholar. He went on later to be dean of the medical school at Yale, and finally he became director of the Sloan Kettering Cancer Center in New York.

Dr. Gronvall seemed to be friendly and helpful, but I became rather leery about his reluctance to be as definite about future support for the Pharmacology Department as he had been when I was being recruited. In the end, this concern was justified; he provided the initial dowry as was promised, in writing, but that was all I ever obtained from his office.

Nearly half of the Pharmacology space was on the seventh floor of Medical Science Building I, and this had, until recently, been large old teaching labs without offices, research equipment, cold rooms or proper electric and other utilities. To transform it into faculty research space, my dowry did not go very far. Bill Pratt built a cheap cold room out of a closet on the seventh floor, and we made do and made the necessary changes as best we could. Our shop team, Bob Austin and Tom Larmee, was very creative and extremely helpful in constructing temporary offices and many of the other facilities we needed.

Fortunately, I had been permitted to bring an enormous amount of equipment, glassware, supplies, centrifuges, desks, tables and lab furniture and instruments from New York that we had accumulated from government grants over the years, thanks to Dean Ivan Bennett. Thus, we had enough extra lab equipment to recruit several new faculty members (Peggy Gnegy, Marshal Shlafer, and Ron Holz), and get them started without further support from the dean.

I found out later that it was not unusual for deans to discuss whatever was needed in recruitment but then be careful not to make any more commitments in writing than they absolutely have to. When I discussed some of these issues later with Dean Gronvall, his answer was that the basic sciences departments at Michigan had done very well over the years, and they had established very strong national reputations. He was now obliged to concentrate his support for the clinical departments, even medicine, because of the many demands being made by the new chairman of medicine, Bill Kelley, and by several others. I believe that Dean Gronvall knew that our department would be able to survive and flourish without any further help from him.

Pharmacology Faculty

I was very impressed by the caliber and diversity of the senior faculty members of the Pharmacology Department at Michigan. This was not only because the Department was well represented in many sub-fields of pharmacology by seasoned veterans, who were both specialists and generalists, but also a number of faculty members were prepared to teach many different pharmacological topics. Hank Swain, for example, could give a whole course by himself, if that were necessary. The Michigan department obviously needed more junior faculty members, and the two additional full professors I brought from New York didn't help to correct this imbalance.

Ed Domino was cranking out very good papers at a phenomenal rate; it seemed to be about as many as the rest of the Department combined. Jim Woods was getting lots of students from the main campus through his appointments in both Psychology and Pharmacology, and he had pigeons training to peck at signals in several of the empty rooms in our Department. Ray Counsell had a joint appointment with Medicinal Chemistry and Fedor Medzihradsky had a joint appointment with Biological Chemistry, both representing unusual and very special links with related academic groups. Of course, the diversity of interests within the Pharmacology faculty represented both a strength, and a weakness, due to the lack of depth of these different areas in the Department. There were also many occasions when protagonists of different sub-fields were at odds and argued with others as to which ones were doing real fundamental science, and who were just doing pedestrian science. Probably the long tenure of Dr. Seevers, followed by a several year hiatus without a formal chairman, contributed to the unusual degree of independence, and limited cooperation and collaboration that existed in the Department when I came.

I had been responsible for the growth of the department at NYU from only three people, and was very lucky to have enjoyed that experience with a high degree of support and productive faculty interaction; I expected to find the same attitudes at Michigan. This turned out to be only partly true; some of the Michigan faculty were indeed very helpful and worked vigorously to take progressive steps in revamping the courses and the research activities, while others were reluctant to change their ways.

I was surprised to find no female or African-American faculty members in the department at Michigan at the time I arrived, nor much religious diversity. From pictures of past faculty groups, I knew that at times, the faculty composition had been broader. I had always assumed that good university science departments would roughly reflect the national composition of these scientists and researchers. Fortunately, good candidates were available for our open faculty appointments and I began to correct this imbalance. I never investigated whether the previous composition had just arisen by chance or intention.

Salary Source for Faculty Members

Coming from a private medical school, which had to raise money every year and depended on the generosity of very loyal alumni and friends of the University to survive, I thought it very unreasonable for the administration of a major state-supported school to expect its faculty to raise a third or more of their salaries from research grants and similar "soft money" sources. Indeed, the UM Medical School basic science faculty taught and did research year round, and I thought they should be paid by the year. It was the system at my arrival that faculty members were paid for only nine or 10 months, with an expectation that they would find their own sources for "summer" salaries.

I managed, against the wishes of Dean Gronvall, to switch the entire regular faculty onto a yearly salary basis from the Departmental budget. This disturbed the dean, who preferred expansion of Departmental size by putting more and more salaries on soft money. I knew that most grantees of NIH funding rarely were successful beyond two rounds of two or three years each, and this meant that academic grantees were not regularly funded after reaching tenure. My preference was to use the equivalent amount of salary money saved by getting grants to support their graduate students and/or postdoctoral trainees in that faculty member's laboratory, but not jeopardize the earnings of the faculty members who failed to get grant funding for a round or two.

Of course, my conservatism was disapproved of as being out of step with the other basic science chairmen's views, and probably a sign of lacking confidence in our faculty's ability to be competitive, nationally. That wasn't true, but I felt depending on such sources places an unfair demand on the faculty that should be avoided. I was concerned that in difficult financial times for the federal and state budgets, grant funding would also be tight, and the chances that the Medical School administration would be able to make up for deficiencies in salary money as such times would be very slim.

Teaching Obligations

The biggest shock coming to Michigan was the heavy teaching load for the faculty. There were a total of 13 courses; each school wanted its own pharmacology course at a time most convenient for that particular school. Funding came through our Medical School, but the Pharmacy School, the Nursing School, the Dental School and the Medical School all had different ideas about the content and emphasis expected in their pharmacology course. In addition, the School of Public Health wanted something related to environmental health and toxicology. We also were expected to send some of our faculty to Flint to teach pharmacology in the late afternoons or nights to nurses who were trying to qualify for a B.S. degree, and needed a solid course in pharmacology to fill part of their requirements.

Looking back, it is a wonder how our faculty was able to meet all of these obligations and did all that work with such good spirits and enthusiasm. There were a few times when I wasn't sure we would make it, but our faculty did pull together when we had to. We began to consolidate some of the courses and gradually reduce the total number of duplicated lectures. The different members didn't always agree about which topics were the most important to teach the students, but they all did a super job in showing how important their particular pharmacological area of interests was in their teaching and their research presentations.

Research Activities

The investigative program started by Dr. Seevers on narcotic drugs and addiction was well respected nationally, and I never questioned whether it should be continued, although I worried about it quite often. A major effort was spent using the morphine-dependent Rhesus monkeys, the "Junky Monkey Colony" (JMC) to test new drugs coming on to the market to see whether any of these had addicting properties that no one had noticed during the standard steps of drug development and approval by the FDA. Although it seemed to be a very worthwhile activity and was supported by the Federal Government, this program contained very little in the way of a research component. I wondered why it needed to be continued at the University of Michigan, and occupy important space and faculty time, as a service unit.

Fortunately, NIDA began to ask the same questions, and started to require that continued support should include some elements of a basic research program. That requirement made a lot of sense and I was pleased to see this expectation from Washington. Later, a similar test facility was established by NIDA at the University of Virginia in Richmond, with Louis Harris. There would now be two places in the country able to test new drugs for addicting properties, and a way to check the results coming from the two labs, if that were needed.

To keep the morphine supply adequate for the JMC, Hank Swain was able to obtain rather large quantities of crude morphine from some special source in NIDA in Washington. Occasionally, Hank would take time out to quietly purify individual lots of it, as needed, for the monkeys. This was a noble task, but it worried me that our supply of crude morphine was being stored in a safe in our Department, and, if this became known, might attract unwanted attention from the wrong people. After discussions with Hank, we arranged to store most of the morphine in a nearby bank vault and only keep on hand a relatively small amount for current needs. As far as I know, no serious consequences ever arose, but this supply of morphine was one of my nagging concerns over several years.

The Woods Safe Episode

Jim Woods had a special safe in his office on the sixth floor of MSB I which was used to hold not only narcotics but the series of new drugs sent to him for testing their addicting potential with the Departmental JMC. Woods' safe was said to weigh about 800 lbs., but was probably considerably lighter than that. However, it wasn't very large, about the size of an orange crate. Jim's office seemed to be a reasonable location for these compounds, and had served that purpose very adequately for many years.

I gave it very little thought until one night in 1976, when the University security guard called me at home with the news that the safe had been carted away, and what did I think should be done about it? I checked with Jim about the large number of potentially dangerous drugs it contained, especially if they were all assumed to be narcotics and were taken either by mouth or intravenously. With that knowledge, I realized that we had no choice but to alert the local police and hope the safe and its contents could be found quickly, before any unfortunate consequences occurred. Many of the compounds were old narcotic samples from the extensive collection of Dr. Seevers that may not all have been labeled, and many were new drugs that were being tested for addictive properties and were identified only by code numbers that would make no sense to the thieves. We distributed a notice via the police, warning that it would be very dangerous to take any of these drugs.

After obtaining the undesired but necessary national publicity about the theft, we found out the next day that the stolen safe had never left the Medical Center. At least, not quite left it. The crooks had carted it down the hall and managed to push it through a door to the top of a shaft leading down to a heating tunnel connecting MSB I with the Old University Hospital. Apparently, the thieves had misjudged the weight of the safe; it had gotten away from them as they were lowering it by ropes, and it crashed to the bottom of the shaft. Unfortunately for them, it fell against a hot water pipeline that contained a sensor that was able to signal any problems like reduced pressure within the line. Aside from the noise that the accidental dropping of the safe must have produced, the thieves apparently realized that the damage to the pipe below would trigger a response in the maintenance department, and this would soon be investigated. They abandoned their prize and also left their acetylene torches and gas tanks in the hospital tunnel, near the safe.

Dr. Woods verified the next day that the safe had not been opened, and all the contents were intact, except that a few of the glass containers had broken inside. The police apparently never found the thieves, but that incident alerted me to the potential dangers for people working in a pharmacology department. We are subject to robbery, like hospital pharmacies and any other places with collections of drugs of abuse and narcotics.

Our Shotgun Marriage with the Pharmacy Graduate Education Program

The Graduate Training Program in the Pharmacology Department, supported by the NIH, underwent a drastic change in 1978 when it was decided by the NIH powers-that-be that each University should have only one training program in the Pharmacological Sciences area. This affected us directly. The Department of Pharmacology had one of the very first training programs in the country that had been operating since the 1950s.

The School of Pharmacy also had a long established program that they were unhappy not to be able to continue. Now, the NIH expected us to graciously merge our two programs and show how they interacted with and were related to each other in some meaningful way. In fact, they were very different programs and were, if anything, competitive, not complimentary to each other. So we had to meet regularly and determine how to make the two into a single entity, and do it quickly.

Some members of the pharmacology department favored just submitting our own application, ignoring any Pharmacy input. That, of course, was not a practical solution, and wouldn't have worked. It is hard to remember how we struggled to put together the academic requirements and course work for students in this new program, and how the trainees would be selected and be divided up between the two components. I remember some very difficult negotiations with Dean Ara Paul and his representatives to get the application acceptable to most of the people involved before we finally sent it off. Yes, it was approved, but, as expected, with some reduction in the total number of student positions. One of the few good things that came out of our forced merger was that we started a yearly joint symposium between the students from the pharmacy program and those in pharmacology.

We held this every spring, for several years at Rackham, and more recently at the Chemistry Building. Leroy Townsend and I worked out the initial details for it with Dean Al Sussman of the graduate school, and I'm happy to report that the program is still continuing today.

Personal History After 1980

In 1980 I quit smoking and resigned as chairman. After serving for 16 years as chairman of pharmacology at NYU and then Michigan, I was ready to return to the laboratory and turn over the departmental administrative duties to someone else. The recent advances being reported using molecular biology techniques excited me, and I wanted to learn how to do this kind of research, clone and sequence genes, make Southern blots and Western blots, do PCR amplifications, and all those kinds of experiments, myself.

It was a great pleasure to be able to concentrate on the research, and to be a part of the daily research going on in my lab. Oksana Lockridge succeeded in sequencing the human serum butyrylcholinesterase protein, and we were then able to clone the BCHE gene and identify a large number of mutations affecting its structure and function during the following years.

In 1990 Ray Ruddon, my successor as chairman of pharmacology, left Michigan to take the position as the director of research at the Eppley Institute for Cancer Research in Omaha, Nebraska, and he invited my scientific colleague of about 16 years, Dr. Lockridge, to go with him. It was a good move for Oksana, and I was seriously thinking of retirement at that time. However, an offer to become acting director of research for the Department of Anesthesiology came from the new chairman of anesthesiology, Dr. Kevin Tremper, and I decided to go ahead in that direction. My academic appointment continued in pharmacology, and I was "assigned to anesthesiology," so I could continue to have graduate students and postdoctoral trainees. Dr. Sergio Primo-Parmo from Brazil joined our Lab. We cloned the paraoxonase gene and we extended our studies on this enzyme as well as on butyrylcholinesterase variants, and were able to obtain continued NIH grant support for both of these projects. Anesthesiology was assigned research space on the seventh floor of MSBI, actually in the same area where I had been before as a member of the Department of Pharmacology. We were permitted the luxury of designing our own lab and office space and we spent several very productive years in that location.

Dr. Tremper kindly established a Chair for Anesthesiology Research in my name, and Dr. Ralph Lydic, an expert on sleep research in the Department of Anesthesiology, has been the first occupant of that endowed position.

In 2000, I returned to pharmacology and moved to MSRB III with Dr. Drago Draganov and a postdoctoral trainee, John Teiber. Since then, we have been able to obtain research funding and continue our research, now primarily on the paraoxonase family of closely related enzymes. It continues to be an interesting and exciting experience to be associated with the University of Michigan Medical School Department of Pharmacology, and I thank all the people I have shared these experiences with, and owe so much to, over such a long time.

4

The Ruddon Years: 1981 – 1990

Raymond W. Ruddon, M.D., Ph.D.

The "Ruddon Years" started on a Saturday, September 1981, as I set out from Frederick, Maryland, in an old Ford pulling a 12-foot trailer that contained crucial lab supplies. In the trailer were various small items of equipment, but most importantly a liquid nitrogen freezer containing frozen cell lines and key antibodies that I didn't think I could trust to anyone else. This turned out to be a mistake because the trailer almost came uncoupled from the car on the steep hills in Pennsylvania.

I was listening to the University of Michigan vs. Wisconsin football game on the radio and became quite depressed as Michigan lost the game— the first home opener that they had lost in years. My spirits were lifted considerably once I finally pulled up behind Medical Science I and saw Bob Austin (now deceased) and Tom Larmee waiting for me. What a pleasant sight they were! Bob and Tom and Mindy Dunn, who had come ahead of me from my lab at the NCI-Frederick Cancer Center, quickly unloaded the trailer and got everything set up in our new lab on the sixth floor of Medical Science I. Their cheerfulness and happy efficiency were a real tonic for a tired old "teamster."

The first few months were very hectic, between trying to set up a new lab, get the departmental office organized, and get my arms around the budget issues, staffing, pharmacology teaching requirements, etc. It was a great help to have key people from my lab in Frederick move with me. Mindy Dunn, Richard Hartle, Barry Peters and Fulvio Perini were all experienced scientists and made the transition go very smoothly. We hit the ground running,

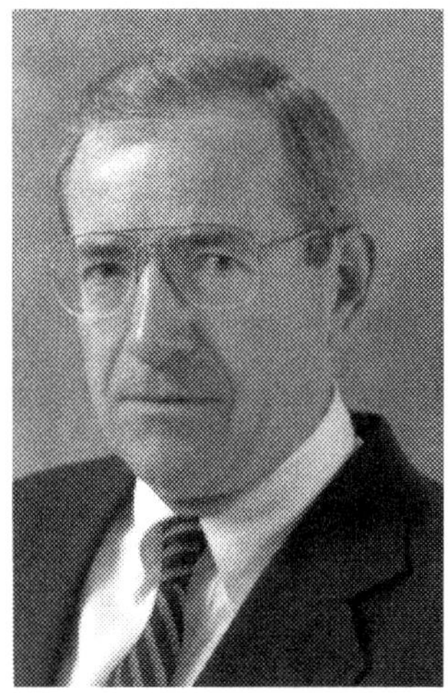

as they say, and soon had the lab cranking out data, which was a good thing since we had to submit an R01 grant to NIH for the next deadline.

Lynne and I had purchased the former Seevers residence from Frankie. It was a delightful experience to move into the house that carried so many happy memories of Pharmacology Department get-togethers in my days as a student and then as a young faculty member. Frankie was very generous in showing us all the ins and outs of our new residence. She spent a great deal of time with Lynne in showing her how to take care of all the exotic plants in the greenhouse, including Moe's wonderful collection of bonsai trees. (Lynne took tender loving care of these for many years, and we donated the bonsai collection to the Matthaei Botanical Gardens before we left Ann Arbor.)

The early years were taken up with some reorganization of the departmental office, faculty recruitment, establishment of new

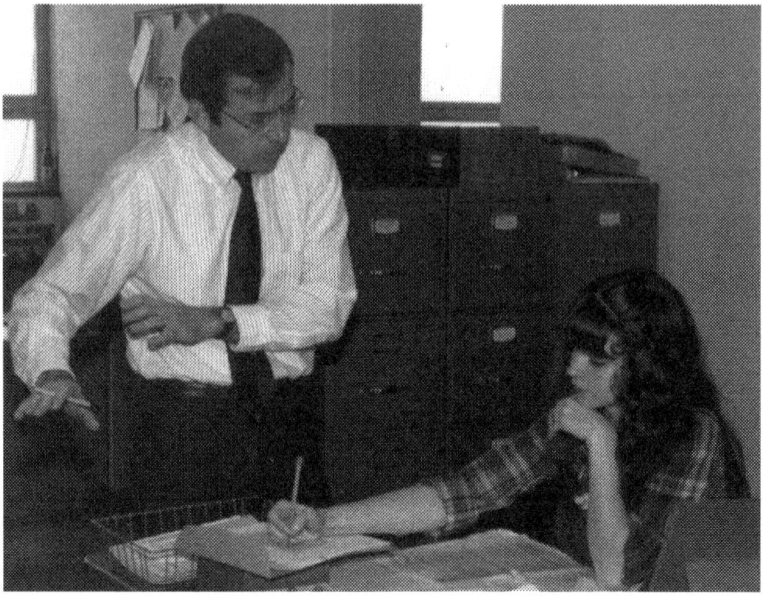

"This is what I want to be done." A young Laura Sell noting it.

budget and planning procedures, review of pharmacology courses, and other administrative and research activities. In the early months, the Department had one word processor (not very functional), one old copying machine, no fax machine, no computers, and generally old typewriters. Hard to believe how we got things done in those days without all the accouterments that we now take for granted in the modern office. I was fortunate to be able to recruit a very capable office staff to go with the holdovers, such as the stalwart Denise Gakle. Jean Razzoog became the departmental administrator and managed the office thoroughly and efficiently, relieving me of many administrative chores so that I could still focus on my research efforts.

One of the most important functions of any new chair is to recruit new faculty. Together with terrific support from the faculty, we set out to recruit "the best and the brightest" young faculty that we could find. This, of course, required many dinners and evenings away from home, what Bill Pratt called "eating for Michigan." We were successful in recruiting top-notch young faculty from various institutions. These included: Jon Maybaum, from the University of California, San Francisco; Rob Simpson, from the University of Wisconsin; Bill Mancini, from Yale University; Rick Neubig of our own University of Michigan; and Steve Fisher from Lederle Laboratories (we recruited him jointly with MHRI). A number of joint faculty appointments also added significantly to the research expertise in the department. These included Bill Ensminger, Marc Longino, Fedor Mezihradsky, Bev Mitchell, Walt Piper, John Wagner, and Donna Shewach (who started as an assistant research scientist in the Department of Internal Medicine and then became a faculty member in Pharmacology).

One of the issues of the early years was the status of the Upjohn Center for Clinical Pharmacology. I had negotiated with Dean Gronvall as part of the recruitment package that the original focus of the Upjohn Center on clinical pharmacology should be reestablished and that the Center should be under the jurisdiction of the Chair of Pharmacology. This was accomplished with some tough negotiations involving space assignment and leadership. In the end, a compromise was worked out with Bill Kelley, then Chair of Internal

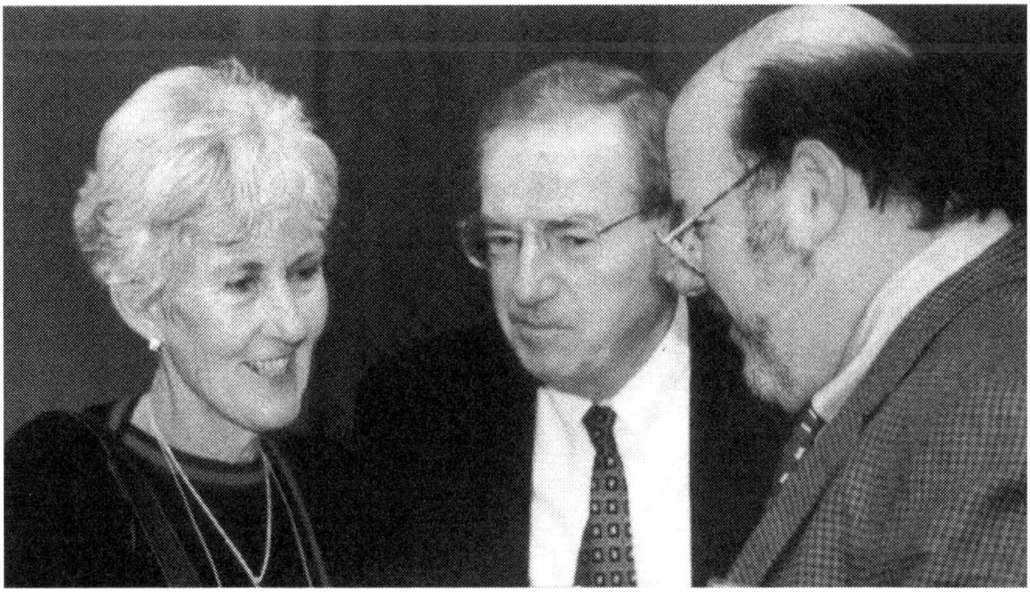

Ray's wife, Lynne, describing how the Department should be run.

Medicine. We agreed that Bill Ensminger, who became a Professor of Pharmacology as well as of Internal Medicine, would become the Director of the Upjohn Center with a focus on cancer clinical pharmacology. For his activities in this role, Bill Ensminger reported to the Chair of Pharmacology.

Another issue that had to be addressed early on was the status of the graduate program and the Pharmacological Sciences NIH training grant. The number of new graduate students coming into the Department had decreased in recent years, and national trends indicated that recruitment of doctoral students into the sciences was going down. The Department launched a vigorous recruitment campaign under the direction of Bill Pratt and later of Peggy Gnegy. The number of new students began to increase and in a few years almost doubled in size, and the departmental program was ranked as one of the top five pharmacology graduate training programs in the US. The Pharmacological Sciences Training Grant was renewed with flying colors for another five years. Because this training grant program is interdisciplinary, a significant effort was initiated to involve representatives from the Biochemistry and Physiology Departments more closely, as well as from departments in the College of Pharmacy. Leroy Townsend, Chair of Medicinal Chemistry, and I shared duties as PI on the grant during alternate grant periods. This appeared to work well, as subsequent renewals of the grant attested.

As the years went on, the Department continued to flourish—not that we didn't have our share of the ups and downs of faculty and funding concerns that plague every academic department. During the 1988-89 academic year, the Department underwent an internal and external review. The positive accomplishments were noted, as well as the issues and concerns that needed to be addressed.

Several points were made by the Internal Review Committee, chaired by Wendell Weber. Among these were the following:

1. ... the Department of Pharmacology is, on a per-capita basis, one of the highest funded departments in the entire Medical School, and is tops in the basic sciences.
2. Compared with eleven other state-sup-

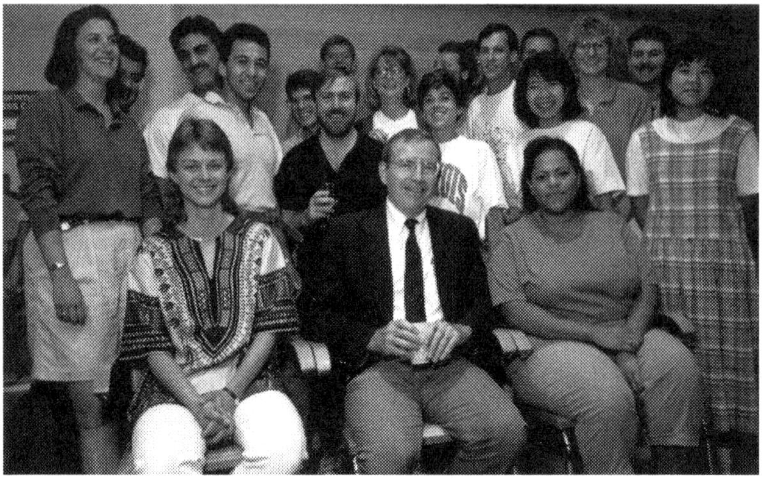

Pharmacology Graduate Students with Ray Ruddon, ca. 1990.
A very impressive group of workers.

ported departments of comparable size, the Department of Pharmacology at the University of Michigan ranked second in total 1986-1987 research dollars, whereas it ranked eighth in terms of institutional support for the same period.

3. New recruits and applicants report that when they ask academic faculty or drug company employees the top choices for pharmacology graduate school, the University of Michigan is always named.

Nevertheless, concerns were noted:

1. Additional institutional support in the form of funds and laboratory space is essential if the Department research programs that have been established are to grow to their full potential within the next decade.
2. Salaries of the instructional faculty of the Department of Pharmacology are well below the 80th percentile of pharmacology departments in the medical schools in the US.
3. The tendency to place increasing reliance on grant support is alarming because it increases the vulnerability of the faculty salaries to decreases in research funding.

The External Review Committee, chaired by Barry Eisenstein, Chair of the Department of Microbiology and Immunology, generally concurred with the findings of the Internal Review Committee. In addition, they noted the outmoded and overcrowded laboratory and office space and the concern that "although salary levels have now been increased to be within 4% of the 80th percentile AAMC levels, there is concern that much of this salary support is derived from research grant 'soft' money." The External Review Committee also found that "The Department is ranked by the American Association for Medical School Pharmacology (AMSP) as seventh among 117 Departments nationally in total research support...." However, they also commented that the Department should strengthen its effort to foster the development of and recruit more research "stars." Nevertheless, the Department did have a number of stars in their research fields. These included Ben Lucchesi (cardiovascular pharmacology), Jim Woods (drug abuse research), Wendell Weber and Bert La Du (pharmacogenetics), Bill Pratt (steroid receptors), Ray Counsell (radiopharmaceuticals), Ed Domino (neuropharmacology) and a number of others.

During the second half of the 1980s, other activities in the Medical School impacted on the Department of Pharmacology. The University of Michigan Comprehensive Cancer Center was established in 1986, and I became the first Associate Director for Basic Science Research. A number of members of the Department became members of the Cancer Center faculty. The Maurice H. Seevers Professorship of Pharmacology was established and I had the privilege of serving as the first Maurice H. Seevers Professor. The Howard Hughes Medical Institute was established and a number of outstanding faculty were recruited to staff it, including Francis Collins, who became head of the Human Genome Project at NIH. During these years, I had the honor of serving two terms on the Medical School Executive Committee and was privileged to participate in some of the decisions that went toward maintaining the Medical School's consistent ranking as one of the top ten Medical Schools in the country (or as one wag put it: "making the Medical School something the football team could be proud of").

Two other events contributed to a positive ambiance of the Department. One was the initiation of planning for the Centennial Celebration of the Department of Pharmacology. This was initiated while I was still Chair, and carried to fruition under the able leadership of Ray Counsell, who became Interim Chair after I left to become Director of the Eppley Institute for Research in Cancer & Allied Diseases at the University of Nebraska Medical Center. In spite of arguments from our colleagues at Johns Hopkins, the University of Michigan had established the first department focused on the science of drugs in the US when John Jacob Abel arrived in Ann Arbor in 1891. Later he moved to Johns Hopkins. Another happy event that started during my tenure was the establishment of the Alumni Steering Committee, chaired initially and to the present by Bob Gussin, Corporate Vice President for Science & Technology at Johnson & Johnson. Bob and his colleagues on the Steering Committee have done much to enrich the spirit of the Department over the years.

I continued to be blessed with excellent staff during the later years of my tenure as Chair. Dennis Ondreyka replaced Jean Razzoog as Departmental Administrator after Jean left to take a position at the Institute for Social Research. Dennis continued the high quality work of that position established by Jean and put his own stamp on the job. He did an outstanding job during my last years as Chair, planning and tracking budgets, overseeing grant submissions, handling faculty and staff issues, directing the office staff, and carrying out innumerable other tasks that made the department run well. Eileen Ferguson became my administrative assistant and was responsible for preparation of my manuscripts, grant proposals, and correspondence (and alleviating general headaches) as well as providing administrative support for the graduate program.

It goes without saying that no departmental chair can continue to carry out all the duties of a chair and still maintain an active research program without great technical staff as well as administrative staff. I was extremely fortunate to have Mindy Dunn and Richard Hartle in the lab during my first years as chair, and later Ray Krzesicki. Ray was an accomplished organist, gourmet cook, wine connoisseur, master carpenter, and a fine draftsman as well as a superb research technician. I have always been fortunate in having outstanding technical staff in the lab, including Cindy Rainey and Donna Lundeen, from my earlier years on the faculty at Michigan.

The Pharmacology Department Shop was the envy of the Medical School during those years. Bob Austin and Tom Larmee could carry out any construction task that was asked of them (and that they were allowed to do by the University of Michigan Plant Department), and they also were experts at lab renovation and small equipment repair and design. They carried out many lab renovations that would have otherwise been beyond the departmental budget. One way to always frighten faculty was to send Bob and Tom into their labs carrying a yardstick and a measuring tape.

Overall, my years as Chair of Pharmacology at Michigan were very rewarding. I had the privilege of serving with an outstanding group of faculty, staff, postdoctoral fellows, and students. My own research prospered, much to the credit of the collaborations that I was able to establish at Michigan, and to the quality of students, postdocs, and technical staff who carried out the research in the lab. The students and postdocs with whom I was privileged to work during those years included: Larry Cole, Ph.D., later on the faculty at Yale University Medical School; Ann Marie Gebhart, Ph.D., who later took a position at Parke Davis; Jean Beebe, Ph.D., now manager of Cancer Biology at Pfizer Central Research Laboratories; Gary Frenette, M.D., Ph.D., now practicing medical oncology; Todd Kroll, M.D., Ph.D., who completed a fellowship in pathology at Brigham and Women's Hospital-Harvard Medical School; and Jeff Huth, Ph.D., Research Scientist at Abbott Laboratories. These postdoctoral fellows and graduate students who trained with me during my "second life" at Michigan joined the ranks of the previous students who were with me during my first life at the University of Michigan: Jim Johnson, Mary Kay Wolpert, Art Cohen, Joe Cranston, Larry Weisenthal, Lora Rikans, John Lazo, Alan Lau, and Mary Bittner. I still keep in touch with most of them and they are a wonderful scientific family. Some of them now have their own scientific "children," who, have become, as one of them put it, my scientific grandchildren. I even have a few scientific great-grandchildren!

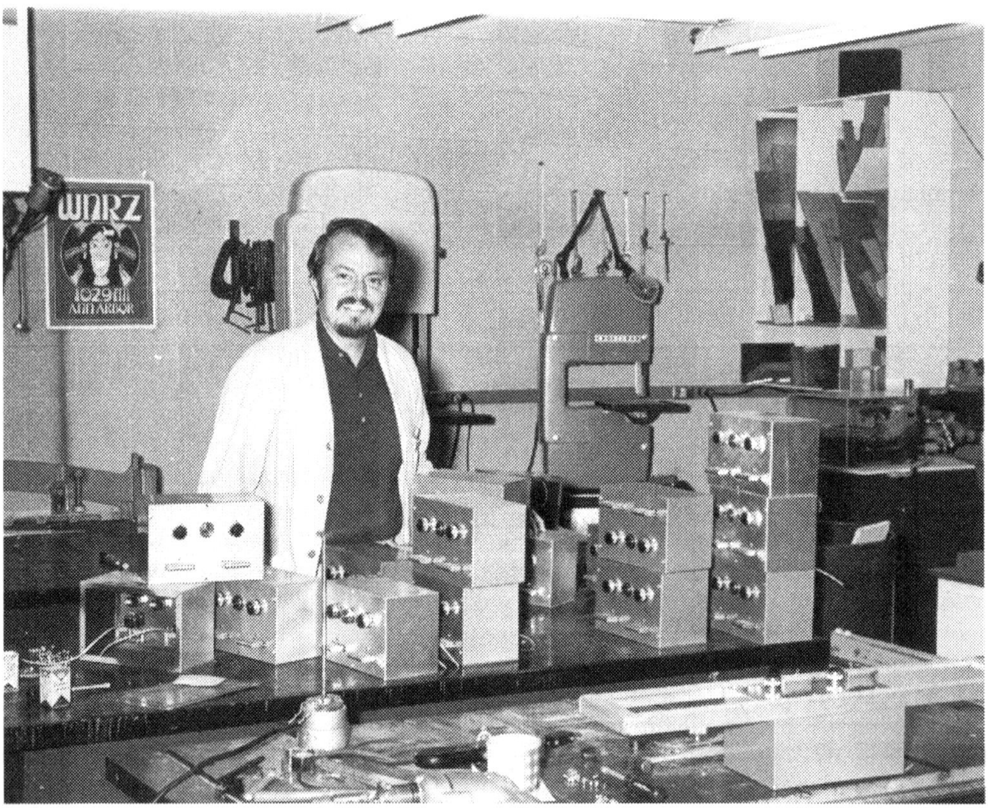

Bob Austin in the Pharmacology Shop, ca. 1980s.

Peter A. Ward, M.D., Interim Dean 1983-1985

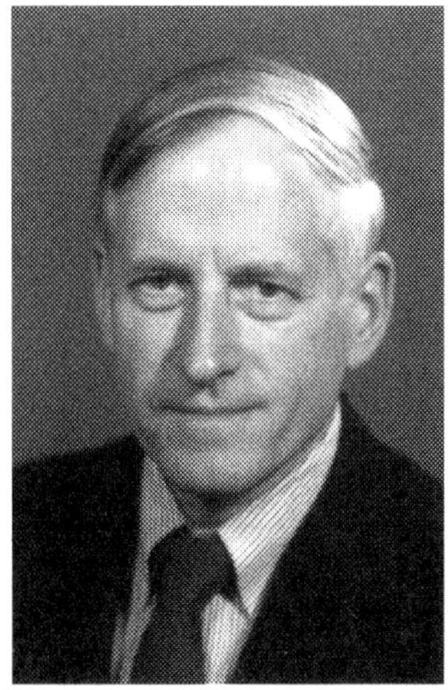

In 1983, Peter A. Ward was appointed Interim Dean of the Medical School. At the same time, a new position was created by the Regents, in which the Dean of the Medical School and the Director of the Medical Center reported to the Vice-Provost for Medical Affairs. This position, as Vice-Provost, was held by George Zuidema, M.D.

In 1958, Dr. Ward earned his B.S. degree from the University of Michigan and in 1960 his M.D. degree. In 1960 he was recipient of the Borden Research Award. He had an internship at Bellevue Hospital from 1960-1961, after which, he completed his residency at the University of Michigan Hospital. He left to become postdoctoral fellow at the Scripps Clinic in La Jolla, California from 1963-1965. Following his fellowship, Dr. Ward became Chief of the Immunobiology Branch at the Armed Forces Institute of Pathology in Washington from 1965-1971. During the years 1971-1980, he was Professor of the Department of Pathology and Chemistry at the University of Connecticut Health Center.

In 1980, Dr. Ward became professor and chairman of the Department of Pathology at the University of Michigan. He was Interim Dean of the Medical School for a three year period. During his tenure, Dean Ward was involved in multiple teaching, legal, and construction initiatives. He was instrumental in the reduction of class sizes in the Medical School. He headed the legal fight in a Supreme Court decision to affirm that universities do not promise the success of each student. Further, under Dean Ward, diversity of the Medical School classes became an important issue, resulting in the creation of a program in education to aid students who were underprivileged.

Dr. Ward's leadership allowed the completion of Medical Science Research Building I and plans for construction of Medical Science Research Building II. Construction also moved forward on the new University Hospital and the Taubman Health Care Center. Dean Ward was instrumental in the Medical School becoming one of a dozen Howard Hughes Medical Institute sites in the United States. The Institute is in Medical Science Research Building I (MSRB I.) In 1985, Dr. Ward stepped down as Interim Dean and resumed his full time responsibilities as chairman of the Department of Pathology, continuing in that position today. Dr. Ward became the first Godfrey D. Stobbe Professor of Pathology here at the Medical School in 1987. In 1996, the Rous-Whipple Award was given to him by the American Society of Investigative Pathology. Dr. Ward was also the Gold Headed Cane Award recipient in 2000 and the 2003 Amberson Lecturer for 35 years of inflammation and lung injury research.

Joseph E. Johnson III, M.D., Dean 1985-1990

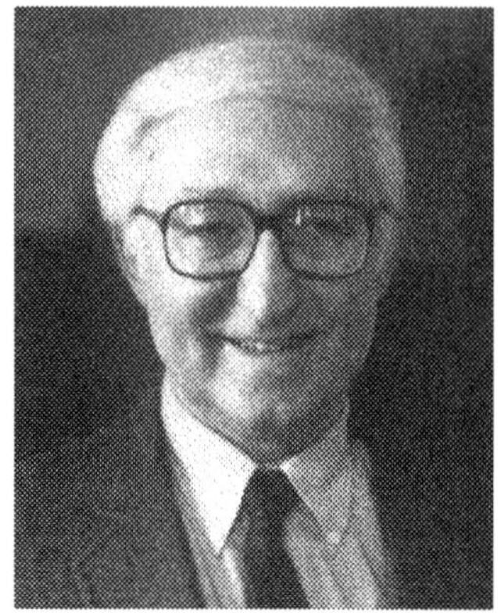

Joseph E. Johnson III was appointed Dean of the University of Michigan Medical School in 1985. He specialized in internal medicine, especially infectious diseases. His early training was at Vanderbilt University in which he received a B.A. in 1951 and an M.D. degree in 1954. After his graduation he had a year of internship at the Johns Hopkins Hospital in Baltimore, Maryland. He then completed his residency there in 1961. From 1961-1966, he was a physician and faculty member of the Johns Hopkins Medical School. He was Assistant Dean for three years at the same institution starting in 1963.

Dr. Johnson left Baltimore to become Chief of Infectious Diseases at the University of Florida College of Medicine in Gainsville from 1966-1972. From 1970-1972, he was Associate Dean. He then was a member of the faculty of the Department of Medicine at Bowman Gray School of Medicine of Wake Forest University.

Dr. Johnson recruited eight new department chairpersons during this period, research funding increased significantly, and nationwide medical school curriculums were changing and developing. In 1986, he recruited Giles G. Bole, who was to be his successor, to join him in the dean's office. The new University Hospital and A. Alfred Taubman Medical Center opened in 1986 as well, while Dr. Johnson was Dean. Medical Science Research Building I opened that same year, and Medical Science Research Building II was finished in 1989; at the same time, plans for developing a Cancer / Geriatrics facility and Medical Science Research Building III were begun.

Dr. Johnson served as Dean until 1990, when he returned to the faculty as a professor of internal medicine. Subsequently, he left the University of Michigan and is currently Senior Vice President of the American College of Physicians in Philadelphia.

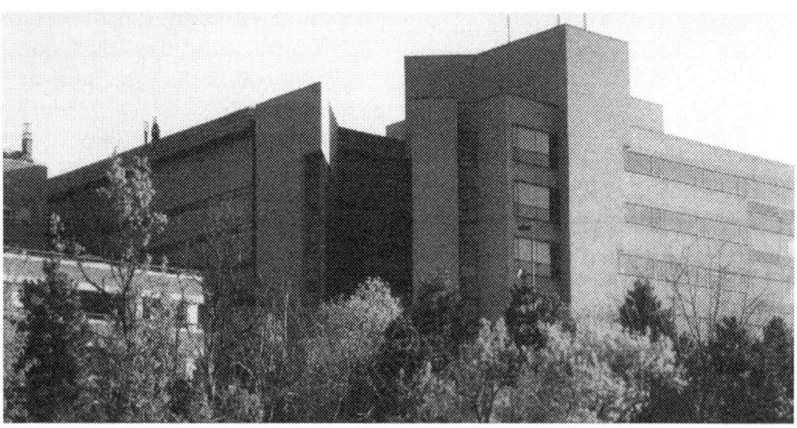

View of Medical Science Research Buildings II (left) and I (right), ca. 2000

5

The Interim Years 1990-1994

Raymond E. Counsell, Ph.D.

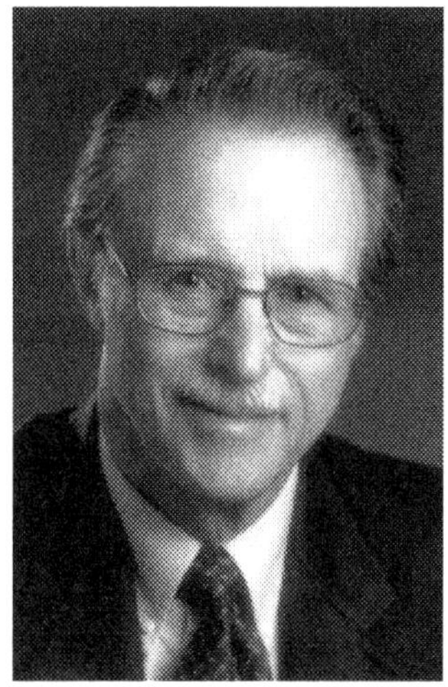

In June of 1990 the Department and members of the Medical School administration, faculty and students assembled to bid farewell to Ray Ruddon, who had provided outstanding leadership to the Department for a period of nine years. His resignation to become director of the Eppley Institute for Research in Cancer and Allied Diseases at the University of Nebraska Medical Center came as a major surprise to those of us in the Department. Even though I had been serving as associate chairman since 1988, I had no inkling of Dr. Ruddon's plans. Certainly, becoming interim chairman was not one of my aspirations. However, Dean Giles Bole had other plans and I agreed to serve in such a capacity on the understanding that it would be only for a period of one year.

Dean Bole very quickly appointed a Chairman's Search Committee composed of Dr. Anne Young, Professor of Neurology as chair and Dr. Leroy Townsend, Professor of Medicinal Chemistry and Chemistry as associate chair. Other members included Thomas D. Gelehrter, Professor and Chair of Human Genetics, Beverly S. Mitchell, Professor of Internal Medicine and Pharmacology, Louis G. D'Alecy, Professor of Physiology, Richard R. Neubig, Associate Professor of Pharmacology and Internal Medicine, and John E. Billi, Associate Dean for Clinical Affairs.

At the same time, the Department established a new arrangement for management. An Advisory Committee was elected, composed of Professors Steve Fisher, Fedor Medzihradsky, Rick Neubig, Marshal Shlafer, and Wendell Weber, with Ben Lucchesi serving as chair. Dennis Ondreyka, the department administrator, and I met regularly with this Committee to review important matters relating to Department governance. Dr. Margaret Gnegy continued to chair the Graduate Programs Committee and Dr. Marshal Shlafer was asked to chair the newly appointed Curriculum Planning Committee.

Other highlights of the year included the presentation of the Distinguished Faculty Lecturer Award to Professor Lucchesi, the Excellence in Teaching Award to Professor Shlafer, the appointment of Professor Woods to the Advisory Board, Drug Policy Research Center of the Rand Corporation, and the presentation of the Outstanding Alumnus/Alumna Award to Dr. Paula Stern, Professor of Pharmacology at Northwestern Medical School. Paula's award presentation was titled "Signal Transduction Mechanisms in Skeletal Tissues." It was also a year when our graduate program numbered 49 students, a record.

On September 21, 1990, Japanese scholars who were associated with the Department in previous years held a meeting in Sapporo,

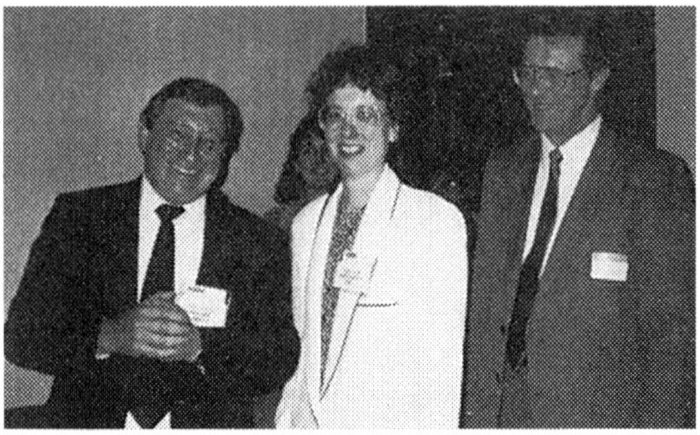

Bob Gussin, Paula Stern and Raymond Counsell

Japan, during the Japanese Clinical Pharmacology Society Meetings. The Michigan Fellows attended a pleasant evening buffet hosted Dr. and Mrs. Lucchesi and Dr. and Mrs. Domino. Dr. Tanabe, the second Japanese Fellow at the University of Michigan, was very active as host.

On a sadder note, it was a year when Bob Austin died unexpectedly at his home in Holder, Florida. Bob was a valued Department employee until he retired in 1988. The Department established in his memory the Bob Austin/ Pharmacology Memorial Fund, which has been used to provide a travel award for graduate students.

There was an air of excitement in the Department as we began 1991. After all, this was the year for our Centennial Celebration. It was a time for us to reflect on our past accomplishments and to plan for the future. It was time to be proud of our tradition and to be part of a heritage that all began in 1891.

Planning for our centennial birthday had begun several years earlier because we wanted it to occur in the fall, hopefully in connection with a football game. This meant that a request for a large block of hard-to-get football tickets had to be made to our Alumni Office. Also, advanced reservations had to be made at local hotels and motels in order to accommodate returning alumni.

To accomplish our goals, a Centennial Celebration Alumni Committee was organized, composed of Robert Gussin, vice president, Johnson & Johnson (who served as chair); Larry Bush, research leader, Hoffmann-LaRoche; Tony Dren, senior clinical research scientist, Burroughs Wellcome Company; Jim Gibb, professor and chairman Department of Pharmacology and Toxicology, University of Utah; John McNeill, dean, Faculty of Pharmaceutical Sciences, University of British Columbia; and Joanne Moore, Professor and Head Department of Pharmacology, University of Oklahoma College of Medicine. This group worked closely with the Departmental Centennial Planning Committee composed of Ed Domino, Harvey Kaplan, Ben Lucchesi, Dennis Ondreyka, Henry Swain, and myself. The overall thrust of the program was to celebrate the accomplishments of our past graduates and to have internationally known leaders, such as Nobel laureate Sir James Black, present their views on the future direction of Pharma-

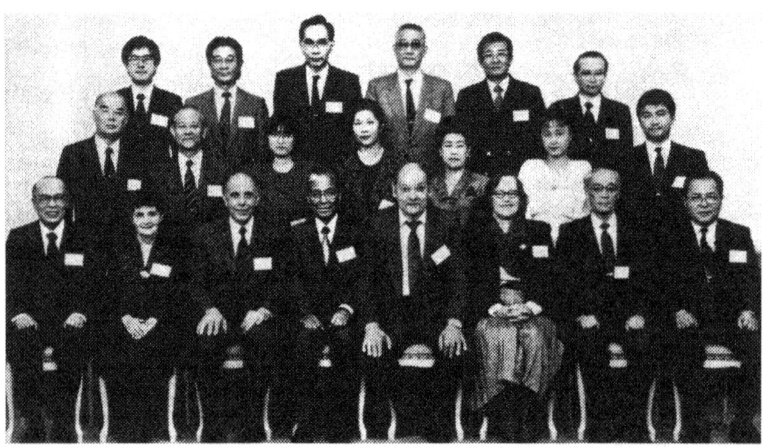

A group shot of a Japaneese Clinical Pharmacology Society meeting.

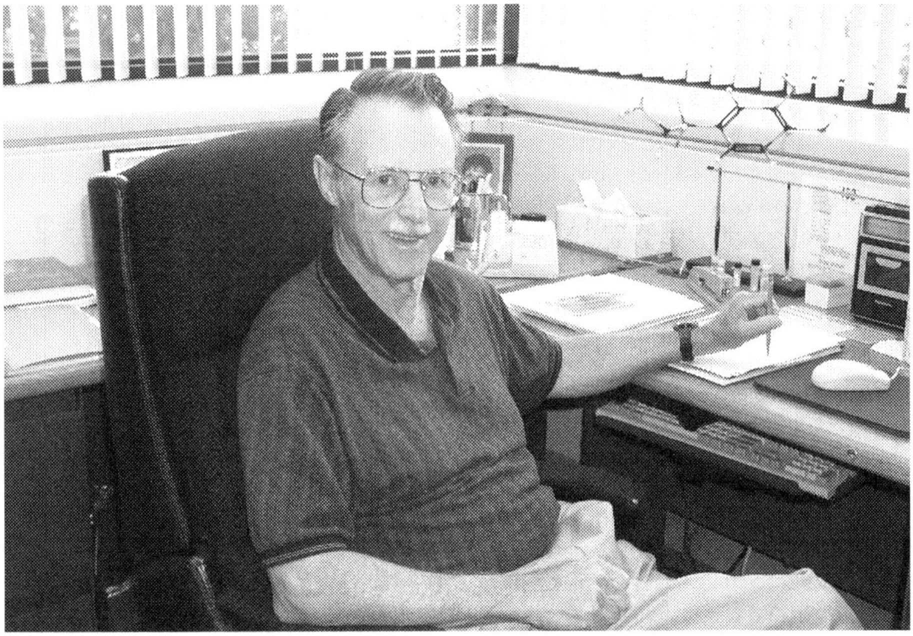

Dr. Raymond E. Counsell— hard at work.

cology.

Some 223 individuals registered for the Celebration and well over 328 people attended many of the activities. Alumni and friends from both the east and the west coasts and as far away as Mexico and Japan participated. They brought with them many fond memories. The program sessions were all well attended, as were the 55 poster displays. The largest gathering took place at the Banquet, where 286 merry-makers enjoyed the stories of Glenn Kiplinger and Hank Swain. On Saturday, 250 alums, faculty, and students saw an exciting football game between Michigan and Florida State from front row seats near the 50-yard line. Everyone enjoyed a terrific game and the opportunity to see Desmond Howard, the Heisman Trophy winner, make some spectacular catches.

Another successful result emanating from our Centennial Celebration was culmination of our Centennial Fund Campaign. This fund raising campaign was initiated a year earlier in order to secure much-needed discretionary funds for the Department. Moreover, the Medical School agreed to match each dollar contributed to the fund on a two for one basis. This effort led to the achievement of our goal of $250,000 which was set aside to support our graduate student program and research efforts.

1991 was also the year that Henry H. "Hank" Swain, M.D. retired and became Professor Emeritus of Pharmacology. Prior to his retirement, however, Dr. Swain completed his history of the Department entitled "One Hundred Years of Pharmacology" in time to be distributed during the Centennial Celebration and mailed to all former graduates, faculty and staff who were unable to attend.

This was also the year in which Dr. Mark Nickerson paid a return visit to the Department. In 1954, at the height of the McCarthy era, three UM faculty members were dismissed. On February 18, 1991, all three returned to Ann Arbor to be present for the first annual Davis, Markert, Nickerson Lecture on Academic and Intellectual Freedom. Dr. Nickerson was then a guest of the Department where he had served as associate professor from 1951-1954. He presented a seminar entitled "The Role of a Pharmacology Department in a Medical School." This was followed by a reception in his honor. After leaving the UM in

1954, Dr. Nickerson served with distinction on the faculties of the University of Manitoba and McGill University. He was also the president of ASPET in 1975-1976.

Honors during the year went to Ed Domino, Peggie Hollingsworth, and Marshal Shlafer. Dr. Domino was elected Life Fellow to the American College of Neuropsychopharmacology. Dr. Hollingsworth received the University President's Medallion in recognition of her contributions to faculty governance during her tenure as chairperson of the Faculty Senate. Dr. Shlafer was the recipient of the Elizabeth Crosby Award given by the Galens Medical Society to a member of the Medical School faculty for outstanding teaching in the basic sciences.

Finally, 1991 saw the Medical School ranked number one among public institutions in its ability to attract research funding. Moreover, our Department continued to lead the basic science departments in the Medical School in terms of total annual research dollars. The faculty, staff and students were congratulated for their achievements.

The spirit of the Centennial Celebration still lingered as we began 1992. The one disappointment was that we were still in search of a chair. For various reasons the earlier search was put on hold and Dean Bole asked me to remain on as interim chair. Dean Bole, however, did appoint a new Search Committee composed of John Williams, M.D., Ph.D., Professor and chair of Physiology (chairman), Jack Dixon, Ph.D., Professor and chair of Biological Chemistry, Tadataka Yamada, M.D., Professor and chair of Internal Medicine, Jeffrey Trent, Ph.D., Professor of Human Genetics and Radiation Oncology, Wendell Weber, M.D., Ph.D., Professor of Pharmacology, and Fred Neidhardt, Ph.D., Associate Dean for Faculty Affairs.

As we began the second century of pharmacology, the Department was heavily involved in changes that were being made in the Medical School curriculum. Benedict Lucchesi and Fedor Medzihradsky served as members of the dean's Committee on Curriculum Improvement. As a result of the deliberations of this committee, significant changes were made in the way Pharmacology would be taught to medical students. In the future, Pharmacology lectures were to be integrated into a totally new organ-based curriculum. This meant that the previous course in Pharmacology taught to both medical and pharmacy students would now be taught only to pharmacy students. There would be no change in the Pharmacology courses offered to nursing and dental students. Unfortunately, the modification of the medical school curriculum increased the Department's teaching responsibilities at a time when we were understaffed and in the midst of a search for a new chairperson.

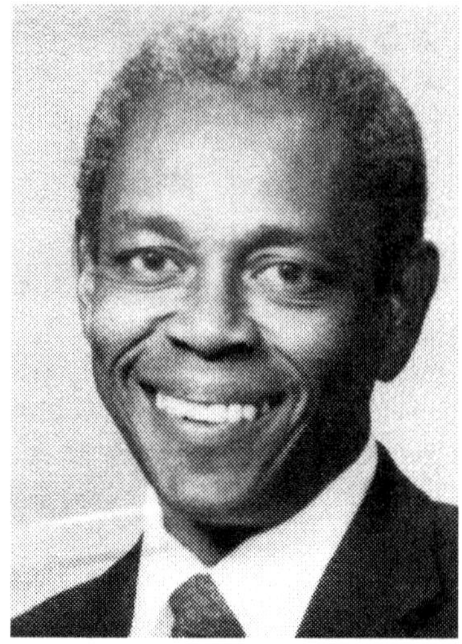

Charles Ross (deceased)

But we survived and our faculty and students continued to excel. Dean Brenner received a special fellowship from the Foundation for the Promotion of Cancer Research in order to undertake a month's study at the National Cancer Center in Tokyo, Japan. In addition, Charles B. Smith was the recipient of a fellowship from the Japan Society for the Promotion of Science Fellowship. Dr. Smith used this fellowship to serve as visiting professor in the first department of pharmacology, Hokkaido University School of Medicine, Sapporo, Japan. Similarly, Benedict Lucchesi was named Sigma Xi National Lecturer for a three-year term. This lectureship program is designed for speakers working at the cutting edge of scientific inquiry to speak to lay groups.

This was the year in which the Charles Ross Fellowship in Pharmacology was established in honor of the late Charles R. Ross, who was one of the first Black Americans to receive a doctoral degree in pharmacology from the University of Michigan. This fellowship was established for the purpose of providing African Americans, like Charles Ross, with an opportunity to obtain a start in a career that otherwise might not be available to them due to socioeconomic circumstances.

Two notable scholars visited the Department in the fall. David G. Nicholls, Ph.D., from the University of Dundee in Scotland was the 1992 Sterling Drug Visiting Professor. Dr. Nicholls' keynote address was entitled "Mechanisms of Neurotransmitter Release." Dr. Nicholls spent a full week in the department meeting with faculty and students. Professor Tetsufumi Ueda served as host for the visit. During the same week Professor Ken Moore was presented with the Department's Outstanding Alumnus/Alumna Award in recognition of his numerous contributions to pharmacology. Dr. Moore received his Ph.D. in 1961 under supervision of Professor Ted Brody. After several years in the Department of Pharmacology at Dartmouth, he joined the faculty at Michigan State University in 1966. Since 1986, he has been professor and chair of the M.S.U. Department of Pharmacology and Toxicology. The title of his seminar was "A Neuropharmacologist's Journey: The Road Less Traveled By."

Nonetheless, the Department continued to be faced with many challenges such as implementation of the new curriculum changes, increased teaching responsibilities, increased competition for grant support and funding, reduced funding for the graduate program, and a continued reduction in teaching faculty. Rightly or wrongly, resolution of many of these concerns was on hold until the naming of a new chairperson. In the meantime, excellent cooperation from the majority of the faculty and an outstanding effort by the office staff under the direction of Dennis Ondreyka allowed the Department to perform its responsibilities. One of the bright spots was receipt of an excellent priority score for renewal of our Pharmacological Sciences Training Program sponsored by the National Institutes of Health. This meant we would continue to receive support for a program that was initiated by the Department in 1958. As noted in the summary statement from the N.I.H., "this is an outstanding program at an outstanding university."

During the year, faculty continued to receive their share of honors and awards. Dr. Domino served as visiting professor in the Department of Pharmacology, University of Hiroshima at the Faculty of Medicine, Hiroshima, Japan. Dr. Fedor Medzihradsky received a Fogarty Senior International Fellowship to carry out sabbatical research on lipid-protein interactions in neural cell membranes at the Universities of Utrecht and Wageningen in the Netherlands. Dr. Richard Neubig was appointed by the American Society of Pharmacology and Experimental Therapeutics as the founding chair of the new section of Molecular Pharmacology. In addition, Dr. Weber was nominated as the 1993 Distinguished Faculty Lecturer by the Medical School for his "outstanding contributions in the areas of research and teaching which have enhanced the Medical School research environment."

Dr. Gunter Schultz, professor and chair at the Institute für Pharmakologie der Freien Univesität Berlin was the Sterling Winthrop Visiting Professor. Dr. Schultz spoke about antisense methods to study the specificity of beta and gamma subunits of G proteins coupling receptors to calcium channels. He presented an overview entitled "The Complexity of the G protein Signaling System" followed by a lecture entitled "Diverse G Proteins Mediate Hormonal Inhibitions and Stimulations of Voltage-dependent Calcium Channels." During his visit Dr. Neubig served as host for Dr. Schultz who enhanced his stay by interacting with many faculty and students.

1993 was also the year that we welcomed the establishment of the Charles W. Edmunds Fund for graduate fellowships. This was through the generous gift of Dr. Edmunds' daughter, Ann Edmunds Avery of Grand Rapids, Michigan. Several years earlier Mrs. Avery had given the University the portrait of her father, which now hangs in the Department library. Dr. Edmunds served as chair of the Department from 1905 until his death in 1941.

On a sad note, the Department lost three close friends during the year. Dr. Gerald A. Deneau, who had received his Ph.D. from our Department in 1957, died in April 1993 after a long illness. Dr. Deneau served as a faculty member in the Department until leaving in 1965 to become a senior pharmacologist at the Southern Research Institute in Birmingham, Alabama.

Dr. Showa Ueki passed away in June of 1993 after a bout with cancer. Dr. Ueki was a postdoctoral fellow in the Department from 1958 to 1959. In addition to serving for many years as chair of the Department of Pharmacology at Kyushu University in Fukuoka, Japan, Dr. Ueki was a key figure in helping enhance the world status of Japanese pharmacology. I had the good fortune of meeting with Dr. Ueki during my sabbatical at his University in 1986.

Frankie Seevers died at home on March 21, 1993. She had been a friend to all pharmacologists associated with Michigan since 1942 when her husband, Dr. Maurice Seevers was appointed chairman. Frankie was unfailingly helpful and welcoming, especially to those

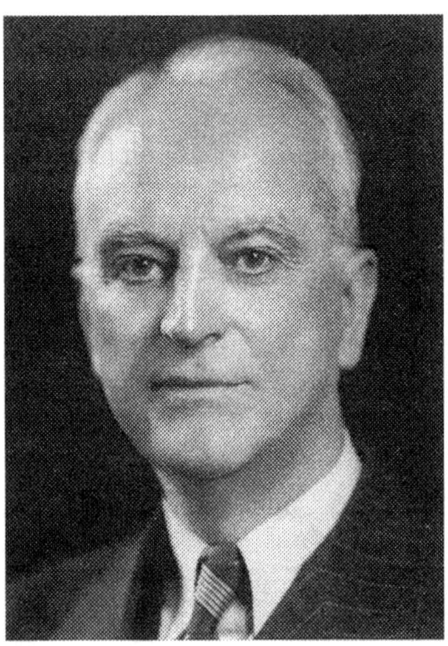

Dr. Edmunds, ca. 1940

who had come a long way to live and work in Ann Arbor. She is survived by her daughter, Pamela, who is a long time resident of Ann Arbor. There was a memorial celebration of her life on April 7 at St. Clare of Assisi Church. She will be fondly remembered by those of us who had the good fortune to know her.

Finally, this was a year that we had to make arrangements for moving our laboratories to a new research building. In consultation with the dean, I suggested that as we search for a new chair, he might consider providing our Department with new space in Medical Research Building III, which was currently under construction. The appeal of this suggestion was that it would allow clinical research faculty to move into our space in Medical Sciences Building I instead of the new building, thus putting them in closer proximity to the hospital. It seemed like a win-win proposition for both parties. The dean ultimately approved this plan.

The year began with the welcome knowledge that Dr. Paul F. Hollenberg would become the chair of our Department effective July 1. This now released the dean's freeze on the search for new faculty to replace those that had retired in previous years. Advertising began immediately for three tenure track faculty. Our goal was to recruit the strongest candidates in terms of pharmacological training, teaching qualifications, and research promise. Plans also continued for relocating the Department to the new Medical Science Research Building III which was due to be ready for occupancy in August.

As I reached the end of my tenure as interim chair it was time to recognize and thank those faculty, staff, and students who supported my efforts for a very busy four years. Despite the lack of a permanent chair, the Department managed to sustain its traditionally strong graduate program and remained among the Nation's leaders in research grant funding. I looked forward to Dr. Hollenberg's arrival and to the excitment and challenges to come.

Giles G. Bole, M.D., Dean 1990-1996

Marshal Shlafer, Ph.D.

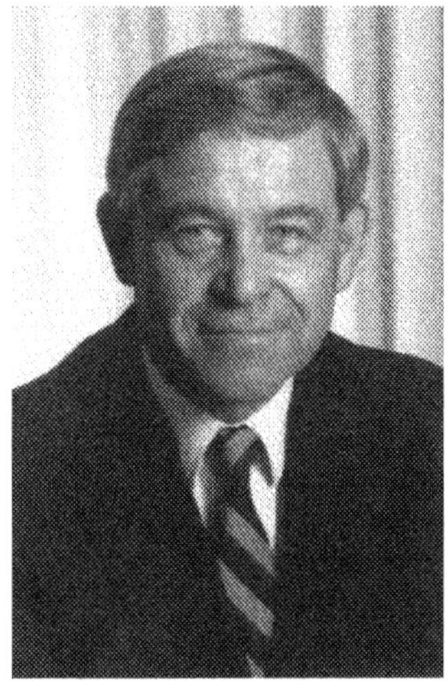

Time flew, the deanships of John Gronvall, Peter Ward, and Joe Johnson came and went (and the glassed-in inner sanctum of the 7th floor suites usually got renovated with each new tenant). In 1990, Giles Bole took the reins (and no renovations). Dr. Bole spent the great majority of his academic career at the University of Michigan. In 1949 he obtained a B.S. and in 1953 an M.D. degree. In 1959 he became a member of the Medical School faculty, then was Director of the Rackham Arthritis Research Unit from 1969-1986. In 1975, he became Chief of the Rheumatology Division in the Department of Internal Medicine and remained until 1986 when he joined the Dean's office.

Early on, one of Dr. Bole's stated goals was to become known as the "education dean," and it became clear he would do what he could to earn that moniker while keeping the rest of the business in good order. He would "look at" teaching quantity and quality just as one would count up the NIH direct costs per square foot of lab space (the bad old Coopers & Lybrand beancounter audit days), and consider teaching when departmental finances were being discussed with the chairs.

Dr. Bole did many things to benefit education and restore a belief in its importance. I learned about him and his plans (and other things) first-hand while I was one of his four associate deans (I was in Student Programs; there was Med Ed, Research and Graduate Studies, and Faculty Affairs, the latter a position that was vacated and left unfilled when Lorris Betz was named senior executive dean right before Dr. Bole bowed-out). I had a direct reporting line to Dr. Bole, met one-on-one with him at least weekly, and participated in lively, insightful, and confidential meetings with the dean's staff for three hours each week, every week, holidays and all. It is from this insider's position that I base my behind-the-scenes stories, spins, and truths that have been generally unknown or misconstrued.

Dr. Bole often appeared gruff but he was more a curmudgeon. Like all deans he got pot shots and second guesses from all sides, all the competing and conflicting interests whether they were about education, money, you name it, even though his associate deans did the best they could to handle problems before they got to the boss. But he had convictions; he was a savvy student of undergraduate and postgraduate medical education, medical schools, and health care systems; and his heart was always in the right place: Michigan.

Dr. Bole was a Michigan man in every sense, in the best sense. To outsiders (and perhaps understandably) he was just another bureaucrat; another dean whose face we wouldn't recognize; another dictator by mere virtue of being dean; and perhaps one who rattled his swords louder than others had, and in plainer sight. But Giles was human in every sense. He could be wounded (he often was) and he showed it to our small circle of staff. We in the dean's staff, and virtually anyone else in the faculty at large (unless they were perpetually narcotized or plain stupid) knew exactly what was on Dr. Bole's mind. It was refreshing, it facilitated our jobs. Once he got rolling on an issue in dean's staff meetings (he always did), eyes around the room rolled too as we held back laughs; or cringed, wondering who'd be next to get reamed or taught a lesson. (His wife Liz once commented "to Giles, a dialogue is two of his monologues put back to back".)

The loyalty to and respect for Dr. Bole among the "7th floor med admin" was unwavering, sincere, and earned, whether you looked at him as the Dean, Dr. Bole, or just Giles. To this day, old-timers in med admin who were around before Dr. Bole and are there still say it was a unique era, in a most positive sense; one with a known direction of where we were heading; and one that is not likely to be repeated any time soon.

Besides spawning the new curriculum, Dr. Bole made major financial commitments to renovating and improving infrastructure in support of teaching and learning. That included equipping the main lecture halls (North, West, and South, Med Sci III) with computers so faculty could use more state-of-the art technology, such as the Internet; and, particularly, computerized PowerPoint teaching slides (which a few faculty used instead of sloppy hand-written overheads that looked like either they were put together years before and never changed, or haphazardly assembled at the last minute before a lecture). He built and equipped new clinical skills teaching labs; he funded a major update to our Learning Resource Center, now stacked to the gills with computers and other technologies for student learning and use, and good support staff. More than giving lip-service to rewarding teaching, he held faculty (and promotions committees) accountable for documenting teaching quantity and quality, and was far more than miffed if serial reports of bad teaching or courses (whether lecture-based or clinical) came to his attention. He looked at who was teaching what, and how well they did.

Most importantly, Dr. Bole articulated his vision of the medical school and its relationship to other entities and people: If it weren't for the medical students, there would be no medical school. If it weren't for the medical school, there'd be no hospital, or basic science departments, or faculty, or grants. This is a public educational institution first and foremost. He was sincere about this, and quite blunt and open about it too.

Dr. Bole ruffled feathers on the teaching issue and many others. He generally favored cuts in federal subsidies for foreign medical graduates, who were the staffing core in many hospitals, particularly in the East, and who were squeezing out US medical school grads for residency positions. He railed against the superspecialization of medical student education, at our superspecialty school, at the expense of turning out more holistic physicians to fill needed primary care roles. (For a long time it seemed as if we were providing the entire US supply of students entering anesthesiology and ophthalmology.) He severed relations with a nearby and quite visible teaching hospital that, for years, took some of our students for virtually the entire M3 year (the core junior clerkships), but did a generally miserable job of educating or keeping tabs on them. (It was a gutsy but needed move, one that opened Dr. Bole to inappropriate but glib criticism, much of it of a political and "societal" nature, totally missing the point that he had a fiduciary responsibility to make sure our students got the best education we could give.)

And it is no coincidence that Giles stepped down not long after John Forsythe ended his job as hospital director. It was clear (at least to our small circle in med admin) that the two became frequently embroiled in what could be called a lengthy and heated contest, if not a war, of conflicting philosophies and priorities. Giles' heart was with top-notch medical education for our students; Forsythe had other priorities, of which money was not the least. Each agreed, privately but with the urging of central campus, to step down if and when the other did. Though he did return to the faculty, Dr. Bole's stepping down as Dean was, in many ways, a sad day for the Medical School.

6

The Years 1994 - Present

Paul F. Hollenberg, Ph.D.

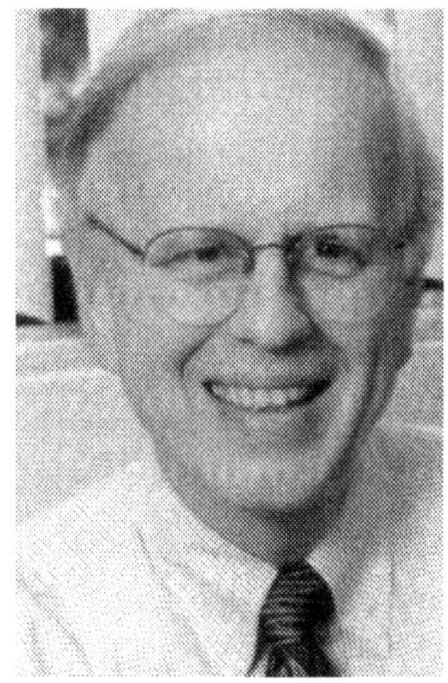

My association with the Department of Pharmacology at the University of Michigan began with a phone call from Dean Giles Bole in July of 1993 inquiring whether I would be interested in interviewing for the position as chair of the Department of Pharmacology. As an alumnus of the University of Michigan, I was well aware of the outstanding tradition and reputation of the Department and was very pleased to be considered as a candidate for the position of chair. Following that phone call, there was an interview followed by a series of visits with members of the faculty and the dean and in October, I was offered the position and accepted. I was very pleased by the opportunity to serve as the chair of a department that had such a great historical tradition and I was well aware of the excellence of its faculty, students, alumni, teaching and research programs.

During the fall of 1993 and winter of 1994, I was busy trying to learn more about the Department of Pharmacology at the University of Michigan, its faculty, students, and staff. Dr. Ray Counsell and Mr. Dennis Ondreyka were particularly helpful in giving me insights into how the Department functioned and the financial operations of the Department. Ray was still functioning as the "interim" chair, which he had been doing for approximately four years, a longer term of service than many "permanent" chairs. During that time, Ray did an excellent job of providing leadership to the Department and dealing with a number of knotty issues.

Prior to my joining the University of Michigan, there had been a major change in the Medical School curriculum which significantly affected the way that we taught pharmacology not only to the medical students, but also to our graduate students and the students in the other health professions, Pharmacy, Nursing, and Dentistry. Therefore, the first couple of years that I was here there was a good deal of adjusting and "fine-tuning" of the curriculum for these various programs. In addition, the approaches to recruiting and training graduate students were changing and we needed to put some effort into revising our approaches to graduate training and recruitment. We were very fortunate to have a group of truly committed faculty working on the curricular and graduate training efforts including Drs. Peggy Gnegy, Ben Lucchesi, Ray Counsell, Rick Neubig, Jonathan Maybaum, Marshal Shlafer, Bill Pratt, Ron Holz, Steve Fisher and Wendell Weber. Another very important teaching activity of our department over the years has been the Senior Clinical Pharmacology and Therapeutics course, which has been very well directed by Drs. Lucchesi and Domino.

As part of the recruitment package, the

Department had been assigned new space in MSRB III. This assignment was to provide us with modern, fully functional space and to allow for the renovation of the departmental space on floors six and seven of Medical Science Building I, so that it could then be assigned to several clinical departments (Anesthesiology, Dermatology, and Ob/Gyn). This would allow them to have newly renovated space in close proximity to the hospital. Although I was very enthusiastic about the thought of the Department moving into brand new space when it was offered as part of the recruitment package, when it came time to start assigning space within the new facilities and plan for the move, I quickly realized what a daunting task this would be. In addition, I realized that it would provide me with an opportunity to immediately alienate almost all of the faculty in the department since it is usually the case that when someone is assigned new space it is never enough or properly configured for what they think they deserve. Fortunately, this task was greatly facilitated by the appointment of a Space Committee consisting of Drs. Bert La Du (who chaired the committee), Jonathan Maybaum, and Stephen Fisher, all of whom were located outside of the departmental space and thus, did not have vested interests in the assignments of space. The spring and summer of 1994 were primarily consumed with plans for moving most of the laboratories from Medical Science Building I to MSRB III as well as plans for moving my own laboratory from Wayne State University to the University of Michigan. These plans were greatly facilitated by the outstanding efforts of the staff in the department (Dennis Ondreyka, Eileen Ferguson, Denise Gakle, Michelle Melis, Brenda Hadley, and Tom Larmee).

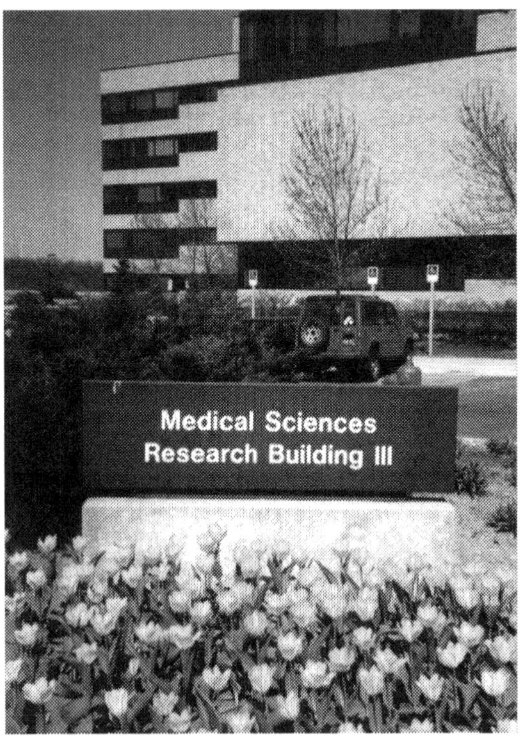

I was also very fortunate to have outstanding people help me in the transition of my laboratory from Wayne State University to the University of Michigan. Key to establishing the new laboratory at Michigan was Dr. Liz Roberts-Kirchhoff, who had been the senior person in my laboratory at Wayne State University. I was fortunate enough to convince her to move to the University of Michigan as a research track faculty member in my laboratory. Although my key technical person at Wayne State University, Dave Putt, did not come for personal reasons, I was very fortunate to be able to hire Hsia-Lien Lin, who had been a member of the Department for some time. She commuted to my laboratory in Detroit for several weeks prior to the move to learn techniques from Dave and also to make preparations for the move. I was also fortunate to have four outstanding graduate students, Liming Shu, Uma Sharma, Imad Hanna, and Xaudong Lu, come with me from Wayne State to help in setting up the laboratory. They were joined here by Dr. Ute Kent, who started as a postdoctoral fellow in the laboratory shortly after the move and made numerous important contributions during the early years. She was promoted to a research investigator fairly quickly and has played a key role in my laboratory for a number of years. In retrospect, the move went better than I could have ever expected or even hoped. Everyone (staff, faculty, postdoctoral fellows, students, etc.) pitched in and did a great job. In addition, since MSRB III was the third in a series of very similar buildings built over a ten-year period, by the time they got to the design and construction of our building, they had identified most of the mistakes they made in the first two buildings and corrected them. Therefore, there were relatively few problems due to occupying a brand new building, and those that occurred were minor.

As part of the recruitment package, Dean Bole had provided the Department with funds to recruit replacements for Drs. Bert La Du, Henry Swain, and Vincent Zannoni, all of whom had retired during the years that they were looking for a chairman of the Department and therefore had not been replaced. In 1994, we initiated a recruitment effort to fill those three positions. This, of course, required lots of meetings of the search committee, as we had more than 300 applications and then many recruitment interviews and dinners. However, the efforts paid off as we were able to recruit three truly outstanding new faculty to the department. Dr. Donna Shewach joined us as an Associate Professor with tenure in March of 1995 and Dr. Lori Isom joined the Department as an Assistant Professor in May of 1995. Dr. Yoichio Osawa came as a faculty member in November of 1995 to complete the first phase of our faculty recruitment efforts. Although a primary concern of the search committee was to identify the best possible candidates involved in molecularly-oriented investigations, it was also essential that these candidates have a strong background in all aspects of pharmacology and that they complement one or more of the six major research areas of strength in the Department (cancer biology and therapeutics, cardiovascular pharmacology, drug disposition and pharmacogenetics, endocrinology and the biochemistry of drug and hormone receptors, neuropharmacology, or site-specific delivery of drugs). As was soon obvious, all three faculty recruits admirably fulfilled all of our criteria and expectations.

Over the years, the Department of Pharmacology at the University of Michigan has had an outstanding reputation for the training that it provides to its graduate students and the quality of the students trained in the Department. The graduate program is truly a rallying point for the Department and it has been important in keeping the Department focused on working together over the years. One critical component of the training in the Department has been the Pharmacological Sciences Training Program which is an interdisciplinary program supported by a training grant from the NIH. For some time, it had been the tradition that the Principal Investigator (PI) of the training grant changed every five years and alternated between the chair of the Department of Pharmacology in the School of Medicine and the head of the Interdepartmental Program in Medicinal Chemistry, which is administered by the Graduate School. Since Dr. Leroy Townsend had been the PI starting in 1992, in 1997 I had the "privilege" of becoming the PI and writing the competing renewal. Although we obtained an outstanding score following the site visit, some concerns were raised regarding the interactions between the members of the two tracks of the training grant during the previous project period and so even though we were funded, I had to write another competing renewal at the end of three years. Fortunately, the site visit went very well and the grant has been funded. One of the most valuable developments to come out of this training program has been the Annual Graduate Student Symposium in the Pharmacological Sciences and Biorelated Chemistry which is supported by the training grant and provides an opportunity for all of the trainees, as well as the other students in the participating departments, to get together and hear some interesting talks and view posters. This is always one of the most enjoyable events of the year for me as I get a chance to meet many of the students in the other programs and find out about their research.

Another long-standing tradition in the department has been our participation in the Annual Pharmacology Research Colloquium that involves graduate students from the Departments of Pharmacology at the University of Michigan as well as the Medical College of Ohio, Michigan State University, and Wayne State University. This has proven to be an excellent opportunity for the students from the participating departments to interact with each other, to learn what's going on in the other departments and to have a chance to get to know the faculty in the other departments and in many cases to line up postdoctoral positions. It has also provided an excellent opportunity for the faculty to meet with each other and set up collaborations and for the chairs to meet and compare notes. It has also provided a great opportunity to visit with some of our alumni such as Drs. Ken Moore and Jay Goodman.

As part of our efforts to recruit graduate students, in 1996 we constructed our first web page and very quickly we found out how rapidly things change and get out of date on the Internet. For those who are interested in checking on the current status of our web page and our Department, the URL is: http://sitemaker.umich.edu/pharmacology.

Our Department has been very fortunate over the years in having good working relationships with a number of the scientists at Parke-Davis including Drs. Harvey Kaplan, Roger Newton, and Kevin Wang, all of whom have had adjunct faculty appointments in the department. In order to foster better relationships between the department and Parke-Davis (now Pfizer), we have held joint poster days on an annual basis with investigators from both units presenting posters. The Ninth Annual Poster Day held in 2002 had more than 80 posters presented, with more than 160 participants. In the spring of 2003, we also co-sponsored a graduate student course with our colleagues at Pfizer entitled "Drug Discovery and Development." We were pleasantly surprised by the enthusiastic reception for this course. We routinely had more than 30 students and postdoctoral fellows at each class.

The Charles Ross Summer Research Fellowship Program for Underrepresented Minority Undergraduate Students was established in 1991 to honor Charles R. Ross, Ph.D., (deceased) one of the first African Americans to receive a doctoral degree in pharmacology. Initial funding for this program was provided by a departmental faculty member and over the years, additional funds were obtained from corporate and alumni donations and Medical School diversity programs. Although the program had been relatively small in the first several years, we were able to identify significant sources of funding and major efforts were put into developing this program starting in approximately 1996. These efforts were done in parallel with the development of a Summer Undergraduate Research Program which was successful in competing for support from the American Society for Pharmacology and Experimental Therapeutics (ASPET), also starting in 1996. As of the summer of 2003, approximately 36 underrepresented minority students had participated in the Charles Ross Summer Research Fellowship Program. This program has been instrumental in increasing the diversity within the Department of Pharmacology and in providing excellent research opportunities for many deserving students. I am particularly grateful to Dr. Benedict Lucchesi who played an instrumental role in the initial development of this program and has continued to make major contributions to its growth and development over the years. I should also acknowledge Laura Sell (deceased) who played a major role in helping to prepare the applications to the ASPET Summer Undergraduate Research Program for many years.

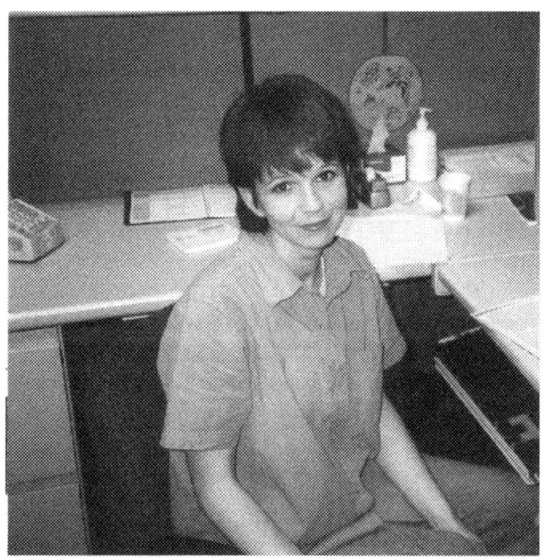

A pensive Laura Sell...

As part of the planning process for the Centennial Celebration of the Department of Pharmacology, the Alumni Steering Committee was established. This was chaired by Bob Gussin, then the corporate vice president for science and technology at Johnson & Johnson. The initial objective of this committee was to help in the planning for the Centennial Celebration and to help raise the funds to support it. However, following the successful completion of the celebration, Dr. Ray Counsell realized the value of this committee and, rather than disbanding it, as had been the original plan, he continued calling on this committee for advice. This committee subsequently played a very important role during the time that Dr. Counsell was the "interim" chair by convincing the dean to make an aggressive search for a new chair and provide that chair with the appropriate package to redevelop the Department. Hence, I was the beneficiary of this committee's work by receiving the funds to make three new recruitments and also to move into the excellent new space in MSRB III.

During the years following my joining the Department, the Alumni Steering Committee has continued to make very important contributions to our department in its role as an external advisory committee. Their visits in the fall of the year are always one of the highlights of the year for the Department and for myself. Each year they review the teaching programs of the Department as well as any other aspects of the Department that they are interested in or feel could be improved. They also are responsible for selecting the recipient of the Outstanding Alumnus/Alumna Award and meet with the graduate students to get their feedback and to provide them with insights into types of careers available following the completion of their graduate degrees. Over the years, this committee has provided an excellent opportunity for some of our alumni to maintain their relationships with the faculty and students in the Department and provide us with invaluable advice. Although the original idea was that members would rotate off after a reasonable time of service, we found some reluctance for people to rotate off and so, instead, the committee slowly increased in size as more members were appointed and no one left. I feel extremely fortunate to have had this group to work with and particularly fortu-

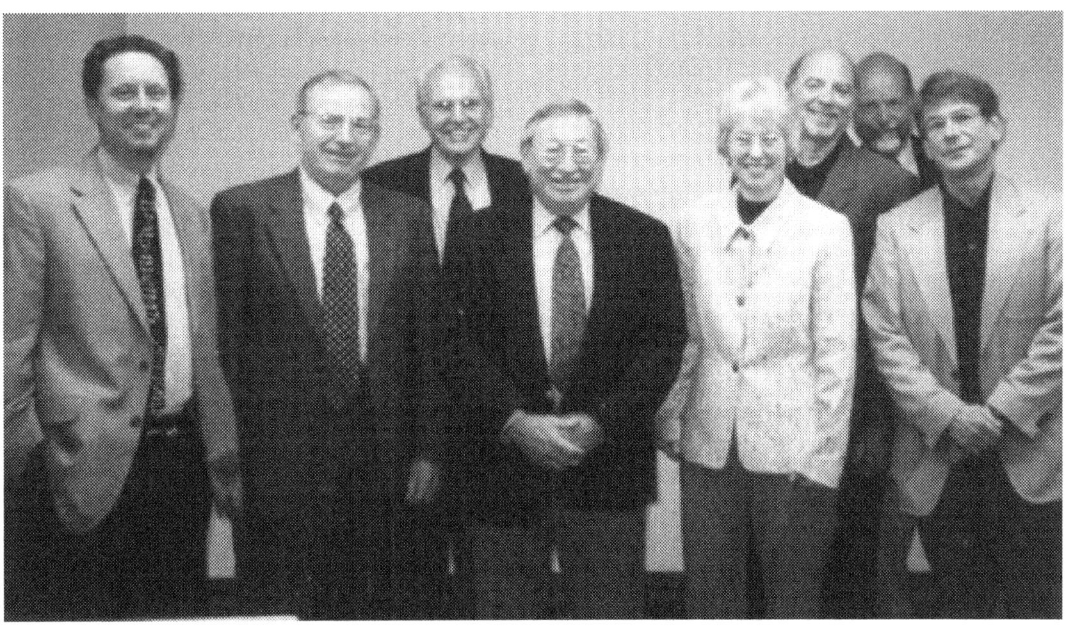

The Alumni Steering Committe Members, September 21, 2001.

nate that Bob Gussin has remained on as chair of this committee and provided outstanding leadership over the years.

It should be noted that another one of their responsibilities, although never stated directly, was to monitor the performance of the University of Michigan football team. Therefore, these meetings are always scheduled for a weekend on which the University of Michigan is playing one of its more interesting opponents and the weather is still reasonably moderate (September or early October). The evaluation normally begins with a tailgate party at the our house. Needless to say we have always enjoyed the visits of the Alumni Steering Committee and think that their efforts have benefited the department and all of its members in many ways. My wife, Emily, and I particularly enjoy the friendship and interactions at the annual meeting.

Although I've only been here ten years, I look back with wonderful memories of the outstanding students that I have had the chance to get to know during this time. I was pleased to note that in the spring of 2000, Dr. Elaine Tanhehco was the 200th student to successfully defend her doctoral thesis and earn a Ph.D. from the Department of Pharmacology. I am very proud of the excellent tradition the department has for training outstanding students.

During the years from 1995-2003, we have had a number of retirements of faculty who have made important contributions to the Department of Pharmacology during their careers. These included Drs. Ray Counsell, Wendell Weber, Fedor Medzihradsky (deceased), and Ed Domino. Although during this time period they all officially became emeritus faculty and were theoretically "retired", the department has been very fortunate to be able to benefit from their continued presence and contributions to our research and teaching programs just as we have from two previous retirees, Drs. Bert La Du and Vince Zannoni, who have also remained active in the Department.

The period from 1995 to 2003 has been a period of great change in the Medical School and the Medical Center. Pressures relating to changes in reimbursements from third party payors and the Federal Government resulted in significant alterations in the way that the Medical Center and the Medical School functioned and put tremendous pressure on the upper level administration. As a result there have been a series of significant changes. Dean Giles Bole, who had hired me, stepped down as dean in 1997. The president of the University, Dr. James Duderstadt, also stepped down at about that time so that early in 1998 the president of the University, the provost, and the dean of the Medical School were all interim appointments. One day Dr. Bill Pratt came to me and said something to the effect that I was the only non-interim person at the University of Michigan between him and God.

Fortunately, that situation was soon remedied by the appointment of Lee C. Bollinger, J.D., as the president of the University and Gilbert S. Omenn, M.D., Ph.D., as the executive vice president for medical affairs. We were very fortunate that following Dean Bole's resignation, A. Lorris Betz, M.D., was appointed as the interim dean and did an excellent job. When Dean Betz was recruited to head up the Medical Center at the University of Utah, he was replaced by Allen S. Lichter, M.D., first as interim dean and subsequently as the dean. We have been very fortunate to have strong support from the dean's office under all three administrations.

The past several years have proven to be very exciting, rewarding, and promising time to be involved in research at the University of Michigan. 1999 saw the completion of the report from the Life Sciences Commission recommending major financial and administrative commitments to increasing the biomedical research enterprise in the life sciences at the University of Michigan. This resulted in the construction of a major new research building, the Life Science Institute and will ultimately lead to the recruitment of between 30 and 40 new faculty. At approximately the same time, all of the graduate programs in the basic biomedical sciences in the Medical School joined together in a combined admissions program, the Program in Biomedical Sciences (PIBS). This resulted in a series of new initiatives that radically changed the curriculum for all of our graduate students. Once again, the faculty of the department pitched in to make the required changes leading to a teaching program for our students which has been very well accepted by the students and we believe will provide them with even better training than they obtained previously. In addition, the faculty members have been very enthusiastic about the changes in our teaching program and the increased opportunities for interactions with other departments. However, as is true in all major medical schools, things continue to change rapidly and our faculty members expect further changes.

In 1998, the Medical School also initiated a recruitment program for outstanding junior faculty known as the Biological Sciences Scholars Program. The Department of Pharmacology has been very fortunate in that it was able to recruit three truly outstanding junior faculty, Jorge Iñiguez-Lluhi, Roger Sunahara and Jose Esteban through this program.

In many ways, this chapter is a "work in progress." During the past ten years there have been many changes and improvements in the Department and yet there is still much to be done. I feel privileged to be a member of a department that has such a remarkable record of contributions to the discipline of Pharmacology, as well as such excellent students, faculty, staff, and alumni. The department is currently ranked eighth nationally in terms of graduate training and is only one of two departments at the Medical School to be ranked in the top ten and only one of four departments at state supported schools in the top ten. However, it is clear that we can, and must, continue to improve ourselves in all areas. I feel very fortunate to have had an outstanding group of students, postdocs, and technical staff in my own laboratory who have continuously provided me with exciting new research observations. The Department has provided me with a truly exceptional environment in which to learn and grow as an administrator and as scientist and I look forward to continuing opportunities to contribute to the department and all of its members—past, present, and future.

During the last 100 years the discipline of Pharmacology has progressed from a relatively descriptive science to a vastly sophisticated discipline. We now have at our disposal the tools and techniques to understand how drugs work at the molecular level, to predict responses of specific individuals to certain drugs based on their genetic profiles, and to determine the blood levels needed of specific chemotherapeutic agents in order to kill bacterial or malignant cells without killing the patient or causing profound morbidity. Diagnostic testing with CR, MRI, and PET scanning have enabled us to target pharmacological as

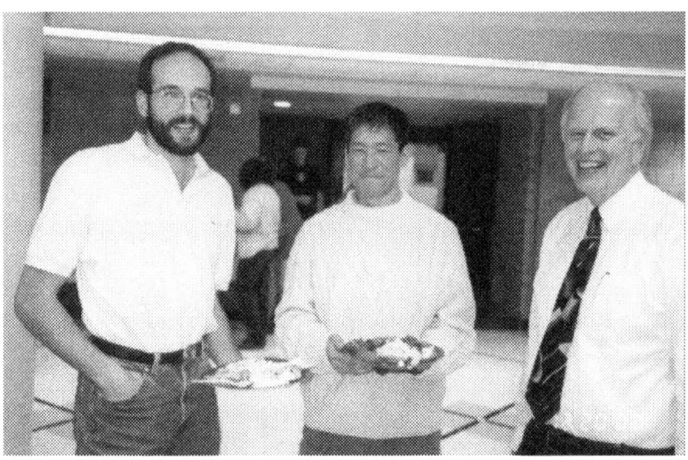

Two of the three successful recruits to the Department Faculty under the Biological Sciences Scholars Program with Dr. Hollenberg.

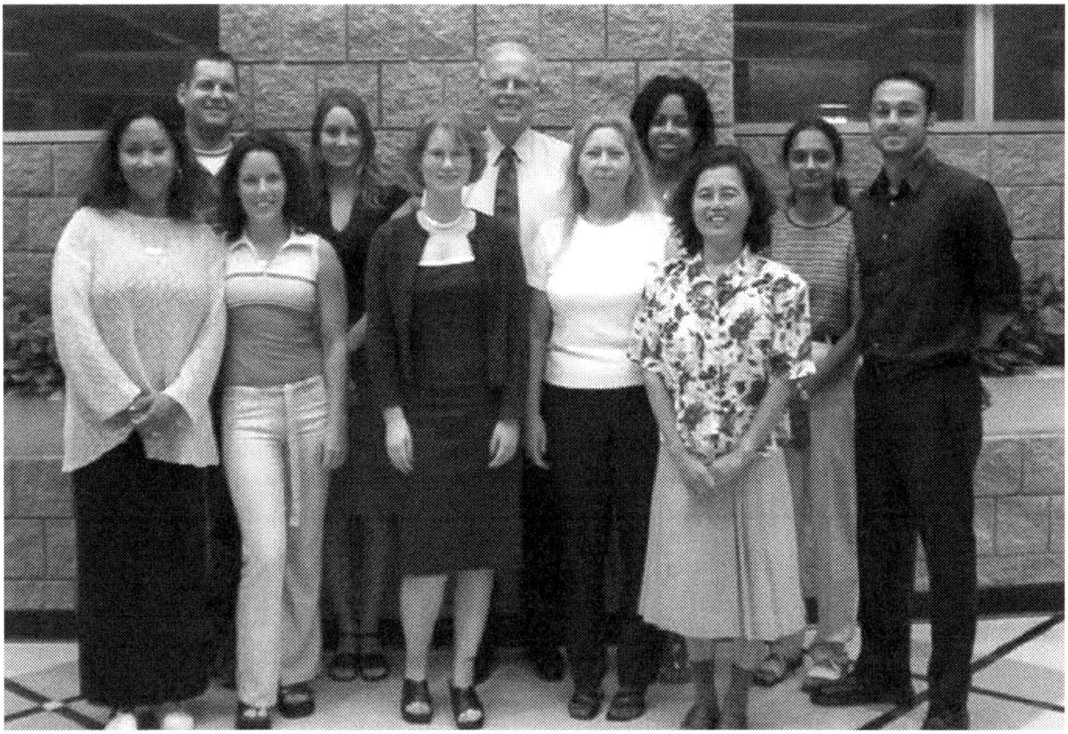

Front Row: Edith Mensah-Osman, Monica Jushchyshyn, Linda VanWeymarn, Ute Kent, Hsia-Lein Lin
Back Row: Gabriel Knudsen, Annie Blobaum, Paul Hollenberg, Namandje Bumpus, Chitra Sridar, Mohamad Shebley

well as surgical interventions. However, the future promises even better pharmacological interventions for the cure or amelioration of various diseases. With the Human Genome Project essentially completed, we are now at the point where researchers will be able to use the information provided to revolutionize human medicine and health care. This "post-genomic" era has now ushered in the application of functional genomics and proteomics. The convergence of these biologically and chemically based approaches with bioinformatics will open exciting new vistas for biomedical research with the potential to produce revolutionary new treatments and diagnostic approaches. Research in pharmacology will benefit greatly from the integrated use of functional genomics, proteomics, pharmacogenomics, and bioinformatics. A major strength of the discipline of pharmacology will continue to be the unique ability of investigators well trained in pharmacology to connect work at the molecular and cellular levels with investigations at the organ system and whole animal levels to provide a basis for the extension of their results into clinical pharmacology with subsequent translation into clinical applications.

I and my colleagues in the Department of Pharmacology are extremely fortunate to be involved in this very exciting enterprise at such an opportune time. In addition to the outstanding possibilities we are presented with for the development of our discipline, we are also currently experiencing a remarkable number of innovative initiatives which are occurring throughout the University of Michigan Medical Center including the Biological Sciences Scholars Program as well as the Life Sciences Institute and the Bioinformatics Institute. This is certainly an exciting time to be involved in pharmacological research at the University of Michigan and I am convinced the best is yet to come.

A. Lorris Betz, M.D., Ph.D., Interim Dean 1996-1998

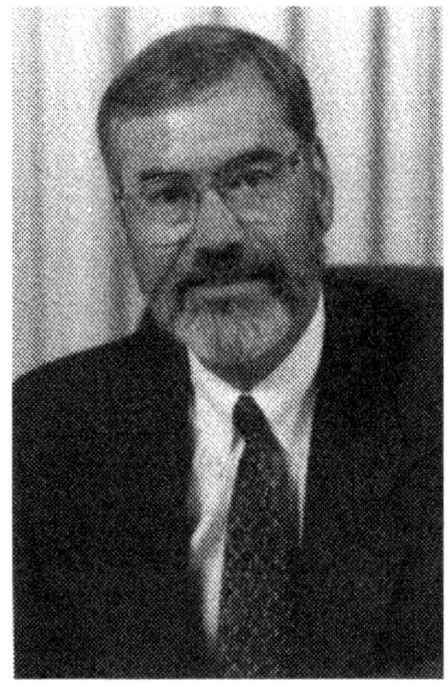

When Dean Bole resigned, A. Lorris Betz was appointed Interim Dean in 1996. Dr. Betz obtained bachelor, medical and graduate degrees at the University of Wisconsin. Subsequently, he completed a residency in pediatrics at the University of California, San Francisco. He was active in studying the mechanisms of brain injury and brain edema formation. His achievements include research in basic mechanisms that are responsible for moving nutrients and electrolytes between the blood and the brain of mammals, and processes that produce brain injury following a stroke.

Dr. Betz's many memberships in various organizations include: The International Society of Cerebral Blood Flow and Metabolism, International Society of Neurochemistry, American Physiology Society, Society for Pediatric Research, American Pediatric Society, Phi Beta Kappa, Sigma Xi, and Alpha Omega Alpha.

In 1983, Dr. Betz became Associate Professor of Pediatrics and Neurology at the University of Michigan. He maintained this postion until 1987 when he was appointed a professor in the University of Michigan Departments of Pediatrics and Communicable Diseases, Neurology, and Surgery. He also became Director of the Crosby Neurological Research Laboratories within the Neurosurgery Section of the Department of Surgery. This is where Dr. Betz was named the first Crosby-Kahn Collegiate Professor of Neurosurgery and Neuroanatomy. In addition, from 1989 to 1993, Dr. Betz was Associate Research Chair in the Department of Pediatrics and Communicable Diseases. In 1993, he was appointed Associate Dean for Faculty Affairs and subsequently Senior Associate Dean for Academic Affairs, and then Executive Associate Dean. Dr. Betz was named Interim Dean of the Medical School in 1996 upon resignation of Dean Bole.

It was during this period that significant changes occurred in the University of Michigan health system. The Regents redesigned the executive structure of the Michigan Health System, and in 1997, Gilbert S. Omenn was appointed as the first Executive Vice President for Medical Affairs. In this position, Omenn was given oversight responsibility for not only the Medical School but also the University Hospital, with both the dean of the Medical School and the Director of University Hospitals reporting directly to him. Also, under Dean Betz, several new programs were started in the Medical School, including the "white coat ceremony" for incoming medical students.

Dr. Betz served as Interim Dean for two years before returning to his faculty position. Almost immediately thereafter, he was appointed Senior Vice President of Health Sciences and Dean of the School of Medicine at the University of Utah in Salt Lake City in 1999.

Michigan's loss was Utah's gain.

Allen S. Lichter, M.D., Dean 1998-Present

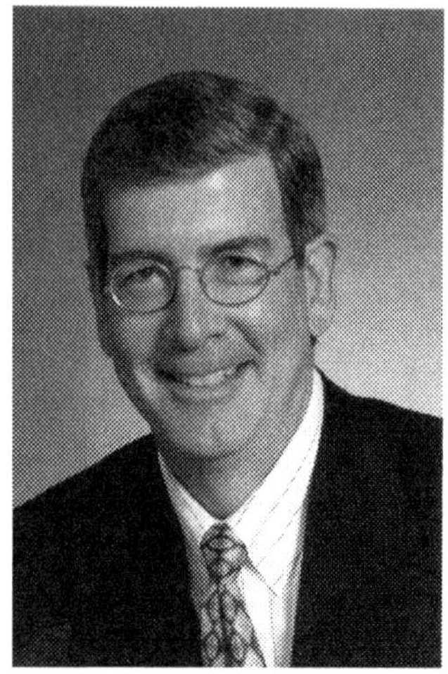

Allen S. Lichter was appointed Interim Dean in 1998. He received a B.S. degree in 1968 and an M.D. degree in 1972 from the University of Michigan. He completed an internship at St. Joseph Hospital in Denver, CO, in 1973 and a residency in radiation oncology at the University of California, San Francisco, in 1976. In 1978, he was Assistant Professor in oncology and radiological sciences at the Johns Hopkins University School of Medicine in Baltimore, Maryland. From 1978 to 1984, he was head of the Radiation Therapy Section of the Radiation Oncology Branch of the National Cancer Institute in Bethesda, Maryland. He was then appointed as a Professor of Radiation Oncology and served as the first chair of that department here at the University of Michigan, between 1984 and 1997.

In 1999, Dr. Lichter was appointed full time Dean of the Medical School where he currently remains. In the long history of the University of Michigan Medical School, Allen S. Lichter is the fifteenth Dean. He views the basic medical sciences to be intergrated with the clinical aspects of teaching medical students.

Thoughts from the Dean

We are extremely proud of the Department of Pharmacology at the University of Michigan. Starting out as our first basic science department, it still holds a place of great prominence in our school. It is difficult to overemphasize the importance of pharmacology education for the medical student and house officer of today and tomorrow. Obviously, medical practitioners must understand the pharmacology of the drugs they and other physicians are using to manage their patients.

But the education of tomorrow's physicians involves far more. We must understand the cost effectiveness of new drugs compared to existing ones. Is a new agent that reduces a toxic side effect from a 2% risk to a 1% risk worth the cost to society if the new agent is ten times more expensive? How can we as academic physicians educate our students and colleagues in the effective use of pharmaceuticals, combating the multi-billion dollar investment that the pharmaceutical industry makes in touting new agents, some of questionable benefit?

And how will pharmacology be affected in the new post-genomic era? Surely we will begin to understand the genomic polymorphism that explain some of the divergent metabolism of drugs, effectiveness of drugs from one patient to the next. In the future, pharmacology education will be tied closely to a variety of molecular diagnostic tests designed to guide practitioners and their patients to the right drugs in the right dose and in the right combinations with other agents to be maximally effective and minimally toxic.

We are entering a most exciting era of pharmacology research, and the University of Michigan Medical School intends to continue to stress the critical importance of pharmacology as a basis for sound medical practice well into the future.

7

The Nickerson Dismissal: An Introduction

Edward F. Domino, M.D.

The McCarthy Years: A Stressful Period in the Early 1950s

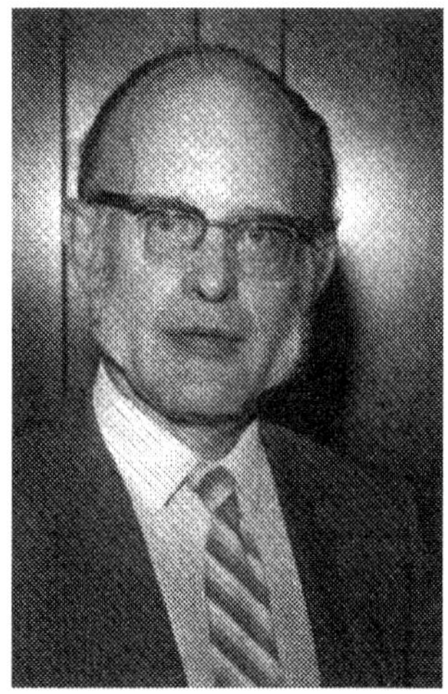

If one were to try and imagine a Shakespearian tragedy that affected all of the characters involved, one would have difficulty surpassing the real life drama of the Nickerson dismissal. The setting was during the 1950s when Senator McCarthy was on a crusade to expose hidden communists in prominent positions in the United States. Specifically, this tragedy took place in our Department. Two extremely strong willed individuals — Moe Seevers as Chairman and Mark Nickerson as a tenured Associate Professor — had very different opinions on how pharmacology should be taught and practiced. In one year, Mark Nickerson flunked one-half of the medical students in pharmacology, earning him the nickname "Black Nick" — to the chagrin of Chairman Seevers and Dean Furstenberg. The time was ripe for a tragedy to begin.

A year after the end of World War II, with the surrender of Germany on May 7, 1945 and the surrender of Japan on August 14, 1945, Winston Churchill warned Americans about communist expansion, in his famous "Iron Curtain" speech. The continuing threats by the USSR led to an ever-increasing concern by some Americans, especially Senator McCarthy of Wisconsin, of communists infiltrating the United States government. The infamous methods of Senator McCarthy and his Subcommittee on Un-American Activities were subsequently used to purge alleged communists from all elements of American society.

Thus, the first half of the 1950s was, politically, a very dangerous period. Even the mere label of being a communist sympathizer, a "pinkie," let alone a "red," placed a person in great jeopardy. Reputations were destroyed and entire families were deprived of their livelihoods, and became outcasts of society because they were "enemies."

Other politicians besides Senator McCarthy joined the select group of "saviors" of America who would expose communists and their sympathizers. This included Congressman Kit Clardy of Michigan, a member of the House Subcommittee on Un-American Activities. He chaired a small group which conducted hearings on communist activities in the State of Michigan on May 10, 1954.

Three University of Michigan faculty members: Chandler Davis, a Mathematics Instructor, Clement Markert, an Assistant Professor of Biology, and Mark Nickerson, an Associate Professor of Pharmacology, as well as two students, were questioned by Congressman Clardy regarding their alleged one-time communist connections. At first, all of them refused to answer questions regarding their own political beliefs. Chandler Davis cited the First Amendment and refused to discuss his politics with anyone, including various University committees. On President Hatcher's recommendation, Chandler Davis was dismissed and actually served time in prison for contempt. He lost all of his appeals including a final one with the United States Supreme Court.

Both Clement Markert and Mark Nickerson subsequently cooperated fully with appropriate University committees regarding their political beliefs. Markert was censured and stayed at Michigan only a short time before leaving for an outstanding career at Johns Hopkins University. Even though University Committees recommended that Nickerson be treated similarly to Markert, with mild censure, Medical School Dean Furstenberg and the Medical School's Executive Committee, at the strong request of Dr. Maurice Seevers, recommended dismissal.

Dr. Seevers officially cited the fact that he was the principal investigator on a secret United States Army contract to support research which was vital to the defense security of the United States. Only those persons that had a Secret clearance on the U.S. Army contract project knew that they were studying a variety of amphetamine analogs of mescaline as hallucinogens and, later, super potent marijuana derivatives. Unofficially, everyone also knew that Seevers and Nickerson disagreed on many administrative, scientific, and other philosophical issues. In spite of the obvious similarity of the specific problem shared by Clement Markert and Mark Nickerson, President Hatcher decided to support the Medical School's recommendation for dismissal, which was subsequently confirmed by the Board of Regents. However, members of the University Senate strongly disagreed, and this action was remembered by some faculty members concerned with academic freedom.

As with any Shakespearian tragedy, all the participants suffered. However, the end result was Regent By-Laws 5.08 and 5.09 clarifying tenured positions at the University of Michigan. Information on the Regent By-Laws can be found at http://www.umich.edu/~regents/bylaws/bylaws05a.html.

What follows in Chapters 8 and 9 describes in more detail the events of those days. Unfortunately, with the death of Dr. Seevers, his perspective is only presented with what has been officially recorded.

Bylaws

Bylaws Table of Contents • Detailed Table of Contents

Chapter V. The Faculties and Academic Staff

- Sec. 5.01. Definitions (revised June 2001)
- Sec. 5.02. Governing Bodies in Schools and Colleges (revised January 1993)
- Sec. 5.03. Powers and Duties of the Governing Faculties
- Sec. 5.04. Faculty Procedure
- Sec. 5.05. Faculty Communications to the Board
- Sec. 5.06. The Deans and Executive Committees
- Sec. 5.07. Administrative Officers of Other University Units (revised July 1997)
- Sec. 5.08. Appointment, Tenure, Promotion, and Resignation of the Staff (revised April 1991)
- Sec. 5.09. Procedures in Cases of Dismissal, Demotion, or Terminal Appointment (revised November 1993)
- Chapter V, part 2. Sec. 5.10-5.24

The outline of the University of Michigan Board of Regents Bylaws Chapter V.

8

An Interview With Mark Nickerson, 1996

Edward F. Domino, M.D.

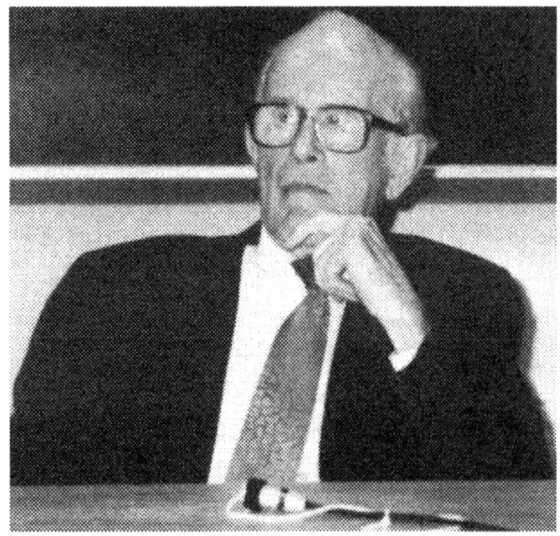

I had the privilege of interviewing Mark Nickerson on August 30, 1996. His resentment toward the University and Dr. Seevers remained unabated over the years. What was a loss to the University and to the United States was Canada's gain. Mark Nickerson became the father of modern Canadian pharmacology and is revered by many Canadian pharmacologists who were influenced and trained by him.

What follows is the telephone conversation between myself (D) and Mark Nickerson (N) now deceased.

D Mark, what are your impressions regarding your stay in the Department of Pharmacology at the University of Michigan?

N I can tell you very succinctly and then give you reasons for what I say. In all my experience, not only in pharmacology but in other academic matters, the three years I spent at Michigan were in the most despotic department that I have ever been in.

D The most despotic? That's saying a lot.

N One of the things that I didn't notice much at first and then started to think more about was that every letter typed in that department had to be typed by someone in Dr. Seevers' office.

D Is that right? For you?

N Yes. There were many people working on the second floor, you remember? Yet we were never allowed to have a secretary on the second floor.

D Mark, I can tell you that in my case as a young instructor, I never had his secretary type any of my mail. I did have someone in the front office type my materials, but they never went through anyone.

N But everything one of the girls in the front office typed he was able to access, if he wanted.

D He had access, I understand.

N I know of other incidents, many of them, but one, in particular, was while I was trying to get another job. I had made arrangements with the Department of Surgery at the University of British Columbia to build a shock program there. The chief of surgery there, Robertson, raised the money and the space and the equipment for me to start as a research professor of surgery, a clinical non-surgical job.

D The University of British Columbia is a strong institution in Vancouver.

N Yes. Robertson subsequently became professor of surgery at McGill and then provost of McGill University. He told me that he had everything worked out. Later, he told me personally that he couldn't do it because Seevers had called the dean of medicine at the University of British Columbia and said, "Don't hire this man." The dean's name was Weaver; he had been with Seevers at Wisconsin. Actually, Robertson was really apologetic to me when we both ended up at McGill. That's just one example. In those days the University operated through one travel agency in Ann Arbor. Seevers had someone there automatically tell him about any member of his department who ordered tickets through the University account. I had several such instances, one of which resulted in not having a contract when I got a job in Manitoba. I didn't have a contract because Seevers had called the president of the University of Manitoba. I think this came about through the travel agency in Ann Arbor. The new president had just taken office a month or so before. Here was my appointment as full professor on his desk, one of the first things to think about, with the note from Seevers and a copy of the Ann Arbor News or at least a clipping from it. Fortunately, that didn't cause me any particular harm. The president asked if there was any question of breaking the law. I said no and he signed my appointment.

D Mark, what about your students and colleagues while you were at Michigan for those three years? When I came I think you had already been there about two years. I think Lloyd Beck was part of your group.

N Yes, and Andy Dontas, you remember him?

D Yes, Andy Dontas was with you.

N Bill Yard. He became professor of anesthesia at the University of Wisconsin.

D I didn't know that. What happened to Andy Dontas?

N Andy Dontas became a professor in a medical school in a city in eastern Greece, not Athens.

D Didn't you have a number of graduate students?

N Yes, Bill Yard came with me to Manitoba and so did Irv Shemano. He got a position at Merrill and then at Dow when Dow and Merrill merged. One of the biggest recollections I have at Michigan is of the special journal club I started.

D I remember that. It was a pretty important thing.

N You wouldn't believe the chewing out I got for that.

D You did, why?

N Because it wasn't done officially through the Department of Pharmacology.

D I remember that when I came, most of the people in the basic sciences of the medical school felt you were the best in the department from a scientific point of view.

N I can tell you one other thing that I learned only some years later. The 1953 International Physiological Congress had one day for pharmacology. Somebody introduced Seevers to Björn Fokow and he said, "Oh you're in Nick's department." Didn't that go over like a lead balloon!

D When you arrived, who else was in the department?

N There was Chenoweth and Shideman. A clinical pharmacologist by the name of Ted Carr was hired very shortly thereafter. He worked over in Kresge.

D Did Ted Brody come maybe a year after you?

N Yes, just about a year later.

D Was that to replace Shideman?

N I don't know, but he was hired very shortly after Shideman left.

D When did Lloyd Beck come?

N I guess about a year after I came. I was trying to get someone else from Western Ontario. Burton, a well-known biophysicist from there, said "I can tell you of a guy with a good brain on him," and that was Lloyd Beck.

D You also got involved with radioactive isotopes at an early stage. Is that correct?

N Yes, that was with a postdoc by the name of Horowitz.

D If I remember, you got an enormous grant from a soap company.

N That was actually from this chemist that I had gotten to know via Lou Goodman. His name was William Gump.

D He was a famous perfume chemist, wasn't he?

N That's right. He was such a good perfume chemist that they just gave him carte blanc to do whatever he wanted with the rest of his time. He synthesized hexachlorophene and I guess I was the first one to test it for a Swiss chemical company in New Jersey.

D Hexachlorophene was then put in soap?

N It was in Dial soap, in surgical scrubs, all kinds of things.

D I remember that you equipped an entire lab in the basement of the old pharmacology building. It was a modern radiochemical facility.

N Yes. That's where Bob Horowitz worked. We were using radioactive carbon. We got some pretty good evidence on hexachlorophene persistence but my interest particularly was in getting radioactive phenoxybenzamine. Gump was the guy who got it.

D He succeeded in getting phenoxybenzamine labeled?

N Oh yes. Gump could do anything with organic chemistry.

D It shows the importance of pharmacologists knowing chemists doesn't it?

N It does. He was absolutely wonderful because what I would do is draw out chemical structures. I combined some of Bovet's compounds with mustard tagging which gave the first proof of covalent binding to receptors. I mixed this combination and turned the chemical structures over to Gump. Anywhere from two or three weeks to two or three months later they would come back as pure crystalline compounds.

D It demonstrates the importance of working with good people and especially good chemists. Was Lauren Woods around at the time?

N Yes, Lauren Woods was in the Department.

D While you were at Michigan you worked in a variety of research areas with other colleagues. Isn't that correct?

N Yes. I did a lot of work with Dave Bohr. He was a good guy to talk with about conditions in the department, even though he wasn't actually in it.

D He knew your situation?

N Yes, he knew it, and so did Sibley Hoobler.

D By the way, Dave Bohr is still at Michigan. He's an emeritus professor. He has a grant and still comes to the Department of Physiology.

N I still get in touch with him whenever I come down for the Davis, Markert, Nickerson lectures.

D Is Lou Goodman still alive? How old is he?

N Yes. He must be 88 to 90. *Editor's note: now deceased.*

D Was he the one who gave you your start in pharmacology?

N No, that was later. My really big pushes in pharmacology came when I was in Baltimore at Johns Hopkins. When I finished my Ph.D. I went to work on chemical warfare. I got to know Gilman who was head of pharmacology at Edgewood Arsenal. There was a chemist who was head of the chemical warfare project at Johns Hopkins. He had told me that I was going to lose my job at Johns Hopkins because a second front had been opened and there was no chemical warfare, etc. I made no bones of it. I took the day off and went out to see Gilman at Edgewood Arsenal. He was pleasant enough but he didn't have any jobs. Chenoweth worked with him. Gilman would have forgotten about it. I was just a young biologist and they're a dime a dozen. The next day the chemist from Johns Hopkins showed up at Edgewood Arsenal and told Gilman "Don't hire this guy Nickerson because he's a red. I can't get my project increased until I get rid of him."

D What year was this?

N I'm not that sure but it would have been about 1944. My degree was in 1944, but my thesis was finished almost a year before.

D Wasn't your Ph.D. thesis on embryology?

N Yes. One of my colleagues sent me a reprint of an interesting publication written by an Italian, if you don't mind me puffing out my cheeks a little bit. It was a big review on the production of patterns in animal feathers, fur, and what not and the evidence for why they get that way. When it came to black and white stripes on feathers he said, "There has been nothing really significant since the definitive work of Nickerson in 1944."

D That's a wonderful compliment.

N Many people have worked on this problem and there were many theories. What I postulated from indirect evidence was that there is a byproduct of the production of melanin that diffuses down through the avascular collar of the growing feather. I could predict the occurrence of a white bar on the basis of the amount of melanin that was produced in the preceding black bar and the thickness of the avascular collar. He said that many people have worked on this, published papers and come up with suggestions of what may be the material, but that nobody doubts that this is what occurs.

D When did you go to Salt Lake City?

N December 1944. After I got dropped from the chemical warfare group at Johns Hopkins, Gilman got me in touch with Goodman who he knew was going to Salt Lake City. Goodman didn't know exactly when so for three or four months he put me on the payroll of the University of Vermont. I then drove Goodman's car out to Salt Lake City while he brought his family and furniture and stuff on the train. So from then on I was a pharmacologist.

D You went to medical school in Salt Lake City, isn't that correct?

N Yes.

D When did you obtain your M.D. there?

N In 1950. I then interned for a year at Salt Lake General Hospital. I was an assistant professor at the time. Goodman said, "You can have $6,000 if you keep your laboratory going while in training. You don't have to be there all of the time and if you get stuck I'll give you a hand." So I would work until about 10 or 11 o'clock at night and then I would leave. I would take a couple of amphetamines, go to bed, get up about 2 o'clock, have a big meal over at the intern's quarters, drive up to the lab which was about five miles away, go over the previous day's results, plan out some experiments for the next day and get back in time for rounds at 8 o'clock in the morning.

D Is this when you developed the phenoxybenzamine story? Was that all in Salt Lake City?

N Most of it was. I did a lot of it there. I also treated some patients with it. I remember treating a pregnant girl with severe pre-eclampsia for four to six weeks. I think that's the longest anyone's taken the drug. At least she had a live and reasonably healthy, although small, baby.

D This was with phenoxybenzamine therapy?

N Yes.

D This was before the days it was clinically approved. Isn't that correct?

N Well, yes. It was never really generally approved because nobody could see a profit if it were sold by Smith Kline and French. Even a big hospital would only be using such a drug a half to a dozen times in a year and no one could afford to make and sell it.

D Then dibenzyline came along. Was it made by Smith Kline and French?

N No. It was synthesized by Gump. He was in on the patent. He pushed pretty hard but he couldn't get anybody to market it. You remember when there was much talk of orphan drugs? Well dibenzyline was an orphan drug. Now in Canada I had permission from the equivalent of the Food and Drug Administration to use it with about three or four of my students. We had a shock team with myself and several M.D.s who were getting their Ph.D.s in pharmacology. We took care of all of the cases that surgeons had given up on. You would be surprised how such patients pile up on long weekends.

D This was your shock team putting practical clinical pharmacology into action, wasn't it?

N Yes. It's a hard thing to prove but we did have over a 50% survival rate of cases that other good physicians had given up on. Nonparametric statistics showed that it was quite a significant effect in that every patient who lived started to get better within four hours after being giving a vasodilator. The ones that hadn't responded within four hours never did.

D Was the major dilator phenoxybenzamine?

N Yes. That's the one we used. Now, it isn't used much because doctors are scared of anything they can't reverse. However, the principle of vasodilatation to get more blood flow rather than vasoconstriction, to get a higher blood pressure, is pretty generally accepted.

D What happened to your people at Manitoba that were part of this wonderful group? You were developing basic as well as clinical pharmacology?

N I have had a minimum (some I don't know about) of 28 of my students become chairmen of one department or another. Vancouver, Alberta, Calgary, Boston, even Nigeria; I've got them scattered all over. But to get back to Michigan. Before the House Un-American Committee Hearings in Ann Arbor, I got a two-and-a-half-hour lecture on what I was to do and not do at the Hearing.

D By whom?

N Seevers. I felt I should tell him what would come out. You know what? The questions that were presented to me at the Hearing were in exactly the same sequence that I told Seevers. That may have been a coincidence but I don't know about that. Anyway he said, "If you don't answer all the questions I'll see to it that you are finished as a pharmacologist."

D Not just at Michigan?

N No. In the field of pharmacology. I didn't need that extra worry when I was questioned at the Hearings in Ann Arbor. Later, I thought it would be sufficient evidence that I wasn't finished if I became president of ASPET.

D You did become president of ASPET. When?

N In 1975. The president of ASPET invites the past presidents to a luncheon. So I decided to send Seevers a special invitation to the past presidents' luncheon with a note that Dr. Nickerson would particularly appreciate Dr. Seevers' attendance at this event.

D You specifically requested that Dr. Seevers attend?

N He was a past president but I wanted to put a special note on his invitation. He was at that meeting but he didn't come to the luncheon.

D What year was that?

N That was 1975.

D I think he died several years after that.

N You're right. I wanted him to know I became president of ASPET before he died. He was still on his feet. It was two or three years before he died.

D What a story!

N Life is made up of people's stories, I guess.

D Mark, in all of us there's a good and a bad; there's a mixture of things and you have seen a dark side of Seevers. However, Canadian pharmacology profited enormously by your coming to Canada. One of the things that impresses me is that when you went to Canada you became a new father of Canadian pharmacology.

N And I profited greatly, too. I think Manitoba, a little measly province with less than a million people in it, is the only place in North America where pharmacology has its own free standing building.

D I didn't know that.

N I raised the money and we built a five-story building, including animal quarters and so on. I think we had the biggest department, about 95 people. Some pretty damn good people. Among the people that came over when we were having trouble with techniques was von Euler. He worked in that building. I don't know how or why but he could make the catecholamine assay work to separate them. At first, we couldn't do it, but after he had been there for a month or so we could always make it work.

D He got a Nobel Prize, didn't he?

N Yes. I'm satisfied with what recognition I got. You know, I have an honorary Doctor of Science. There is something that makes me unique, I think. I am a classmate of my own Professor of Medicine. I was asked if I would give a convocation speech and accept an honorary degree at Medical College of Wisconsin in Milwaukee. I knew that I was sort of a representative of the pre-clinical people and that there would be another person getting a degree as a representative of the clinical departments. There were two speeches, one was the convocation and one was before the honorary degrees. Guess who got the other degree? Dr. Wintrobe, my own Professor of Medicine. We got our honorary degrees at the same convocation.

D What year was that?

N It would have been about 1971.

D When did you leave Manitoba to go to Montreal?

N 1967.

D So you were at McGill for quite a while, weren't you, Mark?

N Yes, 20 years.

D When did you retire from McGill?

N I was officially retired in 1982 but I stayed on until 1987. I am appointed Distinguished Emeritus Professor. They can't fire me and I can't resign. It gives me all the privileges of the University, libraries, etc. I could carry on except for a salary.

D The title but not the salary.

N Yes.

D You left Montreal in 1987, isn't that correct?

N Yes. I got married.

D You remarried about when?

N I married my girlfriend in 1987 and moved out to the country.

D To where?

N Two of my sons from the previous family built us a little four-room cottage. One of them is a computer designer and the other a cabinet maker. As I look out here I see the broad part of the Ottawa River. If I row my boat out to the other side of the river I can write a prescription on my Quebec medical license. I never went through the rigmarole of getting an Ontario license. I do keep in contact with medicine. Ever since I finished my term on the Medical Letter editorial board they have sent me free copies which I read. The Medical Letter is the best way to follow the literature.

D Do you remember that old clinical pharmacology course we taught in the third year at Michigan?

N Yes. I guess I jumped directly into something similar because Manitoba had a five-year medical course with what would be called a captive internship. Pharmacology was a third-year subject and that's where all these guys from the shock team and related areas came from.

D Where do you see pharmacology going, Mark? You have been in the field so long. I am wondering with all the new developments in the basic sciences if you think pharmacology is still going to be with us and stay alive as a scientific discipline.

N My prediction is quite simple. Pharmacology will continue to increase in importance in medicine as long as I can foresee into the future but if they don't take care of the subject, pharmacologists, meaning people practicing it, will become redundant.

D I like the way you put it.

N I mean drugs are bound to become more and more important. A good friend of mine at Duke said, give me the kind of department of medicine I want and you can take all of the rest of the medical school and dump it in the lake. Medicine is going to take over part of pharmacology and biochemistry is going to take over part of pharmacology. Somebody's got to wake up and realize that we pharmacologists are supposed to be the experts on drugs.

D Is there anything else you feel you want to say?

N I appreciate that you probably have some limitations since the book is a history meant to be a demonstration of how great UM pharmacology was.

D I want the truth. I don't think we have to lie about Michigan. I think Michigan has done many things but, as with every university, there's a good and a bad. We all have to learn from the past what we should avoid in the future. You've got to be proud of the fact, Mark, that long after you left, academic freedom is still an important concern of our faculty. The experience that the three of you went through years ago, Markert, Davis, and yourself, is part of our University's growth and development.

N Incidentally, aside from being a classmate of my professor of medicine, another thing that I may be unique in is that I have a lectureship named for me at Michigan because I was fired and a lectureship in my name at McGill for being good.

D I think you're unique in the world in that regard. Mark, maybe on this note we ought to bring things to a close.

N Well I wish the best to you and all of my other friends at Michigan.

9

The Mark Nickerson Affair: Recollections of an Administrative Secretary

Dorothy H. Overbeck, M.A.

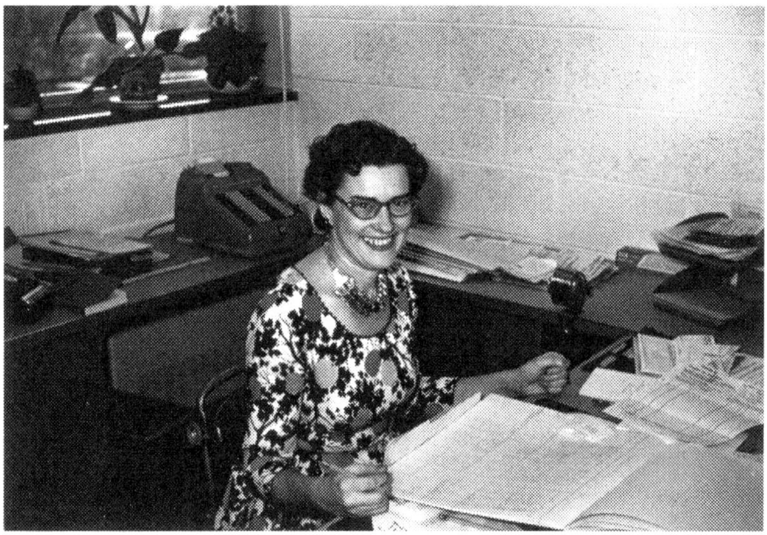

When Mark Nickerson joined the faculty of the Department of Pharmacology in 1951, we were engaged in the Korean War. We had just emerged from World War II and again found ourselves in another time of political anguish. The Department of Pharmacology was almost totally involved in classified research. Dr. Seevers had worked with the US government throughout WWII and he was requested to continue with research for the Army. Our staff was fingerprinted and investigated because of the nature of this research. Representatives from the FBI and CIA were constantly in the departmental office. I know this because I was often the person who met with them and was often requested to assist them in University and local contacts. I felt that federal agents were constantly on guard for possible espionage.

I will never forget the day when Dr. Seevers came into the office and announced to me in a hushed voice that Mark Nickerson was under federal investigation. Both of us were speechless with shock. Dr. Seevers told me that this was confidential and that a Committee had been formed to assess the facts. I felt very sorry for him and for the chairmen of the other two departments involved in the investigation. This was a very difficult position to have forced upon a person. I do not remember anything being discussed about this matter. Business, as usual, was conducted in the Department and until Dr. Seevers told me of the Board of Regents' decision weeks later, the subject was closed.

I understand that accusations have been made against Dr. Seevers of having spied on Dr. Nickerson, including having the secretarial staff inform him regarding Dr. Nickerson's correspondence and having a travel agent at Boersma secretly reporting to him regarding Dr. Nickerson's travel plans. I am appalled at such an accusation because Dr. Seevers would have no reasons to care about Dr. Nickerson's personal business. I understand that Mr. Boersma is also upset about such accusations. If Dr. Nickerson conducted any correspondence through the Department office, Dr. Seevers and I never knew about it. Under the circumstances at that time I doubt that Dr. Nickerson would send any personal correspondence through our office. I wonder if the three faculty members who were under investigation were still under surveillance by the FBI or CIA when these events supposedly occurred. It certainly was unnecessary for Dr. Seevers to spy on anyone with all of the federal agents circulating on campus. When Dr. Nickerson left Michigan in 1954, his personal file was closed. There was never any correspondence regarding him exchanged during my tenure in the Department. It is most interesting to note that almost 40 years went by before there was any attempt to clear the names of the professors involved. By that time, all of members of the University Committee were long since dead. None of the other persons involved were around to speak for themselves. This was most inconvenient for everyone except those who support Dr. Nickerson because we were able to get only one side of the story.

I am totally ignorant of the official accusations that were made against the three faculty members. I am certainly not against efforts to clear their reputations. However, all of this occurred almost 50 years ago. Times were different, people were different and our attitudes and values were definitely different. I do not recall any other institutions requesting information from Dr. Seevers with regard to Dr. Nickerson's qualifications. It would seem doubtful that Dr. Nickerson could have obtained a position anywhere in the US during this period. That was most unfortunate for him. However, it is almost as though Dr. Nickerson attempted to place the blame for the federal investigation on Dr. Seevers.

I do hope that Dr. Nickerson gained some satisfaction in attempts to clear his name. I hope that he was able to find peace with his conscience and within himself.

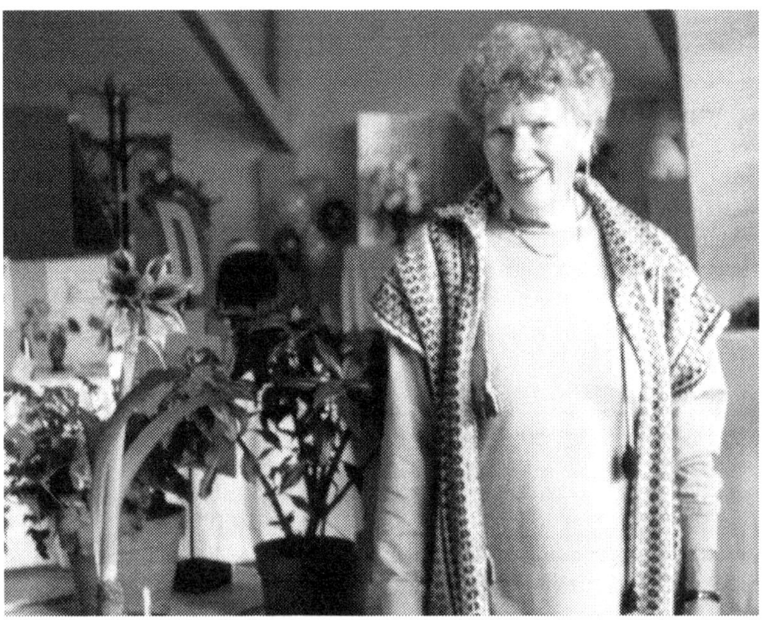

Dotty Overbeck still calling a spade a spade.

10

A History of the Conception, Birth, and Early Years of the Upjohn Center for Clinical Pharmacology

Edward A. Carr, Jr., M.D.

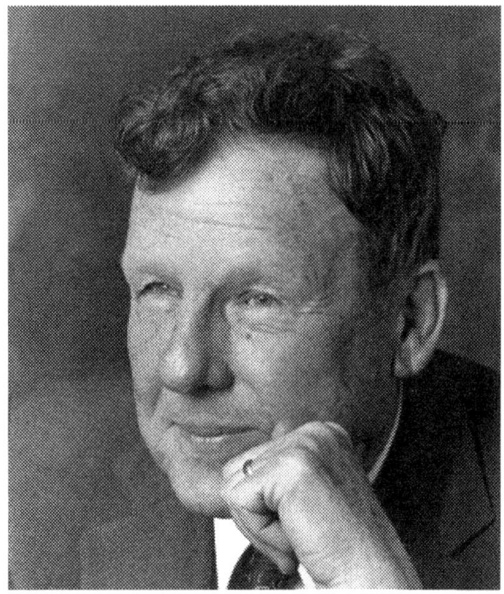

The Scottish writer Thomas Carlyle said that an institution is the lengthened shadow of one man, but the Upjohn Center owes its existence to two. When E. Gifford Upjohn announced the gift of one million dollars to permit the University of Michigan to construct the Center, he indicated that he had several purposes in mind: to express his loyalty to the University, to promote the science of clinical pharmacology, and to honor the Upjohn family. He was also clear on two other points; he wanted the Center to be widely available to qualified investigators from all appropriate University departments, especially in the Medical School, and he gave the full authority for running the Center to the University. He stated, "We (i.e. the donors) do not intend to tell you how to use it but we ask that you use it wisely." He adhered scrupulously to this principle and enabled the Center to operate without a trace of outside interference; he was a man of generosity, foresight and honor.

But the Upjohn Center did not develop in a vacuum. A training program in clinical pharmacology had been in existence at Michigan for several years before the Upjohn gift. It is unlikely that the Center would have arisen, de novo, without the background of this ongoing program and it is even more unlikely that the training program would have existed at all without the constant encouragement and support of Dr. Maurice Seevers. Therefore, it seems appropriate to describe developments that led to the establishment of this training program before discussing the Upjohn Center.

I first met Dr. Seevers briefly in the late 1940s when I was an instructor in pharmacology, working with Dr. Douglas Riggs in Dr. Otto Krayer's department at Harvard. Toward the end of my clinical training at the Pennsylvania Hospital in 1951 I had a more formal interview with him when he came to Washington, D.C. for a meeting. Dr. Seevers subsequently arranged for me to come to Ann Arbor for an interview with Dr. Sturgis, then Chairman of Internal Medicine. I was offered, and gladly accepted, combined assistant professorships in pharmacology and internal medicine at Michigan. These were to begin in July 1953 after I had completed a year's fellowship at St. Bartholomew's Hospital in London, which had already been arranged through the kindness of Dr. Duncan, Chief of Medicine at the Pennsylvania Hospital.

While an instructor at Harvard, I had

observed Doug Riggs giving informal teaching sessions to senior medical students at the Massachusetts General Hospital, in which he blended a review of basic pharmacology with practical examples of the clinical use of various drugs. With his encouragement I began to try similar sessions at the Boston City Hospital. I do not remember whether I used the term "clinical pharmacology" to describe them. Subsequently, after coming to Michigan I suggested to Dr. Sturgis that I try giving such sessions at the University Hospital. He assigned me the hour of 8A.M.-9A.M. on Saturday mornings, before medical rounds, as a good test to see if the senior students would really be interested in such sessions. Thank God, the students "voted with their feet" and attended these sessions regularly.

But clinical pharmacology, like all pharmacology, must have its research as well as its teaching component. Although I had been exposed to some excellent clinical investigators while in medical school and during the fellowship at St. Bartholomew's Hospital, I had had virtually no personal experience in clinical investigation before coming to Michigan. Dr. Seevers gave me a laboratory in his department for the conduct of basic research, but the old pharmacology building was not designed to permit clinical investigations. At this point a chain of events proved fortunate for me. After the end of World War II the first widely available radionuclides emitting gamma rays, and thus permitting non-invasive study by external detectors after injection into humans, were radioisotopes of iodine. I had developed a little familiarity with radio-iodine while doing thyroid research in Doug Riggs' laboratory at Harvard, so at Michigan I gravitated to the Thyroid Clinic, which was directed by Dr. William Beierwaltes. Bill was a go-getter in both the clinic and the laboratory. As other clinically useful radionuclides became available, his clinic developed into a more general Isotope Unit, and eventually into a Division of Nuclear Medicine. Over the years radiopharmaceuticals became a major group of diagnostic drugs, serving as imaging agents. When pursuing a problem in research, Bill was very adept at going back and forth between animals and human studies whenever a new question needed an answer. Thus I was lucky to have an excellent mentor for clinical investigation.

A not-so-fortunate event was a surprise notice from the draft board that Uncle Sam required my services again. After spending a little more than a year at Michigan I was taken in the Korean War's "doctor's draft" in November 1954 and left Ann Arbor for a 15-month tour of military service. I was not sent overseas but all academic plans and arrangements were of course brought to an abrupt halt. The sudden suspension of a very recent dual appointment, one department being based in the University Hospital and the other on the main campus, would have created every kind of problem for me, especially upon my return, if I had not had the aid of Dorothy Overbeck (then Dorothy Norton). Soon after my arrival in Michigan I had realized that anyone appointed to Dr. Seevers' department should consider himself fortunate, for he was joining a faculty of very high caliber, as exemplified by pharmacologists like Dr. Lauren Woods. But now I learned that the department also had, in Mrs. Norton, an administrative assistant with an encyclopedic knowledge of University bureaucracy and procedures. She guided me through the maze of paperwork, showed me how to avoid bureaucratic booby-traps and enlivened it all by her frequent, perceptive and frank— sometimes amazingly frank— comments on University personnel, both high and low! Thanks to Dorothy I was able to rejoin the faculty in February 1956 with a minimum of bureaucratic confusion.

This is not the place to attempt a general history of clinical pharmacology except to note that the clinical trial dates back at least to the eighteenth century with Lind's studies on scurvy, and that the pioneers such as Schmiedeberg and Abel who founded modern pharmacology at the end of the nineteenth and beginning of the twentieth century took a very active interest in therapeutics as well as basic pharmacology. Paul Erlich took an especially keen interest in the clinical success or failure of the compounds he developed. But, at least in the United States, credit for establishing clinical pharmacology as a recognized scientific discipline must go to Drs. Walter Modell, founding editor of "Clinical Pharmacology and Therapeutics," Harry Gold, and Louis Lasagna. After performing studies on analgesics with Dr. Henry Beecher at the Massachusetts General Hospital, Lou established the first American academic training program in clinical pharmacology at Johns Hopkins Medical School. I remember reading with great interest an article on clinical pharmacology that he wrote for "Scientific American" in the 1950s. After 1956 I began to discuss with Dr. Seevers and others the possibility of starting such a training program at Michigan. (Of course, in the area of narcotics and other addicting drugs the work with primates by Dr. Seevers and his associates was already only "one step away" from human studies.) In 1959 the clinical pharmacology training program was formally initiated. Thus I believe Michigan was the second American medical school to have such a program but I am not certain. Dr. Walter Baird, who was already at Michigan, became our first trainee and subsequently became my first associate faculty member in the program. An excellent cardiologist, Wally eventually became Associate Professor of Medicine at Michigan State University, but in the intervening years he was very important in the development of our training program and the early planning of the Upjohn Center. Several years later another individual who was already at Michigan became a trainee and subsequently contributed greatly to the program - Dr. George Bacon, who eventually became a professor of pediatrics. He played a crucial role in the early years of the Center.

In June 1960 we applied to the (then) National Heart Institute (NHI) for a training grant and received a site visit in December 1960. In March 1961 the NHI Council recommended approval but a shortage of funds in the granting agency delayed the actual funding of the grant until 1962. From 1962 to 1974 there were 9 American, 7 European, 2 Asian, 1 Canadian, and 1 South American trainees. Not all were supported by the training grant; other funding was also obtained from various sources, especially for the foreign trainees.

At this point a brief digression is necessary. It would be misleading to imply that all the clinical interests of the pharmacology department were channeled through the program described above. First, independently of that program, Dr. Edward Domino extended his pioneering basic research in neuro- and psychopharmacology to clinical investigations and over the years has produced an impressive body of research that is clinical pharmacology by anybody's definition. Second, although the research on addicting drugs conducted by Dr. Seevers and his associates in monkeys was, of course, not human pharmacology, I believe there was a constant interchange of information between the Michigan group and those conducting clinical investigations with these drugs elsewhere, so the Michigan research had a definite "clinical flavor." Third, some members of the pharmacology department, while conducting most or all of their research in the laboratory, were very careful to keep abreast of clinical literature concerning the drugs in their own areas of special interest. Thus, as teachers of pharmacology, they were very knowledgeable of both basic and clinical aspects of those drugs. Notable examples were Dr. Henry Swain and Dr. Edward Cafruny. Here, as in several other places in this narrative, I have mentioned only a few people who immediately come to mind as examples; others deserve mention but I have neither the space nor the memory to list them all and can only apologize to those omitted from mention.

Returning to the subject of training programs, several other schools also initiated them and in June 1965 a score of interested individuals came together in Basin Harbor, Vermont, to discuss the status of American clinical pharmacology. As the weather was fine, at least one of the sessions was held outdoors on the shores of Lake Champlain, with Lou Lasagna presiding over us like a Seneca chieftain reviewing his braves. Lou published a report of the entire conference in Science (vol. 152, p. 388, 1966). One of the main conclusions was that "lack of space currently limits the adequate staffing of most clinical pharmacology centers." Michigan was no exception although, paradoxically, another potential problem in the Michigan program slightly mitigated the space problem for a time. In addition to the didactic parts of the program, each trainee was given research experience, including, whenever possible, participation in a clinical investigation. My own research interest centered on radiopharmaceuticals, which at that time were almost exclusively diagnostic rather than therapeutic drugs. Diagnostic drugs have their place in pharmacology but it is far from a central place and most trainees were, quite understandably, interested in therapeutic drugs. Fortunately, other faculty members in several departments, especially internal medicine, were willing to serve as mentors of the clinical pharmacology trainees. While participating in clinical research in these departments, the trainees had the temporary use of some of the mentor's clinical facilities. But these arrangements still left clinical pharmacology as a Blanche Dubois, dependent on "the kindness of strangers," for much of its space. More space had to be found...or else created.

The clinical pharmacology program certainly did not have funds to pay a professional architect to design a whole new unit for us, or the funds to construct such a unit if it were designed. And without new space it seemed very unlikely that the program would ever be large enough to get such grant funds. Impasse. Therefore, in the autumn of 1963 I made a telephone call to the head of the University's School of Architecture, asking him if he might have some senior architecture student who would like to get a bit of practical experience by designing a clinical pharmacology unit. The discretionary grant funds available to me at that time were very limited and I could only offer the princely sum of 100 dollars. But an architecture student, Mr. Lewis Dickens, subsequently called me and indicated his interest. We met many times during the 1963 Christmas recess. He had a very serious, professional attitude and first asked for some reprints of clinical pharmacology publications that would give him an idea of the field. He then listened to my rather inchoate ideas about the proposed unit and suggested making a three-dimensional model instead of a set of blueprints. At that time a separate building seemed completely out of the question so the design envisioned a unit to be created by renovation of part of one story of an existing building— we had no idea which building (if any). As I was still working in the Department of Medicine's Nuclear Medicine division and Bill Beierwaltes had assembled a staff very active in clinical investigations, there was the vague hope that the proposed clinical pharmacology unit - if it ever came to exist— might be near Nuclear Medicine. About half of the new space was designed to permit clinical work with radionuclides.

Mr. Dickens suggested a portable model. As the plan at that time envisioned a one-story unit, he was able to make the model on a flat surface with a hinged cover that folded up to make a portable case resembling a long, thin suitcase. Mr. Dickens spent the entire $100 on the supplies needed to make this model and took nothing himself. Dr. Seevers and Dean William Hubbard saw the model and made useful suggestions about modifications. I then rose, or sank (as you wish), to the level of traveling salesman, taking the model to show to appropriate people at the NIH. They expressed interest but it was impossible to tell how many were impressed and how many were simply amused. My former mentor, Doug Riggs, was by then Chairman of Pharmacology at Buffalo and, at his invitation, I also showed the model to his dean at Buffalo.

In 1965 Dean Hubbard informed me that Dr. E. Gifford Upjohn had expressed interest in making a sizable gift to the University of Michigan at the time of the upcoming sesquicentennial of the founding of the University. I do not know if the gift was from the outset destined for the Medical School as opposed to other areas in the University but in any event the Medical School was a logical site, in view of the Upjohn Company's long and honorable history of providing useful drugs for the medical profession. Although the clinical pharmacology program was certainly not the only good candidate, the ongoing program's focus on pharmacology and therapeutics plus one other advantage suggested that a strong proposal could be submitted to Upjohn. This other advantage was the fact that the program not only had a great need for space but also had a specific plan, already developed, that identified in some detail the type of space needed and the way it would be used. By this time suggestions by Drs. Seevers and Hubbard had already modified the original design in several important ways, e.g., increasing the number of "wet" laboratories, decreasing somewhat the amount of space for radiopharmaceutical studies and providing more space for trainees.

Dean Hubbard suggested that I write a three-tiered proposal. The first tier would request a grant large enough to permit construction of a building that would not only house the clinical pharmacology group but would also provide many facilities for other investigators in the University to use on an ad-hoc basis. The third tier would be a proposal that envisaged a much smaller amount of space, devoted solely to the clinical pharmacology program. The second tier would be intermediate, both in its aims and in the amount requested.

With Dr. Seevers' strong encouragement I wrote a first draft of the three-part proposal and after he had reviewed this, a second draft. Enthusiasm is a two-edged sword. I was very happy to write the first draft but adopted an evangelical style that brought a clear (and justified) warning from Dr. Seevers, who told me to stop trying to write (in his words) "like a cross between Billy Sunday and the epistles of St. Paul."

Dean Hubbard modified the proposal further in a third and then a fourth draft. He and Dr. Seevers then took the proposal to Dr. Upjohn in Kalamazoo. A formal request for a specific gift of this type could of course come only from the President of the University. In November 1965 Dean Hubbard asked President Hatcher to make such a request and in December 1965 President Hatcher did so. At the end of January 1966 Dr. Upjohn announced the gift in a letter to President Hatcher.

Dr. Upjohn accepted the first tier proposal, i.e. agreed to make the largest of the three suggested gifts. The amount given was one million dollars, a considerable sum even today and a very generous sum in 1966 dollars. An important stipulation of the donor was that the University attempt to obtain a grant for matching funds from the National Institute of Health. If obtained, these additional funds from the NIH would approximately double the size of the proposed building.

The proposal for matching funds, submitted to the NIH in June 1966, contained, inter alia, a sort of "constitution" (i.e., a set of governing rules) for the Center. A "core program" conducted by investigators "whose principal career effort (was) in clinical pharmacology" was to be the focal point of the Center. Drs. Baird, Domino and I were among the 10 in this group. A "broad access" program was to allow "all qualified investigators in the faculty to undertake specific research projects in clinical pharmacology." Twenty-five investigators, including Drs. Benedict Lucchesi and Charles Schuster from Pharmacology, as well as Dr. Arthur French, Director of the Clinical Research Unit in the University Hospital, were listed in this program. A total of 10 departments were represented. Dr. Seevers wrote several important rules for the Center. Although primarily designed for clinical studies, the Center's programs also envisaged basic science research in support of such studies but no animals would be housed in the Center. As the hospital's Clinical Research Unit already provided facilities for bed patients, studies in the Upjohn Center would be confined to ambulatory patients. The Center could have its own technical and secretarial staff but every investigator in the Center had to hold an appointment in some University Department.

Dean Hubbard appointed a Policy Committee to oversee the Center. Dr. Seevers and he were co-chairmen, the other members being the chairmen of Internal Medicine, Pediatrics, Psychiatry and Surgery, Mr. John Zugich (Associate Director of the University Hospital), and me (at that time Chairman of the Planning Committee for the Center). Although Dr. William Robinson, Chairman of Internal Medicine, was clearly supportive of clinical pharmacology, he did not, to my knowledge, at any time raise objections to the Pharmacology Department's role as administrative base for the Center. Yet Internal Medicine supplied the largest number of proposed investigators for the Center and my own clinical research program had been developed in a division of Dr. Robinson's department. I believe there were at least three reasons for Dr. Robinson' s position regarding the Center. First, although an experienced investigator and careful teacher, he was above all a superb clinician — one of the best I have ever known — who took extremely seriously his department's extensive responsibilities for patient care. The Center would not have a major role in patient care. Second, I believe he recognized and respected the primary role that Dr. Seevers had already played in the development of clinical pharmacology. Third, Dr. Robinson was in charge of a large and vigorous, but sometimes rambunctious, academic department, interacting constantly with a hospital administration that had its own concerns, e.g. financial stability. Dr. Robinson already had a surplus of major responsibilities. Whereas pediatricians and psychiatrists logically have an important interest in clinical pharmacology, surgeons may be expected to have less interest, as they are so heavily occupied with another form of treatment. But the appointment of Dr. Child, Chief of Surgery, to the Policy Committee proved a great boon to me. He was a sound counselor and an effective supporter of the Center.

Dean Hubbard wanted the application for matching funds to go to the NIH as quickly as possible. At that time the NIH subjected requests for construction funds to especially rigorous scrutiny. We were warned, "The brick is the hardest buck to get from the NIH". I believe the Dean felt, correctly as events proved, that NIH construction funds would become even more limited as time went on, so any delay was unacceptable. But we had to develop and describe, starting in February, a detailed plan for a building twice the size of the structure originally planned and different in many aspects from the latter, for a larger building would offer the possibility of special facilities not present in the smaller building. The application also had to request and list in detail all furnishings and equipment, both scientific and otherwise. These physical details had to be interwoven with an extensive scientific proposal involving about three dozen investigators who were to conduct a wide and varied array of research projects, to be organized and administered in such a way as to form a coherent whole rather than a fragmented collection. Despite the fact that these investigators' time was already heavily committed because of their academic duties, the application had to be completed and forwarded to the NIH in June. If we had not had the tireless assistance of Mr. Joseph Diana, the Dean's financial officer, I doubt that we could have met the deadline at all. Even though we did meet the deadline, the application, for $800,000, still had many loose ends. When a grant application leads to a site visit from a group of experienced scientists, especially if their review is to be very stringent, then haste in the preparation of the application is like a bucket of dead fish. Its odor simply cannot be concealed. The site visit led to rejection of the application.

In December 1966 I was appointed director of the proposed Center, on the recommendation of an ad-hoc search committee, consisting of the members of the Policy Committee minus me. I strongly believe Dr. Robinson's support and, even more, Dr. Seevers' support were major factors in the Committee's decision. Unfortunately, a casualty of the hectic period of preparation of the first NIH application had been my personal relationship with Dean Hubbard. Given the enormous disparity in our positions in the academic hierarchy, this change could obviously cause more problems for me than for him. If the choice had been his alone, it seems likely that the Dean would have preferred to look outside as well as inside the University and, in any event, appoint someone else as first director. But after my appointment the Dean continued to work as hard as before to make the Center a reality, his contributions being entirely positive.

In February 1967 we applied to the

National Institute of General Medical Sciences (NIGMS) for $700,000 to support, over a period of five years, a research and training effort. This would first use existing facilities at Michigan, including space in the Kresge building assigned by Dean Hubbard, from 1967 to 1969. We would then move into the Upjohn Center. From 1967 to 1969 the Center would be under construction, using the Upjohn gift. The application noted that we hoped eventually to increase the size of the building but such a future increase would depend on our obtaining additional funds later. The February 1967 application requested no construction funds but requested equipment and furniture for the Center, salaries for technical and secretarial staff, supplies, etc. As before, both clinicians and basic scientists were included among the 20 investigators named and provision was made to base some investigators in the Center. Most of the 20 had participated in the 1966 application but two important additions in 1967 were Drs. Raymond Ruddon and Thomas Tephly from Pharmacology. The proposed research was centered around four themes: 1) allergic and other adverse reactions to drugs, 2) quantification of drug effects (in cardiology, rheumatology and anesthesiology), 3) drug metabolism and drug effects on endocrine-metabolic processes, 4) therapy in special age groups (e.g. children) and special conditions (e.g. organ transplants). The February 1967 application has been described here in some detail because its approval by the NIGMS, after a March 1967 site visit, set the initial course for the Center. Later in 1967 a second attempt was made to obtain additional construction funds from the NIH. We were warned, even before the site visit, that NIH construction funds had now become exceedingly limited. Thus we were disappointed but not really surprised when our application was again rejected. Therefore at the end of 1967 construction of the Center in its present size began, funded by the Upjohn gift, with equipment and initial operations assured by the NIGMS funds from the successful February 1967 application. The National Heart Institute had also approved a five-year renewal of the training grant. Because of construction delays the Center did not open until June 4, 1970. In the name of the University, President Fleming formally accepted the building at a ceremony attended by many Upjohn representatives, including Dr. E. Gifford Upjohn and the (then) President, Mr. Robert Boudeman, and Chairman of the Board, Mr. R. T. Parfet, Jr. Guest speakers at an afternoon scientific symposium were Drs. Walter Modell, Thomas Maren, Thomas Durant and, from Upjohn, Dr. Norman Marshall. Though a strong supporter of the Center, Dr. Seevers was certainly never a yes-man. As some of the Center's research would involve children, I had worked with the University decorator to put very bright colors on interior walls in a certain area. When I took Dr. Seevers on a tour of the new building, I proudly showed him this area. He gave it one glance and said, "This looks as if it was designed by a half-wit."

Dr. Donald Kay, a rheumatologist already at Michigan in 1970, moved into the Center as a faculty member shortly after its opening. At a later time our last trainee, Dr. Donald Weidler, also became based in the Center after completion of his training. Three others, coming from outside the University of Michigan, joined its faculty and were based in the Center. Dr. William Murray, an anesthesiologist with a Ph.D. degree in pharmacology, was recruited from his position with the U.S. Food and Drug Administration to become Associate Director of the Center. With basic scientists we struck gold twice: Dr. John Wagner, who had an international reputation as a pioneer investigator in pharmacokinetics and biopharmaceutics, moved from the Upjohn Co. to the University, where he became a Professor of Pharmacy based in the Upjohn Center. With the aid of Drs. Christensen and Coon in Biochemistry, Dr. Fedor Medzihradsky was recruited. Fedor's arrival was one of the most fortunate events in the Center's history. He had a very enthusiastic outlook and was at the same time a meticulously careful investigator in the laboratory. Among the many members of the supporting staff who also contributed to the functioning of the Center the names of Ms. Carroll and Ms. Bassett, Research Associate and Research Nurse, respectively, come to mind, as well as the Administrative Secretaries, Mrs. Farkas and Mrs. Jallad. An Operating Committee, consisting of Drs. French, Murray, Ruddon and me, reviewed all proposals for use of the Center in research, including the many projects in which investigators not based in the Center used its facilities on an ad-hoc basis.

In 1974 I became Chairman of Pharmacology at the University of Louisville and in 1976 Chairman of Pharmacology and Therapeutics at the State University of New York at Buffalo. As the Upjohn Center had been developed through the efforts of many individuals, neither I nor any one else was indispensable in 1974 and my departure was no crucial event. But we are concerned here with the early history of the Center and I am not competent to serve as its historian for the years after 1974. As of 1974 this Upjohn Co.-University of Michigan collaboration had accomplished several things. The first (to our knowledge) building specifically devoted to clinical pharmacology in an American University had been constructed. An administrative arrangement whereby the Department of Pharmacology took a primary but not exclusive role, with "bridges" not only to the Department of Medicine but also to several other departments, had proven to be not just idealistic talk but a functioning interdisciplinary reality. Collaboration extended even beyond the clinical departments of the Medical School to the Department of Biochemistry and to the School of Pharmacy. Ongoing research in the Center involved investigators based in the Center but also many based elsewhere in the school. Several major research themes had been identified and each was being pursued in a number of ways. The requirement that every investigator based in the Center also hold a regular appointment in an established academic department avoided the risk of having "orphan" members, dependent entirely on the Center. The Center's operations had proved fundable, with an initial five-year NIH grant in 1967 and a second, three-year grant in 1972.

But interdisciplinary organizations of this type, with broad goals, face certain potential problems. Although a broad range of research projects does not preclude the possibility of a striking discovery by one of the investigators, the likelihood of such a dramatic success is probably less than in a program where all efforts are concentrated in a single area. Moreover, as times change, academic departments often change their priorities and a Center that depends on interdepartmental collaboration must adapt to changes in several, not just one, departments. This may cause problems for the Center director in recruiting and retaining faculty members, each of whom must find a niche in some department. All these problems converge, of course, in the problem of funding.

A major concern in 1974 was the future of the training program in clinical pharmacology. Dr. Murray would have been a logical choice to direct the program. But, although his strong background and congenial personality had made him a valuable member of the Center, his own research program was unfortunately slow to develop at Michigan and he elected, in 1973, to move to Duke University, where he eventually became a Professor of Anesthesiology. Dr. Bacon, another qualified individual, remained at Michigan but had already begun to make his mark as a pediatric endocrinologist and had a very heavy academic load of teaching, research and clinical care. Fortunately he agreed in 1974 to take on the administrative task of directing the Center but it would have been unreasonable to ask him also to run the training program. Other qualified faculty members in the Medical School presented the same problem, i.e. they were already fully occupied with their own academic duties. So, ironically, the training program, which had been the embryo from which the Center developed, languished. A recent partial review of the eventual careers, in the U.S. and abroad, of the 1962-74 trainees show that one became the director of a scientific foundation, at least eight became professors and two, associate professors in various Universities, and at least two took full-time positions in the pharmaceutical industry.

In closing, I wish long life to the Center and success to those who work in it.

11

The Upjohn Center for Clinical Pharmacology

Benedict R. Lucchesi, M.D., Ph.D.

Dr. Seevers firmly believed that the discipline of pharmacology was to be involved in both basic and clinical research. In the mid-1950s, he had the foresight to recruit Dr. Edward Carr to develop a program in Clinical Pharmacology. Initially, the program was housed on a lower level in University Hospital. Under Dr. Carr's direction a training grant proposal was submitted to the National Institutes of Health. At the time of the grant submission, I was a graduate student in the Department of Pharmacology. I was working on my dissertation research that involved the study of the recently introduced class of drugs known as beta-adrenoceptor antagonists. The members of my Dissertation Committee included both clinical and basic science faculty since the research focused on the study of beta-receptor antagonists as antiarrhythmic agents and the potential to use this new class of compounds for the management of patients with cardiac rhythm disorders. Dr. Carr selected my research project as an example of how the clinical pharmacology program at Michigan would combine the basic and clinical sciences in the training components of the program. I was asked to present my project before the site-visitors during the review of the training grant proposal. After several revisions, the training grant was funded with successful renewals in the subsequent periods. Thus the beginning of a formal research and training program in Clinical Pharmacology at the University of Michigan that for many years thereafter, remained as one of the premier programs in the United States. Under Dr. Carr's leadership, physicians from many parts of the world received formal training in Clinical Pharmacology. Many went forward to academic positions or to appointments in the pharmaceutical industry. Most important was the fact that Dr. Seevers had a profound influence in the development of clinical pharmacology in Japan.

Dean William Hubbard, Dr. Maurice Seevers and Dr. Edward Carr (Professor of Internal Medicine and Professor of Pharmacology) were successful in obtaining private funding to establish the Upjohn Center for Clinical Pharmacology. Dr. Carr was appointed Director of the Upjohn Center. He reported to the Dean of the Medical School and to an Executive Committee consisting of chairpersons from clinical and basic departments and the dean of the College of Pharmacy. The Upjohn Center was interdepartmental and multidisciplinary. The Director of the Center had the responsibility for appointing members from among the basic and clinical departments in the Medical School along with selected faculty from the College of Pharmacy. Among the original appointees there were faculty from Internal Medicine, Anesthesiology, Pharmacology, Biochemistry and the College of Pharmacy. The appointed faculty were provided office and laboratory spaces within the Upjohn Center, which also housed fellows in the Clinical Pharmacology Training Program. The facilities allowed for the conduct of studies in clinical and basic research. The main level of the Center had a clinic area and fully staffed nursing station, reception area and patient treatment rooms plus administrative office space, a conference room and the Director's office. The upper level of the Center had office space and laboratories for the appointed faculty and research fellows. Within a relatively short time Dr. Carr established a training program in Clinical Pharmacology that launched the careers of many clinical pharmacologists.

It should be noted that the Department of Pharmacology placed a heavy emphasis on clinical pharmacology in the medical curriculum. A faculty was assembled to conduct a formal, one semester, required course in Clinical Pharmacology and Therapeutics for third year medical students. In later years, as the medical school curriculum underwent successive modifications, the Clinical Pharmacology course became a fourth year elective. Dr. Carr, and later Dr. Swain, continued to administer the senior course with the assistance of faculty from many departments. Some 40-plus years later, the course remains within the Department of Pharmacology as one of the most successful fourth year electives and served as a model for the development of other fourth year courses referred to as "science in the clinics." The focus of the course remains largely unchanged and is to review elements of basic science as they relate to the development and appropriate use of pharmacologic agents for the management of human clinical problems.

With the retirement of Dr. Seevers and eventually the departure of Dr. Carr, the Upjohn Center was placed in the "care" of successive interim directors. The excellent clinical and laboratory facilities once a part of the Department of Pharmacology were being viewed with envy and would serve in an important way in recruiting the successor to Dr. Seevers. Needless to say, a "turf-war" was imminent. I was called to meet with Dr. John Gronvall, then Dean of the Medical School. He asked if I would be willing to serve as Interim Director of the Upjohn Center until a new chair for the Department of Pharmacology could be recruited. The term "interim" was not too appealing. However, I recognized the importance of preserving the facility as an integral part of the Department of Pharmacology and agreed to accept the responsibility to serve as requested. This was to be a harrowing time. The Center had been without leadership for an extended period. The faculty who had laboratory and clinic space in The Center had developed their own means of survival using "creative" approaches to fund their research activities. I became aware that there was a total lack of financial records, grant accounts and approved protocols for the ongoing studies. The reason was obvious. The indirect charge to industry at that time was approximately 110% of the direct costs. At this rate, the Upjohn Center could not be competitive. Thus, to remain viable, creative individuals accepted "monetary gifts" placed in accounts in the cashier's office from which they supported their investigative activities. The overhead charges were bypassed.

It was apparent that the indirect rate put us at a great disadvantage. Thus, I conducted a brief survey of the major pharmaceutical companies in the United States as well as a survey of the few existing clinical pharmacology centers at major medical schools. The purpose was to determine what indirect rate would be acceptable to the industry and what rate would be considered equitable for the academic institutions. The figure I arrived at was 15%. The information was provided to the leadership at the Division for Research Development and Administration (DRDA) and a policy was established whereby the new indirect charge for "clinical" studies would be 15%. The agreement was to be in effect for three years after which the policy would be reviewed to determine if the new rate placed the institution in a more competitive position to attract clinical trials. The fact that the rate continues to exist speaks for itself. However, as of 2000, there is a directive indicating that the overhead rate for clinical studies is to be increased to 25%. In many ways, this remains a "bargain" and an attractive incentive for sponsors of clinical studies to place clinical trials at the University of Michigan.

The Upjohn Center, as well as other areas (e.g. Dermatology), began to experience an increase in funded clinical studies. Among the studies conducted in the Department of Pharmacology and the Upjohn Center was one that I did in conjunction with Bertram Pitt, M.D., who had recently joined the faculty as Director of Cardiology. Bert and I had known each other for many years and I played a small part in recruiting him to Michigan by submitting his name to Dr. William Kelley, Chairman of Internal Medicine.

Dr. Pitt had many interactions with the pharmaceutical industry. Among his contacts was a small company in Miami, Florida, Key Pharmaceutical Company. During an informal meeting at my home arranged by Dr. Pitt, our discussion focused on the need for drug development in the area of cardiology. It was suggested that a device like a band-aid impregnated with nitroglycerin would be a convenient way to administer the drug to patients with ischemic heart disease. The suggestion seemed to arouse the interests of the company president, who was an attorney by training. Within a relatively short time, limited funding was obtained and the initial studies were conducted in experimental animals. There was the need to develop a sensitive assay for monitoring the plasma concentration of nitroglycerin to prove that a topical device impregnated with nitroglycerin would deliver the drug across the skin in a dose capable of sustaining a therapeutic response. The blood assay for nitroglycerin was developed by Dr. Philip Stetson, whom I had appointed as Director of the Core Laboratory in the Upjohn Center. Dr. Stetson developed a unique HPLC assay that was approved by the US Food and Drug Administration and served to demonstrate for the first time that nitroglycerin could be delivered to the systemic circulation when applied topically to the skin. Although nitroglycerin ointment had been available for clinical use, the bioavailability had never been established by direct determination of a blood concentration of the active substance.

The time came to apply what was learned in the basic laboratory to a clinical situation. The clinical device for administration of nitroglycerin consisted of a unique polymer impregnated with nitroglycerin. The polymer design allowed zero order release of the drug thereby establishing and maintaining a continuous plasma concentration of the drug. The absolute value of the blood concentration would be dependent upon the size of the polymer patch applied to the skin. Dr. Pitt was the first "volunteer" to receive a nitroglycerin patch. The size of the patch was over estimated slightly and the subsequent hypotensive response was reversed rapidly by placing him in the recumbent position and removing the patch. There was no doubt that we could deliver a sufficient amount of nitroglycerin by the transcutaneous route.

The clinical studies were done in the cardiac catheterization laboratory and in the Clinical Research Center as patients were to be kept over night. Dr. Joseph Walton and research nurses participated in the project. Patients with ischemic heart disease were subjected to cardiac pacing to the point of experiencing symptoms of angina pectoris and/or electrocardiographic evidence (ST-segment change) of myocardial ischemia. Once the threshold for induction of ischemia had been determined, the nitroglycerin patch was applied and the pacing protocol was repeated over the course of several hours and again on the next morning. The results indicated that the nitroglycerin patch was effective in reducing signs and symptoms of myocardial ischemia and that prolonged exposure to nitroglycerin would result in the development of tolerance. After months of study, the data were presented to the FDA and the first nitroglycerin patch was approved for clinical use.

The Upjohn Center was becoming self-sustaining. The opening of the Pain Clinic in conjunction with the Department of Anesthesiology provided a valuable source of operating revenue. The Phase I study of a drug believed to be an inhibitor of platelet aggregation provided an unanticipated surprise when it was discovered to produce thrombocytopenia after two weeks of administration to normal volunteers. Instead of being a grave disappointment to the sponsor, the drug subsequently was approved by the FDA for the management of thrombophilia and is currently marketed under the trade name of Anegrelide.

With the recruitment of Raymond Ruddon, M.D., Ph.D. as Chairman of Pharmacology, my interim-stewardship over the Upjohn Center came to an end. Part of the agreement under which Dr. Ruddon accepted the Chair of Pharmacology included a change in the focus of the Upjohn Center. The Center, originally organized to be multidisciplinary in its activities, was to become aligned towards the cancer clinical pharmacology. Dr. William Kelley, Chairman of Internal Medicine, negotiated with Dr. Ruddon to ensure that William Ensminger, M.D., Ph.D., was to become the new director of the Upjohn Center and in conjuction with Dr. Ruddon, the Center was to focus its efforts on basic research in cancer chemotherapy. The outpatient clinic and the patient treatment rooms were renovated into wet laboratory space. The Upjohn Center for Clinical Pharmacology was to undergo a complete change in its direction and departure from the intent under which the original donors had provided funding for the construction of the building. In the end, the Cancer Center was established in the newly constructed Cancer and Geriatrics Center.

Dr. Ruddon's subsequent departure from the University of Michigan and a protracted search for his replacement allowed the Upjohn Center to drift further away from its original relationship with the Department of Pharmacology. As a result, the Department of Pharmacology lost the clinical component of the discipline; the one feature that set it apart from the other basic sciences in the Medical School. This unfortunate sequence of events came at a time when there is a pressing need for centers of excellence devoted to the conduct of well-supervised clinical studies and programs for the training of clinical pharmacologists. It is evident today in the year 2003 that a critical shortage exists in the field of trained clinical pharmacologists. The shortage of qualified personnel has reached the crisis stage. There are some, including me, who believe that the University of Michigan can regain its leadership role in clinical pharmacology. This may be accomplished by returning to the structure first envisioned by Drs. Seevers and Carr in which the program in clinical pharmacology was multidisciplinary and included basic as well as clinical research along with a vibrant training program for clinicians from all medical disciplines and for doctoral and postdoctoral fellows in the basic medical sciences.

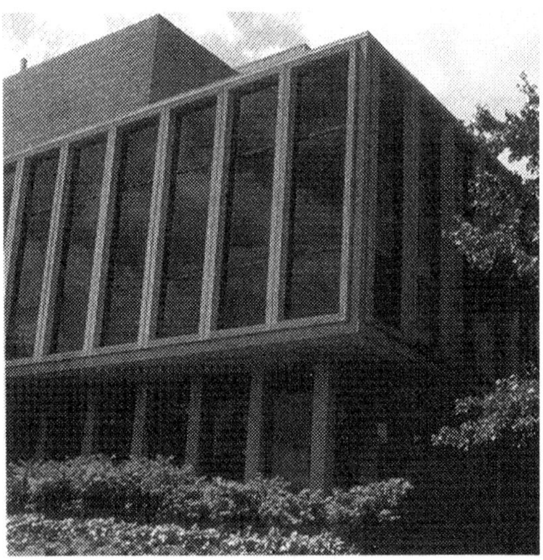

The Upjohn Center

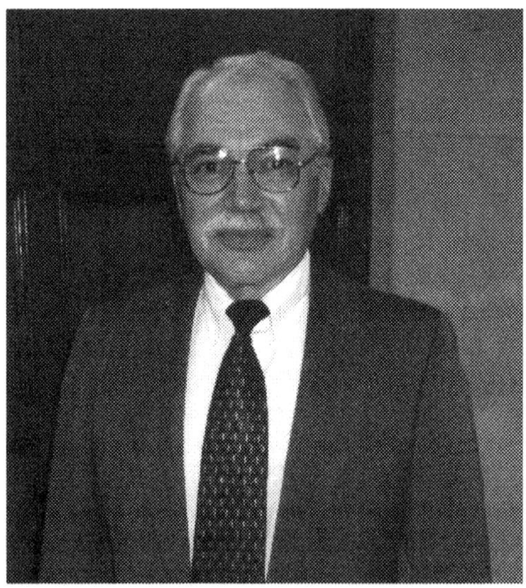

Dr. Walter Baird, one of the early Clinical Pharmacology Fellows.

12

Current Thoughts on the Upjohn Center

William D. Ensminger, M.D., Ph.D.

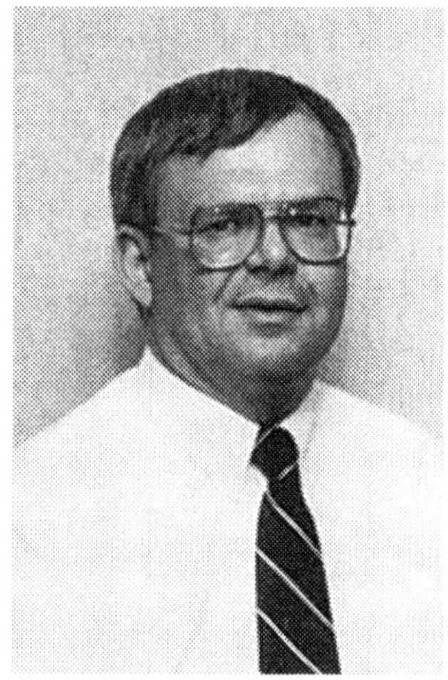

The early history of the Upjohn Center is described in previous chapters. A review of the Center as of 1981 reveals a deficiency of focus and difficult financial times due to the lack of a training grant or program project grant. The space within the Center and the Core Lab were increasingly being utilized by the Anesthesia Department for projects unrelated to all other efforts by Upjohn Center members. The new chair of Pharmacology, the Medical School Dean, and the Dean of the College of Pharmacy recognized that the Center needed an area of focus. Due in large part to Dr. Ruddon's personal research interests and to the increasing attention given locally to cancer research, the Upjohn Center was chosen as the home for a new program in cancer pharmacology.

A Search Committee was selected to choose a director for the Upjohn Center and for the cancer pharmacology program. I had recently received the Burroughs Wellcome Clinical Pharmacology Award, having been chosen as one of two nationally selected Scholars in 1980. I also had my laboratory in the Upjohn Center. I was selected by the committee and approved as director of the Upjohn Center and the Cancer Pharmacology Program in 1982.

As part of the package, the Center received recurring financial support from the dean's office for administrative services. The Pharmacology Department obtained two new tenure track faculty positions.

Subsequently, Dr. Jonathan Maybaum and Dr. William Mancini (now deceased), both biochemical pharmacologists with expertise in nucleic acid processor/antimetabolite metabolism, were recruited to those positions within the Department, Program, and Center. Dr. Ronald Natale, an Internal Medicine faculty member with an interest in tumor clonogenic assays and, Dr. Dean Brenner, an Internal Medicine faculty member with interests in anthracyclines and chemoprevention, also joined the Center. Dr. John Wagner, internationally renowned pharmacokineticist and member of the College of Pharmacy, was also an active member of the Center until his retirement in the early 1990s.

Dr. David E. Smith replaced Dr. Wagner as a representative of the College of Pharmacy. Dr. Smith provides pharmacokinetic expertise to the Center and to the medical school complex as well. Around 1990, Dr. Natale moved to join the faculty at the University of Southern California and Dr. Brenner relocated his laboratory and office to the Veteran's Hospital. Dr. Donna Shewach joined the Department and the Center at that time, providing further focus on nucleic acid/antimetabolite biochemical pharmacology. Dr. Shewach also later became associate director of the Center.

In 1983, I received a substantial contribution from a grateful cancer patient. A portion of those funds was put to use in a much-needed renovation of the interior and laboratories of the Center and the purchase of important core equipment, such as a GC mass spectrometer. These funds also provided for pilot studies which subsequently led to a successful program project application in regional chemotherapy and radiosensitization. The renovation of the Center's facilities and rejuvenation of its program played a role in obtaining an endowment from the Upjohn Company in 1984. Due to the efforts of Dr. Ara Paul, dean of the College of Pharmacy, and the assistance of Dr. Ruddon, Upjohn Company representatives visited the Center. As a result, a $1,000,000 endowment to provide for the maintenance, renovations, and equipment, as necessary, the Center was then established.

The close proximity of the Center to the Radiation Oncology Department has facilitated extensive interactions and collaboration over the years. In 1987, Dr. Theodore Lawrence joined the Radiation Oncology Department. Over the years, he and his associates have worked closely with Drs. Ensminger, Maybaum, Shewach, Smith, and Mancini. Multiple publications and grants (including a program project grant) have been generated by these joint efforts in the areas of radiosensitization, halogenated pyrimidine metabolism, regional chemotherapy with conformal radiotherapy, radioprotection and, most recently, in suicide gene therapy. Dr. Lawrence is now Chair of Radiation Oncology and the collaborations continue unabated.

The research efforts of the Center have had meaningful impact on cancer therapy. The totally implanted pump for intraarterial infusion and the totally implanted ports for vascular access were developed in the Center and have impacted upon the lives of thousands of patients. Studies in the regional pharmacokinetics and pharmacodynamics of halogenated pyrimidines have been seminal in the field. The application of radiosensitizers such as hepatic arterial floxuridine and intravenous gemcitabine has been developed and examined both in preclinical models and in patients. Yttrium 90 glass microspheres, a novel form of brachyradiation therapy, were first administered to patients in a study coming from the Center. Currently, suicide gene therapy is being examined as a way to target cancer cells selectively with antimetabolites.

The clinic space within the Center has been utilized at only partial capacity over the years. Many pharmaceutical company-sponsored studies otherwise suitable for the Center have been conducted instead within the General Clinical Research Center (GCRC) Outpatient Clinic due to the GCRC nursing coverage and close proximity to medical coverage (house officers), and to an indirect subsidy provided through the NIH grant. Currently the Upjohn Clinic houses pharmaceutical company studies emanating from the GI and Endocrinology Divisions of Internal Medicine and the Department of Neurology. It appears likely that clinic space will be converted to research laboratories in the long run. A number of offices within the ground floor of the Center house research assistants/data managers of the Center for Clinical Investigation and Therapeutics.

As the Center is now in its fourth decade, investigators within the Center are productive and well funded, in large part due to the synergy caused by the continued focus on cancer pharmacology. It is at this point unclear whether future construction of large research buildings in the medical complex will lead in the long run to the loss of the current building and resultant changes in the configuration of the Center and its program.

13

One Hundred Years of Pharmacology Centennial Celebration September 26-28, 1991

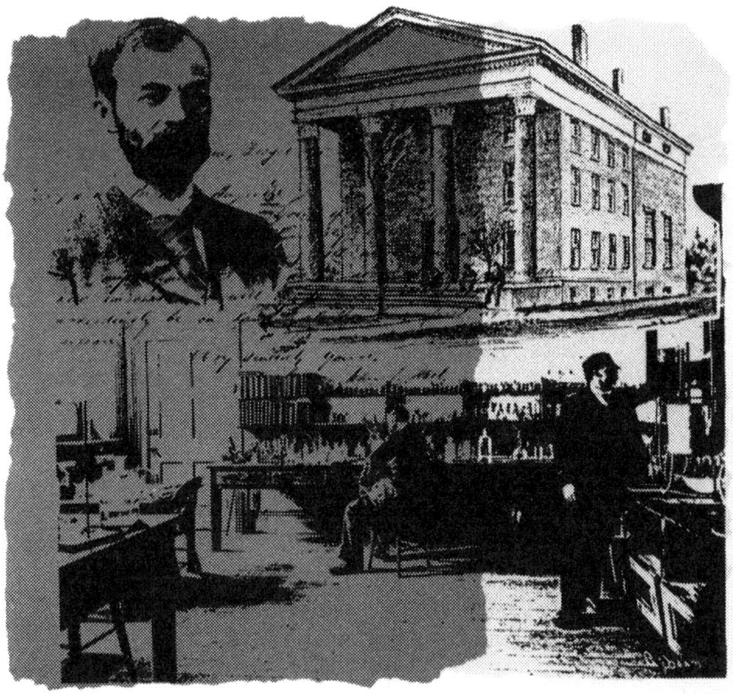

Advances in Cardiovascular Pharmacology
Ben G. Zimmerman, Ph.D.
Session Chairman
Professor, Department of Pharmacology
University of Minnesota

Advances in Neuropharmacology
Kenneth E. Moore, Ph.D.
Session Chairman
Professor and Chairman, Department of Pharmacology and Toxicology, Michigan State University

Pharmacology of Substance Abuse
Charles R. Schuster, Ph.D.
Session Chairman
Director, National Institute on Drug Abuse

Pharmacology—A Look to the Future
Robert Z. Gussin, Ph.D.
Session Chairman
Vice President, Johnson & Johnson

Sir James Black, FRS, FRCP
Nobel Laureate
King's College School of Medicine

Hale Auditorium
The University of Michigan
Ann Arbor, Michigan

sponsored by
The Department of Pharmacology

PROGRAM

Thursday, September 26 7:00-9:00pm	**Registration and Reception** University of Michigan Museum of Art
Friday, September 27 8:00am	**Symposium – Hale Auditorium** Welcome: James Duderstadt, President, The University of Michigan; George D. Zuidema, Vice Provost for Medical Affairs; Giles G. Bole, Interim Dean, Medical School; Raymond E. Counsell, Interim Chairman, Department of Pharmacology
8:30-12:00 noon	Advances in Cardiovascular Pharmacology Tribute to Michael J. Brody Chairman: Ben G. Zimmerman, Ph.D. Professor, Department of Pharmacology, University of Minnesota *Influence of ACE inhibitors on the renal rennin-angiotensin system* Gerard L. Gebber, Ph.D. Professor, Department of Pharmacology, Michigan State University *Central determinants of sympathetic nerve discharge* John H. McNeill, Ph.D. Dean, Faculty of Pharmaceutical Science, University of British Columbia *Treatment of experimentally induced diabetic cardiomyopathy* Donald W. DuCharme, Ph.D. Associate Director, Cardiovascular Disease Research, The Upjohn Company *Purification, identification, and characterization of a sodium pump inhibitor isolated from human plasma* Paul Simpson, Ph.D. Senior Pharmacologist, Lilly Research Laboratories *Advances in the pharmacological modification of tissue necrosis after ischemia and reperfusion*
12:30pm	Luncheon – Executive Residence Dining Room Posters – Phelps Lounge, Executive Residence
1:30-3:00pm	**Advances in Neuropharmacology** Chairman: Kenneth E. Moore, Ph.D. Professor and Chairman, Department of Pharmacology and Toxicology, Michigan State University *Regulation of different dopaminergic neuronal systems in the brain* Lindsay B. Hough, Ph.D. Professor and Vice-Chairman, Department of Pharmacology and Toxicology, The Albany Medical College *Histaminergic modulation of antinociceptive responses* Michael R. Vasko, Ph.D. Associate Professor, Department of Pharmacology and Toxicology, Indiana University School of Medicine
3:30-5:00pm	**Pharmacology of Substance Abuse** Chairman: Charles R. Schuster, Ph.D. Director, National Institute on Drug Abuse *Role of the University of Michigan in the development of the behavioral pharmacology of*

substance abuse

Tomoji Yanagita, M.D., Ph.D.
Director, Preclinical Research Laboratories, Central Institute for Experimental Animals, Kawasaki, Japan
Assessment of pharmacological determinants of abuse liability of drugs

Julian E. Villarreal, M.D., Ph.D.
Director, Department of Pharmacology and Toxicology, CINVESTAV-Inst. Polytech National, Mexico City, Mexico
Opiate abstinence produced by specific antagonists as a special type of pharmacological response

Steven R. Goldberg, Ph.D.
Chief, Preclinical Branch, National Institute on Drug Abuse, Addiction Research
Behavioral pharmacology of nicotine

Stephen G. Holtzman, Ph.D.
Professor, Department of Pharmacology, Emory University
Discriminative effects of drugs: relationships to potential for abuse

7:00-10:00pm — Banquet – Michigan Union Ballroom
Glenn F. Kiplinger, M.D., Ph.D., Emcee Henry H. Swain, M.D., Speaker

Saturday, September 28
8:00-11:00am — **Symposium – Hale Auditorium**

Pharmacology – A Look to the Future
Chairman: Robert Z. Gussin, Ph.D.
Vice President, Johnson & Johnson

Sir James Black, FRS, FRCP, Nobel Laureate
King's College School of Medicine

William L. Dewey, Ph.D.
Past President, Federation of American Societies for Experimental Biology
Associate Provost and Professor, Departments of Research and Graduate Affairs and Pharmacology, Medical College of Virginia

Christine K. Carrico, Ph.D.
Director, Pharmacological Sciences Program
National Institutes of General Medical Sciences

Pedro Cuatrecasas, M.D.
President, Parke-Davis Pharmaceutical Research Division of Warner-Lambert

Theodore Cooper, M.D., Ph.D.
President and Chief Executive Officer, The Upjohn Company

Robert L. Volle, Ph.D.
President, National Board of Medical Examiners

11:00am — Tailgate Luncheon in the Courtyard

12:00 noon — Depart for Stadium: Football game, U of M vs. Florida State

5:00pm — Faculty Open Houses

Pharmacology and Biostatistics at The University of Michigan, 1950-1961

Harold F. Hardman, M.D., Ph.D.

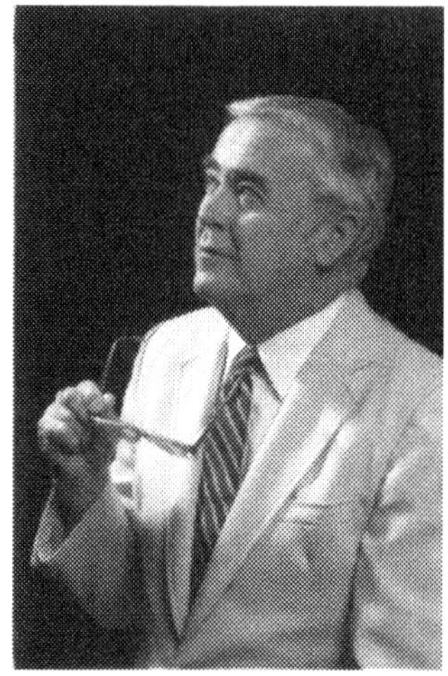

At the Centennial Celebration of the Department in September 1991, we talked about the use of statistical methods in the evaluation of pharmacological data. The use of "t tables" and "P values" represented the beginning of quantitative pharmacology. Michigan was considered to be one of the leading pharmacology departments in the United States and this reputation was based upon the faculty that Dr. Seevers had brought together in Ann Arbor during the period of 1945 through 1960.

I wished to determine when the Michigan faculty in pharmacology began using P values in their publications. I restricted my library search to the Journal of Pharmacology and Experimental Therapeutics (JPET) and began the search with the year 1950. I used the P value as a measure of the level of sophistication indicating a basic understanding of biostatistical methods. I also required a reference to some book or article that was utilized in calculating the P value presented in each article.

In 1950 there were 161 articles published in JPET; 23 of these met the criteria I just described. Only 14% of the manuscripts included calculations of the P value. Michigan was represented by one paper and that was the publication by James Weeks, Chenoweth and Fred Shideman (JPET 98:224, 1950). I included this paper even though it does not technically list a P value. It is clear that they knew how to calculate it and that is verified by their reference to the 1937 work Biological Standardization by J.H. Burn.

The next publication from Michigan to contain a P value occurred in 1952. The authors were again Weeks and Chenoweth, JPET 104:187, 1952. The reference to statistical analyses included: S.S. Wilks' 1949 Elementary Statistical Analysis and R.A. Fisher's Statistical Methods for Research Workers of 1941. Chenoweth and I authored the third publication from Michigan containing P values, JPET: 109: 461, 1953. The reference to statistics was to Statistical Methods, by G.W. Snedecor in 1946.

The next publication from Michigan that met the criteria for inclusion in this study was authored by Hendershot and Chenoweth, JPET: 110:344, 1954. There were several references to P values in the tables but no reference was included in the bibliography. Chenoweth had moved to the Dow Chemical Company in Midland, Michigan, before this paper was submitted to JPET for publication, and I suspect that some of the people at Dow helped him out with the statistical calculations of the P values. Hendershot joined Chenoweth at Dow, and his next publication in JPET 123, 1958 contained both P values and a bibliography reference to O.L. Davies' 1949 Statistical Methods in Research and Production.

To the casual observer it would appear that Chenoweth was the common factor in the use of statistics in the four papers listed above. In reality it was the three students who worked for Chenoweth who were the motivating force to incorporate the use of statistical methods in their pharmacological data.

The next factor that aided in the adoption of statistical methods in the publications of the Michigan group was the movement of Ted Brody, Ed Domino and Hank Swain from the University of Illinois to the University of Michigan in 1952, 1953, and 1954, respectively. Brody, Domino, Swain, and I had been graduate students together at the University of Illinois and had taken a graduate course in biostatistics in which the textbook employed was the 1946 fourth edition of Statistical Methods by George W. Snedecor. The course in biostatistics at Illinois was taught by Dr. Jules Last, an internist who held the rank of Associate Professor of Pharmacology. His wife, Muriel R. Last, worked with Dr. Earl R. Loew, the discoverer of the antihistaminic actions of diphenhydramine. Earl Loew had worked at Parke Davis (located in Detroit at that time) and he was conversant with biostatistical methods. Carl Pfeiffer had worked at Parke Davis (1941-1943) as head of pharmacology at the same time that Earl Loew worked there and when he accepted the chairmanship of pharmacology at the University of Illinois in 1945, he invited Dr. Loew to come to Chicago. In addition to Dr. Loew, Carl Pfeiffer also hired Dr. Klaus Unna to come to Chicago in 1945. Dr. Unna had been with the Merck Institute for Therapeutic Research from 1937 to 1944. Unna was also well acquainted with the use of statistical methods in biomedical research. The Department of Pharmacology at the University of Illinois was well staffed with senior faculty who taught biostatistical methods to the junior faculty and the graduate students in the department. This sophistication spread to other departments within the medical college and the primary reference to statistical methods seen in publications from the University of Illinois Medical School was to our biostatistics textbook.

The research publications from the Department of Pharmacology at the University of Michigan began to show the influence of junior faculty trained at the University of Illinois. The next paper citing biostatistics in JPET from the Michigan Department of Pharmacology was co-authored by Domino, Fox, and Brody 114:473,1955. The statistical method reference was to Statistical Methods. The following JPET publication with statistical analysis from Michigan was by T.M.Brody 117:39, 1956. Once again the statistical methods reference was to Statistical Methods. In 1957 Domino and Richard Rech published a JPET paper (121:171, 1957) in which P values were calculated but no reference was given for the source of information concerning the statistical methods utilized in the calculation of the P values.

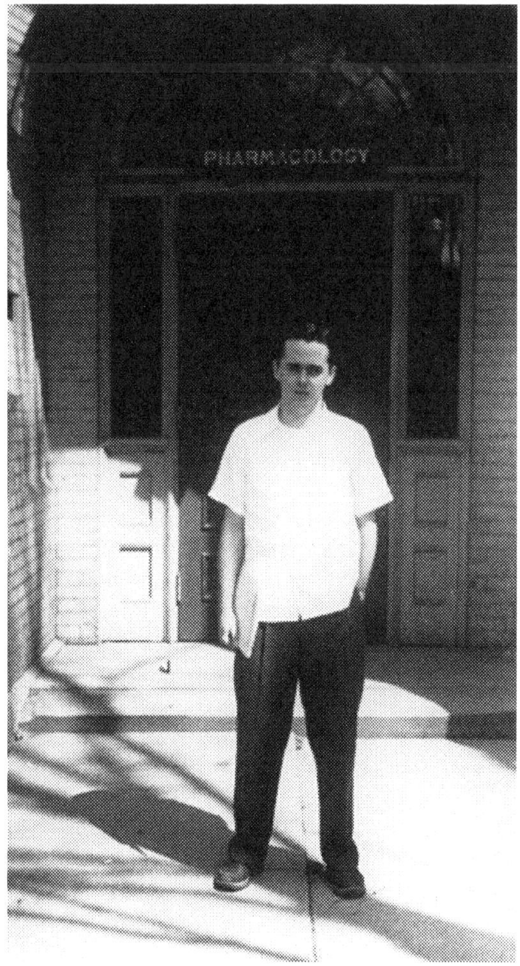

A young Harry in front of the old building.

A new instructor, Edward J. Cafruny, who had received his Ph.D. training in the Pharmacology Department at Syracuse University, began at Michigan in 1957. His first publication while at Michigan contains P values. However, he did not list a reference to statistical methods in his bibliography (Cafruny 121:225, 1957). The next publication from Michigan published in JPET that contained P values was by Domino and Roy Hudson 127: 305, 1959. This paper did have a reference to statistical methods in the bibliography, however, it was different from the previous Snedecor references. For the first time we see a reference to the 5th edition, 1956.

There are two publications in 1961 from the Pharmacology Department at Michigan in which reference is made to P values. The first is by Cafruny and Palmer, JPET 131:250, 1961, which lists P values but does not have a reference to statistical methods listed in the bibliography. The second paper is by Baird and myself, JPET 132:382, 1961, which presents P values and a reference to the fourth edition of Statistical Methods.

The occasion of celebrating the 100th birthday of the Department of Pharmacology at the University of Michigan raised some questions about how good the Department was in relation to other departments of pharmacology while I was a student and faculty member in the Department (1950-1961). This period was characterized by several new developments that might have served as indices of excellence. The development and expansion of the National Institutes of Health extramural research programs could have been compared for departments of pharmacology. The introduction of new items of equipment that were developed during World War II and modified for use in biomedical research such as spectrophotometers, oscilloscopes, polygraphs, etc., were acquired during the period of 1950-1961, and many of the pharmacology laboratories were completely re-equipped during this period. I did not feel that a comparison of laboratory equipment would provide a suitable basis for ranking departments. I decided to look at the adoption of a method for analyzing data as a criterion of intellectual curiosity and advancing sophistication in biomedical science. All one needed was a slide rule and a calculator to carry out the statistical analysis needed to determine a P value (the slide rule was used to determine square root).

The unexpected revelation observed in the above study was that three graduate students and three junior faculty were responsible for the introduction of biostatistical methods in the evaluation of their data. What we saw was a case of new blood bringing new ideas to an older established faculty.

If we go back to the 1950 edition of JPET and list the institutions that were employing statistical methods and calculating P values, we find six medical schools, four pharmaceutical companies, and two federal government laboratories. Only 14% of the papers published in JPET in 1950 contained P values and bibliographic references to statistical methodology. In 1960 eight out of 64 papers from Michigan's Department of Pharmacology that were published in JPET cited P values and bibliographic references (about 13%). The routine use of statistical methods developed very slowly at Michigan and required the sustained efforts of several faculty working together simultaneously to bring about the general acceptance of the new technology.

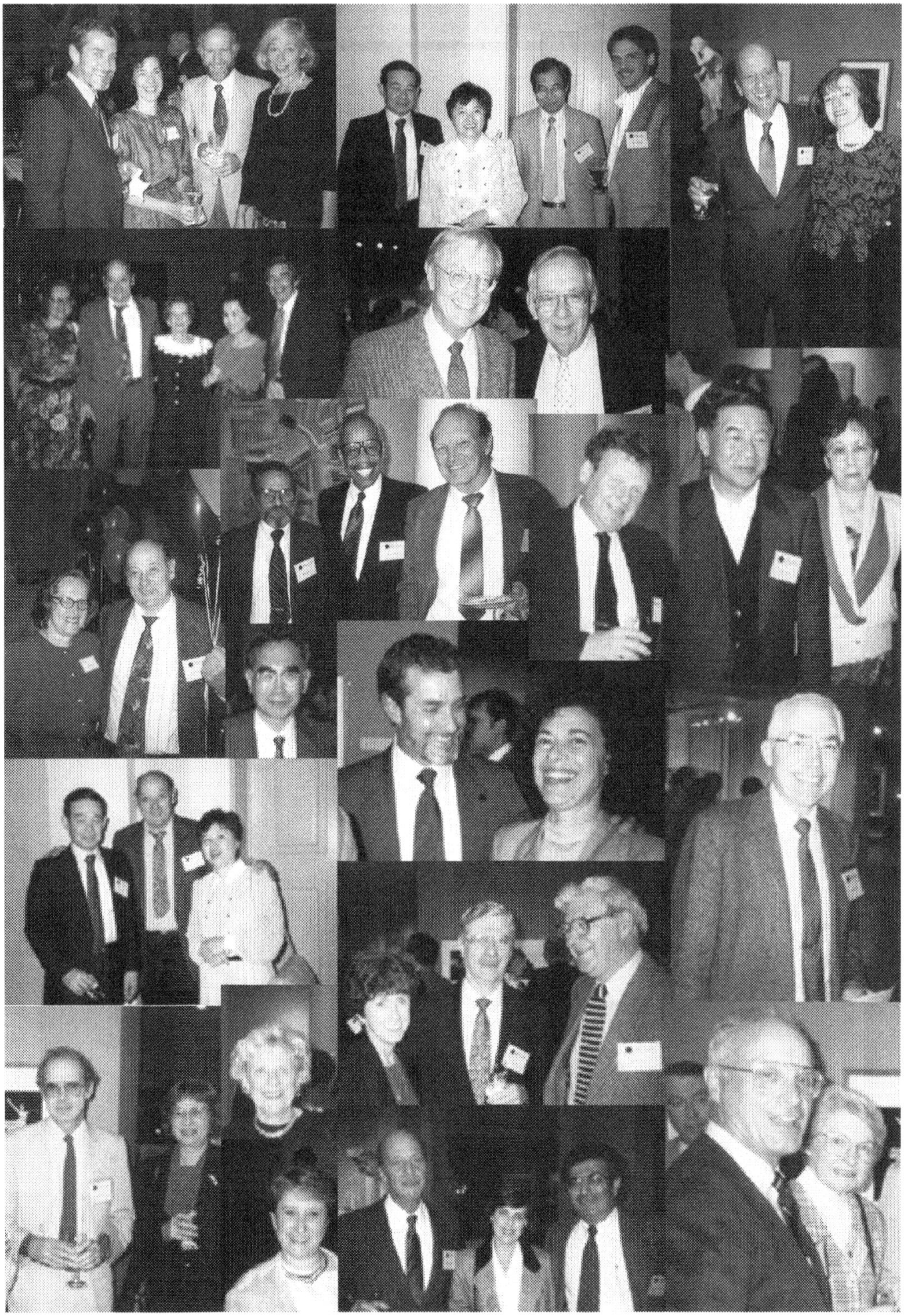

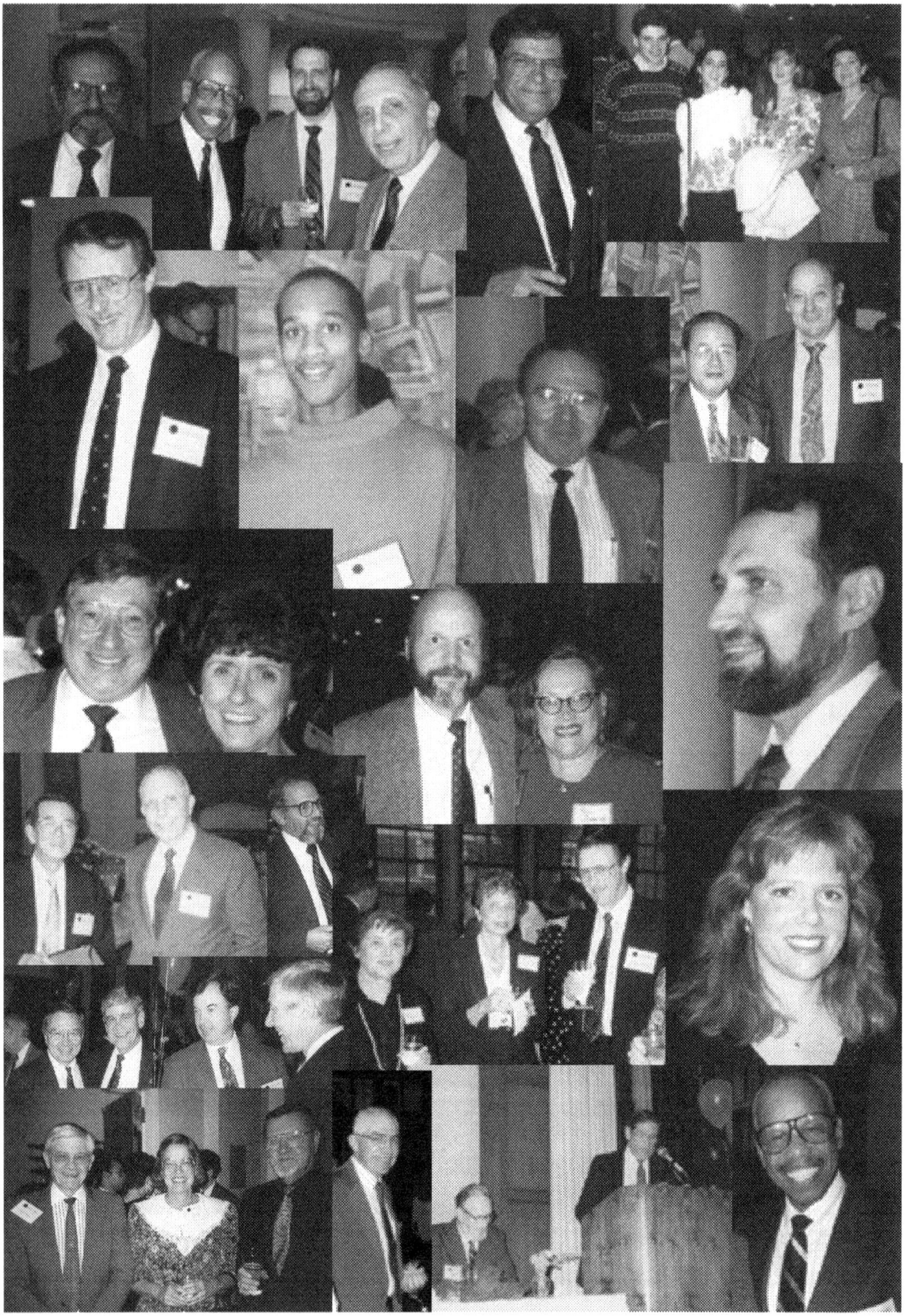

14

Training and Research in the Pharmacology of Drug Abuse and Dependence

Gail Winger, Ph.D., and James H. Woods, Ph.D.

The primary objective of this chapter is to describe, in terms of people and time, the longstanding and continuing emphasis on research on drug abuse and drug dependence in the Department of Pharmacology, with particular focus on developments since our arrival in the Department in the mid-1960s. But first a little, even more ancient, history. Departmental involvement in drug abuse studies dates from the chairmanship of Dr. Charles W. Edmunds, who was appointed to the expanded membership of the "Temporary Advisory Committee on Drug Addiction" in June, 1929. This Committee was constituted by the National Research Council of the National Academy of Sciences (NRC-NAS) to identify or carry out critical research on drug abuse, with funds provided by the Bureau of Social Hygiene in New York City. The Committee had several research concerns, but the one that has most influenced studies at the University of Michigan was the possibility that all "addicting alkaloids" could be replaced by substitutes having no problems of abuse potential. This possibility set the tone of much of the opioid abuse research that was carried out over the next several decades once the laboratory became involved in "screening" large numbers of opioid compounds for their dependence potential in the quest to identify an abuse-free opioid analgesic.

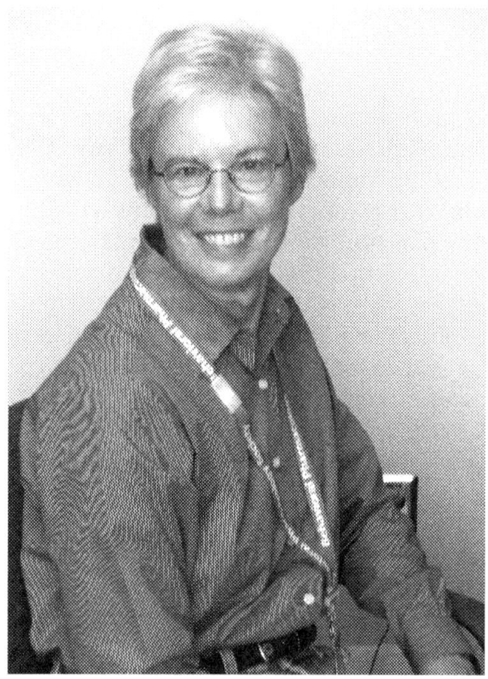

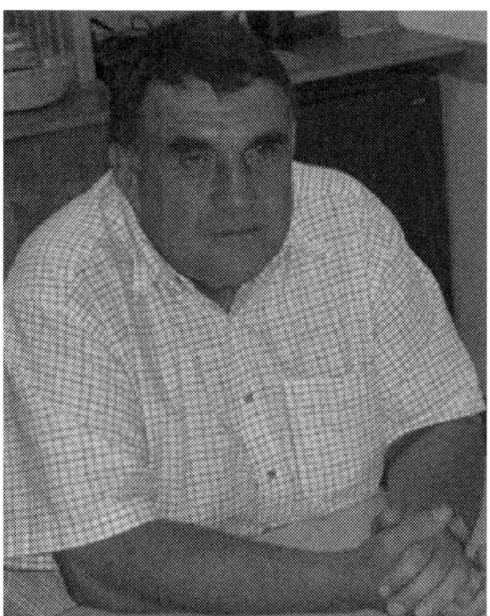

Dr. Edmunds hired Dr. Nathan B. Eddy to conduct research on drugs of abuse at the

University, and Dr. Eddy began a series of studies comparing the effects of morphine and codeine in laboratory rats. In addition, the effects of a variety of novel opioid compounds, particularly those synthesized specifically as possible abuse-free analgesics, were evaluated in the laboratory as well as in prisoner addicts in facilities at the Public Health Hospital at Lexington, Kentucky.

The aim of identifying an analgesic drug that had little abuse liability appeared within reach in 1939 because some drugs had been synthesized by then that appeared to move closer to this goal. However, much of the activity of the Committee was halted at this time, due to loss of funding and to the diversions produced by the Second World War. Following the war, however, and in part as a result of the war effort in Germany, where several opioid drugs, including meperidine and methadone had been synthesized, a new committee was constituted to continue to evaluate the abuse liability of synthetic opioid drugs and search for a non-addicting opioid compound. This committee, established in 1947, was called the Committee on Drug Addiction and Narcotics (CDAN), and Dr. Eddy was the principal pharmacologist and medical officer. Another member of this committee was Dr. Maurice Seevers, the Chairman of Pharmacology at the University of Michigan.

Dr. Seevers had become Chairman of Pharmacology at the University of Michigan in 1942. He brought with him from the University of Chicago via the University of Wisconsin an emphasis on research into drug abuse liability assessment and the use of rhesus monkeys as experimental subjects in this research. Dr. Seevers first proposed to CDAN in 1948 that monkeys be used for preliminary evaluation of the dependence potential of synthetic opioids that were being made in academic and industrial laboratories through out the United States and abroad. He recognized that monkeys had responses to drugs of abuse that were manifestly similar to those observed in humans, particularly signs of cocaine and opioid intoxication and opioid withdrawal. This focus persists to the current time; use of rhesus monkeys to evaluate various behavioral and pharmacological aspects of drugs of abuse is one of the most noteworthy attributes of drug abuse research at the University of Michigan.

When we came to the department (JHW as a research assistant in 1965 and GW as a graduate student in psychology in 1966), Dr. Seevers was chairman of a large, dynamic department. The faculty was interested in classical subjects in the field of pharmacology: drug metabolism, cardiovascular pharmacology, central and sympathetic nervous system pharmacology, and drug dependence. There was lively, casual, and supportive intellectual camaraderie among faculty members. Groups of faculty would attend each other's lectures to medical students, and then go together for coffee afterwards and critique the recent presentation.

Apart from the leadership that Professor Seevers provided for the Department as a whole, his own primary research interest was the laboratory on opioid dependence assessment located on the third level of Medical Science Building I and headed by Gerald Deneau. A great deal of the research done in this laboratory continued to focus on obtaining information that could be used to identify opioid analgesics that were devoid of abuse potential. As stated by Dr. Seevers in his acceptance of the first Nathan B. Eddy award by the Committee on Problems on Drug Dependence (CPDD, the name given to the CDAN in 1965) in 1976, "The concept was gradually formulated that opiate dependence could be virtually eliminated if a potent, non-addicting analgesic of the morphine-type were to be found."

In these early stages of the development of a science of drug abuse, physiological dependence on drugs of abuse, particularly opioid drugs, was thought to reflect the most dangerous aspect of these drugs. The withdrawal signs that occurred when physiologically dependent monkeys were deprived of opioids were easily observed and measured and thus could be used to screen large numbers of compounds. Through this monitoring, it would be possible to identify compounds that lacked the "addictive" or dependence-inducing potential

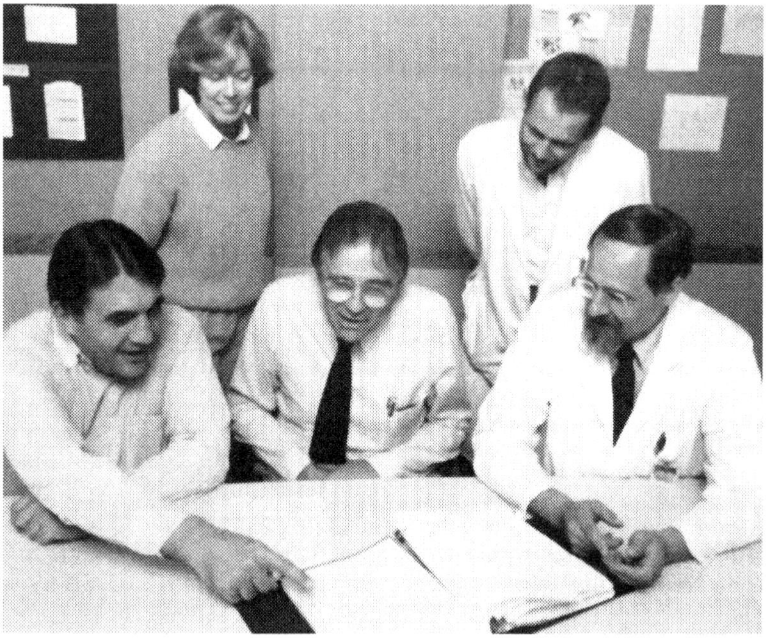

In the foreground Jim Woods, Fedor Medzihradsky, C.B. Smith with Gail Winger and Charles France in back, ca. 1987.

of morphine and might therefore be the hoped-for non-addictive analgesic. In Dr. Deneau's laboratory, groups of rhesus monkeys were given injections of morphine every six hours throughout the day. The dose of morphine was sufficient (3 mg/kg four times per day) to produce profound opioid physiological dependence. Part of the research effort involved giving these monkeys a test drug rather than their usual morphine injection and observing the effects. Drugs that acted through the same mechanism as morphine would prevent morphine withdrawal signs from developing, whereas drugs that blocked the effects of morphine would produce morphine withdrawal signs. Among the more interesting compounds were those that were then termed "mixed agonist-antagonists." These drugs precipitated withdrawal in the morphine-dependent monkeys, but produced sedation and perhaps morphine-like dependence themselves when given chronically to monkeys with no history of morphine administration.

On the second level of "Med Sci I," Dr. Seevers encouraged Dr. Tomoji Yanagita to establish a rhesus monkey self-administration laboratory. There is an interesting side light to this founding of this laboratory by Dr. Yanagita, who went on to become a preminent scholar and researcher in drug self-administration in monkeys in Kawasaki, Japan. Having come to the Pharmacology Department as a Japanese scholar in 1960, he was searching for research topics that he might pursue during his time here. He went into Dr. Seevers' office and suggested a line of research, perhaps an acetylcholine project. Dr. Seevers' response was noticeably lukewarm. Perhaps a cardiovascular project, then. Again a supportive but less than enthusiastic reply. Dr. Yanagita tried a few other ideas which were met with a similar response. Then, almost in desperation, he mentioned the possibility that he could work with Dr. Deneau in the monkey dependence colony. This time Seevers responded with an enthusiastic "That's a very good idea, Tomoji," and a new drug dependence researcher was born. It is a tribute to Dr. Seevers' judge of character that he encouraged Dr. Yanagita in this line of work. Although Dr. Yanagita worked first with an oral self-administration model in monkeys, his superb technical and intellectual skills allowed him soon to set up a laboratory in which minimally restrained monkeys could demonstrate the reinforcing effects of drugs by making responses that initiated an injection through a chronically indwelling intravenous catheter. This laboratory was the first of its kind, has been emulated in a number of other settings, and continues to produce uniquely relevant data on drugs of abuse to this day, in its original setting.

Adjacent to the self-administration laboratory, another behavioral laboratory was established for the most recent addition to the faculty, C. R. Schuster, a psychologist who had also been studying narcotic self-administration in rhesus monkeys at the University of Maryland. Dr. Uriel Estrada was briefly in charge of the original self-administration laboratory after Dr. Yanagita resumed his research in Japan, and Dr. Seevers turned this laboratory over to Dr. Schuster as well after Dr. Estrada returned to Mexico. It was there in the behavioral and self-administration laboratories, with Dr. Schuster, that we began our initial work on drugs as reinforcers in the late 1960s.

There was, at the time— the infamous 60s with its hippy counterculture, war protesters, and wide spread use of marijuana and other drugs of abuse — a very strong public interest in drug abuse, and this was reflected in the activities within the research community in the Department and throughout the country. Students were interested in learning more about drug abuse, and Dr. Domino had just obtained a training grant from NIMH to fund graduate training in psychopharmacology. Graduate students could obtain a Ph.D. in Pharmacology and an M.S. in Psychology, or a Ph.D. in Psychology and an M.S. in Pharmacology. Among those that took the former route were Steve Goldberg and Marvin Wilson who took their degrees with Dr. Schuster, while Maxine Stitzer and Gail Winger took their higher degrees in Psychology, mentored by Dr. Woods. Dr. Goldberg was interested in the profound behavioral changes that resulted when opioid antagonists were given to monkeys following chronic administration of opioid agonists. He found that some of these effects could be classically conditioned to light signals with resulting changes in heart rate, respiration, temperature, and food- and opioid- maintained responding. Dr. Wilson investigated in rhesus monkeys the ability of a number of compounds to modify behavior maintained by intravenous cocaine, finding some interesting interactions using dopamine antagonists as well as cholinergic antagonists. Dr. Stitzer evaluated the effects of psychoactive drugs on punished behavior in pigeons, and went on to work with Dr. Domino in the Pharmacology Department where she worked on the behavioral effects of nicotine in rats, and later the effects of psychoactive drugs in human volunteers. Dr. Winger's thesis was related to the ability of intravenous ethanol to maintain behavior in rhesus monkeys, a finding first reported by Drs. Deneau, Yanagita, and Seevers in 1965. In 1968, Dr. Fumio Ikomi, the 27th Seevers Japanese-Michigan Fellow, and soon thereafter, Dr. Andrew Karoly, on sabbatical from Humbolt University in California, joined Dr. Winger in further research on ethanol.

A young Mexican physician, Jullian Villarreal, took over from Dr. Deneau the scientific and administrative guidance of what was known as the dependence colony in 1966. Dr. Villarreal had come to Michigan as a graduate student in Pharmacology, mentored first by Dr. Domino, and then by Dr. Seevers. His thesis on the behavioral effects of mixed agonist-antagonist opiate drugs was extremely appropriate given the focus this laboratory was taking at this time. Dr. Steven Holtzman was a graduate student with Dr. Villarreal, completing his thesis work titled "Body Temperature and Operant Behavior as Baselines for the Evolution of Morphine-like Physical Dependence Capacity" in 1969. The 19th Japanese fellow, Dr. Sakutaro Tadokoro also worked with Dr. Villarreal from 1965-1967 and was involved in some very interesting studies on the effects of drugs on social aggression in rhesus monkeys.

When Dr. Schuster left Michigan for the University of Chicago in 1969, Dr. Seevers gave Jim Woods the responsibility for the self-administration laboratory and the behavior laboratory on the second floor of Med Sci I. Dr. Villarreal remained in charge of the dependence laboratory on the floor above at that time and this was the general situation when Dr. Seevers retired in 1971. Under Dr. Woods' influence, and that of his first postdoctoral student, David Downs, the second floor laboratories took an even more behavioral approach to drug abuse. The effects of different schedules of drug delivery were evaluated in monkeys in self-administration research projects. Pharmacology graduate student John Carney and Psychology graduate student Seymore Herling were both involved in projects in which the effects of various psychoactive drugs on behavior maintained by opioids or cocaine were compared with the effects of these drugs on behavior maintained by food. Carol Iglauer received her Ph.D. in Psychology based on her work on the relative reinforcing effects of different doses of cocaine. Rita Valentino was a Pharmacology graduate student shared by Dr. Woods and Dr. C.B. Smith, and she developed a project studying the discriminative stimulus effects of opioid antagonists in pigeons. Dr. Alice Young was a second postdoctoral student with Dr. Woods, and she was responsible for the general screening activities of the self-administration laboratory. She evaluated the reinforcing effects of ketamine and ketamine-like compounds in Macaca nemistrina, and also studied the ability of a number of mixed agonist-antagonists to maintain responding and to serve as discriminative stimuli.

The 1970s were a very productive period for opioid research in general. Additional sums of money were made available for basic research on drug abuse, thanks to President Nixon's initiative on drugs of abuse. The Department submitted a large grant, a Center of Excellence on opioid research with Acting Departmental Chairman Henry Swain as the principal investigator. Dr. Villarreal was responsible for the opioid dependence research, and Dr. Woods asked for support for his investigation of opioids as reinforcing stimuli. Dr. Charles B. Smith had the task of studying in vitro pharmacology of the opioid drugs, including measures of their effects in the principal smooth muscle preparation, the guinea pig ileum. Dr. Fedor Medzihradsky was involved in studying the molecular aspects of opioid action. This grant, which included a function of screening opioids for their abuse liability in each of these laboratories, was originally funded by the National Institute on Drug Abuse in 1972.

At that time, the source of drugs to be screened by the Center continued to be industrial and academic laboratories as it had been in the past, as well as governmental and other regulatory agencies. The CPDD continued to contribute some support for the drug evaluation activities of the members of the center. Their descriptions of the profiles of opioid activity of the synthetic opioids submitted by a variety of chemical laboratories continue to be used in the search for abuse-free analgesics. Although the vast majority of this effort was now financed by the NIH, the thread of financial support and the rope of administrative involvement continued to tie this research effort tightly to the CPDD, as it does today. The administrative mechanism was one in which chemical compounds that were thought to have opioid activity, typically synthesized in academic or industrial laboratories, were submitted to the CPDD where they were coded by the biological coordinator and sent to the various laboratories that were participating in the program. Dr. Eddy had been the first biological coordinator, followed in 1967 by Dr. Everett May at the Medical College of Virginia, and then in 1976, by Dr. Arthur Jacobson at the NIH (Arthur first shows up on the CPDD membership in 1975). The current biological coordinator, appointed in 2000, is Dr. Andrew Coop. Data on the activity of the coded compounds are returned to the biological coordinator, who then provides them to the submitting organization. These organizations have agreed that the chemical structure of their drugs, as well as our findings on their biological activity can be released within three years of their submission.

In addition to determining whether various opioid drugs might have potential as non-addictive analgesics, the Michigan laboratories are also able to screen drugs for their potential as drugs of abuse. This information was of considerable interest to regulatory bodies such as the Food and Drug Administration and the World Health Organization, which are responsible for scheduling therapeutic drugs at the national and international levels respectively. This scheduling is designed to restrict the access of drugs that appear likely to be diverted to illicit use, and data from animal models, particularly models of the reinforcing effects of drugs, are particularly relevant. When the CPDD was originally constituted, it was part of the NAS-NRC, which was then responsible for making the decisions as to whether particular compounds were likely to be abused. This arrangement ensured that laboratory data from Michigan and other venues was included in the decision-making process. Two changes developed that reduced the direct flow of information from the laboratories to the decision-making committees. One was the Controlled Substances Act of 1970 that established the Food and Drug Administration as the body that was responsible for making decisions about the categorization and scheduling drugs with therapeutic usefulness but potential for abuse. The other was the separation of the CPDD and the NAS-NRC. Although the Controlled Substances Act of 1970 still vests the National Institute of Drug Abuse with the task of supplying data relevant to the scheduling of drugs, and our laboratory receives some authority for supplying these data through its funding by the NIDA and its connection with CPDD, the contribution of laboratory animal data to the decision as to whether a particular drug should be restricted through the scheduling process has become frighteningly small in recent years.

Opioid research made some gigantic leaps during the 1970s, which necessarily impacted the research at Michigan. In 1973, Dr. William Martin published a paper in which the existence of multiple opioid receptors was postulated. Although his sigma receptor was eventually discounted as a true opioid receptor, the mu opioid receptor, the substrate for the actions of morphine and morphine-like opioids, and the kappa opioid receptor, the substrate for a number of opioid drugs including ethylketocyclazocine, and ketocyclazocine, have retained and gained significance as two of the three classes of opioid receptors. In 1974, the mu opioid receptor was identified biochemically using a new procedure, a binding assay, in the laboratory of Dr. Solomon Snyder and co-workers at Johns Hopkins University. In 1975, endogenous opioids were discovered in brain tissue by Dr. Hans Kosterlitz and colleagues at Aberdeen University in Scotland. The identification of a second type of opioid receptor, the kappa opioid receptor, has had particular impact on the behavioral research done in the Department, and interest in the effects of these types of agonists continues to the present time.

Dr. Winger returned to the laboratory in 1975 after a stint at the Downstate Medical Center in Brooklyn, NY and at the Johns Hopkins University in Baltimore. She continued her research on the reinforcing effects of ethanol and sedative hypnotics. She was assigned to space on the third level of Med Sci I, next to Dr. Villarreal's physical dependence laboratory. Dr. Villarreal returned to Mexico in 1972, and the dependence laboratory was placed under the supervision of Dr. Henry Swain.

The principal investigatorship of the opioid center grant was given to Dr. Woods in 1979 when Dr. Bert La Du became Chairman of the Department and Dr. Swain stepped down from his role as acting chairman. Dr. Woods hired Dr. Jon Katz in 1979 to take over responsibility for the physical dependence laboratory, and moved Dr. Winger into a supervisory role in the self-administration laboratory when Dr. Young took a faculty position in Psychology at Wayne State University. Dr. Katz's tenure was followed by that of Dr. Debra Gmerek in 1981. Dr. Gmerek completed a series of studies on kappa agonists in monkeys, demonstrating that the physical dependence produced by these drugs was markedly different from that produced by drugs that act on mu opioid receptors. Kappa receptor agonists were of particular interest as potential solutions to the long-standing issue question of development of abuse-free analgesics. Kappa receptor agonists produced an analgesic response through activation of opioid receptors (the analgesia was blocked by the opioid antagonist, naloxone) , but they did not produce dependence of the morphine type, as demonstrated clearly by Dr. Gmerek. Unfortunately, the hope for these drugs as clinical analgesics was dashed by the finding that the dysphoric responses in humans to a mixed agonist-antagonist, nalorphine, was due to the agonist effects of nalorphine on kappa receptors. Rhesus monkeys reported no positive reinforcing effects of kappa opioids, and, although aversive effects of these agents were difficult to establish in the monkey, they seemed clearly present in the few clinical situations where they were examined.

While Dr. Gmerek was administering the dependence laboratory under Dr. Woods' supervision, a decision was made to begin to dismantle this laboratory as it was originally designed. One reason was the concern raised about the frequent wounding of monkeys that were housed together in this facility. Another was that a similar dependence colony existed at the Medical College of Virginia under the auspices of Dr. Louis Harris, and there did not seem to be sufficient demand for the screening of novel opioids for their dependence liability to warrant the expense of maintaining two large laboratories for this purpose. A third reason was the growing realization that physical dependence, although an important sequala to chronic opioid administration, was less important to the development and maintenance of drug abuse than were the reinforcing effects of these drugs. There was therefore a shift in emphasis from physiological dependence to studies of these drugs as reinforcers and to experimental investigation of their primary clincial indication, analgesia, and their most dangerous effect, respiratory depression.

The physical dependence laboratory was replaced by cages of individually housed monkeys, and much of the work began to involve the more clinically relevant studies on the analgesic effects of opioid drugs. This work on analgesia in rhesus monkeys was initiated by Dr. Linda Dykstra when she took a sabbatical leave at the University of Michigan in 1986 to work with Dr. Woods. To this research effort was added studies on the respiratory depressant effects of opioid drugs.

To replace the research on physiological dependence, a psychology graduate student, Charles France, developed a protocol in which pigeons reported the discriminative stimulus effects of opioid withdrawal. This was accomplished by daily administration of a single dose of morphine, and teaching the animals to report the subsequent administration of the opioid analgesic, naloxone. Dr. France spent a postdoctoral year at Harvard University and then returned to the Pharmacology Department to continue to develop and refine this sophisticated approach to testing for physiological dependence development to opioid drugs and apply it to monkeys.

There was then a rather complete set of behavioral tools for the evaluation of novel drugs as they were sent to the Department by the CPDD. A given drug could be evaluated for its reinforcing effects, its ability to produce analgesia, its potency in suppressing respiration, and its ability to produce or reverse morphine withdrawal. In addition, it could be tested for binding to the opioid receptor, for its effects on the guinea pig illeum and on the rat vas deferens in studies of in vitro pharmacology.

The opioid research supported by the center grant was supplemented by grant support into the activities of phencyclidine and other NMDA agonists during much of the 1970s. Dr. Wouter Koek arrived from the Netherlands to provide a great deal of assistance with these studies. Although the hopes of identifying an antagonist of phencyclidine were dimmed to darkness by the finding that this hallucinogenic drug acted by blocking the ion channel that underlies the effects of the excitatory neurotransmitter glutamate, there was still plenty of interesting research done in the laboratory to characterize the effects of this compound and others drugs that blocked this channel. Along with several other projects, Dr. Koek evaluated the behavioral effects of a series of glutamate antagonists in monkeys, and found that they had much in common, suggesting that these behavioral effects were due to similar biochemical mechanisms, including blockade of NMDA. Dr. Ying Lu, then a graduate student in Pharmacology, studied the effects of glycine site antagonists on NMDA-induced convulsions in mice. Dr. Cory Campbell, who earned a Ph.D. in Pharmacology and then an M.D. at Case Western Reserve University, evaluated the effects of some of these drugs on learning and memory in pigeons. These hallucinogens, which are abused by some groups of people, have clear reinforcing effects when delivered intravenously to rhesus monkeys, and this effect was studied as a number of NMDA antagonists in the self-administration laboratory. Those with rapid onsets of action, such as ketamine and PCP, served well as reinforcers, whereas those with slow onsets of action such as dizocilpine and the competitive antagonist, CGS 19755, did not maintain high rates of responding.

During the late 1970s and early 1980s, one of the opioid research emphases of the center grant continued to be on more thorough characterization of kappa agonists and comparing their effects with those of mu agonists in the various preparations. Their dependence and withdrawal profiles were shown to be quite different from those of mu agonists as described earlier; they produced discriminative stimulus effects that did not overlap with those produced by mu agonists; they did not reduce respiration rates; and they had no reinforcing effects. Kappa agonists did, however, produce analgesia, but the pA2 that resulted when this analgesia was blocked by quadazocine, indicated that kappa analgesia was through a different receptor mechanism than that produced by mu agonists. A graduate student in Psychology, Albert Bertalmio, was instrumental in applying the concepts of pA2 analysis to in vivo data, particularly that obtained in self-administration and drug discrimination studies. Some detractors feel that it is inappropriate to apply pA2 analysis to behavioral data, but Dr. Bertalmio was among those who showed that the assumptions of in vitro analysis appear to be well met when opioids are used in these analyses. Dr. Bertalmio's enthusiasm for opioid pharmacology was sufficiently strong that he continues to monitor the progress of the laboratory, although he has another job in Ann Arbor.

Dr. Eduardo Butelman, who received his Ph.D. degree in Psychology from the University of London, joined the laboratory as a postdoctoral fellow in 1990, along with Dr. Paul Skjoldager, from Dr. Fowler's laboratory at the University of Mississippi. Dr. Skjoldager assisted Dr. Winger in the self-administration laboratory, evaluating and comparing the reinforcing effects of opioids, cocaine, and NMDA antagonists. Dr. Butelman developed an interest in the ongoing studies of kappa opioid agonists and their effects relative to mu opioid agonists. Joining in the study of opioid drugs was Ellen Walker, a psychology Ph.D. student who made some critical observations of the analgesic agonist and antagonist effects of the partial mu agonist, buprenorphine. William Essman was a Psychology graduate student in the laboratory during this time as well. Bill attempted to identify the behavioral effects of sigma agonists so that it would be possible to determine whether a drug was producing its effects through the sigma receptor. The conclusion was that no characteristic effect of sigma agonists could be easily identified.

When Dr. France left the laboratory in 1991 to take a position at Louisiana State University, Dr. Steve Negus, trained by Dr. Dykstra at North Carolina and by Dr. George Koob at the Salk Institute in San Diego, joined the laboratory. Dr. Negus continued the research effort in kappa agonist effects, and also branched out into the behavioral effects of delta opioid agonists. Sandra Comer, a graduate student in psychology, studied the convulsive effects of delta agonists in mice, and the behavioral effects of delta agonists in pigeons. Dr. Comer, following a post-doctoral term with Dr. Marilyn Carroll at the University of Minnesota, took a research position with Dr. Marian Fischman at Columbia University, where she is evaluating critical aspects of drug abuse in humans. The research that started when Dr. France was

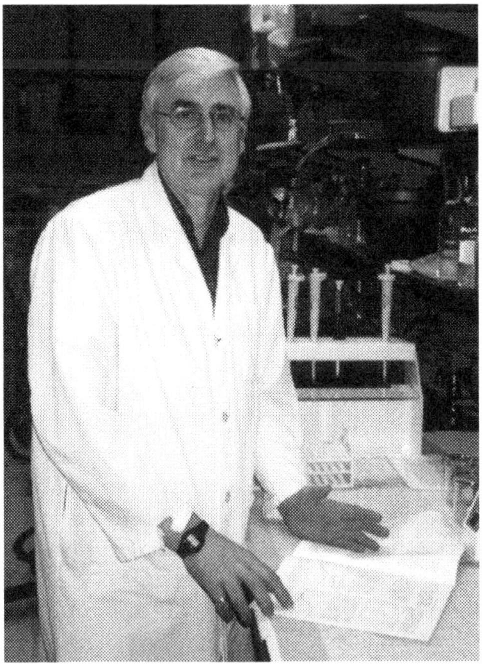

Dr. John Traynor replaced Dr. C.B. Smith on the opioid project in 1995.

in the laboratory, on how efficacy at each of the opioid receptor can be accurately translated into distinct behavioral effects, continued.

The aims of the center grant also expanded to include the development of drugs that could be evaluated for their therapeutic potential for the treatment of opioid abuse. This was encouraged when John Lewis, then of Reckitt-Coleman, and later of Bristol University, joined the research team in the mid 1990s as a member of the Center grant. Dr. Lewis had developed buprenorphine as a partial mu opioid agonist analgesic for Reckitt-Coleman during the late 1970s, and was aware of the potential usefulness of this drug in the treatment of opioid abusers. Buprenorphine, as a partial agonist, did not produce dangerous respiratory depression, and had reduced reinforcing effects compared with mu agonists with greater efficacy such as heroin and morphine. Its agonist effects were also followed by prolonged antagonist effects that could effectively block the reinforcing effects of opioid drugs in drug abusers. Buprenorphine is currently used for the treatment of opioid abuse, and Dr. Lewis was interested in synthesizing other drugs that might mimic and improve on the interesting pharmacological profile presented by buprenorphine. In addition, the availability of Dr. Lewis's chemical skills allowed the center grant to consider the synthesis and evaluation of more selective antagonists at each of the opioid receptors, and irreversible antagonists at the opioid receptors. Among the most exciting results of Dr. Lewis' chemical synthesis program are MCCAM, a mu partial agonist with long lasting mu antagonist effects, and CCAM and MCAM, both pseudo- irreversible, mu-selective antagonists.

Dr. John Traynor replaced Dr. C.B. Smith on the opioid center project in 1995. Dr. Traynor also brought molecular skills to add to those of Dr. Medzihradsky who retired from the Department in 1999. Dr. Traynor's interest in inverse opioid agonists has focused on the delta opioid receptor, where these agonists appear most easily recognized. He directly supervised the thesis of Dr. Andrew Alt, who obtained his degree in Pharmacology, completed postgraduate work with Dr. Mike Vasko in Indianapolis.

Delta opioid agonists continue to provide interesting therapeutic leads in the laboratory. Daniel Broom and Emily Jutkiewicz, both predoctoral students in pharmacology, evaluated potential uses of delta agonists in behavioral disorders such as depression and schizophrenia. Their promising results have encouraged Mary Torregrossa, a graduate student in neuroscience, to evaluate delta-opioid induced changes in brain derived neurotropic factor, an endogenous substance that has been shown to be increased by administration of therapeutically active antidepressant drugs.

When Dr. Negus moved to Harvard University in 1993, Dr. Butelman took his place as the person in charge of the analgesia, respiratory depression, and discrimination studies in monkeys. Dr. Carol Paronis, a postdoctoral student of Dr. Steve Holtzman at Emory University, and Dr. Shiroh Kishioka, the Seevers Fellow, were both active participants in this program, particularly as it related to evaluation of the respiratory depressant effects of opioids. They found that, whereas marked tolerance developed to the analgesic effects of mu opioid agonists, there is no tolerance to the respiratory depressant effects of these drugs. In addition, dependence, as indicated by naltrexone-induced stimulation of respiration, developed within two to three days of morphine administration.

Dr. Gerald Zernig, an Austrian physician with an interest in drugs of abuse, came to Ann Arbor in 1993 to participate in the research here. Dr. Zernig was most helpful in working out mathematical characterizations of the ability of irreversible opioid antagonists such as CCAM to eliminate mu opioid receptors and alter the efficacy of opioid agonists. He worked with data obtained from studies of analgesia and self-administration to characterize the relationship between efficacy and effect in behavioral experiments. This research focus continues at present, supervised primarily by Dr. Mei-Chuan Ko, a Taiwanese postdoctoral student, who obtained his Ph.D. in psychology in this laboratory in 1998. Dr. Ko was particularly interested in identifying sub-types of kappa opioid receptors using selective antagonists in studies of analgesia and respiratory depression. He has added an interest in the effects of intrathecal morphine, an analgesic preparation given frequently to women during child birth that has itching as an important side-effect.

A decision was made to approach the abuse liability of stimulant and depressant drugs in much the same fashion as was being done with opioid drugs. Rather than limit the profiling of these drugs to investigators at the University of Michigan, however, individuals from other institutions were encouraged to participate in this endeavor. The original group consisted of Drs. Woods and Winger, looking at the reinforcing effects of drugs in these classifications, Dr. Graham Patrick at the Medical College of Virginia, who studied physical dependence development to pentobarbital in rats, and the ability of test compounds to substitute for pentobarbital in this model, Dr. William Woolverton, first at the University of Chicago and then at the University of Mississippi, who evaluated the ability of drugs to produce an interoceptive stimulus like that of either amphetamine or pentobarbital in rhesus monkeys, and Dr. Charles France, at LSU and then at the University of Texas at San Antonio, who developed a physical dependence model for benzodiazepines that was much like the model for opioids that he had established earlier at Michigan. Initial financial support for this group effort was obtained through NIDA through a grant with Dr. Theodore Cicero as P.I. Although NIDA has continued to provide the funds that maintain this research, it has been through grants to the individual investigators rather than funds for the group as a whole.

Although the evaluation of novel opioid drugs for their activity in the various preparations in the laboratory continues to be an important focus of the work done in the laboratory at the present time, and a source of interesting new compounds for research and potential therapeutics, the basic research aspects of the laboratory effort maintains most of the enthusiasm of the investigators. There has been a tempering of the earlier anticipation that a novel opioid analgesic will soon be forthcoming that will replace the more traditional compounds as an effective analgesic with reduce capacity for abuse. Basic research has shown that the same receptor that mediates analgesia also mediates the reinforcing and dependence-producing effects of morphine-like agonists, making it less likely that these functions can be separated pharmacologically. This realization was probably clear to pharmaceutical companies sooner than it was obvious to academic researchers, because there is virtually no pharmaceutical push for the development of "better" opioid analgesics at the present time. Morphine continues to be among the most satisfactory and widely-used analgesics for moderate to severe pain.

In concert with this de-emphasis on the search for an abuse-free analgesic has come the realization that people who use opioids for pain relief are at relatively low risk of altering their patterns of use to patterns of abuse of these drugs. Abuse of most psychoactive drugs occurs in individuals who, perhaps for a combination of genetic and environmental reasons, are vulnerable to this behavior. This vulnerability, for reasons that are not entirely clear, does not present itself in animal models of intravenous drug self-administration, but our laboratory, with the assistance first of postdoctoral student Eric Pakarinen from Dr. Joe Moerschbaecher's laboratory at LSU and then Jeffery Vivian from Dr. Klaus Miczek's laboratory at Tufts University, attempted to model patterns of individual differences in the tendency to abuse drugs by studying abuse of orally available drugs, particularly ethanol. This research indicated to us, at least, that orally available ethanol may be quite a different reinforcer than intravenously available ethanol. Whether that difference is qualitative or quantitative is a question currently being raised by psychology predoctoral student Graham Flory.

The research on oral ethanol consumption led naturally to evaluation of the effects of opioid antagonists in the treatment of overconsumption of alcohol, and this has proved to be a fruitful area of research. Keith Williams earned his Ph.D. in psychology in 1998 by studying the ability of naltrexone and other opioid antagonists to decrease oral ethanol consumption in rhesus monkeys, and he remained in the laboratory as a postdoctoral fellow, continuing his interest in opioid antagonists, until taking a position at Grand Valley State University.

Studies in the self-administration laboratory have had several foci. One is the evaluation of the relative reinforcing effects of drugs of abuse, including opioids, stimulants, and NMDA antagonists, using a behavioral economic approach. Dr. Chad Galuska joined the laboratory as a postdoctoral student in 2003 from a strong behavioral training at West Virginia University. He is providing valuable support in the complex behavioral studies in monkeys. Another is the evaluation of the reinforcing effects of hallucinogens such as (-) and (+) MDMA. William Fantigrossi, as a predoctoral student in Psychology, studied the reinforcing effects of the isomers of MDMA, finding both isomers to support self-administration. The data currently suggest that one isomer is maintaining behavior through an action at the serotonin site, which is a novel mechanism for reinforcing effects.

Evaluation of potential pharmacotherapeutic approaches to the treatment of cocaine abuse has been another important aspect of the laboratory. Dr. Shaomeng Wang in the Department of Internal Medicine is a chemist who is interested in synthesizing selective dopamine antagonists as potential treatments for cocaine abuse. Pharmacology graduate student Greg Collins is undertaking the task of evaluating Dr. Wang's compounds using cocaine-stimulated locomotor activity in rodents.

We became very interested in another approach to treatment of cocaine abuse and overdose, when we heard in 1993 of the successful synthesis of a cocaine catalytic antibody by Dr. Donald Landry at Columbia University. We contacted Dr. Landry and worked out a collaboration in which we evaluate the ability of his antibodies, which both bind to and break down cocaine before it can reach the brain in pharmacologically active amounts, to modify the behavioral effects of cocaine. Although the goal is to evaluate the most effective of these antibodies in rhesus monkeys that are self-administering cocaine, the antigenic effect of the antibodies in the monkey preclude this approach until the antibodies have been modified to reduce this effect. It was recognized that a rodent self-administration laboratory was the best way to evaluate these compounds, and the question of how best to set up a rodent self-administration laboratory was answered by the arrival of Dr. Richard Briscoe as a postdoctoral student from Dr. David Gauvin's laboratory at the University of Oklahoma. Dr. Briscoe provided us with the techniques for rat self-administration studies as well as those for blood pressure assays in unanesthetized rats and mice. These procedures have proven to be extremely useful for studying the interaction between the catalytic antibody and cocaine, as well as between cocaine and another potential treatment for cocaine abuse and overdose, butyrylcholinesterase.

Dr. Ted Baird, also a postdoctoral student from Dr. Gauvin's laboratory, ably carried on these studies after Dr. Briscoe's departure, generating data that suggested that both of these protein-based approaches to cocaine toxicity may have promise. Dr. Felipe Gomez is currently working on the rat self-administration paradigm and has found that a genetically modified version of butyrylcholinesterase is able to reduce the potency of cocaine as a reinforcer in these rats. Ziva Cooper, a graduate student in psychology, hopes to use the rat self-administration procedure to understand more about the effects of stress on the reinforcing effects of opioid drugs.

Yet another self-administration focus involves studies of the relation between cocaine self-administration and release of ACTH and cortisol in the monkeys. The availability of intravenous catheters for drug administration has proven extremely useful for non-stressful blood withdrawal studies, so that the influence of cocaine self-administration as well as the effects of passive cocaine administration on the HPA axis can be evaluated. This research effort was made by Jillian Broadbear in her psychology Ph.D. She found that, whereas cocaine does increase the activity of the HPA axis as indicated by dose-related increases in ACTH and cortisol in the monkeys, these increases occur as well when cocaine is passively infused. Furthermore, blocking ACTH and cortisol increases at a number of different levels prevents cocaine from boosting these levels, but does not alter the ability of cocaine to maintain self-administration behavior. Dr. Broadbear also remained as a postdoctoral fellow, continuing to evaluate the relation between stimulant self-administration and HPA axis activity, until she returned to her native Australia.

Our increased interest in the HPA axis, combined with our long-term interest in opioid abuse and dependence attracted the attention of Hani Houshyar, who obtained her Ph.D. in Pharmacology in 2000. Her thesis involved observations of the effects of development of morphine dependence and withdrawal in rats on the HPA axis and temperature. Although originally based on the work of Dr. Steve Holtzman in Dr. Villarreal's laboratory years earlier, Dr. Houshyar found that the temperature effects of combined opioid withdrawal and stress were quite different in the rat than Dr. Holtzman had found in the monkey. Morphine dependence in the rat also produced profound alterations in the HPA axis that may serve as a model for other disruptions in the HPA axis as well as form the beginning of a better understanding of the stress effects of drug abuse. Dr. Houshyar is continuing this line of investigation under the mentorship of Dr. Mary Dallman at the University of California at San Francisco. Susan Wood, a graduate student in pharmacology has undertaken some of the studies of stress and the effects of CRH antagonists on stress in a rat model.

The working of the laboratory would be impossible without the assistance of an able technical staff over the years, and the long-term assistance of Dr. Woods' secretary, Rebecca McLaughlin. Ms. Tiffany Bass, as our animal manager, has kept us minding our P's and Q's and SOP's for the past several years.

While this brings the effort of the behavioral pharmacology laboratory up to the present time, we feel that the past continues to impose a strong framework to the science that we do. The laboratory continues to be strongly influenced by Dr. Seevers and his position that science should impact policy, and that scientists should participate in policy making and regulatory activities. In addition, as a physician, Dr. Seevers was strongly interested in patient care and what is now termed "harm reduction." We continue to be very involved in the identification of clinical therapeutics, be they drugs that can be used in the treatment of drug abuse, or opioids or other psychoactive drugs that may have been overlooked as potentially useful therapeutic agents.

15

Life at Michigan During the Seevers Era, 1944 and Beyond

Lauren A. Woods, M.D., Ph.D.

I am providing background and describing life experiences that molded my personality as I moved through life. They determined my work ethic, honesty and interaction with other personalities. Thus was developed my ability to accept responsibility and perform effectively in teaching, research, and administration.

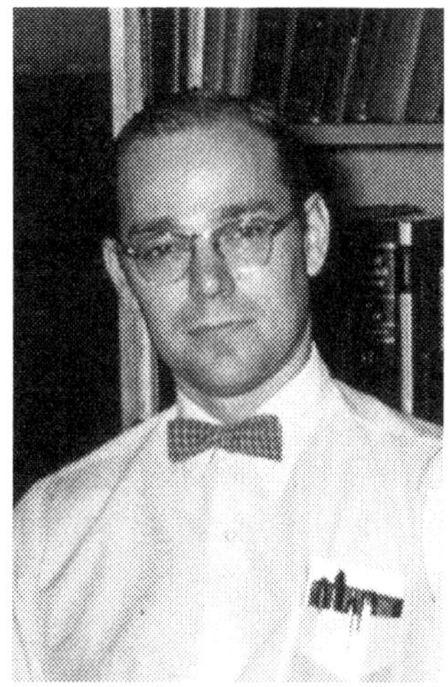

I was born September 10, 1919, and was raised on a farm 30 miles northwest of Mitchell, SD, and, out of necessity, at age 10 was driving a car, truck, tractor or team of horses pulling a plow or cultivator. When I was 11 my father was killed in an accident and as a result my brother (9 years older than I) tried to continue but there resulted a foreclosure on the farm and all the livestock and farm equipment was sold to pay off debt. At age 13 I recall vividly the shocking of wheat in 100°F (in the shade) weather, the bundles weighing more than I. Then in 2 years came the drought and dust storms of the early '30s, and poverty, an experience one never forgets. I was lucky to have a few pennies occasionally. That environment was certainly no better than that of the migrant workers of California, Oregon and Washington.

During 1934 my mother attended summer school at a teacher's college and then passed the examination for a state teaching certificate for elementary schools. In 1935 she paid $25, on the installment plan, for my tuition at Dakota Wesleyan University in Mitchell, SD. At age 15 I was the youngest male student. From that time on I earned all expenses for all of my education. For four years as one of two men working in a 140-bed hospital, I did every job but taking care of patients, and for them I provided a number of blood transfusions (for money) since I am O-negative. I swept the patient corridors every day and wet-mopped and waxed the floors every week, shoveled coal in the boiler, washed all windows in fall and spring, and installed storm windows in the fall and removed them in the spring. I shoveled snow from the sidewalks in the winter and did the landscaping in the summer.

Graduating with a B.S. degree in 1939 and a dual major in math-physics and chemistry, I wished to continue my education but needed enough income to exist. I applied to chemistry departments of a number of well known schools in the middle west and was admitted to all, but only the University of Detroit (a Jesuit institution; I was not Catholic) offered me $125 a month and free tuition. U of D only had two-year master's programs but this offered me an opportunity. And so to Detroit.

Entering the office of Father George J. Shiple, the chairman of Chemistry and a Ph.D. graduate in Biochemistry from Fordham Univ. (with Dr. Sherwin, a very well-known researcher), Father Shiple greeted me with a jovial handshake and said, "Guess what, Lauren, you will be teaching trigonometry to engineering freshmen next semester!" and handed me a copy of the text: my introduction to teaching. All of this with my regular courses. During the next 10 days before classes began, I worked every problem in the text. It turned out to be an enjoyable experience. There were about 54 students in the class; most if not all were older than I, working to complete degrees on a part-time program. They were employed in Chrysler, Ford, and General Motors Engineering Research and were very good students. The second semester was more relaxing.

In August of 1940, the Annual Meeting of the American Chemical Society was held in Detroit and grad students from U of D participated in handling registration, etc. I operated the cash register and helped with other matters. Some of the Chemistry faculty at U of D were very anxious to get students of their program accepted by Dr. Henry Gilman, a world-renowned organometallic chemist at Iowa State University in Ames, Iowa. U of D faculty introduced me to Dr. Gilman and somehow persuaded him to give me a fellowship; he wanted me to come immediately. And so with Father Shiple's blessing I was in Ames in about two days staying the first night in a rooming house with many of Dr. Gilman's students and listening to how I should try to outwit him. I promptly found another rooming house (with breakfast and dinner) which was a pleasant walk (except in winter and snow) to the Chemistry Building.

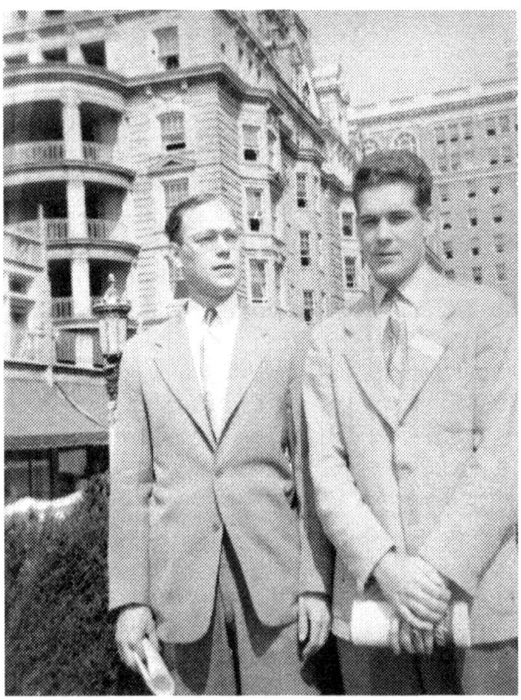

Lauren Woods and F. Gilbert McMahon in Atlantic City, ca. 1950.

Dr. Gilman had about 26 graduate students; how was he able to supervise them all? He was checking in the labs morning, afternoon and night, six days a week, as well as Sunday mornings. Many of the students would have done C, H, N and metal analyses on new compounds during the week and then on Saturday set up stirred reflux reactions and go out for the evening. Sunday morning they would have the analytic results for Dr. Gilman. One Saturday afternoon I showed Dr. Gilman a beautiful new crystalline compound (nothing pleases a chemist more than crystallizing a new compound never seen by man before) and he asked me if I would have the analysis the next morning. I said no because I had a date that night. He appreciated my honesty. After a year I was assigned an office laboratory next to his office. The rumor around the university campus was that I was Gilman's "fair-haired boy."

I received my Ph.D. degree in organic chemistry on July 14 (Bastille day), 1943. I had synthesized compounds containing antimony, lead, mercury, lithium, sodium, potassium, or gold and had performed many chemical reactivity studies on them. Then Dr. Gilman assigned me with three other chemists to work on a special National Defense Research Program associated with the Manhattan Project at Ames. Our task was to study a variety of chelating agents that would permit the volatilization of uranium thus permitting the separation

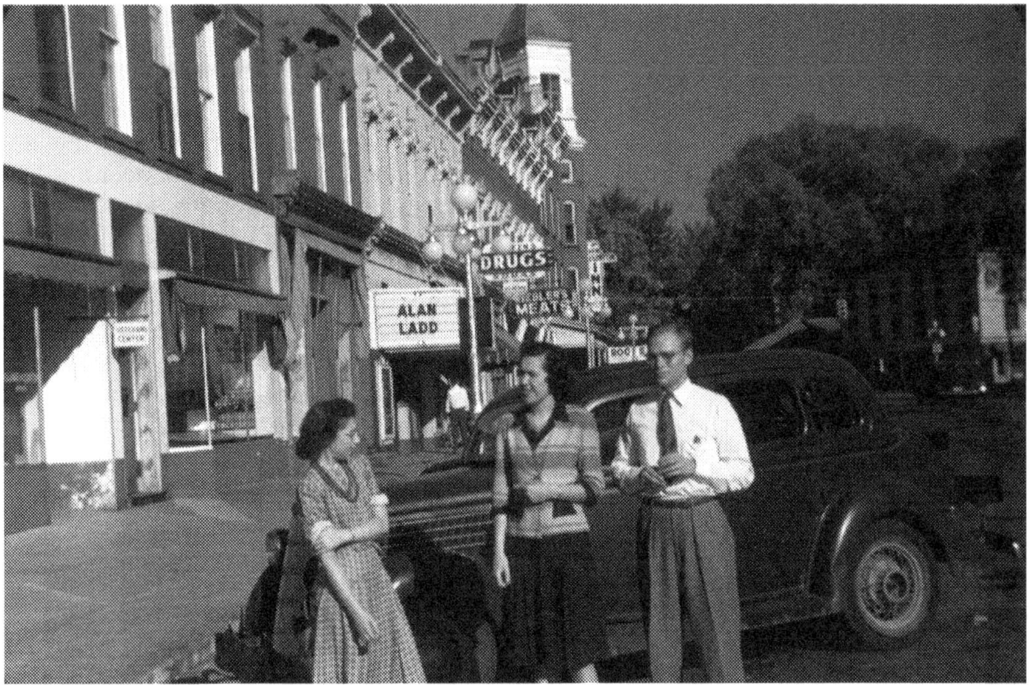

Carol and Lauren Woods stand with Mary Lou Page (far left) in front of their second-hand Ford in Ann Arbor, 1946.

of its isotopes.

The Manhattan Project at Iowa State University was headed by Dr. Frank Spedding, a professor of physical chemistry and thermodynamics (trained at the University of California-Berkeley) but the most important member of the team was Dr. Harley Wilhelm, a professor of chemical engineering and metallurgy who developed the technology to separate plutonium from uranium. The plutonium used for the atomic pile, which demonstrated the first sustained nuclear chain reaction, underneath the old football stadium at the University of Chicago, and the first atomic bomb at Alamogordo, NM, was purified by the Chemistry Department at Iowa State University. Incidentally, the Atomic Energy Commission built a magnificent Research Institute, with operating funds, for Iowa State in recognition of its great contribution to the atomic energy program.

The Chemistry Building had restricted access with armed guards at the entrance and required sign-in and sign-out. I had the first of probably half a dozen FBI clearances before beginning work. The security measures of the Manhattan Project at Iowa State were interesting. A number of technical employees had been imported from the east coast and among the group was circulation of the Daily Worker and common discussion of very liberal ideas, in my mind. Hindsight suggested that Stalin was informed of significant developments of the Ames project within days or weeks. In 1993, taking advantage of the end of the Cold War, the president of Random House negotiated access to sections of the KGB archives in the Soviet Union for a small group of scholars. Weinstein, an American historian, and Vassiliev, a former KGB agent, were among them and authored the "The Haunted Wood." This publication describes, from the early 1930s to the beginning of the Cold War, intensive and pervasive Soviet intelligence operations in the United States that reached up into the American government. The book implies that the Roosevelt and Truman Administrations were not vigilant enough, although the main focus of the book is on individual American spies for the Soviet Union. (This and companion publications are discussed in pp. B4-B6 of the June 25, 1999, issue of "The Chronicle of Higher Education").

One of the other chemists on the uranium chelation program was a close friend, Dennis Blume, from Dakota Wesleyan University (Mitchell, SD), who followed me to the University of Detroit and than to Iowa State. One afternoon in the winter of 1944 Dennis performed a reaction in a Carius tube, a three-foot long, thick-walled glass tube with a stricture at the end (for sealing with a torch) in a 250°C oven for several hours. After turning off the oven and allowing cooling, he unfortunately, without working behind an explosion shield, used a file to scratch the seal, allowing the breaking of the glass tip. The reaction mixture detonated and blew a hole in his abdomen, killing him instantly. A few weeks later another member of the four-man group had a lab explosion that left a splinter of glass in his eye and hand. I then asked Dr. Gilman if I could change to synthesizing anti-malarial drugs.

Following my change in research direction, I prepared a number of sulphide and sulfone amino quinoline derivatives that were submitted to the University of Michigan for testing of efficacy and toxicity in the School of Public Health and in the Department of Pharmacology. Several years earlier we had submitted gold compounds to the Rackham Arthritis Institute at the U of M (they were not useful). As a consequence of this experience I decided to seek training in biomedical research. I wrote to the deans of a number of medical schools with enclosures of my publication and academic records. Only Dean Furstenberg at the University of Michigan responded positively by informing me that he had sent my records to Dr. Maurice H. Seevers, the new Chairman of Pharmacology, who promptly invited me to visit Ann Arbor. So in late August 1944, I stopped off in Ann Arbor on the way to be married to Carol Ogle in Ithaca, NY, and then to attend the annual meeting of the American Chemical Society in New York City.

The visit to Ann Arbor was very positive. Dr. Seevers, like Henry Gilman, expected honesty and discipline and told me that when he was interviewing for the job at U of M he had asked President Ruthven what the limits were to developing the Department of Pharmacology and the answer was none. Dr. Seevers introduced me to the few departmental faculty and took me to the School of Public Health. And then I was on my way east.

When Carol and I returned to Ames, Iowa, in September 1944, a letter from Dr. Seevers was awaiting us offering me a position as Research Associate and Instructor but also insisting that I enter medical school. I promptly responded and we packed our meager belongings and arranged to move to Ann Arbor. Leaving my many friends in Ames, and especially Dr. Gilman, was difficult. He believed strongly in quality and integrity and I felt I had his trust and respect. He helped me in many ways. When my mother was dying in 1942, he loaned me the money to travel to Mitchell, SD, to see her in the hospital. Dr. Gilman had planned on my pursuing additional work with Louis Fieser at Harvard and he called Dr. Seevers to tell him he was ruining my career. Later Seevers told me that he informed Gilman, "Cut the crap. He can decide what he wants to do."

Carol and I took a cab from the train station to the Michigan Memorial Union and with our little baggage barreled through the front door to the registration desk with the "doorman" panting after us saying, "Ladies can't come through the front door!" I had arrived a week late for the beginning of medical classes, but Miss Vera Cummings, the Registrar in the Dean's Office, would not let me register until we had a definite address. She obviously disapproved of the situation, my being admitted only the week before without any MCAT tests. So we bought a paper to look for ads and found a room on Oakland Street, sharing a refrigerator and a bathroom. The room had a sofa to be made up at night for sleeping and a fireplace, which we found was an entryway for bats. One morning Carol screamed at me for putting a mouse in her overcoat pocket! It was a bat that had crawled in during the night.

So Miss Cummings let me register. Her attitude toward me softened after I had finished the first two years at the top of the class. For this accomplishment Dean Furstenberg awarded me a year's subscription to the Journal of Obstetrics and Gynecology; I suggested that someone else deserved it more.

After several weeks of catching up on the subjects of histology and gross anatomy, I began planning my lab on the first floor of the old Pharmacology building. Dr. Seevers, of course, financed all the equipment, supplies and remodeling from department funds. A hood and laboratory islands were installed and much glassware, centrifuges, etc., purchased. After about six months the lab was functioning.

During the winter of 1944-45 I recall giving lectures at night on chemistry to a few graduate students in pharmacology. My emphasis was on the importance of chemical structure on biological activity. Because of my experience at Iowa State University I also emphasized the immense power of fission energy and the potential of fusion energy. The lectures were also attended by rats (laboratory, wild and mixes) peering out of the holes high in the wall of the second floor lecture room. The holes were the result of the removal of steam, drain, etc., pipes during many past renovations.

During the 1944-45 period, after Sherwood Lawrence left, the individuals considered teaching and research faculty were Fred Shideman, Gordon Moe (a physiologist), Dr. Seevers and I. So there were the four of us until Maynard Chenoweth joined us about 1948 and Mark Nickerson in 1950. The early group exhibited an unusual "esprit de corps" under Dr. Seevers' leadership. Dr. Seevers expected quality, integrity and complete candor. I was privileged to be exposed to two such individuals.

Until VJ (Victory over Japan) day the Medical School was on an accelerated schedule, almost three semesters a year so it was not until late 1946 or early 1947 that I matriculated in the medical course in pharmacology. Also, during this time one of my classmates in pathology expressed an interest in research. I suggested to Jim Wyngaarden that he visit Seevers in Pharmacology and as a consequence Jim and I had several research projects together. One was the addiction liability of methadone in the Rhesus monkey. We were injecting the drug two times a day; about once a month on the weekend Jim went to Grand Rapids, MI, to court his wife, and I injected the animals. Jim and I also had intensive training from Gordon Moe on the dog heart-lung preparation. We all learned a great deal in Seevers' department, since he had a tremendous breadth of experience in studies on laboratory animals and human subjects.

During the time I was getting set up in my laboratory and progressing in medical school, Carol was looking for better living quarters and for jobs since she was too energetic to sit at home. She worked in sequence at the University Hospital, the main library (next to the Pharmacology building), and as a dietitian at the Michigan League. Then she read an article in the newspaper that there was a need for overflow housing for sorority girls

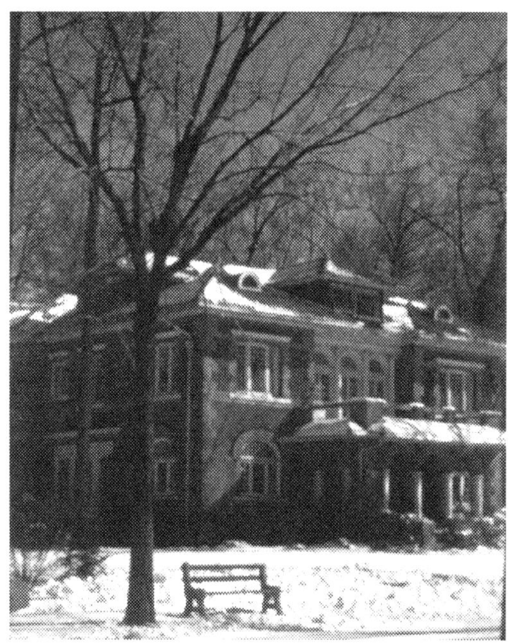

The Woods family rented this house at 1315 Hill. Now an empty lot, soon, an apartment complex.

enrolled in undergraduate programs at the University of Michigan. So she went to the Dean of Women to propose locating a house to rent and providing housing, breakfast, and dinner for the overflow students. The Dean's reaction was, "My dear, the girls are older than you are." However, the Dean gave Carol the name of Mrs. Maddy (the divorced wife of the professor who established the Interlocken Music Camp) who owned the building at 1315 Hill Street, which we promptly leased. It was an ideal setup housing 31 girls, and we had a separate apartment on the first floor. The basement had an apartment for a graduate couple (who monitored the closing hours at night), a room for two girls (who helped serve the meals) and the kitchen. All food was carried by a dumb waiter to the first floor and served at a table that could seat 50. Two male students earned their meals washing dishes, pots and pans. The living room had about a 50-foot ceiling and walk-in fireplace, the entryway for numerous bats.

Within 18 months we adopted our oldest son, Douglas. Carol flew to Provincetown, Prince Edward Island, to get him and I met them in Windsor, Ontario, to go through immigration. Little did we know that Carol was pregnant with David. So we had to change our housing plans, to finish out the lease on the house on Hill Street and to lease a smaller house at 1502 Cambridge Road. The girls at the latter address ate meals at the Hill Street location for about a year. Law and graduate students lived with us on Cambridge Road, many of whom we maintained contact with for many years.

By 1945-46 I was developing specific procedures for morphine and derivatives and later on for cocaine, mescaline and myanesin. Initially, Dr. Seevers paid for my technician, and of course for animals and supplies. We were working with mice, rats, occasionally rabbits, dogs, monkeys, and rarely humans, using UV or colorimetric procedures. About 1952 I isolated and purified crystalline morphine-3-glucuronide from dog bile and dog urine and later from monkey samples, the first time ever for this metabolite of morphine. Later on I sent samples of my pure product to Eddy Way and several others in the field. By the early 1950s I had my own research grants and was soon developing radioactive tracer procedures with ^{14}C and ^{3}H. Usually we synthesized our own derivatives and developed chromatographic techniques for separation of impurities and metabolites and establishment of the specificity of the procedures.

After the first semester of my junior year in medical school I took a leave of absence because I felt I should be doing more of the teaching. Dr. Seevers did not ask me to do this and I had a feeling he wanted me not to do it. But my guilty feelings supervened and I taught the pharmacy class that year. I enjoyed it but returned to the next year's medical class to finish. Later on I taught the nursing course in pharmacology after Fred Shideman left for Wisconsin. Ultimately I taught in and organized every course offered in pharmacology at Michigan.

By 1948 Dr. Seevers had been contacted by Don Irish, Director of the Division of Biochemistry at Dow Chemical Co., in Midland, MI, for a group of us in Pharmacology to give lectures on biochemical mechanisms, toxicity, metabolism and fate of chemicals, including much discussion. Chenoweth was on these early trips and as a result he moved to Dow Chemical later on. Dehydroacetic acid was at that time of great interest as a preservative for wine, there being a big market in California. Fred Shideman and I were intensively involved in the DHA studies. Some faculty and students participated in consumption of controlled amounts of wine, as well as ad lib, with analysis of blood levels and excretion of the additive. The work on DHA was published in some four or five papers in JPET. One early benefit of the Dow relationship was their donating supplies of chlordane to remove the cockroach population in the old building. During the 1950s Dr. Seevers and I continued consulting with Dow three or four times a year until I left Ann Arbor in 1960.

Being on the first floor of the Pharmacology Building had some advantages and some disadvantages. I was readily available to Dr.

Seevers but I was more aware than others as to what was going on in the building. His voice could be heard calling for various individuals. On one occasion Sam Irwin let a monkey loose in the hallway and someone let it get into Dr. Seevers' office then closed a door on it. The monkey circled the room, the windowsills, the bookshelves, and the desks, scattering papers, books and documents all over. Finally, the animal was corralled and I thought Sam was lucky to be awarded his Ph.D.

Because of my background in organic chemistry I was asked to serve on several thesis committees for Bob Elderfield, Professor of Chemistry, and Fritz Blicke, Professor of Pharmaceutical Chemistry. This experience always renewed my chemical knowledge and expanded my contacts in the University. Indeed, in the 1950s I hired in sequence two Ph.D. graduates of Bob Elderfield's program to develop some structure-activity studies as well as synthesize radioactive drugs.

About 1954 I was asked by the National Cancer Institute to initiate metabolism studies on several cancer chemotherapeutic agents and the result was a continuous program under my supervision until I left Iowa in 1970. Bruce Mellett continued the projects at Michigan. I was appointed to several committees of the American Cancer Society and also served on the NIH Cancer Chemotherapy Study Section of which I was chairman for several sessions. This exposure brought me into contact with about seven individuals who were Nobel Laureates at that time or would be so designated a few years later.

As I recall Joe Cochin was my first graduate student. He was from Detroit and I believe attended Wayne State University. Some graduate students were referred to me from the University of Detroit. Carol and I visited there occasionally and chatted with Father Shiple, who was a really wonderful person. I think Gil McMahon, Trieste Vitte, and Bruce Mellett came via this route. The last was Ray Ruddon who arrived about the time I was leaving for Iowa and finished his Ph. D. work with Bruce Mellett. Other students included Jane Haggart, Harvey Muehlenbeck, Sukru Kaymakcalan, M.D. (he received a M.S. degree), Don Blaney, Carl Hug, Jr., Sal Mulé, and Jane Heng (who was primarily with Ed Domino). There were also several medical students who worked with me during the summer. I might have missed others.

I must not neglect Anand Misra. About 1956 Seevers asked me if Anand would be welcomed in my lab since he was on an international fellowship. He had completed a doctorate in medicinal chemistry, I believe, in a university in Scotland. He was a gem. Later, for a variety of reasons, he joined me at Iowa.

Sukru and his wife, Sabahat (an M.D., pediatrician), returned to Turkey where Sukru became Chairman of Pharmacology at the University of Ankara Medical School and was a member of the WHO Committee on Drug Dependence. Their oldest son was born in Ann Arbor's St. Joseph Hospital. Their children were brilliant, the son attending MIT and the daughter the equivalent in top women's colleges. About 1977 Carol and I visited the Kaymakcalans in Istanbul, their home, and were royally entertained. The son accepted an engineering position with General Electric in mid-New York State and about 10 years ago took his father to Roswell Park and Sloan Kettering for treatment of a malignancy. This was not successful and Sukru died in this country. His son died a short time later, of what we never learned.

In the early 1950s we had a very productive faculty group. Most of us had our own research grants but Dr. Seevers attracted by far the bulk of funding in the department. He was involved in classified research for the armed services and I had access to special safes since I participated in some of the studies. Of course this required FBI clearance again. Dr. Seevers was very particular about the candor, quality and integrity of his faculty (and graduate students). This was the problem that Mark Nickerson had with Dr. Seevers. As I recall we had a "journal club" which met frequently, and "social" gatherings in the department. I remember Nick as being very liberal in nonscientific discussions, to the point of my feeling uncomfortable, perhaps because of my experience with the Manhattan Project at Iowa State University. One interesting episode occurred at one of the meetings. Chenoweth came into the meeting and mentioned that one of the faculty was noted for contributions to the advancement of science in a British Annual Review publication. Everyone thought it would be Nick since he had won the Abel Award, but Chen then said I was the one based on my work at Iowa State on trimethylgold. When Nick was scheduled to meet with the House Un-American Activities Committee, Carol and I invited Nick and the family to our home in Barton Hills, the first building phase of which had been completed. With all the publicity we felt sympathy for their son, Steve. Mark and the family also took us fishing. Dr. Seevers could not forgive the lack of candor of Nick in this whole episode. Nick's handling of this affair was ill-advised, either by himself or by others, since a forthright approach could have settled the matter very quickly. I learned very early that in dealing with other people the approach of "I know better than you or anyone else—" does not work. Over the years I was blessed by exposure to Father Shiple, Henry Gilman and Mose Seevers. It is shameful that the university has allowed the contributions of Seevers to the reputation of the medical school, the university, and the science of pharmacology and toxicology, to be besmirched by activities of recent years.

Dr. Seevers and I worked very closely together. In 1952 the Quaker Oats Co. brought a very serious toxicological problem to Seevers. The company had been preparing furfuryl alcohol in bulk amounts by catalytic reduction of furfural which was derived from oat grain. Quaker Oats sold the alcohol to an engineering firm which mixed the chemical with carbon, sulfuric acid and an accelerator and then troweled the product quickly as a liner of paper pulp digestors. The result was a resin lining which was resistant to caustic chemicals. All worked fine for many months but then several workers who were troweling the mixture died from severe acute pulmonary edema. With the help of Brownie Hendershot, I very quickly set up a crude exposure system with a three-foot high glass cylinder as a "generator" and large desiccators as exposure chambers for mice and rats. If commercial exposure chambers existed at that time we could not afford to wait to order them. Bill Sheldon who operated the shop in the building helped with the fabrication. He made a holder for about a dozen plates that could be quickly inserted into the large glass cylinder. We bought boxes of plates from the "dime" store on North University Street. Air flow was controlled with a flowmeter, the air entering the bottom of the cylinder and out the top into the desiccators (all was a closed system inside a hood). We tested all the starting materials (including by putting drops in rabbit eyes which is no longer permitted) and then made the resin using their recipe with materials that had been OK and then with materials which were causing toxicity. We identified with the help of the Quaker Oats Co. that a specific substance was the toxic agent and the company became aware that it had changed catalytic procedures in the reduction of furfural to furfuryl alcohol. The pulmonary intoxicant was 2-methyl, 2-3 dihydrofuran. This experience reinforced my awareness of the importance of toxicology and relationship of chemical structure to biological activity.

Dr. Seevers and I did studies on the effect of mescaline in former drug addicts at the Public Health Service Hospital, Lexington, KY, and included blood levels and excretion of the substance. This work was done with the help of Harris Isbell and others. Seevers and I also did some animal studies on marijuana products supported by the armed services and we visited Edgewood Arsenal in Maryland several times.

Seevers and I planned the Pharmacology space in Medical Sciences I, with input from other faculty, and we made some mistakes that I never repeated in subsequent planning. We did better in that building than Biochemistry did. Hal Christensen, the new chairman of biochemistry, perhaps with help of some faculty, had lab benches, islands, and wall cabinets, etc., built into all labs so when they began to move in floor centrifuges, refrigerators, etc., there was no room. The building budget had

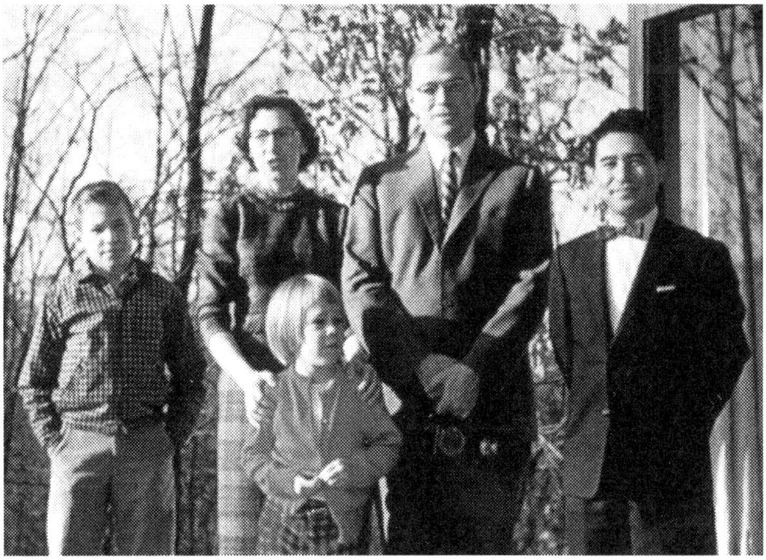

Woods and family with Dr. Showa Ueki, ca. 1960.

to provide $600,000 to rip out benches, etc. Incidentally, I was appointed chairman of the building committee for Medical Sciences Building II by Dean Hubbard, but left for Iowa before it got off the ground.

I progressed to full professor in 1957 and served on many of the usual committees. The most important committees on which I served were the ad hoc review committees for faculty promotions and new appointments. These review committees were appointed by Dean Furstenberg and reported to the Executive Committee of the Medical School. One committee I served on, which saved the University much trouble later on, collected information (mostly by phone) about the integrity, personality, etc., of the individual up for appointment and we recommended disapproval. The department chairman was furious but the appointment was denied.

Seevers' philosophy was always to train a successor and, since Fred Shideman had moved to Wisconsin following a plan to succeed Dr. Tatum, Seevers for one reason or another focused on me. As is obvious we did spend a great deal of time together and I am sure he expected me to succeed him. In addition, I had considerable support among the medical faculty and the new Dean of the Medical School, Dr. Hubbard. We had finished our home in Barton Hills and we intended to live there for the rest of our lives.

In the late fall of 1959 I received an inquiry from the search committee for pharmacology at the University of Iowa. I had looked at the chairs of several universities and a number of positions in drug companies, but I had perceived problems without real opportunities or challenges. Seevers did not think much of the set-up at Iowa but he did not discourage me from visiting. The committee at Iowa included both clinical and basic science chairmen and it was obvious that the basic science departments were considered second-class citizens by the dean.

Following my visit I wrote an approximately four-page letter to the chairman of the committee describing what needed to be done. Included was my plan to establish a toxicology program and a clinical pharmacology program, including internal medicine and anesthesia, and other departments as desired. Residents with two years of experience would enroll in a two-year master's program in pharmacology; they would take graduate courses and do research in pharmacology labs, the objective being to learn experimental design and laboratory techniques.

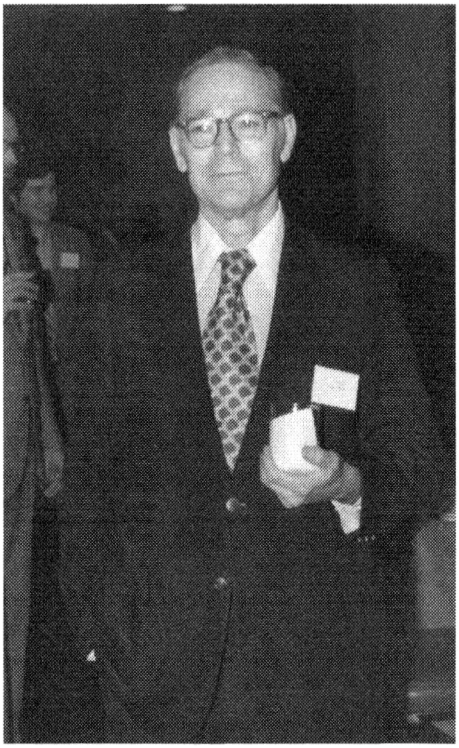

Lauren Woods, ca. 1977

I heard nothing for four weeks and then received a telephone call from the associate dean, Dr. Robert Hardin, then acting dean, inviting me to return for further discussions. The dean had had a heart attack, and I have always believed that my letter and discussions thereof contributed to the situation. Following detailed negotiations, including meeting with President Hatcher, I decided to accept the position. We hated to leave Ann Arbor and the adjustment for Carol and the children was very difficult. I looked upon the move as a great challenge and opportunity to apply many of the skills and ideas I had acquired from the several universities with which I had been associated. Also, the pharmacology program at Michigan was well established and I realized how fickle search committees could be.

After leaving Michigan I am sure that Dr. Seevers was responsible for my appointments to the Council on Drugs of the American Medical Association and related councils. In addition, he must have arranged for my joining the Expert Panel of the Flavoring Extracts Manufacturing Association with which I consulted for 38 years, resigning in the year 1997. The activities of this panel continuously utilized my experience in chemistry and toxicology.

As to what happened at Iowa. With the assistance of Fred Stone, Director of the Institute of General Medical Sciences at NIH, I established the first Toxicology Center in the United States. Ph.D. graduates of this toxicology program dominated the Toxicology Society for a number of years. In 10 years the Pharmacology Department moved from almost inactivity to one ranked by peer pharmacologists throughout the country (American Council on Education and reported in 1970 by US News and World Report) as second to none in the US (tied with Fred Shideman's Minnesota and Arnold Welch's Yale). Michigan was in the next lower level and Harvard not at all. When I was leaving Iowa for Richmond in 1970, President Sandy Boyd came to the pharmacology chairman's office to ask me to please stay at Iowa.

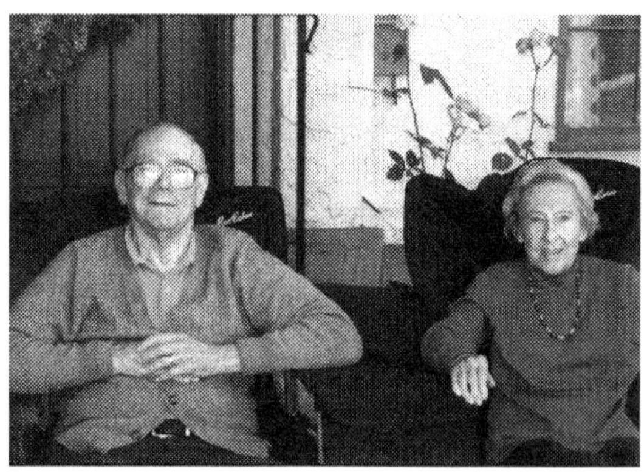

Woods and wife Carol, ca. 2003

Recollections, 1945-1949

John R. Lewis, Ph.D.

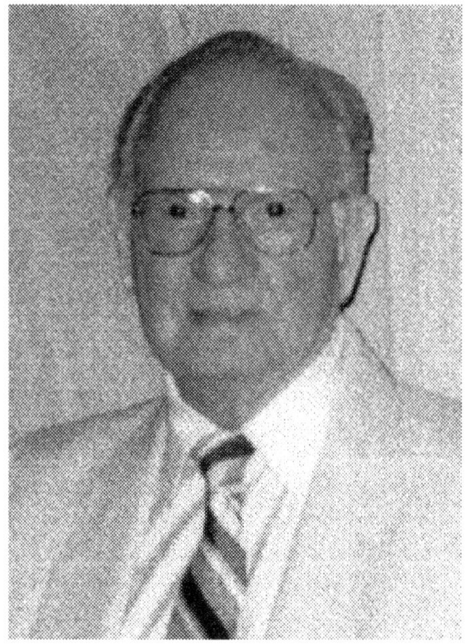

After receiving an M.S. degree in Biochemistry from Michigan State College in 1940, I was employed by Frederick Stearns & Co. in Detroit as Supervisor of Biological Control. Dr. Al Lands, who was director of pharmacology in the same laboratory encouraged me to study pharmacology. He arranged for me to take courses in the medical school of Wayne State University. The company allowed me to take time from my work to complete courses in physiology and pharmacology in the Medical School. After I completed these courses, Dr. Lands recommended that I be given a fellowship to work toward a doctoral degree in pharmacology. This was approved by Dr. Heibert, president of the company. Therefore, Dr. Sayhoun, Director of Biology, took me to the University of Michigan for an interview with Dr. Seevers. This interview was favorable and Dr. Seevers accepted me as a graduate student in his department. Accordingly, the company awarded me a two-year fellowship to work toward a doctorate. However, the terms of the fellowship stipulated that I would do screening of compounds supplied by Stearns for analgesic activity, and at the end of the two-year fellowship period I would continue to work for Stearns for an additional two years.

Thus, in the Fall of 1945, I enrolled as a graduate student in the Pharmacology Department of the University of Michigan. Dr. Seevers decided that I should take most of the courses a medical student would take except I did not take gross anatomy. However, my life as a graduate student was complicated since I was married and had two children. To further complicate the situation, I was unable to find a place to live in Ann Arbor because all available homes had been taken by students returning from military service at the end of the war in 1945. Since I had a home in Farmington about 30 miles east of Ann Arbor, I chose to keep it and commute to Ann Arbor. This distance, however, gave me a sense of isolation from the other students, except on those occasions when I decided to stay late on the campus to study or conduct some experiments. Other graduate students who joined the Department while I was there included Joseph Cochin, Walter Freyberger, Jim Weeks, and Barbara Rennick (there may have been others whose names I don't recall). Incidentally, I missed only one day, which was due to bad weather, during the two years I commuted. There were a few times when I was driving home late at night that I fell asleep and missed some of my turns, but fortunately I did not have an accident.

The arrangement of taking classes and doing some analgesic testing of the Stearns compounds worked fairly well so that at the end of my two-year fellowship period, I had completed all of the assigned class work, but I had done little work for my thesis. At this time, an unexpected event occurred: Frederick Stea-

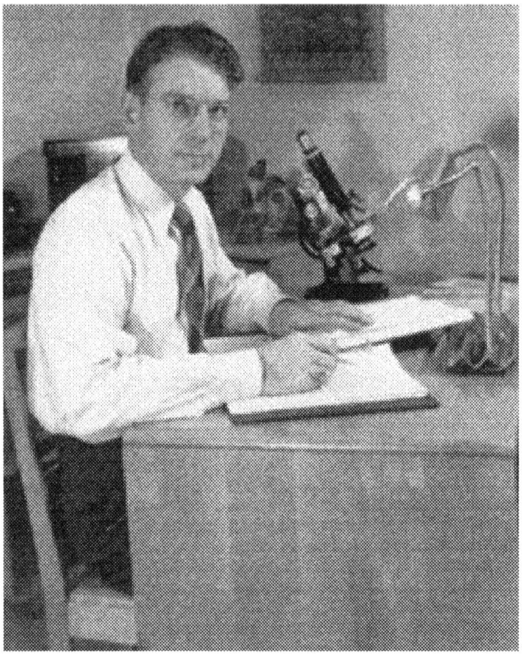

A young John Lewis as a student at U of M studying pathology, 1947.

rns & Co. was purchased by Winthrop Laboratories in Rensselaer, NY. These companies were merged into a new Sterling-Winthrop Research Institute in the fall of 1947 and the staff of Stearns was moved from Detroit to Rensselaer. This move necessitated a reevaluation of my status with regard to my fellowship and work on my degree. An agreement was worked out between Dr. Seevers and Dr. Tainter, the director of the newly formed Institute, whereby I was to join the Pharmacology Department of the Institute and be allowed to complete the work for my thesis at the Institute. At the same time, I would be working on projects for the Institute.

My principal assignment for my thesis was to work on the pharmacology of the analgesic, ketobemidone (1-Methyl-4-3-hydroxyphenyl-4-piperidyl ethyl ketone). I completed the laboratory studies and wrote my thesis under the guidance of Dr. Seevers, with whom I met several times during its preparation. The work for my thesis was divided into two sections: an analysis of algesimetric methods, and the pharmacology of ketobemidone. I was given my final exam by my graduate committee plus some other members of the Department and I was awarded a Ph.D. degree in February, 1949. The studies of analgesic methods were continued by others who followed me in the Department, namely, Sam Irwin and Ray Houde. The results of my studies on ketobemidone were the subject of several publications in pharmacology journals.

After several years of research in the pharmacology laboratories of the Institute, I was transferred to Administration where my principal work involved writing, which I enjoyed more than laboratory work. However, after several years I became unhappy with some of my assignments; so I decided to make a change. Thus, in 1960, I resigned from Sterling-Winthrop Research Institute and joined the American Medical Association as Assistant Director of the Department of Drugs and Assistant Secretary of the Council on Drugs. I also served as Acting Director of the Department for two years. Inasmuch as Dr. Seevers was a member of the Council on Drugs, this association provided me the opportunity to work with him again as my mentor. This relationship continued until the AMA reorganized the staff and Council. I remained in the Department of Drugs as Senior Scientist until I retired in 1980.

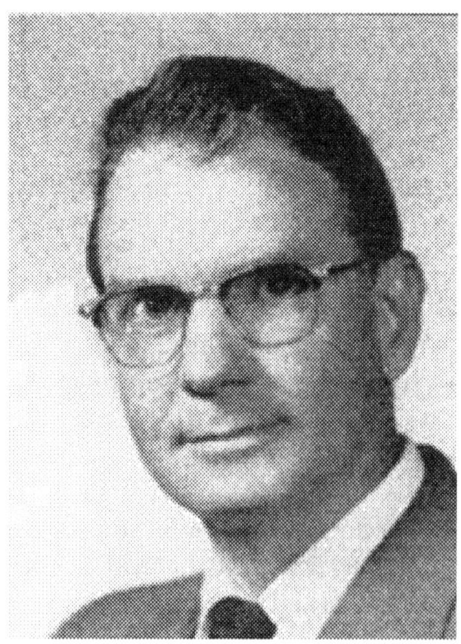

The Making of a Pharmacologist — From Childhood to Ph.D.

James R. Weeks, Ph.D.

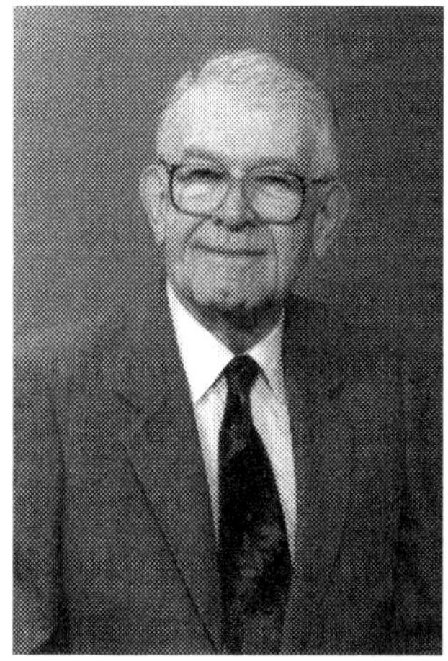

I was always interested in science, from astronomy to electricity. On completing high school, I still did not know what field of science to enter. My father owned a small "over-the-counter" drug company. He had studied pharmacy for one year of the then two-year program. His advice was to study pharmacy, even if I never planned to practice pharmacy. Pharmacy embraces several sciences, and thus could serve not only as an orientation but also give me another profession that might sometime be useful. At first I thought it would be biochemistry, then virology, which was then splitting off from bacteriology as a separate discipline.

The turning point was at the end of my sophomore year of college, when Dr. Harald Holck, who taught pharmacology, demonstrated the action of alcohol on rats to a class on public health. He showed that a small dose caused ataxia and a large dose, loss of consciousness. I was fascinated. The decision for pharmacology was clinched later that year when I observed an open-chest dog preparation with recording of auricular and ventricular activity and blood pressure. Remember, this was in the late 1930s — recording was on a smoked paper kymograph, using a mercury manometer with a float for blood pressure, and pulleys and levers for heart movements.

Pharmacology was taught in the junior year, and bioassay in the senior year. At the end of my junior year the George A. Breon Company offered a graduate fellowship in pharmacology. It would cover tuition, a small stipend, and support research on an extract of Convallaria majalis (Lily of the Valley) leaves. This plant contains the cardiac glycoside convallatoxin. They wanted a complete literature search, some studies on oral absorption, and relative potency to digitalis by four assay methods (frog lethality, pigeon emesis, intravenous cat, and isolated cat papillary muscle). But there were no qualified students available. Dr. Holck apparently thought that I had some promise, and he convinced the Breon research director to accept a senior instead of a graduate student. Since fellowships could not be granted to undergraduates, the stipend was payment for research by time ($0.35/hr). The following year I did get a fellowship.

The varied nature of the research gave me a lot of valuable experience. I soon discovered that much of the early literature on convallaria was in German. The plant was a folk remedy in eastern Europe, and comparative studies on cardiac glycosides, including convallaria, were generally from continental Europe. I had to learn German to complete the literature survey. In addition to the convallaria studies, I helped Dr. Holck with his research on sex difference and development of tolerance to barbiturates in rats. These were heroic experiments — rats were injected every 90 minutes with geometrically increasing doses until death (most normal females died after a few hours, but it sometimes took over two days for males). We did 60 rats at a time — one a minute for an hour and then 30 minutes to calculate doses, make up solutions, start new rats, eat, etc.

In preparing for and conducting research, Dr. Holck not only worked personally in the laboratory; he also explained how the experiments were organized and interpreted and the importance of controls, avoidance of bias in observations, and application of appropriate statistics. Dr. Holck was far ahead of his time in this last respect. In my work, he allowed me freedom to solve problems on my own, but at the same time was always ready with advice.

College undergraduates do not usually attend scientific meetings, but Dr. Holck made an exception for me. I attended both the 1941 (Chicago) and 1942 (Boston) Federation of American Societies for Experimental Biology (FASEB) meetings (these were small then; it was possible to say, "I'll see you at the mixer," and then be able to do it!) He thought, as Dr. Seevers did, that one needs to have faces to tie into names in books and journals. I was introduced to men famous at the time (Otto Loewi, Henrik Dam, Torald Sollmann, K. K. Chen, Harry Gold, McKeen Cattell) and others "likely to be" (Otto Krayer and John C. Krantz). One thing, regretfully, I did not fully appreciate at the time. At the 1942 Boston meeting, Dr. Holck arranged for me to share a hotel room with his Ph.D. mentor, Anton J. Carlson, Professor of Physiology at the University of Chicago. I was too young to realize the stature of the man who was my roommate. Alas, only a student of the history of physiology could appreciate this story.

I had an especially interesting experience at the 1941 Chicago FASEB meeting. The first edition of Goodman and Gilman's Pharmacological Basis of Therapeutics had just appeared. At the banquet chance seated me at the same table as the authors. They predicted (correctly so) that the response would be overwhelming. The publisher considered the number to be outrageous. A bet followed, with the prize being a case of Scotch. The prize had just been delivered to their room and they had been making sure that the quality met expectations. They were a bit boisterous and certainly feeling no pain!

Because my research was so varied, and being a co-author on one of Dr. Holck's barbiturate studies, my publications were rather short papers. By 1943, at the tender age of 23, I had five publications, one in the Journal of Pharmacology and Experimental Therapeutics. The first paper appeared in 1942. A call to active duty in World War II meant that the last four manuscripts were written while in the service. Writing my thesis was postponed until after the war. The diploma is dated 1945, but all work was completed in 1942.

I then went to the University of Michigan for my Ph.D. Because of my unusual research experiences at University of Nebraska and excellent training with Dr. Holck, in some ways I was picking up at Michigan where I left off at Nebraska. Course work was different and more demanding, but the physical surroundings were familiar. The central part of the Michigan building was the original chemistry building and the pharmacy college at Nebraska was the original chemistry building and of nearly the same vintage.

The first group of graduate students took biochemistry, physiology and pathology with medical students. To do this, we had to get permission from the head of each department. When I asked Dr. Weller for permission to take pathology, he was very concerned that I had not had gross anatomy. I had studied both comparative anatomy and physiology. He accepted me reluctantly with an admonition that I might have a problem in the laboratory (I got an "A"). Joe Cochin, an undergraduate chemistry major who had had neither anatomy nor physiology, had even more difficulty. Joe persevered, and grudgingly got permission with a strong warning that he was doing it at his own risk. Joe asked me "Who else — HIS?" It was hard, but he still made the required "B" for graduate credit. Dr. Weller hadn't considered Joe's brilliant mind.

Several of us gathered for brown bag

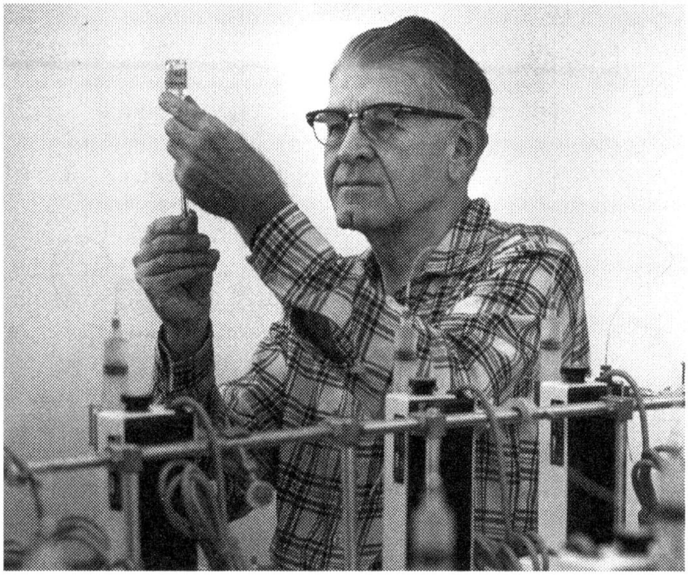

A young Dr. Weeks at work

lunches. There we would discuss our research and sometimes stories about our mentors. Dr. Gordon Moe worked with students in setting up experiments and gathering data. Isolated dog heart/lung preparations are exceedingly bloody things, leaving a lot of dirty equipment. At the end of the day, the experiment was done. Dr. Moe looked around, said, "I already know how to clean up," and went home.

Dr. Moe had a talent that I envied. One time we asked Dr. Moe if he would give a lecture or two on renal physiology some evening. He said he would on one condition: "I will not do any preparation." His lecture was a joy to hear — a perfectly organized, clear presentation of a difficult subject. If I didn't know better, I would have thought he had spent hours of preparation.

Dr. Chenoweth was my mentor. My first project was to record the spontaneous contractions of segments of rabbit intestine on a smoked paper kymograph. We were studying the effect of various substances on the magnitude of their contractions. Here I first encountered the "Whooopsss phenomenon." It takes many forms. All start out with a straightforward, simple experiment, but when one looks at the result, one exclaims, "Whooopsss, this can't be!!!" After confirming the observation, one moans in anguish, "What in hell is going on?"

This straight forward experiment was: set up the muscle, then after the size of the contractions are constant, draw off the bath fluid and replace it with fluid containing the test compound. We did a few experiments and results were as we had anticipated. Then a voice came to me from the past, "James, have you forgotten what I taught you — CONTROLS!!" I suggested that I try just draining the bath and replacing it with fresh saline medium. We were anxious to try more compounds so decided to continue on awhile and do the controls later. We did, but the voice came on stronger so I did a control anyway. Whoooopsss! The contractions were much smaller in the fresh saline, and 30 minutes later had regained only 75% of their initial value. Replacing the bath fluid with saline in which a piece of intestine had been soaking restored full activity immediately. Something had been released by the intestine, which stimulated its activity. To avoid the problem I merely drained the saline from the muscle bath, added test compound, and returned it to the bath. I spent a long weekend repeating everything I had done.

After that, nobody said anything when I

wanted to run blank controls. What about this stimulant coming out of the intestine? While I was doing this work, Walter Vogt had a paper in press in a German journal describing it and naming it Darmstoff. Many years later it was shown to be a prostaglandin. It is well that I did not try to isolate darmstoff. Prostaglandins are unstable and can stimulate isolated rabbit intestine at 10 ng/ml!

Chenoweth and Shideman had a small grant for comparing the effects of compounds on metabolic rate (oxygen consumption) of isolated muscle at rest and working. Strips of rat diaphragm had been used extensively in Warburg flasks and when stimulated electrically while recording strength of contractions, but never simultaneously. Resting and working metabolism could be very different. The grant was to devise a suitable instrument and to demonstrate its usefulness.

While working with the rabbit intestine I made such a device, but it needed refinement and in any case it was far too large to use with rat diaphragm strips. I had already been accused of having the questionable virtue of being a gadgeteer , and had acquired a modest skill in laboratory glass blowing. Dr. Chenoweth thought I would be a natural candidate to use this project as doctoral thesis research. I accepted. In principle, I did not think it would be too difficult. Warburg's method would be used to measure oxygen consumption. One would need a small gas-tight vessel with a means of introducing a muscle strip, stimulating electrodes, some sort of packing for a thread to a recorder, and some means of circulating the oxygen in the bath fluid to ensure oxygenation of the muscle strip and equilibrium with the gas phase. Accomplishing these things proved far more difficult than listing them.

One aspect was a little different for this project. There was nobody around who had had any experience with such a thing. I had encouragement and sympathy but concrete helpful advice was scarce. A couple of months were wasted showing that a roller-style pump described in the literature would not work. Early stages worked on straightforward mechanical problems. We would measure oxygen consumption during isometric twitches of stimulated muscle and contracture (sustained contraction without stimulation). Recording these actions posed no problem. For twitches we used crystal phonograph pickups and a penwriting galvanometer. Resting length changes were recorded on the smoked paper kymograph. How to get the mechanical activity out of the vessel was suggested by a clinical thermometer — a small chamber in glass tubing with capillary constrictions on each side to trap a droplet of mercury. I passed a human hair through the constrictions. Thelma Gould had two-foot long straight hair. I was accused of chasing her with scissors.

Someone, I think Starling in his original isolated heart-lung preparation, made a blood pump by squeezing rubber tubing mechanically to act as a piston and two one-way valves. My adaptation was two valves using ball bearings ground into thick-walled glass tubing and a short segment of gum rubber (hemocytometer) tubing between them. Pumping was hydraulic by a water-filled jacket around the rubber and pulsatile pressure applied. One hydraulic line served four vessels. The idea was derived from the hydraulic brake system on automobiles.

After making sure joints were air tight, all was ready to test the mechanics of the vessel. Oxygen circulated nicely. Whooopsss! Oxygen was still being lost from the vessel. It was diffusing through the rubber tubing. Chen's brother was a research polymer chemist who said that all elastomers would pass the minute amounts with which we were dealing. Before I started working with Chenoweth, I did some blood gas assays for Shideman using the Van Slyke method. Never mind the details, but the apparatus used a short length of very thick walled rubber tubing that would not pass minute amounts of gas. I had read Van Slyke's original publication. He used two sizes of rubber tubing, the space between the larger and smaller filled with mercury. Filling the jacket over my tubing with mercury solved the first "whooopsss."

Now came mounting and stimulating a

muscle strip. All instructions on the use of isolated tissue for metabolism studies emphasize the necessity of keeping prepared tissue cold (in an ice bath) until used. During rest, the oxygen consumption was what would have been expected. Whooopsss! The muscles didn't twitch when stimulated. Freshly cut strips lying in a dish contracted nicely. This problem was easy to solve. I found that they still respired normally if left at room temperature. I have no explanation of what is damaged by chilling, and have found nothing in the literature, although I did not do an exhaustive search.

A preliminary experiment showed that isometric twitches increased oxygen consumption. At this point I did the control — everything except the muscle. I presumed the electric current from the stimulus would lead to electrolysis and liberation of a small amount of oxygen and a correction of observed values. Whooopsss! The volume of gas in the vessel decreased. I repeated this several times. It was always there, but the magnitude varied unpredictably, precluding using a correction factor. Sometimes it was as much as half the increased oxygen consumption due to contraction. Everybody was perplexed. At this time, Dr. George Mangun, then at Henry Ford Hospital in Detroit, was studying tissue oxygen levels using the recently developed oxygen electrode. Chen thought it worthwhile to pay him a visit. At the end of the day, somewhat as a joke, I said, "You know everything about electrodes and oxygen uptake, what do you make of this weird thing I just encountered?" He thought a few moments, and said, "Could it possibly be formation of hydrogen peroxide from nascent oxygen on the platinum electrode?" On our return to Ann Arbor I visited a professor in the physical chemistry department. His assessment was that it was "thermodynamically possible but very unlikely to occur."

There were no other explanations, so I set about to test this one. First, how could I detect traces of hydrogen peroxide? From somewhere, I remembered that a forensic test for blood on clothing, etc., was the benzidine/peroxide test. An enzyme in blood catalyzed changing benzidine to a colored compound. So I turned it around and made one of the reagents fresh hemolyzed dog blood (1:100 in water). Hydrogen peroxide, in a concentration of 1:1,000,000 had a detectable color. I set up four vessels, containing a Krebs-Ringer phosphate solution, ran the stimulator in two of them, and then added the blood/benzidine reagent. I thought I saw color in the two with the stimulator, but did not trust my senses (I am red/green color blind). I called someone in the next lab to come in (he knew nothing of what I was doing), and asked if he saw any color in any of the four vessels. Without hesitation, he pointed out the two that had been "stimulated."

Now I knew what had happened, but what to do about it? One suggestion was adding sodium azide to neutralize the peroxide. No good, sodium azide was one of the compounds we were to test. Another was to platinize the electrode so it would possibly alter the surface so the peroxide formation would not occur. No good, oxygen was consumed even without stimulation — apparently the platinum black catalyzed oxidation of the glucose in the saline medium. My reasoning now was that the peroxide formation must have been a surface phenomenon, therefore would be reduced if surface area were reduced. I coated the platinum wire stimulating electrodes with polystyrene coil dope (used in electrical components) except at the very tip. No hydrogen peroxide formed and the volume in the vessel increased with stimulation. The last problem had now been solved.

I had started this project in the fall of 1948. About the fall of 1949, a decision had to be made whether to drop this project and select another thesis project. At the end of the summer of 1950 my GI bill benefits would terminate and I had accepted a position at Drake University. Chen and I agreed that if all problems had not been solved by December, we would find a new thesis project. December arrived and I was "virtually certain" all would be solved within about a month. It wasn't until April that I had all the solutions.

I hurriedly did enough experiments for

the thesis and a publication in the Journal of Pharmacology and Experimental Therapeutics. One significant discovery: it was known that muscles in contracture had increased oxygen consumption, therefore the contracture caused the increase. We showed that the increase occurred before the onset of contracture. As doctoral dissertations go, it was very slim. Committees and journal editors are not interested in the work done to get the data, only the results. The last two weeks or so were spent calculating many means and standard errors. I sat at the Friden calculator whenever it was not in use. (There were then no computers). The Friden could add, subtract, multiply and divide, but not print. One had to do all calculations twice, and even more if the answers did not agree.

During my stay at Michigan there was research in progress on addiction using monkeys. I frequently helped by catching and holding the monkeys for their injections. This kindled an interest in addiction. I mentioned earlier that I held rats for some of Dr. Holck's barbiturate research. This kindled an interest in tolerance. Tolerance and dependence are hallmarks of drug addiction.

When I joined The Upjohn Company about 10 years later, there was an unwritten policy that senior scientists could devote a nominal 10 percent of their time to "personal research," which need not be related to their assigned projects. Having an animal take its own drug seemed to be a good method for studying addiction. Upjohn then paid for parts, I built the apparatus at home, and used it on Upjohn rats. Mine was the first publication on intravenous self-administration of drugs by an animal. If history shows that this work was a lasting contribution to science, it will be my only one and it was only a scientific hobby.

I left the University of Michigan for Drake University at the end of the summer of 1950. I had a heavy teaching schedule, so I postponed writing my thesis until the summer of 1951. I could not finish the thesis and oral defense in time for the summer 1951 commencement, so my diploma is dated 1952. By the date degrees were granted, the early Seevers graduates were: John Lewis '49, Walter Freyburger '51, and then Grace Gray, Thelma Gould, Alexander Kandel and I in '52. I still feel like I was the second Ph.D. graduate in the Seevers Years.

I have presented this detailed account of my thesis research problems as an example of what a candidate might encounter. Many others have met equally challenging tasks. I think my problems and my arrival at solutions can be grasped by readers not familiar with laboratory studies. At the very least it might show that being a "gadgeteer" might not be completely without virtue!

Editor's note: Jim Weeks' demonstration of the fact that drugs are reinforcing via his rat self-administration techniques cannot be overestimated. He did it first! His advice to Tomoji Yanagita and Gerry Deneau, who did similar studies in monkeys, was crucial. Only a person with Jim's unique talents, which he describes as "the questionable virtue of being a gadgeteer," could have accomplished this. In Dr. Tomoji Yanagita's chapter of the Japanese Fellows in Pharmacology (1999), on page 55, he refers to his visit to see Dr. Weeks in Kalamazoo, MI, and in particular to the i.v. catheter problems that Jim solved before the invention of silicone rubber tubing. This allowed Dr. Yanagita to proceed with his research as shown below.

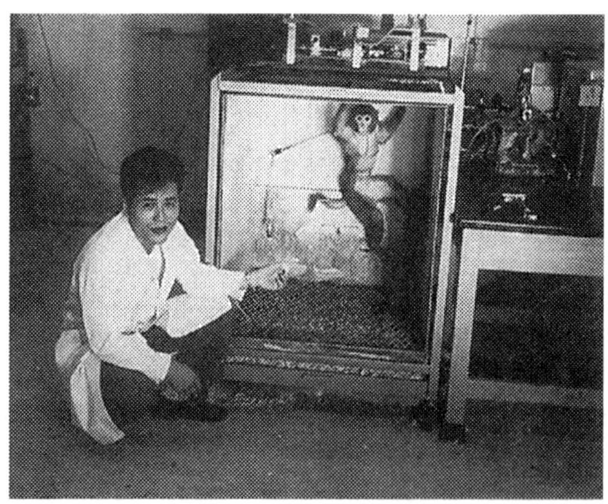

Dr. T. Yanagita with his new set-up for self-administration of drugs in a Rhesus monkey.

My Memoirs of Staff and Students, 1949-1965

Donald R. Bennett, M.D., Ph.D.

At the end of 1948, after three years in the army (1943-1946), three full years as an undergraduate at the University of Michigan, being married two years with a one-year-old infant living in Willow Run Village, a B.S. in zoology, and a rejection in hand from the University of Michigan Medical School as an out-of-state student, I was wondering what to do with my life. Fortunately, I had a friend, Leland "Brownie" C. Hendershot, who was in the same situation as I. Brownie had met James Weeks in a course on differential equations; Jim met with us on the campus Diag and suggested that we might like to join him in pharmacology. I at least knew about the discipline of pharmacology, because I had taken a course in pharmaceutical chemistry from renowned Professor Blicke in the School of Pharmacy, and a course on the History of Medicine in which I had written a history of pharmacology as a term paper. I also became interested in pharmacology as a result of reading a good part of Goodman and Gilman's first edition (1941) in Professor Blicke's course.

We submitted applications and were invited for a group interview with Dr. Seevers along with another rejected medical school applicant, Robert M. René. The first thing Dr. Seevers asked us was whether each of us might be interested in a combined seven- to eight-year M.D./Ph.D. program; he also had work for us that would provide some financial support ($600 to $900/year). We all thought it was a splendid offer and we accepted it immediately!

We were not disappointed when we began graduate work in January 1949, because we met some fascinating people. We had just missed James Wyngaarden, an assistant in pharmacology, who received his M.D. degree in 1948 and ultimately went on to greater heights, like director of NIH for eight years. John Lewis had just received his Ph.D. working for Dr. Seevers and had gone on to the Sterling-Winthrop Research Institute. Dr. Lewis was to serve as a mentor for me later in life when I joined the Department of Drugs at the American Medical Association in 1976. Dr. Lewis was also one of the early presidents of the Drug Information Association. The other graduate students and assistants included Joseph Cochin, Mylapore Guruswami, and Gilbert McMahon (Dr. Lauren Woods' lab); Walter Freyberger, Carl Gruhzit, Barbara Rennick, and Walter Veldkamp (Dr. Gordon Moe's lab); Linares B. Johnson, Alex Kandel, Komol Pengsritong and Jim Weeks (Dr. Chenoweth's lab); Thelma Gould and Leonard Procita (Dr. Shideman's lab); I believe Samuel Irwin and Grace Gray worked directly for Dr. Seevers.

Except for Drs. Moe and Seevers, even the faculty seemed like older, but smarter, graduate students. Dr. Lauren Woods was a senior medical student; Dr. Frederick Shideman had graduated from medical school in 1946; and Dr. Chenoweth had graduated from Cornell University medical school in 1942. Dr. Chenoweth spent three years in The Chemical Warfare Center at Edgewood Arsenal, and he returned to Cornell as faculty before accepting a faculty position in 1946 at Michigan.

All of these faculty and students could not have been more friendly or helpful in furthering our education. For the first time, René, Hendershot, and myself really felt like we were part of a team rather than just faceless students in a big university. If you were willing, all of the pharmacology graduate students and assistants would let you participate in setting up their experiments; therefore, there was considerable opportunity to learn various techniques.

Raymond Houde, M.D., had arrived as a National Cancer Institute postdoctoral fellow in the fall of 1948. Dr. Houde was visiting for one year at Michigan to learn more about analgesic methodology. He went on for a second postdoctoral year to the US government's Narcotic Research Facility in Lexington, Kentucky. Fortunately for all of us, he met a young lady technician (whom he later married) in Dr. Woods' laboratory; therefore, Dr. Seevers would find an excuse to bring Ray back from Lexington for short visits. Ray contributed greatly to educating all of us about analgesia, and he went on to a distinguished career in clinical pharmacology in the area of analgesiology at Sloan Kettering Memorial Cancer Center in New York.

Sam Irwin was working for Dr. Houde who was using the Wolff-Hardy-Goodell Thermal-Induced Pain apparatus on the spinal rat preparation; however, Dr. Houde was also interested in conducting studies in humans utilizing not only that apparatus, but also comparing it with pain induced by the 1) Seevers-Shideman variable-weighted needle-on-eyelid technique, 2) electrical stimulation of metallic tooth fillings, and 3) ischemic pain induced by maintaining blood pressure midway between systolic and diastolic pressures in one arm for up to 45 minutes. Since René, Hendershot, and myself were principally taking courses, we were assigned to Dr. Houde as clinical trial subjects to help him with these experiments. René and Hendershot, but not Irwin and myself, always had a bout of emesis after receiving a parenteral narcotic, usually weekly, in these studies. Irwin and I rather enjoyed the experience, and I always seemed to be less tense and to do better on the microbiology and biochemistry quizzes the following morning after the usual weekly evening injection. Personal involvement in drug-taking studies by staff and students was common at that time. In fact, Dr. Seevers insisted that a day be designated in the medical school pharmacology course in which all of the students took one of many different drugs or placebo to gain personal experience about taking drugs. I always felt it was a very instructive laboratory session, but unfortunately, probably for liability reasons, it was terminated in later years.

By 1950, Hendershot and I were working in the laboratory of Dr. Chenoweth on sodium monofluoroacetate along with "Johnny" Johnson, Alex Kandel, Komol Pengsritong and Jim Weeks. Those were exciting, and also exhausting, times. I wrote the following in the acknowledgement section of my Ph.D. thesis: "The author wishes to thank Dr. Maynard B. Chenoweth for his guidance, aid, and the pleasure of having worked in a pleasant and stimulating environment which he instills into all of his research problems". For the kindness, advice and support he extended to me during the next thirty years, that acknowledgement turned out to be a prologue rather than an epilogue.

Attendance at ASPET and FASEB meetings was strongly encouraged by Drs. Seevers and Chenoweth— if you could cover most of

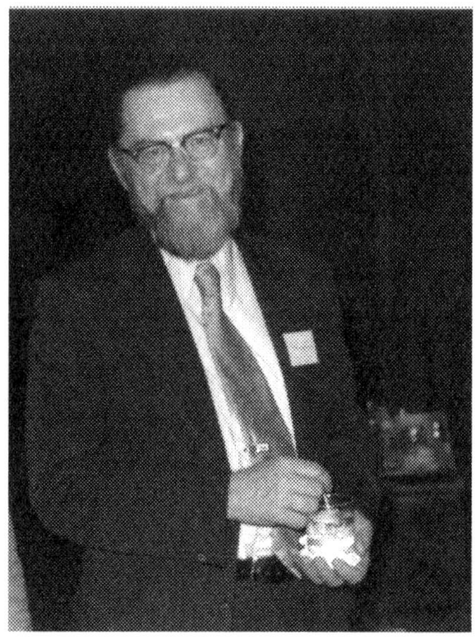

Maynard B. Chenoweth (deceased), was born in Chicago, IL., on November 25, 1917. He obtained an A.B. degree from Columbia University in 1938. He was a Pharmacology Fellow from 1942-1943 at Cornell University, later becomming an associate professor. In 1953, Dr. Chenoweth started working as a pharmacologist at the Biochemistry Research Lab in the Dow Chemical Company. Some of Dr. Chenoweth's multiple interests were pharmacodynamics of fluoroacetate and 2-3 dimercaptopropanol, cardiac and anesthetic agents.

your expenses. I got to my first FASEB meeting in Atlantic City traveling non-stop all night in the middle of the back seat of Carl Gruhzit's car as one of five other graduate students. Older graduate students got the window seats. We found "rooms" for five dollars a night. You hoped to make as many friends as possible, particularly in the pharmaceutical industry, to cover expenses for a few meals. Those trips were great life, as well as pharmacology, learning experiences. Later we became more sophisticated. For 20 dollars each and gas, Dr. Dick Jolly and I would pick up new cadillacs or oldsmobiles in East Lansing or Detroit and drive them to their new owners in or close to cities where pharmacology meetings were going to be held.

We attended some great departmental seminars given by outside speakers. Those that come to mind were chromotography, chelation, lysergic acid diethylamide, sparteine, and rauwolfia alkaloids (before Ciba marketed the product for hypertension and psychoses).

1950 and 1951 were years of change and adjustment. Dr. Moe took his excellent cardiovascular lectures and Barbara Rennick, who had just completed her M.D. degree, with him to the University of Syracuse. Walt Freyberger took his Ph.D., and Bill Veldkamp his M.S. degree, to Upjohn. Carl Gruhzit went to teach pharmacology in Hong Kong. Dr. Komol Pengsritong finished his M.S. degree and returned to Bangkok. Dr. Nickerson arrived to fill the void in Dr. Moe's lab. Dorothy Norton (later Overbeck) arrived to keep the Department functioning initially as departmental secretary while Dr. Seevers began his many trips to Japan, and to make tea for those marvelous late afternoon all-faculty-and-student discussion sessions in the departmental library. René accepted a position as a first-year medical student at another medical school, as did Johnson to attend medical school in the West. Guruswami, McMahon and I got our M.S. degrees. Gil McMahon had just completed his sophomore year in Medical school. I had turned down an acceptance to medical school in 1950 from the University of Indiana, my home state, because when I interviewed, that Department of Pharmacology did not have a formally defined combined M.D./Ph.D, program. By this time, I was really enjoying research in pharmacology at Michigan, and I wanted to combine those interests with a career in medicine. By not registering as a student and working full-time for six months in the Department of Pharmacology, I met the residency requirement for the state of Michigan. Then, I was accepted to the University of Michigan Medical School in 1951.

New arrivals in 1951 included Bob Rathbun, Annetta Kelly and Harry Hardman. Harry was the first of the University of Illinois contingent. He had just received a M.S. degree in pharmacology and began work on his Ph.D. Harry brought a bright and organized mind and a sense of work ethic, as well as a wonderful sense of humor and enthusiasm to the graduate student body. Like Jim Weeks, he also brought a perspective of pharmacy to the department. All three initially worked directly for Dr. Seevers and ultimately received their Ph.D.s in 1954. Jane Haggard also arrived in this year and worked for Dr. Woods, receiving her Ph.D. in 1955. Bob Rathbun and I lived in Willow Run Village just a few doors apart, and our families became good friends. The friendship persisted in spite of the fact that I burned a hole in the oil line of his now-classic two-door Plymouth coupe with a rumble seat while inadvertently grounding one of the battery cables.

In 1952, Jim Weeks and Alex Kandel received their doctoral degrees and left for pharmaceutical company positions; this left a large void in Dr. Chenoweth's group. Hendershot and I were glad to share the exhaustion with Harry Hardman who was assigned to work part-time with Dr. Chenoweth. When Grace Gray received her doctoral degree and went on to veterinary school at the University of Minnesota, the department lost its best teacher and resource in the preparation of Thirry-Vella loops and pharmacology of the GI tract. A faculty arrival that year included the second of the University of Illinois contingent, Ted Brody. Dr. Brody immediately filled the "metabolic and cellular pharmacology" void created when Dr. Shideman left for the University of Wisconsin, and Dr. Brody helped to maintain the Department's young faculty appearance. Ken Cochran, a pharmacologist who received a Ph.D. from the University of Chicago in 1950, was appointed as a part-time instructor. His major appointment was in the Department of Epidemiology. Ken's perspective in epidemiology was often greatly appreciated at our seminars in pharmacology.

Graduate student arrivals in 1952 included Gerald Deneau, who was assigned to work in the narcotic-evaluation monkey colony for Dr. Sam Irwin who had just been appointed as an instructor, as well as Bruce Mellett who was assigned to work on analgesics for Dr. Woods. A part-time instructor arrival was Archie Miller, a recent Ph.D. from the University of Virginia who was also a part-time medical student. Archie ultimately went on into the specialty of endocrinology. Drs. Gerry Deneau, Harry Hardman, Bob Rathbun, Bruce Mellett, Brownie Hendershot, Jim Miller (a veterinarian working for Dr. Seevers), John Kissell (a student of Dr. Domino), and myself had a special relationship for the next three to four years, because we often took courses together, shared information and studied together for our Ph.D. preliminary examinations.

The Illinois contingent expanded with the selection of Dr. Domino and Dr. Swain as faculty in 1953 and 1954 respectively following their internships at Presbyterian— St. Luke's and Cook County hospitals, respectively. Both immediately carried on the tradition of a young, enthusiastic faculty interested in both teaching and new areas of research. Dr. Ted Carr came on the faculty as an assistant professor in 1953. Dr. Carr was to provide a perspective on and training in clinical pharmacology. It was largely through his encouragement that I began my long-standing association with the American Society of Clinical Pharmacology and Therapeutics. Dr. Lloyd Beck also arrived as a research associate in 1953. By 1954, it was clear that Dr. Beck would assume the role of "Critic in Residence" for the Department. Lloyd earned that title, because he had an extremely analytical mind, was a clear thinker, and always wanted to be helpful, even if it meant assaulting the basic tenants of your research project, scientific beliefs or personal opinions. Years later as editor-in-chief of AMA-Drug Evaluations for ten years, I, and my staff, depended heavily on critics like Lloyd for accuracy in our writing. I counted Lloyd as one of my best friends, and I was honored that he was on my doctoral committee along with Drs. Seevers, Chenoweth, Woods, and David Bohr (Physiology). Our friendship persisted after each of us had left the University. I provided lectures for him in toxicology when he was chairman of the Pharmacology Department at Duluth. I believe Dr. Beck's first graduate student was Bert Lum, who arrived from Hawaii during 1953 or 1954.

The years 1953 and 1954 had their downside as well. Dr. Chenoweth left to take a position with the Dow Chemical Company. Few knew that Dr. Chenoweth and his wife had an additional financial burden due to the fact that one of their children had to be institutionalized for health reasons. We all understood the reason for the change from academia to industry, but it didn't make it any easier to accept his departure. He was a taskmaster, but always even-handed and fair. He loved placing light on the darkly lit sectors of scientific knowledge. When he was helping us to finish up a long and tiring experiment at 2 a.m., and was asked why he chose this research career path rather than the practice of medicine, he reminded us that we had the potential to save many more lives working in research than we might hope to save even after years of practice.

The dismissal of Dr. Mark Nickerson in 1954 was especially difficult for me. I always arrived at work early, and so did Nick. He loved teaching and was a master at it. Over that first cup of coffee in the morning, I still remember many personal discussions with him about pharmacology, science, policy, and politics. At the brown bag lunch in the Department for the faculty-student group, Drs. Nickerson, Chenoweth, Woods, Domino, and Swain would all add to our general fund of knowledge, particularly information that one can't find in textbooks. Although an excellent researcher, Dr. Nickerson was best at teaching in the clinic. He initiated the first course in clinical pharmacology at the University of Michigan for the third or fourth year medical students. With only a year's internship of clinical experience, a good working knowledge of pharmacology and a brilliant analytical mind, he could hold his own in discussions about therapy with any clinical departmental chairperson who anecdotally had been there, done that, seen that! He was a marvelous representative for our Department in the clinical sciences. I always felt that Nick's conferences were as good as those published by Drs. Harry Gold and McKeen Cattell in their clinical pharmacology conferences at Cornell, which were so widely and rightfully acclaimed at the time.

Needless to say, I also greatly respected Dr. Seevers for the opportunities he made available to the development of my career, as well as the common sense approach to teaching and practicing pharmacology that he provided to all of his colleagues and students. His knowledge about the field, politics and probable future of pharmacology as well as his capabilities in teaching and research in pharmacology were legendary. His kindness was also legendary. No staff or graduate students missed the opportunity to attend a party hosted by Dr. Seevers and his wife at their home, not because it was politically correct, but because each person was made to feel special by "Mose" and Frankie.

I never knew who was most right in the dispute that occurred between Drs. Seevers and Nickerson; however, like most students at that time, I also knew that I did not know all the facts on either side.

After I had received the M.D. degree in 1955, the years between 1955 and 1958 were filled with part-time teaching pharmacology to graduate, medical and nursing students, thesis research, and a full-time internship (1956-1957) until I received my Ph.D. degree in February 1958. Many students and part-time instructors on the combined M.D./Ph.D. program were doing the same activities or going to medical school if they had already completed their Ph.D. degree, i.e., Drs. Ed Cafruny, Joe Cochin, Harry Hardman, Brownie Hendershot (Dentistry), Dick Jolly, and Archie Miller.

After receiving the D.D.S. in 1953 and the Ph.D. in 1955, my closest friend and fellow graduate student, Brownie Hendershot, went to work with Dr. Chenoweth at Dow Chemical's Biomedical Research Laboratory in Midland, Michigan. He conducted considerable dental and other research for four years before he accepted a staff position at the American Dental Association (ADA). He served as assistant secretary of the Council on Dental Therapeutics and associate editor of the ADA until 1963 when he was appointed as editor of the ADA, a position he held for ten years. His untimely death in 1980 cut short his contributions to dental therapeutics and ended an accomplished career.

Dr. Lauren Woods was especially helpful to me and other faculty involved in teaching medical and nursing students during this period. Dr. Woods was an excellent administrator and teacher in addition to continuing his research in the narcotic field. As supervisor of the medical and nursing courses, he taught a number of faculty members how to organize their lectures and provide an excellent course in pharmacology to many different types of students. Dr. Woods always had a number of outside interests: 1) He contributed to Dr. Drill's book in pharmacology. 2) He was very active as a volunteer in the United States Pharmacopeial Convention (USPC). Both Drs. Shideman and Woods were elected president and vice president of USPC, Inc., for five years respectively, but not concurrently. Dr. Woods was very active in the United States Adopted Names (USAN) organization as well. Later, I also was an active volunteer for USPC for 15 years as well as for USAN. When I was elected as vice president of the USPC, I remember distinctly that the staff still spoke highly of the contributions of both Drs. Shideman and Woods to USPC.

Dorothy Overbeck remained with the Department until her retirement in 1973. As is true for many long-term Departmental

Secretaries in a University, she was especially helpful to graduate students and developing faculty during their early formative years. She always responded to reasonable requests whether the issue was a research grant, presentation of lecture material, publication of manuscripts, one's paycheck, or a need to see Dr. Seevers promptly in a crisis.

Another contingent of graduate students had arrived during the mid-'50s (1954-1958) and were busy taking courses, preliminary doctoral examinations, and helping with the considerable research that was being conducted in the Department. They were: Dick Rech and Jane Heng (with Dr. Domino), Duncan McCarthy (with Dr. Seevers), Joanne Moore (with Dr. Swain), and Glenn Kiplinger, Deane Calvert and Ken Moore (with Dr. Brody). The Department was further enriched with new graduate students during the late '50s: Paula Stern and Roger Hornbrook (Dr. Brody), Michael Brody and Ben Zimmerman (Dr. Beck), Carl Hug and Sal Mulé (Dr. Woods), Ben Lucchesi and Bob Reynolds (Dr. Hardman), Don Knapp, Roy Hudson and Gareth Owen (Dr. Domino). The contribution to the field of pharmacology made by most of these students in their ensuing careers is remarkable. The early, untimely deaths of Drs. Mike Brody, McCarthy, Calvert, and Owen undoubtedly limited that contribution.

Dr. Carr was expanding the discipline of clinical pharmacology. Wally Baird had worked with Dr. Carr while attending medical school. Upon graduation in 1958 and following an internship year, he accepted a position as a clinical pharmacology trainee in 1959. Ultimately, Dr. Baird also was appointed as an assistant professor in both the Departments of Medicine and Pharmacology, until he left in 1969 to assume a position as director of the Critical Care Unit at Ingham Medical Hospital in Lansing, Michigan, as well as to hold a position as clinical associate professor at the Michigan State University College of Medicine. Following receipt of the M.D. degree, Dr. Ron Chipps began a postdoctoral fellowship with Dr. Carr in 1961, and he also became a clinical pharmacology trainee, receiving a M.S. degree in pharmacology in 1965 prior to returning to the practice of medicine.

Dr. Seevers decided that one of the faculty should serve as a single administrative mechanism for communication where all graduate students could express their successes, concerns and requests for faculty assignments or transfers. I was appointed as the administrative assistant to fulfill this function. I was indeed privileged, because I got to know each of these students a bit better than I would have otherwise as a faculty member. Each student's needs, management of their hopes and frustrations, and expectations were a wonderful learning experience for me in the management of others who worked for me later in my career. Compared to the denominator, few transfers were requested, and were almost always based on changing interests rather than personal conflicts.

I'm sure that all of the faculty and students of that period would want to recognize the contributions of Bill Sheldon and Bob Shepherd. Bill was in charge of the drug supply and equipment room, and Bob was in charge of the carpenter shop. You did not teach effectively in any course with a pharmacology laboratory or use any chemical in your research project(s) without the help of Bill Sheldon. Likewise, Bob Shepherd was usually the major facilitator in constructing any apparatus required for a research project. In addition, Bob, a Type I diabetic, taught all of us a lot about how to recognize and manage hypoglycemic symptoms when his food input and workload didn't quite match his insulin intake. At that time, we were also blessed with good animal caretakers, like Art Riggs, who taught us city boys how to handle frogs, monkeys, opossums, dogs, rats, mice, guinea pigs, turtles and pigeons.

During the latter '50s, Dr. Seevers offered a number of his graduates an opportunity to remain on the faculty. These included Drs. Deneau, Hardman, Mellett, Cafruny and me. Dr. Seevers offered me a position as instructor on the faculty in 1958, but only after I turned down his first suggestion. He had contacted the Michigan Law School and determined that the Law School Admissions Committee would seriously consider an application from one of Dr. Seevers' students who had successfully completed a combined M.D./Ph.D. program. Dr. Seevers felt that we were going to need lawyers trained in pharmacology and medicine. I remember telling Dr. Seevers that I had been a college student for 14 years, that I was 31 years old and had not paid any income tax yet, that I was somewhat worried about my English composition skills, and that my own children already in elementary school treated me as just another student. He reluctantly accepted my decision. The "old man" simply had an innate sense of what was going to be needed in our profession in later years.

Actually, I thought his idea about law school might be his method of retribution to repay me for the time a few monkeys got loose from me in the basement of the old pharmacology building, scurried up to his office, relieved themselves on his desk, and then went to the third floor. Unfortunately, the attic door was open and they hid in the attic between the outside stone wall and the inner wooden wall about two feet out of our reach. I can't remember, but I would like to think it was Gerry Deneau rather than me, who suggested that we pour some diethyl ether into the space, wait for the monkeys to become sleepy or anesthetized and then lift them out with the aid of a stick and rope. We did just that, although it took more ether than anticipated. Some one called the University fireman and when they arrived, they were not at all impressed with our cleverness. Instead they kept reminding Dr. Seevers that we could have easily created an open-air instead of a closed attic. Oddly enough, other than a few expletives, Dr. Seevers was quite calm about the incident. It was only later that Dr. Deneau learned from an article with pictures in the University of Wisconsin school newspaper that "Mose" had inadvertently also let a monkey loose at that facility that went into a nearby park where the police had to recapture the animal.

My own Ph.D. thesis work entailed cardiovascular research. Dr. Seevers would often ask the faculty to help in the development of data on compounds for which the Department had signed a contract with various pharmaceutical firms. The first such endeavor for my lab involved a Sterling Winthrop compound. Dr. Woods informed me that I would be responsible for the cardiovascular and the gastrointestinal data; he stressed that the company was particularly interested in the GI actions of the compound in the intact animal rather than the Thirry-Vella loop preparation or use of in vitro methodology. That latter request began a whole new GI research project that served as Ph.D. theses for a number of other graduate students. A fellow medical student in my class, Robert Biggs, was now completing a residency in ophthalmology. He and his research mentor, Dr. Matt Alpern, requested some help from me in their study of sympathetic innervation on the amplitude of accommodation. That study stimulated our interest in the eye and it ultimately served as a Ph.D. thesis project for another graduate student and completed the three major areas of research in my lab, CV, GI and the Eye.

I got to know those students who worked directly for me even better than those for whom I served as a part-time counselor. In my laboratory from the period of 1957 to 1965, I served as mentor for four Ph.D. and two M.S. candidates. The first graduate student assigned to me was Thomas Baum. He arrived in the fall of 1956 from the Long Island University's School of Pharmacy to begin course work. Tom had left Brno, Czechoslovakia at the age of 11 and spent three years in England during World War II before emigrating to the US. He had also spent three years as a detail man for Ayerst before entering the Department. Obviously, he was a bit more mature than the average graduate student, and better equipped to suffer through my first teaching experience as a Ph.D. mentor. Although we were able to determine the cardiac actions of compounds, Dr. Beck and his students, Mike Brody and Ben Zimmerman, were particularly helpful to Tom Baum in determining vascular actions. Tom went on to develop a thesis project based on the cardiovascular actions of simple aliphatic amines, especially t-butylamine. Tom received his Ph.D. in 1961. He accepted a research position at Wyeth in cardiovascular research, a position that he held for 17 years. He then took a position as head of cardiovascular research for Schering, which he held until his untimely death in 1981.

During 1957, Ed Alpert had been working part-time as a first year graduate student for Dr. Hardman on the Army research project. In 1958, he was assigned to my laboratory to prepare for prelims and work on his Ph.D. thesis. Both Tom Baum and Ed Alpert helped me move the laboratory from the main campus building to the new quarters in the Medical Science Building I. Neither complained about the work involved, because now we didn't have to waste time every morning suspending our lunch on a string from the ceiling in order to protect it from the cockroaches in the old building. Ed showed an initial interest in the eye project, and ultimately completed a thesis in that area in 1964. Ed was in the combined program and received his M.D. degree in 1965. As a first lieutenant in the Public Health Service, he was assigned for two years to work on a malaria project at the federal prison in Atlanta, Georgia. He returned to Ann Arbor to complete his residency in internal medicine as well as completing subspecialty work in allergy. He has been in the practice of allergy and immunology in Detroit since that time; in 1995-1996 he served as president of the Michigan Allergy and Asthma Society.

Roger Hornbrook was assigned to my lab in 1958. Initially, Roger was very helpful to me in developing information on the pharmacology of a group of phenoxyethylamines that the Dow Chemical Company had requested the Department to evaluate. Roger was also helpful in the early development of strain gauge technology in order to assess gastrointestinal motor function in the intact animal. Ultimately, Roger became more interested in the research work in Dr. Brody's lab. He received his Ph.D. degree under the tutelage of Dr. Brody in 1963. He accepted a position at the Department of Pharmacology at the University of Oklahoma, and ultimately became chairperson of the Department of Pharmacology in the Pharmacy School at that University. Another graduate student, Jerome Levin, spent some time in our lab before transferring to Dr. Beck's lab to acquire his Ph.D. in vascular research.

A new graduate student, Henry Jacoby, having recently completed his pharmacy degree at the Philadelphia College of Pharmacy and Science, was assigned to work in my lab in 1959. Hank arrived having just purchased a new car (a Corvette convertible). Dr. Seevers drove a car to work at that time that looked as if it were at least ten years old. Dr. Seevers observed the Corvette at the departmental picnic, and he wondered who owned the car. Hank promptly sold the Corvette; however, he purchased a similar new car within two weeks after receiving the Ph.D. degree in 1963. Hank selected the GI area for his thesis work. That area has remained a life-long commitment. He worked for many years at Merck and McNeil in GI research before finally helping his first supervisor at Merck, Dr. Dave Brodie, initiate and develop a pharmacology contract organization. Hank has created many reports and publications as a result of this work. After Dr. Brodie left to become a full-time consultant for an Israeli pharmaceutical company, Hank became president of his own pharmacology contract organization in Brigantine, New Jersey, not far from the Atlantic City Boardwalk and site of many past Federation meetings.

Tom and I needed a technician to help complete all of our commitments. In 1959, David Reinke lived next door to me. He was completing his studies towards an M.B.A., and he was bagging groceries at the A&P grocery to make ends meet until he became a chief executive officer. We could pay a bit more than the A&P job; Dave accepted our offer and worked on every project in the lab. A year later, he applied as a graduate student and completed his Ph.D. in 1964, investing most of his research productivity in the GI area. On graduation, Dave accepted a position with the Physiology and Pharmacology Department of Michigan State University (MSU). In 1966, Dave joined Dr. Brody's then newly-developing Department of Pharmacology at MSU. For his entire scientific career, Dave has been principally involved with teaching pharmacology in the MSU Colleges of Nursing, Human Medicine, Veterinary Medicine, and Osteopathic Medicine. He became vice chairperson of the Department of Pharmacology and Toxicology that is shared by the three schools of medicine.

Three additional graduate students worked in my laboratory; two received the M.S. degree in pharmacology. The first was Hector Vasquez Leon, M.D. Our laboratory was fortunate to have Hector who was from the district of Michoacan, Mexico. He was assigned to work on a M.S. degree in conjunction with the eye project. Hector was immensely popular with both students and faculty during his stay from 1958 to 1960. He had just completed his government service, which meant that he had been dropped off by airplane in a remote Mexican rural area with a Doctor's bag and a pistol and then he was picked up two years later. His clinical accounts of that experience were absolutely fascinating. When Hector left, he accepted a position in pharmacology in the Department of Science Functions in Zulia, Venezuela.

I would be remiss not to mention the contribution of Dr. Paul Bass to the effort in our laboratory. In 1960, we contacted Paul who was a research pharmacologist at Parke-Davis in Ann Arbor in charge of GI pharmacology. Paul was a great help to me, and to those graduate students who worked in that area in my lab. He and I had a number of publications together. He later was appointed as a lecturer in the Department of Pharmacology in 1966; he kept that position until 1970 when he went to the Department of Pharmacology in the Pharmacy School at the University of Wisconsin, where he ultimately became a professor of pharmacology.

The Department is now fortunate to have a historical written record of the Japanese Michigan Fellows (Japanese Michigan Fellows in Pharmacology: 50 years of Cooperation, edited by Drs. Edward Domino and Tomoji Yanagita, NPP Books, 1999). Our laboratory's experience with Hector is a good reminder that Dr. Seevers extended that opportunity to trainees from numerous countries other than Japan as well. During the Seevers' years, Dr. Komol Pensritong from Thailand was the first of nine off-shore candidates to receive the M.S. degree in pharmacology in 1950 followed by Mylapore Guruswami from India (1951); Ennio Vivaldi from Chile (1954); Sukru Kaymakcalan (1954) from Turkey; Ligia Ybarra Falcon(1958) from Venezuela; Adawia Al-Alousia (1958) and Khadid Salman (1960) from Iraq; Pojana Bukhamana (1960), also from Thailand; and Suleyman Kaayalp (1962) from Turkey. Drs. Roberto Vargas-Escheverria and Julian Villareal, also from Mexico, received their Ph.D. degrees in 1965 and 1969 respectively. Like the Japanese Michigan Fellows, these foreign graduate students also contributed greatly to research and teaching in the Department during the years from 1948 through 1969.

Alan Rosenbaum came to our lab as a second-year medical student to explore an interest in research before deciding on a final career path. His principal work was on the GI project; he received an M.S. degree in 1965 and his M.D. degree in 1966. He ultimately combined his pharmacology training with a career in psychiatry serving on the faculties of Mayo Clinic and Wayne State University; he always has been interested in conducting and publishing clinical research. Two other medical students, Marvin Anderson and Paul Turner, spent some time in our lab, but chose not to seek formal degree certification in pharmacology.

Like Tom Baum, Elliot Piperno was also a graduate of the Long Island University's School of Pharmacy and he began a program in the fall of 1961 to obtain a Ph.D. degree and was assigned to Dr. Domino initially; however, he came to work in my lab in 1963 working principally in the GI area. It soon became obvious that his major interest involved a clinical orientation, especially involving animals; therefore, after spending the summer working as a wild game biologist in northern Michigan, he enrolled in Michigan State University's Veterinary College beginning in the fall of 1965. His pharmacology training benefited him well during his long career in toxicology at Merck and McNeil Pharmaceutical companies, joint teaching appointment at the University of Pennsylvania's Veterinary College, and independent consulting.

During this period of the first half of the 1960s, the Department's selection process for excellent graduate students seeking the Ph.D. continued to be eminently successful. If not then, certainly now, currently well-recognized names in the field of pharmacology included Don Knapp ('62-Dr. Domino), Carl Hug ('63-Dr. Woods), Paula Stern ('63-Dr. Brody), Bob Reynolds ('63-Dr. Hardman), Gerry Gebber ('64-Dr. Beck), Ray Ruddon ('64-Dr. Woods), Bob Gussin and Dr. Roberto Vargas-Escheverria ('65-Dr. Cafruny), Don Ducharme ('65-Dr. Beck), Jim Gibb ('65-Dr Brody), Jack Diamond ('65-Dr. Brody), Morris Zedeck ('65-Dr. Mellett), John McNeill ('67-Dr Brody), Charlie Ross ('66-Dr. Cafruny), Jerry Levin ('66-Dr. Beck), Tony Dren ('66-Dr. Domino), Richard Dean ('66-Dr. Lucchesi), Sharon Valley ('67-Dr. Swain), Janice Stickney ('67-Dr. Lucchesi), Jim Johnson ('67-Dr. Ruddon) and Julian Villareal ('69-Dr. Seevers). This was the last group of graduate students that I knew personally. I have listed their thesis advisor and the year in which they received their Ph.D. degree in chronological order that also approximately defines their order of entry into the graduate program. Again, early deaths cut short the contribution to pharmacology made by Drs. Charles Ross and Donald Knapp.

Not all students went on for the Ph.D degree. Fred Schiattarella (now Scott) and Joe Luciano received their M.S. degrees in 1962 and 1964, respectively, and left to complete a medical degree elsewhere. After completing their master's degrees in 1963 and 1965 respectively, Jack Davitt and Al Small accepted positions at the Food and Drug Administration in Rockville, MD.

In my opinion, the Seevers' years can be best described as visionary and transitional. "Mose" recognized opportunities and the need for change in our field; he met that challenge. There was an old joke in clinical circles that I heard when I was completing my Family Medicine residency. It asked, "What does it say in the preface of the Emergency Room Guide for Doctors?" The answer is, "What to do until the molecular biologist arrives!" Dr. Seevers was not only a classical (traditional) pharmacologist but also a clinical pharmacologist. The opportunity to learn the techniques of both these fields was available to any graduate student beginning in the fifties. While some faculty and students were debating whether clinical or traditional subsets of pharmacology would be most important, Dr. Seevers was already encouraging the development of faculty and techniques associated with the discipline of biochemical pharmacology as well. He was a strong proponent of selecting a mix of graduate students with medical, veterinary, pharmacy, biology and chemical backgrounds. He set the stage for the molecular biologist to arrive in our field, but without diminishing the importance of clinical and classical pharmacological studies, because he believed the scope of pharmacology at the University of Michigan should extend from the patient to the molecular level.

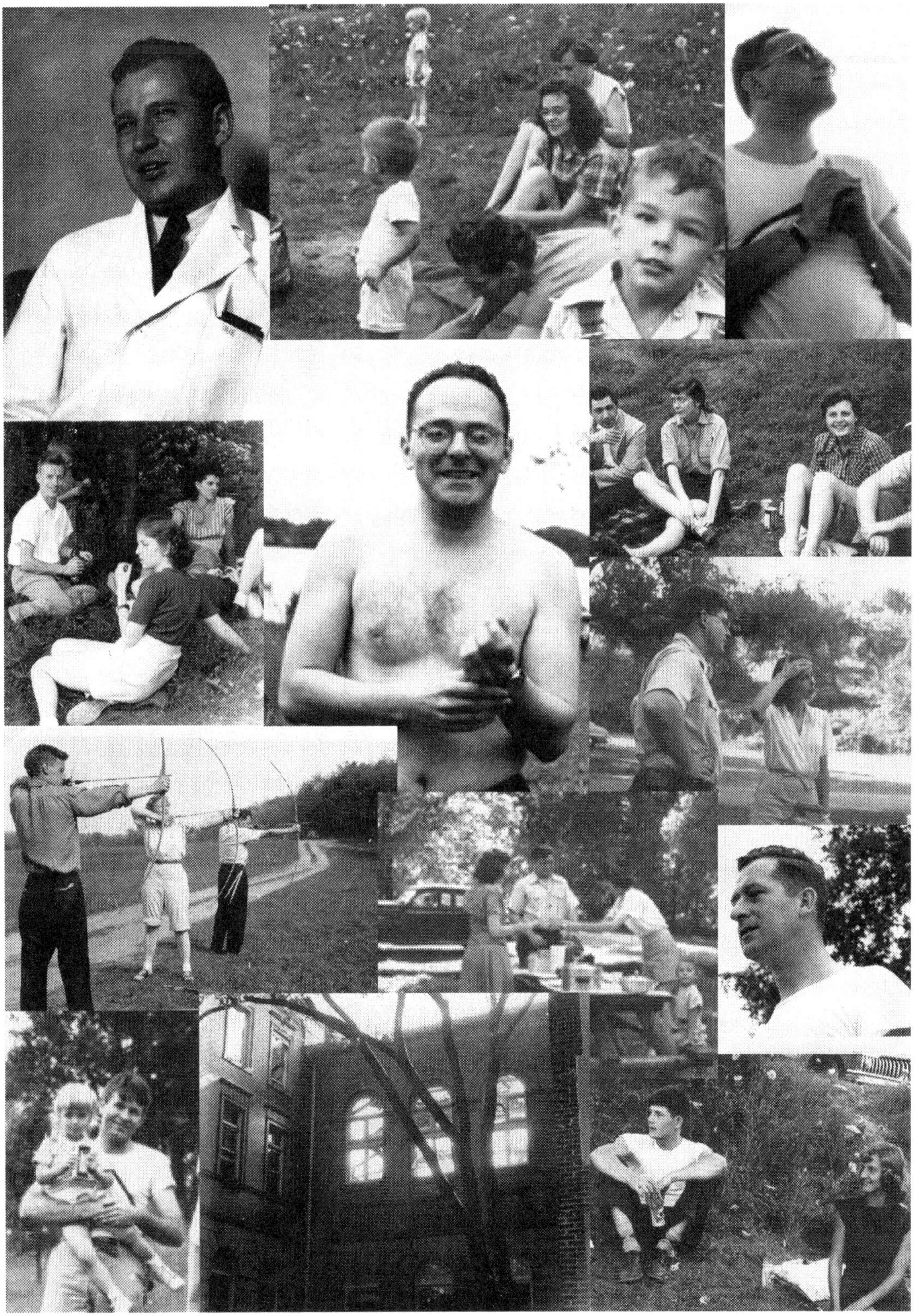

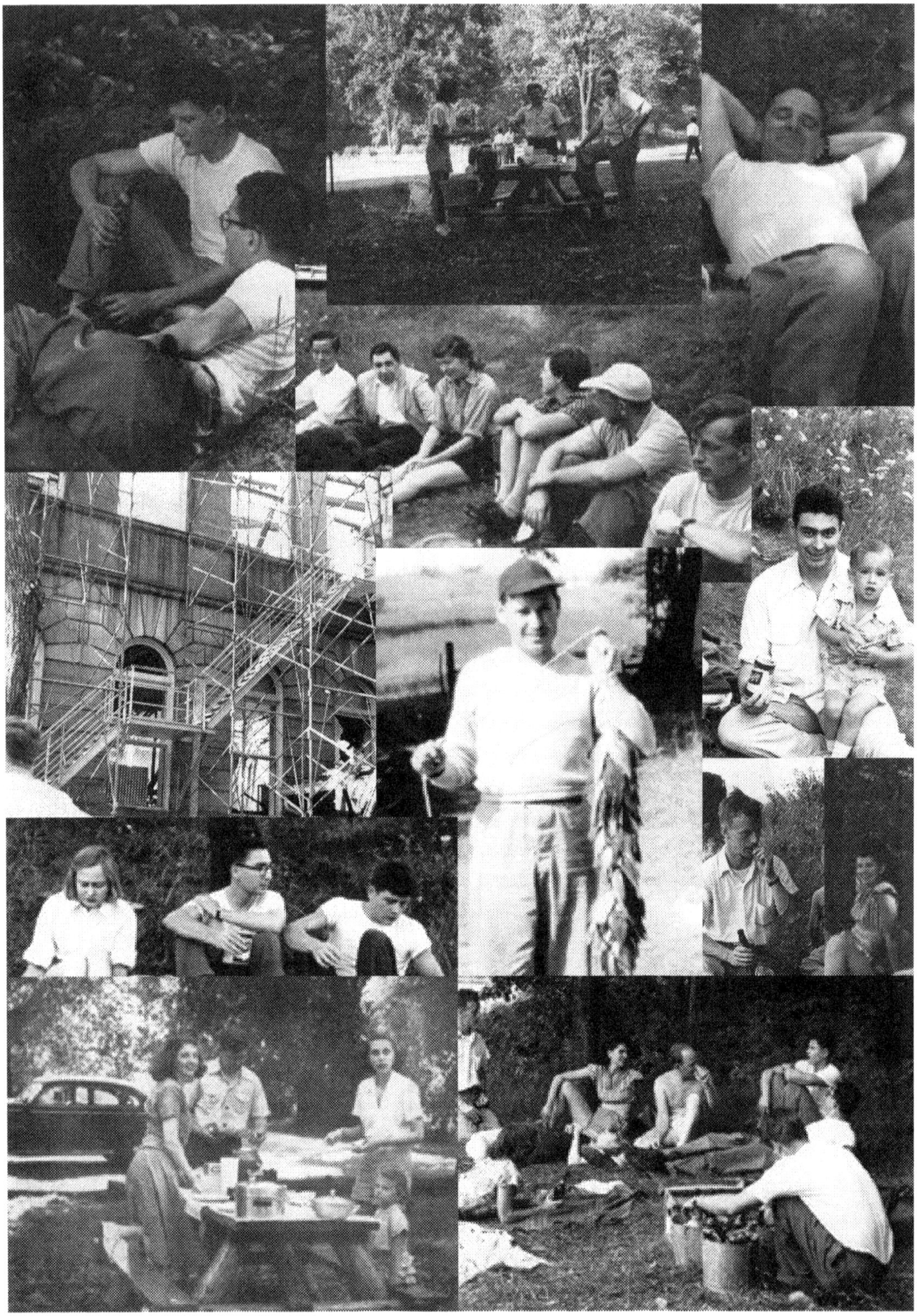

*My Memoirs of Frederick E. Shideman, M.D., Ph.D.**

Al Quebbemann, M.D., Ph.D.

Editor's note: Fred Shideman was a key member of the Department in the early 1940s after Dr. Seevers became chairman. I asked Dr. Quebemann to add his memories of Fred after he left Ann Arbor, MI for Madison, WI for his appointment at the University of Minnesota.

Dr. Shideman was a pharmacologist and educator. He was born on October 16, 1915 in Albion, Michigan. He was member of the Royal Society of Medicine, Japanese Pharmacology Society, Peruvian Pharmacology Society, Korean Medical Association. He was president of American Society for Pharmacology and Experimental Therapeutics from 1963-1964. Dr. Shideman was recipient of the travel award of the American Physiology Society to the XVIII International Physiology Congress in Copenhagen, Denmark in 1950.

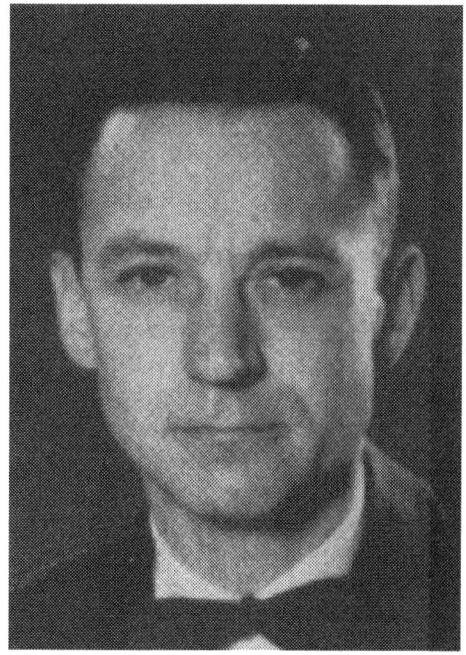

Frederick E. Shideman, ca. 1964

Dr. Frederick E. Shideman, M.D., Ph.D., Head of the Pharmacology Department, University of Minnesota, was drawn to what was noble in life, his family, his work and his friends. Photos in his office revealed what he especially valued and shaped his career. They included that of his wife, Margaret, and their wonderful family and grandchildren. He and Mrs. Shideman took tremendous pride in their family's success and happiness. His office also contained photos of his mentor Maurice Seevers.

On back of the door to his office were posted schedules of lectures to be given that day by the Department. He checked these off with a pen every day on arriving at the office. His sense of mission for the department was unstinting devotion to teaching as well as uncompromising excellence in research.

In the summer of 1962, Dr. Shideman, then Chairman of the Department of Pharmacology and Toxicology at the University of Wisconsin, was offered the headship of the Department of Pharmacology at the University of Minnesota. He assumed his duties at Minnesota on September 1, 1962. While at Wisconsin, Dr. Shideman had pursued research on renal drugs and examined the role of catecholamines as mediators of cardiac drug effects. He continued these studies throughout his tenure at Minnesota.

Dr. Shideman brought with him from Wisconsin Drs. Gilbert Mannering and Jack Miller. He decided that the Department should not focus on a single discipline, but encompass all the major areas of pharmacology. Staff members added by Dr. Shideman include Drs. Akira Takemori, Ben Zimmerman, Amedeo Marrazzi, Nelson Goldberg, Edward Cafruny, Harvey Kupferberg, Bernard Merkin, Faruk Abuzzahab, James Cumming, Donald Hun-

*Deceased

ninghake, Sheldon Sparber, Norman E. Sladek, Marion W. (Drag) Anders, Patrick E. Hanna, Aloysius Quebbemann, Xenia Machne, Earl W. Dunham, Jordan L. Holtzman, Alan R. Sinaiko, George L. Wilcox, Robert F. O'Dea, Thomas P. Green, Gustav Graff, Mark Montgomery, Elizabeth Jeffery, John A. Babson, Rita B. Messing, Timothy F. Walseth, among others. Ms. Ramona Schwasinger, who started as departmental secretary in 1962, was Dr. Shideman's first hire in Minnesota. In 2002 she continues as Executive Secretary. Jim Burak, who became the Department's first Executive Officer in 1969, continues in that role today.

Dr. Shideman added a Division of Clinical Pharmacology within the Department. With broad expertise in basic pharmacology and toxicology, and in clinical pharmacology, the Department saw remarkable growth during his tenure, developing into an internationally recognized center of excellence in pharmacology teaching and research.

Dr. Shideman was an outstanding administrator and had a social conscience which made him a friend to all in the Department. He never gave a glib answer. He respected those who disagreed with him. He often received letters or post cards from lay people commenting on some medication or theory. All such communications were posted on the departmental bulletin board.

Dr. Shideman's legacy to science will have been his success in the training and inspiration he imparted to young students. He was committed to medical student education and to the training of promising pre- and postdoctoral scientists. In 1962 he revised the courses offered by the Department. The fall of 1962 also saw the initiation of six new federally supported research programs in the Department. In addition, a grant was procured from the NIH that provided stipends for 18 predoctoral and 3 postdoctoral trainees. When the grant was activated in the spring of 1963, there were 25 predoctoral and 4 postdoctoral students in the Department. In 1976 there were 30 predoctoral students supported by the training grant and an additional 14 predoctoral students supported by other sources. The number of graduate students remained between 37 and 44 through the mid-1980s. In addition, at the time of Dr. Shideman's retirement as Professor Emeritus in 1986 the Department also had 13 postoctoral trainees and 22 faculty members. He placed great emphasis on clarity of thought and expression and imparted this to his children and his students. Dr. Shideman's son, Jeffrey R. Shideman, received his Ph.D. from the Department. When Jeff entered the graduate program, he had over 120 publications, including over 40 full-length publications, a record at Minnesota. Frederick Shideman, III is currently a M.D./Ph.D. student in the Department.

As head of the Department of Pharmacology, Dr. Shideman taught many noted pupils. He was Lou Ignarro's major advisor. After Lou submitted what he hoped would be his first publication, Dr. Shideman called him in, asked him to sit down, and told Lou that he would show him what he thought of the paper. He tore up the manuscript and threw it in the garbage. He then instructed Lou on how to properly obtain and organize his research data for scientific publication. In 1998 Lou won the Nobel Prize in Physiology or Medicine.

Vignettes: "I Remember When..."

Staff and Students of the 1940s and Beyond

My memoirs of my husband
Walter Freyburger, Ph.D.
Jeannette Freyburger

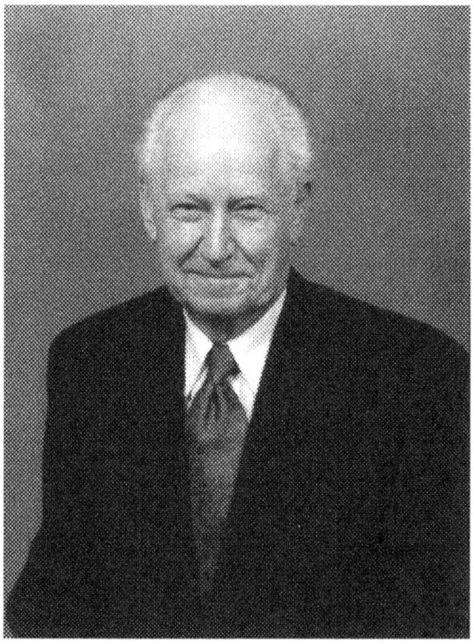

Walter was a dedicated pharmacologist and loved his work. He was a great person to have as a friend and husband. I am proud of his early research on the heart - lung machine and of his later dedication to the field of new drugs. He was also a good naturalist and wanted to leave the earth a good place for the next generation.

The University of Michigan Pharmacology Department in the late 40s delighted Walter. It was a challenging group that he thrived in.

F. Gilbert McMahon, M.D., 1947-1951

I was most fortunate in 1947 when I joined Dr. Seevers' department as a US Public Health Fellow. At that time the Department was arguably at its peak academically. I was under the tutelage of Lauren Woods, with Jim Weeks, Joe Cochin and Ray Houde in the same lab. Gordon Moe, Fred Shideman, Barbara Rennick, Leonard Procita, and Maynard Chenoweth also had their research teams, and

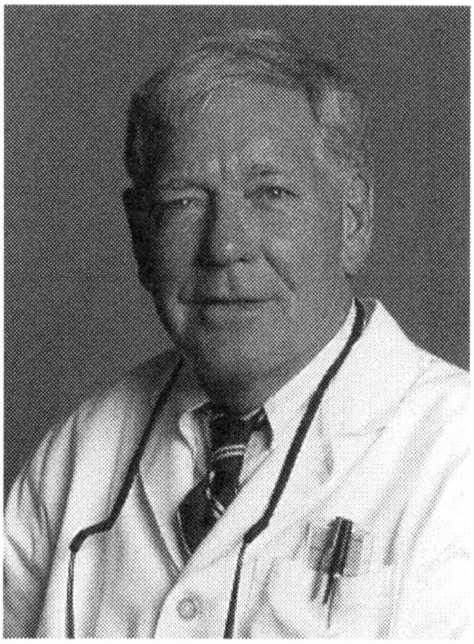

were publishing prolifically in the late 40s and early '50s.

At the end of my first year, Dr. Seevers called me into his office and told me to go across campus and apply to the medical school. My initial reaction was one of disappointment and I asked him whether he was dissatisfied with my work. He reassured me by saying, "We all get M.D.s with our Ph.D.s, and you should go for both degrees." In any event, in 1949 I entered medical school, which, certainly, profoundly influenced my life's activities. I spent weekends and vacations in Lauren Woods' lab, ending with a Masters in Pharmacology, and another year to go for my doctorate.

After I had interned, Fred Shideman, who was then chairman of Pharmacology at the University of Wisconsin, invited me to Madison where he had expected I could complete my thesis and do some teaching in his department as well as becoming a resident in internal medicine. When he took me into the Medicine chairman's office to make the arrangements, the Medicine chairman said, "My residents are full time for three years and McMahon has to decide between internal medicine and pharmacology." I chose internal medicine, but my training in pharmacology soon led to a keen interest in clinical pharmacology. Most of my professional life has been in that field. I certainly consider what successes I have had professionally to be the result of having been exposed to such a dynamic and supportive group at Michigan.

My memories of Gordon K. Moe, M.D.

Barbara Rennick, M.D. 1947-1951

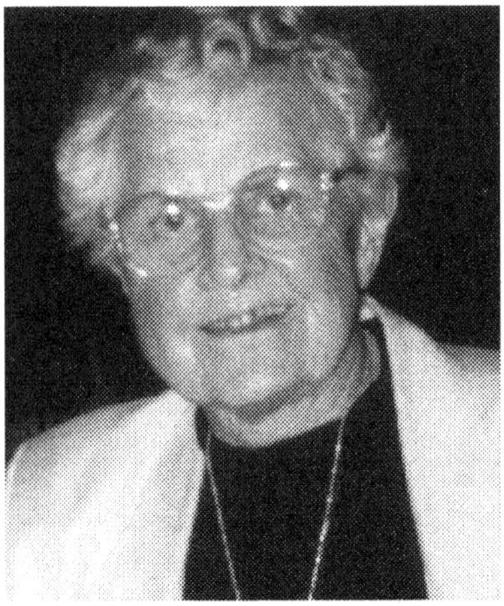

I came to the Pharmacology Department in 1946 and was accepted as a medical student and teaching fellow on a Parke-Davis stipend for two years. I worked with Gordon Moe on his research during the four years I was in Moe Seevers' department. Grace Gray came at about the same time.

Gordon was working with tetraethylammoniuim (TEA) as a ganglion blocking agent. He collaborated with Richard Lyons, an internist in the department of medicine. The rapid departure of TEA from the blood was studied, and the kidney proved to be a big factor. I continued to evaluate the kidney role and made a major study of the renal tubular active transport of organic cations, such as TEA, for 30 years. Gordon moved to chair the Department of Physiology at the new State University of New York at Syracuse; Richard Lyons also moved to Syracuse. I joined Gordon's department in my first faculty position.

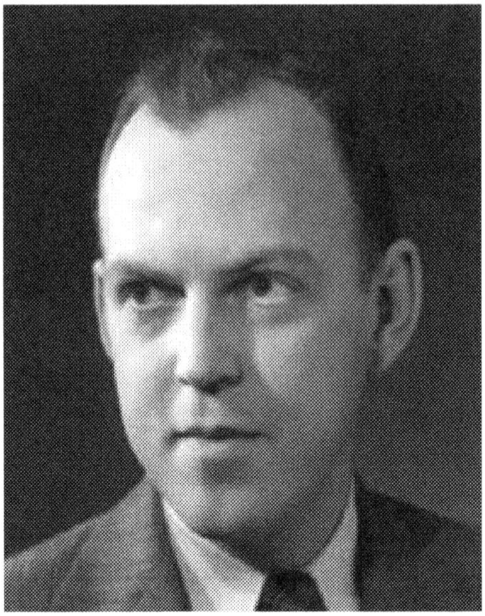

Dr. Gordon K. Moe

Gordon gave up studying TEA as a clinical tool. He advanced to study electophysiology of the heart and became prominent in the field. He accepted an accessory position as director of a research institute in Utica, NY, which was a function of the Masonic Order. He preferred this role and continued there for the rest of his life. He had national and international symposia dedicated to his work.

Editor's note: Gordon K. Moe received a Ph.D. degree in physiology from the University of Minnesota in 1940. He then was an instructor in pharmacology at Harvard while pursing a M.D. degree at that institution from 1941-1943. In 1944 he joined the Department of Pharmacology at the University of Michigan as an assistant professor. He was promoted to associate professor of pharmacology in 1946 and left the Department in 1950 to become professor and chairperson of the Physiology Department at State University of New York College of Medicine in Syracuse. In 1960 he became Director of Research of the Masonic Medical Research Laboratory in Utica, NY for the next 25 years.

16

Memoirs of Dr. Seevers' Administrative Associate, 1950-1973

Dorothy H. Overbeck, M.A.

I began my tenure as secretary in the Department of Pharmacology on July 1, 1950. I transferred from the Department of Dermatology after working for Doctor Arthur Curtis for five years on a research project. At that time, the Department of Pharmacology was small, with just Drs. Maurice H. Seevers, Maynard B. Chenoweth, Gordon K. Moe, Frederick E. Shideman, and Lauren A. Woods. Chen, Gordon, and Fred were associate professors, and Lauren was an assistant professor. I always called Chen, Fred, and Gordon the "Three Musketeers," because they remained close friends until they died. Chen and I kept in touch with annual Christmas letters until his death. Over the years, he mentioned that he, Fred, and Gordon would occasionally get together for reunions. Lauren may have been included in later years, but in 1950, he was only a junior faculty member.

The graduate students that I remember being there in 1950 were Walter Freyburger, Grace Gray, Jane Haggart, Alexander Kandel, Annetta Kelly, and Thelma Gould. We had two secretaries at that time who fulfilled all of the stenographic requirements. There were also two employees, Arthur and David, who took care of the animals. The monkey quarters were off limits to everyone except those who were working for Dr. Seevers. As I recall, Sam Irwin was about to join the Department and Dr. Seevers was his mentor. Gordon Moe was departing for the State University of New York at Syracuse in September and Walter Freyburger had accepted a position with the Upjohn Company in Kalamazoo. Walter completed his Ph.D. in 1951.

Our professional association was very informal and close-knit. When Dr. Seevers wanted to talk to someone on the third floor, he would not use the telephone. He would walk out into the front hall and yell in a booming voice for a particular faculty member or for one of the graduate students. Lauren, on the first floor, was available for personal walk-in calls.

Dr. Seevers had just resigned his position as associate dean of the medical school. He had been doing double duty as associate dean and as chairman of the Department of Pharmacology for three years. Provost Adams was urging him to reconsider his resignation as associate dean because he had done such an outstanding job of reorganizing much of the medical school administrative procedures during his tenure. Dr. Seevers expressed his sincere regrets to Provost Adams. However, he felt that all of his energy had to be directed exclusively toward the development of the Department of Pharmacology.

During the preliminary discussion regarding my duties as secretary, Dr. Seevers stressed the need for me to establish my presence and authority as the individual responsible for managing the office. This was the introduction for me to be ready and prepared to defend my position. I had not been working in the Department for more than a couple of days when Dr. Seevers spoke to me about Bill Sheldon. William Sheldon, Jr., was our laboratory technician who was in charge of the stockroom. He was responsible for setting up all of the laboratory experiments for the Medical School classes in pharmacology. He was an excellent carpenter and could design and adapt special equipment for almost any research project that the faculty devised. However, Bill was a bully and he enjoyed antagonizing people. Dr. Seevers told me to be prepared to defend my territory because Bill would certainly try to assert himself. The former secretary had been unable to stand up to him and had suffered the consequences. I was ready and able when Bill walked into the office and began to assert himself. He was introduced to a very spirited confrontation. The new secretary stood her ground, and after a few harsh words, Bill stormed out of the office. From that moment on, we were the best of friends. Dr. Seevers was very relieved and pleased that I had taken care of Bill. It was very difficult for Dr. Seevers to reprimand anyone among the graduate students or the non-academic personnel. When I "stepped up to the plate" and solved the problem with Bill, he knew that I would be able to follow through on most of the personnel problems.

It was also my job in the Department of Pharmacology to be a mind-reader. One morning Dr. Seevers wandered into the office and said that his driver's license had expired and that he had forgotten to have it renewed before his birthday. Then he proceeded to ask me why I had not reminded him that it had to be renewed! The buck stopped at my desk for a variety of things.

Dr. Seevers always parked his car at the dock entrance when we worked in the old building. He could come and go as he pleased and most importantly, he always knew where his car was parked. After the demolition of the old Economics Building, our dock space was cut in half and Dr. Seevers' car was not welcome at the dock location. He steamed and fretted and steamed some more. However, he had to move his car over to the parking garage, and that is when the fun began! He never could remember where he parked his car. I finally made a point of asking him every morning or afternoon where he had parked and I would dutifully write it down to remind him later. Otherwise, we would have a real swearing contest on his part about how he could not find his vehicle and how unfair it was that he had to park in a parking garage.

Lloyd Beck was the other person who used to lose his car. Lloyd usually came into the laboratory around 9A.M. or later and worked very late into the day. By the time he arrived, all of the choice parking spaces were taken and he had to drive around before finding a very inconvenient spot quite a distance from Medical Science I. He would be furious, of course, feeling very sorry for himself, and by the time he left for home he could not remember where his car was parked. I wonder how much time in the evenings he spent trying to find his car. I used to ask him if he wanted me to keep track of where he had parked on a day-to-day basis, as I did for Dr. Seevers. That did not always please him!

World War II had recently concluded and the Korean War had just begun. Dr. Seevers had been conducting research projects for the US government all during the war and the Army and was to continue classified research for several more years. This required all personnel who had anything to do with these projects to be fingerprinted. We probably were all screened and investigated. The monkey addiction program was gathering momentum and, therefore, we had many visits from the FBI and CIA. The University had many research projects that were under surveillance. Therefore, it did not seem unusual to be constantly visited by federal agents.

Parke-Davis and Dow Chemical were mainstays of our research programs. Quaker Oats and several government grants soon followed.

The Department really began to expand in 1951. With the addition of more faculty members and the growth in research funds, individual researchers began to acquire their own funding. The Department had a great deal of money; because of the quality and integrity of our research, Dr. Seevers and his staff had no trouble finding funds. The Department was ready for expansion and Dr. Seevers was contemplating hiring faculty and admitting more graduate students. Dr. Robert Horowitz and Dr. Mark Nickerson were the first faculty

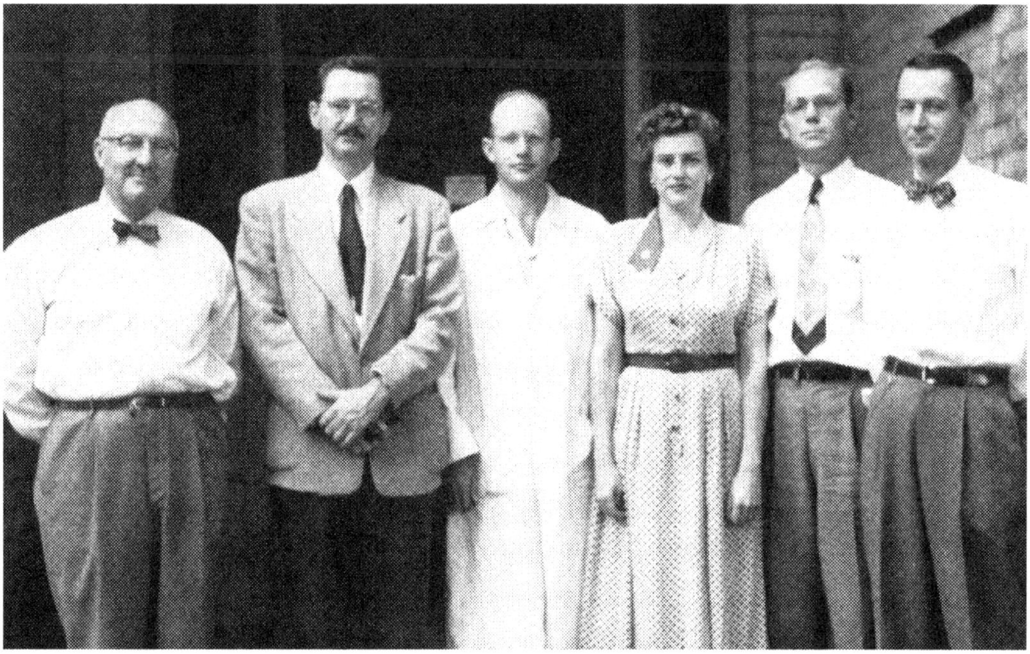

The Pharmacology faculty in 1951— Maurice Seevers, Maynard B. Chenoweth, Mark Nickerson, Dotty Norton, Lauren Woods and Frederick E. Shideman.

members to be recruited in 1951.

In May of 1951 the Second US Medical Mission was scheduled to visit Japan. All of the chairmen from the basic sciences in the Medical School went along. This was the beginning of a most extraordinary relationship between our Department and the Japanese pharmacologists who visited and studied here at Michigan. Dr. Seevers was the "goose that laid the gold egg" to improve the competency of the Japanese pharmacology. It was always a pleasure to have the Japanese as guests and students. We benefited greatly by having the opportunity to live and work together over so many years.

Fred Shideman left for the University of Wisconsin in 1952. Chen moved on to Dow Chemical in 1953 and Mark Nickerson moved to Winnipeg in 1954. During the next five years more graduate students and faculty were added. We were bulging at the seams in the old building. By that time, we were looking forward to moving into the new Medical Science Building adjacent to University Hospital. Another secretary was added and it became obvious that we needed a bookkeeper to keep track of the many research grants that were being awarded to our faculty. Events were moving along at a rapid pace. Dr. Seevers was deeply involved in teaching, lecturing, writing, supervising his research sponsored by the Committee on Drug Addiction and Narcotics, serving as an expert witness in court cases, attending board meetings, maintaining personal contacts with his associates in the pharmaceutical industry, and searching for competent pharmacologists to join the Department. He was constantly investigating avenues for research funds for his faculty. He had a national reputation for his integrity in research as well as his impeccable personal honesty. His past reputation as an outstanding scientist enhanced his ability to attract research funds from a variety of sources. Many of the faculty members and incoming graduate students had served in World War II and the Korean War. They were young and just beginning their professional careers.

We still remained a very close-knit department. Every afternoon about three o'clock we rang an old school bell announcing our tea break. Faculty, graduate students and technicians joined together in the library if it was possible to get away from their research. We moved to our new quarters in Medical Science Building I in the summer of 1958. At that time, the faculty consisted of two professors, one associate professor, two assistant professors, five instructors, and three lecturers. Dr. Seevers was chomping at the bit to move. He was driving all of us "up the wall" to get packed and ready. The new building was not completed but he toured our new quarters almost daily. We finally moved and unpacked but things were in a state of chaos. There were a great number of misplaced boxes and many complaints. If Dr. Seevers could have waited just another few weeks, the move would have been much smoother.

There were only three times during my tenure of 23 years when I was ready to resign. The 1958 move was the ultimate! The buck stopped in my office with all of the complaints. Poor Lauren Woods was one of the frustrated movers. He discovered that all of the gas and air jets on his laboratory benches were reversed. The laboratory tables had been designed by architects and not scientists. He appeared in my office late one afternoon and wanted something to be done about this problem. Somehow, his complaint was the last straw. I remember that I was very unpleasant and told him if I heard just one more complaint from anybody that I was going to quit. He looked at me with a startled expression, turned around and walked out of the office. I believe that I apologized to him the next day.

Most of the faculty and staff were delighted with their new quarters. We had all the room in the world for research and especially for storage. With so much storage room, Dr. Seevers, who tended to be a "pack rat" of sorts, had the seventh level storeroom loaded with all kinds of useless equipment that he could not bear to throw away. One of the few times in our long association when he was really furious with me concerned throwing away some of his precious "junk." While he was away on one of his frequent extended trips during the late 1960s, Bill Sheldon was trying to make room for important supplies and he consulted with me about getting rid of some of the useless equipment that we had trucked over from the old building. We decided that it would never be missed because Dr. Seevers rarely went to the storage area and did not know what was there. Bill carefully selected what was to be discarded. While it was still piled up on the loading dock, Dr. Seevers returned home several days ahead of schedule. He parked his car beside the dock and saw the evidence. He flew into the air, and Bill and I were in the doghouse. He had Bill haul all of that junk back to the storage room. Luckily, Dr. Seevers never held a grudge and after he had spoken his piece, the air always cleared with no hard feelings.

The move to Medical Science Building I signaled the acceleration of acceptance of graduate students for the Master of Science and Ph.D. degrees in Pharmacology. Several of our graduate students chose to study for Ph.D./M.D. degrees. We had been awarded a substantial sum of money from the USPHS for graduate support and this grant was still in effect when I retired in 1973. We had support from the Kellogg Foundation since the early 1950s. Kellogg concentrated their funding on South and Central American students. The students were required to attend the English Language Institute at Michigan before they could be admitted to the curriculum. Miles Laboratories supported our Mexican students. Some support was forthcoming from grants from Parke-Davis and Dow Chemical, provided a student was doing grant-related research. I recall that Ben Lucchesi and Ray Ruddon were awarded support grants from the American Cancer Society Foundation. These were outstanding awards.

Dr. Edward Carr began developing his program in clinical pharmacology, and by 1966 the Upjohn Company agreed to fund the program. Dr. Carr became the first director of the Upjohn Center for Clinical Pharmacology in 1966, which was completed in 1970. Dr. Carr held a joint appointment in the Departments of Pharmacology and Internal Medicine.

Dr. Seevers' drug addiction and narcotics program began to expand. Dr. Charles Schuster arrived in 1963 to join this program, as did Dr. James Woods in 1965. Both of these scientists were trained psychologists. Dr. Gerald Deneau received his Ph.D. in Pharmacology in 1957 and was in charge of the narcotics program under Dr. Seevers until he left the Department in 1965.

Dr. Seevers hired Bob Shepherd as carpenter and shop person to share Bill Sheldon's duties. Two laboratory assistants were hired to care for the monkeys. Our secretarial staff increased to three full time secretaries and a bookkeeper. I was not greatly involved in the regular secretarial work. We were very fortunate over the years to have had excellent secretaries. Our very best secretary over those years was Ellen Benner Howard, who is still working with Dr. Domino. Rosalind Arbour was our bookkeeper for 13 years and was another of the best.

On the whole, the Department ran very smoothly. Our faculty and staff were fortunate because Dr. Seevers' philosophy was that as long as you did your teaching and research and produced a high standard of results in both areas, your personal life was your own business. He did not burden his faculty with extra assignments and meetings. We had very few problems throughout my 20-year stay. The ones which did arise, Dr. Seevers managed to solve quite satisfactorily. He was traveling a great deal of the time and he loved the challenges that these important assignments offered to him.

The student unrest during the 1960s did not concern us except that we made a rule that none of the secretaries should work at any time except between 8:00 a.m. and 5:00 p.m. We felt that the riot on South University in the mid-60s and the subsequent camping of students and other persons all over the Diag on central campus and the sit-ins being carried on in the churches around campus perhaps made for unsafe and unstable conditions.

Dr. Seevers was scheduled to retire in 1971. According to University procedures, a search committee was appointed three years before the retirement of a departmental chairman in order to find a replacement. As usual, the time passed and the committee could not agree on a candidate. Dr. Seevers retired on schedule and Dr. Henry Swain was appointed as acting chairman. I had planned to retire with Dr. Seevers. We were then to move to the offices across the hall from the Departmental office. This did not occur and I agreed to stay on until a new administrative assistant could be hired. I retired in 1973.

I would like to add that working for Dr. Seevers and for the Department of Pharmacology was one of the most important chapters in my life. Dr. Seevers was a brilliant person. He was intelligent, a scholar, a true "bench man" in research, possessed with tremendous energy to give of himself in all of his numerous professional activities. He was a person of impeccable integrity whether it related to his research, the decisions he was called on to make in departmental matters, and as a member of the many important committees to which he was elected. He could be very blunt and freely gave his honest opinion on the subject at hand. He never held a grudge, always apologized and admitted if he was in error. He had a delightful sense of humor and you always felt his total lack of self-importance. I could never understand why so many graduate students were scared of him. He often mentioned that he wished the students would come into his office and talk to him. The faculty felt free to do that and he was always pleased to see them.

The Department of Pharmacology under Dr. Seevers' chairmanship produced many outstanding pharmacologists during his tenure. The "old man," as we affectionately called him, was so proud of all of his "boys." He was always sorry to see them leave Michigan but he knew that all of them were on the thresholds of important careers.

Even after all of these years, many happy memories remain with me. Given the opportunity, I would repeat all those years with Dr. Seevers in the Department.

Memoirs: Before, At Michigan, and After

Harold F. Hardman, M.D., Ph.D.

I grew up in the town of Bloomfield, NJ, where I could see the Empire State Building located 13 miles east of my bedroom window. Two miles south was the Schering Pharmaceutical Company and two miles north was the Hoffmann-LaRoche Pharmaceutical Company. So, I was always exposed to either vitamins or hormones, depending upon which way the wind was blowing.

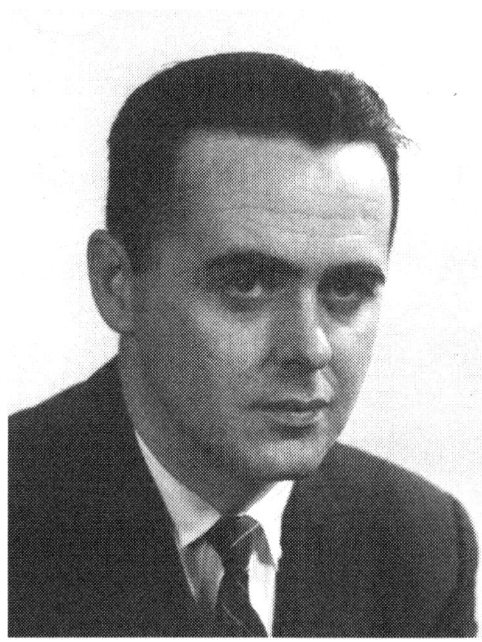

I had an uncle who was a pharmacist; he stimulated my interest in drugs and medicine. I worked with him from 1941-1946, and I enrolled in Rutgers College of Pharmacy in 1944. It was close to home which permitted me to commute, save money, and keep my job in the drug store. I applied for and was granted a scholarship from the American Foundation for Pharmaceutical Education, which I maintained until I received the Ph.D. degree in 1954.

I was drafted into the Army at 19, after I had completed two years of college. I functioned as a pharmacist in Tokyo in the Army of Occupation. When I returned from army duty, I enrolled in pharmacy again but I had decided not to become a pharmacist. I wanted to go to graduate school and get a Ph.D. I then visited Schering, Hoffmann LaRoche, and Ortho Pharmaceutical companies to gain their advice about where to study pharmacology. The University of Illinois and the University of Michigan were the most attractive suggestions to me. I chose Illinois because the program started in September, whereas the Michigan program started in June. I wanted the summer of 1949 to take additional courses in biology; my background was strong in chemistry but weak in biology.

I interviewed at the University of Illinois in Chicago and met Ted Brody, who was completing his M.Sc. degree in the College of Pharmacy. He had decided to switch to the medical school to get his Ph.D. in pharmacology, and he advised me to plan the same. I was accepted and Dr. Theodore Sherrod was assigned as my mentor. He was serving an internship and had very little time to spend with me. Mostly I got help from fellow students who were further along in their training; Keith Killam and John Adams were most helpful. My second year was filled with course work and laboratory work on dogs and rabbits. Dr. Sherrod worked patiently with me to evaluate the coronary vasodilator action of several drugs on isolated perfused rabbit hearts and on intact dog hearts. The highlight of the year was the presentation of my first 10 minute paper at the Federation meetings in Cleveland (1951).

My modest research efforts were not considered good enough to be published, and I began to think about transferring to a department where there was a more active program in cardiovascular research. I chose Michigan because they were using the dog-heart-lung preparation with frequent publications by Dr. Gordon Moe and Dr. Maynard Chenoweth. It was a technique I wanted to learn. I made the move to Michigan in 1951 with the blessings of Dr. Sherrod and the chairman of the department, Dr. Carl Pfeiffer.

When I arrived at Michigan, Dr. Gordon Moe had left; he was replaced by Dr. Mark Nickerson. I was assigned to Dr. Chenoweth and incorporated into a program studying chelation as a mechanism of drug action. Chenoweth proposed that the chelation of copper by the cardiac glycosides was responsible for the positive inotropic action of digitalis. I spent a year and a half on this project, but we failed to put together a publishable paper.

Dr. Chenoweth next proposed that I go to work on the dog-heart-lung preparation, comparing the inotropic activity of theophylline and aminophylline. Numerous anecdotal reports claimed aminophylline to be the superior cardiac stimulant. This advantage was attributed to the ethylenediamine solubilizing agent. When injected rapidly, aminophylline causes a rapid fall in blood pressure and sometimes cardiac arrest. This response is not seen with theophylline alone and is apparently related to the chelate structure of ethylenediamine. Calcium ions appear to be the substance being chelated. This was my first attempt to get a paper published, and it was accepted just as submitted by the Journal of Pharmacology and Experimental Therapeutics (JPET). Dr. Chenoweth said I was lucky to have a first attempt accepted immediately; he doubted that it would ever happen again. He was right— it never did.

Dr. Chenoweth left the Department of Pharmacology to work at the Dow Chemical Company in 1953, and I expanded my studies on theophylline to include a series of substituted purine derivatives. The amino substituted purine derivative, 2,6-diaminopurine sulfate, appeared to be superior to the methylated xanthines as a cardiac stimulant.

My thesis defense was scheduled for April 12, 1954. Dr. Mark Nickerson, a member of my thesis committee, failed to appear. It was reported that the President of the University of Michigan had suspended him because he was being investigated by the House Unamerican Activities Committee and he was not cooperating with them. The president subsequently fired him despite the fact that he held tenure. Nickerson pleaded protection under the First and Fifth Amendments. He acknowledged that he had supported organizing lumbermen in a union to gain health benefits, but he refused to testify against his friends and colleagues. I knew him as a friend with whom I worked and I admired his skills as a scientist. I also went fishing with him on rare occasions. The chairman of pharmacology at Michigan, Dr. Maurice Seevers, wanted to get rid of Nickerson but blocked him from getting another job in the US. Under the cover of darkness he drove to Winnipeg for a waiting position as Professor and Chairman of Pharmacology at the University of Manitoba. I bought his Penn-Yan fishing boat and kept it until the mid-70s when I sold it to a graduate student who named it "Phenoxy." It may still be afloat. Dr. Nickerson offered me the opportunity to move to Canada and work with him, but I declined the offer with regrets.

The American Association of University Professors (AAUP) investigated the firing of Dr. Nickerson and censured the University of Michigan. The censure subsequently was revoked when the university agreed to recognize the constitutional rights and tenure of the faculty. The local AAUP requested compensation be given to Dr. Nickerson. He was invited to return to the campus and meet with students and faculty to discuss academic freedom. Now the University holds an annual lecture on academic freedom named after Davis, Markert, and Nickerson.

My support of Dr. Nickerson, who never discussed communism with me, did not go unnoticed in the Department. There were no significant pay raises for several years, and I eventually left the department at the first convenient opportunity. I was later proud to propose Dr. Nickerson for an honorary D. Sc. degree from the Medical College of Wisconsin in 1974. This was his main honorary degree. My assignments in the Pharmacology Department increased in 1955 when I was given the responsibility for a contract with the Army Chemical Center at Edgewood Arsenal. They were interested in the pharmacology of a series of eight delta 3-tetrahydrocannabinols to determine if they had any potential value as incapacitating agents. The contract was worth $25,000 per year. I hired several medical students to work with me on this project. The outstanding response we observed in unanesthetized dogs and monkeys was a profound central nervous system depression that lasted for several hours or days, depending upon the dose of drug employed. Some dogs remained unconscious for periods up to six days following a single intravenous injection of 10mg/kg of EA 1476. During this period of CNS depression the mean heart rate of the dogs was reduced from control values of 100 to 20 beats per minute; mean respiratory rates were reduced from control values of 30 to three per minute and deep rectal temperatures were reduced from mean control values of 39.1 degrees C to 29.6 degrees C. The dogs appeared to be in a state of hibernation, and yet they could be aroused by picking them up, shaking them and placing them on their feet in an upright position.

The Army Chemical Center was very interested in the potential usefulness of these chemical agents. Our work became classified security information and remained classified unti1 August 1970. The army thought that EA 1476 might be administered to injured personnel so that definitive treatment could be delayed for several days while the personnel were transported to treatment centers.

We were impressed with the outstanding pharmacological activity of the delta 3-tetra-3 hydrocannabinols and their relative lack of toxic effects. These synthetic marijuana derivatives produced a state of sleep unlike that induced by the barbiturates since the animals could be aroused readily with minimal stimulation. In many ways this class of compounds resembled the newly introduced tranquilizers reserpine and chlorpromazine. The animals also exhibited an indifference to painful stimuli, which suggested that the delta 3-tetra-3 hydrocannabinols possessed analgesic activity. Further studies indicated that this class of compounds produced outstanding effects upon the cardiovascular system and were capable of lowering the blood pressure of dogs to a significant degree. There is a prolonged latent period (two hours) before the fall in blood pressure becomes statistically significant. The hypotensive response appears to result from an action of the drug within the central nervous system resulting in a decreased outflow of sympathetic nerve impulses. If one sections the spinal cord at C-1 in the dog or cat, the hypotensive action of EA 1476 is prevented. Another pharmacological action of the tetrahydrocannabinols is that they lower deep rectal temperature when the environmental temperature is maintained at 25 degrees C. With doses of 1mg/kg., i.v. of EA 1476 the average fall in deep rectal temperature 12 hours later was 2.9 degrees C. and it progressed to 9.2 degrees C. at 24 hours. Significant changes in rectal temperature can be seen as soon as two hours after intravenous administration.

When this contract was declassified in 1970 I applied for a grant from the National Institute of Drug Abuse in order to expand my studies on the hypotensive and hypothermic actions of the tetrahydrocannabinols. This grant was funded from 1972 to 1984, at which time I stepped down as principal investigator. Drs. Domino, Seevers, and I published two review articles on the synthetic tetrahydrocannabinols in Pharmacological Reviews in 1971.

Another part of the Army Chemical Center contract was to examine mescaline and related analogs to determine their behavioral effect and toxicity in five species of laboratory animals. The effect of mescaline and seven mescaline analogs was studied in the mouse, rat, and guinea pig following intraperitoneal administration. The LD50 value was determined for each of the above species. For seven of the eight drugs tested the LD50 value is significantly lower in the rat than in mouse or guinea pig, The LD50 values for the above drugs were also determined in the mongrel dog and rhesus monkey following intravenous administration. A comparison of the observable signs of drug action in the dog and monkey shows the dog to be the preferred species for evaluating the behavioral effects of this class of drugs. The superiority of the dog as a species for evaluating these compounds was shown by the fact that specific effects consistently observed with mescaline and its analogs in the dog but not in the monkey include: ataxia, clonic convulsions, salivation, emesis, apprehension or fright, and apparent hallucinations. This work was reported to the Army Chemical Center at Edgewood Arsenal in 1953-54, declassified in October 1969, and accepted for publication in 1972.

In 1954 my mentor, Maynard Chenoweth, was established in his new position at Dow Chemical. He was studying general anesthetic compounds. Our colaboration was completed and I was searching for a project of my own. I had been given full responsibility for the army contract relating to the pharmacology of the tetrahydrocannabinoids, but that work was classified. I needed a project that I could publish. I had been impressed by a publication in Pharmacological Reviews by Adrian Albert titled "Ionization, pH and Biological Activity" (Pharmacol. Rev. 1.136-168.1952). I bought a copy of his first textbook, titled Selective Toxicity, published in 1951 (with a price of $1.75), as well as subsequent editions up to the seventh, published in 1985. The first edition was a small monograph (6-1/2 x 4"), totaling 227 pages. It was the only book that I ever wore out by handling. I was prepared for a surprise in the student physiology laboratory where we were perfusing the heart of a turtle with Ringer's solution. I tested the pH of the perfusate and found it to be 10.0. The turtle heart continued to beat in a regular manner without loss of the amplitude of contraction. I realized that I had made a discovery that I could use in studying drug ionization and pH in a biological system. You can't vary the pH of perfused mamalian hearts over the range of 6.5 to 10.5, but you can do this with a turtle heart. I maintained an active research program studying the effect of drug ionization upon pharmacological activity for the next 19 years. I felt that Adrian Albert was my real mentor in pharmacology.

The move from Michigan to Marquette was exciting in several ways. I was asked to improve the performance of the medical students on the National Board examination in pharmacology by the medical school dean. The graduate school dean also asked me to establish a graduate program in pharmacology.

Dr. Harry Beckman, the Chairman of Pharmacology at Marquette, was president of ASPET in 1957. He was one of the key figures in convincing the National Institute of General Medical Sciences to fund training grants in pharmacology. A few years later, in 1960, he applied to the NIGMS for a small grant to train clinical pharmacologists. The plan was to recruit medical students who had completed the first two years and would then complete the Ph.D. and M.D. degree over a five-year period. The program was unique and a forerunner of the Medical Scientist Training Program (MSTP 1964). It was designed to accept one student per year for five years and then graduate one student per year. The grant was approved and funded when I arrived at Marquette.

Dr. Beckman named me director of the grant in 1961 and I applied for a supplement to fund straight Ph.D. programs also. The supplement was approved and funded. The chairman of the site visit team told me that we should have asked for more money. We concentrated on developing the graduate training-programs over the next several years and were shocked when our training grant was not recommended for renewal (1966). We tried to determine what was wrong with our program, but were not able to gain any information from NIH about the reasons for not renewing our grant. Out of a sense of desperation I contacted my congressional representative, Henry Reuss, who was chairman of the House Appropriations Committee. With his help we were able to negotiate a five-year phase out program. I raised additional funds from several pharmaceutical companies and we were able to fund all the graduate students in the program at that time. We decided to reduce our graduate program from 20 to 10 full time students. We also put increased effort into gaining more research grants and used technician salaries to support graduate students.

In October of 1969 I distributed a paper I had written about training grants to a meeting of NIGMS directors of pharmacology training grants. The paper was critical of the distribution of training grants where several training grants in pharmacology were awarded to the same university, i.e., medical school, pharmacy school, and veterinary school. This happened in several states, when my grant was being phased out. The state of Wisconsin was not being treated fairly, since the pharmacology training grant at Marquette was superior to the paramedical pharmacology training grants in the neighboring states of Minnesota and Iowa. I gained considerable support from my colleagues in pharmacology, many of whom were losing their training grants and were anxious to maintain graduate training in their departments. I had proposed a reduction in the size of the individual training grants so that some funds could be assigned to all approved programs. The NIGMS did change the rules for funding training grants a few years later. They decided to fund only one pharmacological sciences training grant per institution.

I was elected secretary of the Association of Medical School Pharmacologists (AMSP) for the period 1970-1972. Dr. George Acheson was elected president of AMSP for that time. I inherited the position of acting president during 1971-72 while Dr. Acheson was on sabbatical leave in England; I felt like one of the founding fathers of AMSP.

My exposure to the movers and shakers of pharmacology provided many opportunities to get involved in the various aspects of ASPET. One of the purposes of AMSP was to bring together the chairmen of pharmacology departments, many of whom were not graduates of classical pharmacology departments. The group was small, averaging about 30-40 chairmen per meeting. The emphasis was built around academic problems related to teaching, medical school administration, and graduate student training. We encouraged regional meetings and expanded scheduled meetings (spring FASEB and fall ASPET) to include winter AMSP meetings. We also got involved in the problems relating to the funding of research grants.

My contributions to pharmacology as secretary and acting president of AMSP involved the collection of vital statistics. It was difficult for me to understand why so many chairmen did not want to participate in sharing data about space and finances. Dr. Elliot Vesell was asked to survey US and Canadian departments of pharmacology in 1973. AMSP voted 19 yes and 10 no to ask for information on space and finances. Dr. Vesell's survey was the first effort to begin the collection and dissemination of vital statistics. This beginning evolved into the yearly report on salaries, faculty distribution, space, number of graduate students, research grant income, etc. The Hardman-Brody questionnaire was completed in the 1978-80 period, while I was president of AMSP. Another project initiated in that 1970-72 period was the encouragement of regional meetings. They have continued to grow in size and value.

In 1971 as acting president of AMSP, I met with ASPET Council and suggested that we publish in the Pharmacologist a list of available positions in medical school departments. The ASPET Council granted unanimous approval and directed Dr. Cook, our executive officer, to circulate a questionnaire to pharmacology chairmen to collect the data. At the next meeting of ASPET Council the suggestion to share information on open positions was turned down because it was felt that the list would be incomplete and inaccurate. I concluded that some chairmen were embarrassed by their riches and preferred to keep their good fortune confidential.

Another role for the president of AMSP was to offer help to deans searching for pharmacology chairmen. In addition, while president of AMSP, I served on several extramural pharmacology review committees. My contribution as president of AMSP (1978-80) included my presentation of how various medical schools utilized indirect costs from federal grants. I appointed a committee to explore this important mechanism to supplement research support. I developed a draft of a questionnaire to determine whether and how indirect cost revenues from grants are reallocated to departments of pharmacology. The Executive Committee wanted to rework the draft questionnaire with me. I suggested that each pharmacology department gather the data that is needed for a departmental review. We could then share these data with one another and computerize them. I also agreed to continue to search for the mechanisms that permitted some indirect costs to be returned to the earning department. Dr. Walaszek conducted a survey over a period of four years and showed that over this time period the number of departments receiving a share of indirect costs increased from zero to 34. The magnitude of the amount received by the department varied from 2.5% to 22% of the total indirect costs. Now departmental chairmen could negotiate a new source of income with their deans. I introduced the concept at MCW and we negotiated a 15% return for all departments. I recall my presidency of AMSP as a time when we were very productive in upgrading pharmacology.

I was chosen as a member of the review team for Central Academic Administration at MCW. The AAMC provided a database on all aspects of medical schools administration, which included the database on pharmacology. We had all the information we needed relating to faculty salaries. We were surprised to find that the AAMC data was a year old because of the medical schools' delays in sending the information to the AAMC. We were able to generate the same data and distribute it within a few months so that it was current and not a year old when we negotiated budgets with our deans. My interaction with Dr. Paul Jolly, director of the Division of Operational Studies of the AAMC, opened the door for extensive information about various databases relating to medical school administration and finances. Creating the AMSP Questionnaire (Annual Report) provided key information to departmental chairmen in the direction of their departments.

Dr. John Burns, president of ASPET, appointed me as Chairman of the Program Committee in 1973. This was a good assignment that provided an opportunity to become familiar with the research programs of many members of ASPET. During the three years that I was Chairman of the Committee the emphasis was to increase the number and quality of the symposia.

Another goal was to introduce poster sessions. The problem we faced was a lack of rooms for oral presentations of the 10-minute papers at the Hotel Dennis, our headquarters hotel. I met a lot of resistance from ASPET members who were opposed to poster sessions. Several ASPET members threatened to resign from the society if their papers were assigned to a poster session. Dr. Arnold Schwartz was of great help to the committee because at my request he gave demonstrations of poster sessions at the spring FASEB meetings in Atlantic City. Gradually the poster session gained acceptance, and today many members of ASPET find it to be the preferred method for presentation.

I moved from Chairman of the Program Committee to the elected position of Councillor for the period 1976-79. I chaired several award committees (the ASPET award and the Sollmann award) and learned that in selecting referees to judge the candidates those judges closest to the field of a given candidate were generally more critical than judges from other fields of interest. One had to be careful to choose an equal variety of judges for each candidate.

I was elected president of ASPET from 1982-84 and completed the transition from oral presentations to posters as the primary method for presenting our research. Another project was the development of the Corporate Associates Program. The income from this source had remained level for the previous five years (1978-83). I took a direct solicitation of the major pharmaceutical companies asking them to pledge $6000 per year. My goal was to obtain 10 pledges in this amount and designate them as Major Benefactors. We also gained increased numbers of contributors with more modest pledges. The result was an income that was twice as large as the ones received during the previous five years. I initiated a dinner meeting for council and representatives from the major benefactors category so we could tell them how we were spending their contributions. This program has continued to grow each year and now represents a major source of income.

On my watch as president the nominating committee brought me the first all-female slate for the office of president of ASPET. Marjorie Horning was elected as our first female president. During the years when I held elected office in ASPET, I also participated in professional activities such as editorial boards and review panels. These included: Journal of Medicinal & Pharmaceutical Chemistry, Wisconsin Medical Journal, Journal of Pharmacology & Experimental Therapeutics, Research Communications in Substance Abuse, Journal of Cardiovascular Pharmacology, National Institute on Drug Abuse, National Institute of General Medical Sciences Pharmacology Study Section, Chairman of Joint Food and Drug Administration National Institute of Mental Health Drug Abuse Advisory Committee, and Basic Pharmacology Advisory Committee of the Pharmaceutical Manufacturers Association Foundation.

Walter Ellis was the public affairs officer for FASEB when I took office as president in 1984. Ellis then died and was replaced by Gar Gaganovitch. Gar was chosen by me and Executive Officer Robert Krausst because he was the Chief Staffer for Senator Lowell Weicker's Senate Appropriations Committee. Gar guided us and arranged for me to be the first FASEB president to testify before the chairman of the Senate Appropriations Committee. I asked for a 25% increase over the 5000 RO-1 grants proposed by Dr. Friedrickson, Director of NIH. The strategy behind this request was that the younger investigators, having more modest grant requests, would be favored in funding and the very large grants would be more limited than in the past. The proposal for 6250 RO-1 grants was supported by Senator Weicker and his committee and subsequently approved by Congress.

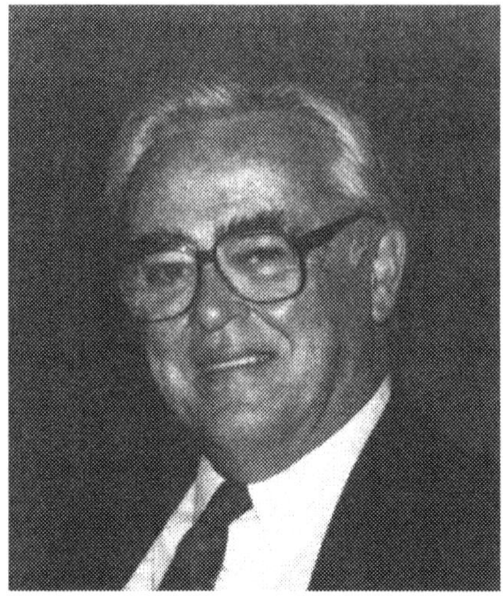

A distinguished Harry Hardman.

In addition to interacting with the chairmen of key congressional committees, we urged members of FASEB to contact their congressional representatives and tell them what we are doing to improve health through biomedical research.

A project that I endorsed over the objections of ASPET Council was the creation of a new journal to replace Federation Proceedings (FP). The biochemists in particular were critical of the scientific quality of the articles published. The pharmacologists and pathologists used FP to publish synposia which were not considered to be acceptable for publication in the best review journals. I voted to move this project forward and convinced the biochemists that they had to take an active role in developing the new replacement journal, which we called The FASEB Journal. Today our journal is ranked the third most prestigous biomedical journal, after Nature and Science.

The new conference center and the wings on the Milton O. Lee building provided expansion space for the member societies. Pharmacology was the only society that did not want any additional space. I hope we will not regret our decision in the future as ASPET thrives within a growing FASEB.

Memoirs: 1952-Present

Theodore M. Brody, Ph.D.

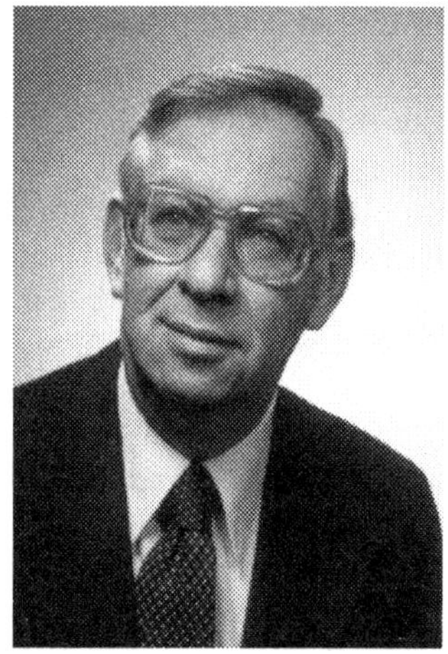

The Early Years

My education in pharmacology began in 1947 at the University of Illinois Medical Center, Chicago. Prior to that time I had received a B.S. degree from Rutgers University and spent three years in the US Army during World War II with service in the South Pacific. Five years at Illinois were exciting under the dynamic leadership of Dr. Carl Pfeiffer, and with Dr. James Bain as my mentor. Both Pfeiffer and Bain later served as presidents of the American Society for Pharmacology and Experimental Therapeutics (ASPET). The graduate students were a hard-driving group of bright individuals who provided me with more than an adequate challenge. In addition to the usual Ph.D. candidates, the program at Illinois offered research training and M.S. degrees to medical students interested in careers in pharmacology. This resulted in a significant number of potential medical practitioners selecting teaching and research as their life's work. Many in the group were later to make seminal contributions to the discipline and to public health. Several also served as presidents of ASPET (Drs. Steven Mayer, Eva and Keith Killam and Harold Hardman). Of the student group, Edward Domino, Henry Swain, and Hardman also became faculty members at the U of M.

Pharmacology was just beginning its growth phase at this time, so during the late 1940s and early 1950s there were no special courses in pharmacology available for graduate students because the information base was still fairly limited. The standard medical course in pharmacology provided just about all that was pertinent. During the first two years, Ph.D. candidates took the same basic science courses offered to medical students, did research, and wrote a thesis. Mine was "On the possible role of oxidative phosphorylation as a mechanism of drug action," an early foray into the new and exciting field of biochemical pharmacology.

I was awarded the Ph.D. degree in 1952, at which time my mentor, Dr. Bain, suggested postdoctoral training. He recommended Dr. Albert Lehninger, then at the University of Chicago, and Dr. Van Potter at Wisconsin. I visited with them at their respective institutions. Unfortunately, Lehninger was leaving for Cambridge on sabbatical, but Van Potter offered me a fellowship. I had just about decided on Madison when Carl Pfeiffer suggested I visit Dr. Maurice Seevers, Chair of Pharmacology at The University of Michigan. (A close relationship existed between Pfeiffer and Seevers since the latter had been Pfeiffer's mentor at the University of Wisconsin.) Apparently there was the possibility of a position. An opening had occurred because Associate Professor Dr. Fred Shideman had left for Wisconsin to become Professor and Chair.

The Ann Arbor Days

I drove to Ann Arbor, discussed the position with Dr. Seevers, dined with Mose and his wife Frankie, and was offered the position as Instructor of Pharmacology at a salary of $5,500 per annum, which I accepted. My wife Ethel and I moved to Ann Arbor and I began my academic career on September 1, 1952. I will always be grateful for this opportunity; a beginning, which in no small part profoundly shaped the direction of my life.

Prior to my arrival, there were five pharmacology faculty at UM, including Fred Shideman. All (Seevers, Nickerson, Shideman, Woods and Chenoweth) had either M.D./ Ph.D. or M.D. degrees, and I became the only faculty member without a professional degree, although I felt that I had a reasonable background in the basic medical sciences. Interestingly, a similar situation had existed at Illinois, where my mentor, Dr. Bain, was the only faculty member without a medical degree. Both Seevers and Pfeiffer believed it to be advantagous for faculty to have the M.D. degree, in addition to a Ph.D., which at that time was not unusual for most departments of pharmacology. (In the 1950s, more than sixty percent of academic pharmacologists were M.D.'s while currently less than five percent of faculty in this country possess the M.D. degree).

The UM Department of Pharmacology was housed in an old building which was originally the Chemistry Building erected in 1855, and remodeled many times. The building on the Diag and across from the Undergraduate Library housed the Department from 1910 until 1958, when the Department moved into the new Medical Science I, adjacent to the University Hospital. The old pharmacology building was finally razed in 1969, after being set afire by an arsonist.

It was from Mose Seevers that I became familiar with the do's and don'ts of department administration, and my fourteen years at Michigan were a significant learning experience, enabling me to survive as a Chair in the years ahead. Mose was an extremely colorful individual, dedicated to Michigan and to his discipline. He worked hard, partied hard, wrote extremely well, had a good command of the spoken word and was successful in almost all he set his sights on. He characteristically used salty language liberally sprinkled with memorable barnyard metaphors. A graduate of Washburn College in Topeka, Kansas, he was president of his class and captain of the football team. He worked his way through college, graduate and medical schools, receiving the Ph.D. in Pharmacology in 1928 and the M.D. in 1930 from the University of Chicago. He accompanied his mentor, Arthur Tatum to the University of Wisconsin, took a two-year internship, and subsequently achieved the rank of Associate Professor in the Department of Pharmacology. He left Madison for Ann Arbor to become Professor and Chair in 1942. Seevers' contributions to pharmacology, both nationally and internationally, have been well-documented. He served as president of ASPET twice, founded its Board of Publications Trustees, was instrumental in the organizing of IUPHAR, served on many editorial boards, NIH study sections, national and international commissions, and was considered a world expert on narcotic dependence and tolerance development.

Seevers was a vigorous supporter of the Ph.D. program in pharmacology, and the Department produced a large number of Ph.D.s during his tenure. He also encouraged all Ph.D. recipients to continue on to the M.D. degree, convinced that medical training was essential to establishing credibility with medical students and rapport with clinical faculty. His tour de force was in providing Japanese physicians with training in the Department of Pharmacology at Michigan, since no pharmacology graduate training programs were available in Japan at the time. A large number of Japanese spent several years at UM and returned to Japan to occupy pre-eminent positions in the field, both in academia and industry. Seevers' influence on Japanese pharmacology will undoubtedly be felt for decades.

The major blemish on the Seevers escutcheon was the Mark Nickerson incident during the infamous McCarthy era and the Un-American Activities Committee hearings in 1954. In my view, Dr. Nickerson's firing by the University resulted primarily from the

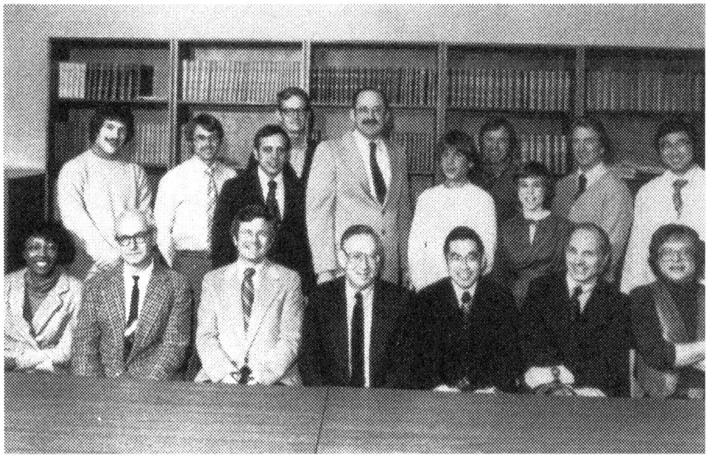

The pharmacology faculty of Michigan State University, ca. 1978.

failure of Seevers to support him. Nickerson had announced to the medical faculty that he had once been, but was no longer, a member of the Communist Party. Nickerson, who was a tenured associate professor, and had joined the faculty a year before I had, was nationally known as an outstanding young pharmacologist and had been the recipient of the John Jacob Abel Award in 1949. After he was dismissed, he and his family fled to Canada where he became Professor and Chair of the Department of Pharmacology at the University of Manitoba. Later he held a similar post at McGill. Nickerson and I had been jointly responsible for a large part of the laboratory instruction in the medical pharmacology course. I vigorously defended Nickerson's actions both publicly and privately, and as a result found myself in the proverbial doghouse. It is my perception that my job was no longer in jeopardy when I received ASPET's John Jacob Abel Award in 1955.

My years at Ann Arbor were happy and productive. Our four children were born there. Research efforts went well. In the early 1950s I was fortunate to obtain an NIH grant of $8,000 per year, which was later supplemented by a similar amount from the Office of Naval Research. This was a time when one could hire a technician for $2,500! Publications appeared, grant support grew, and I was further fortunate to have a number of outstanding graduate students who chose to work in my laboratory. This included a significent contingent from the University of Alberta. I also had a talented group of postdoctoral fellows and technicians. Superior students, adequate funding, time to think, and departmental support are truly the keys to a successful scientific career. I really appreciated the practice of the department chair in allowing me to have complete freedom in my scientific endeavors, and later attempted to follow that example. As with many departments during that period, pharmacology at Michigan grew in size and thrived.

Some of my doctoral graduates at Ann Arbor included: Drs. James Miller '54, Glenn Kiplinger '59, Deane Calvert and Kenneth Moore '60, Paula Stern and Roger Hornbrook '63, James Gibb and Jack Diamond '65, and John McNeill '67. Among Japanese postdoctoral fellows were Drs. Eikichi Hosoya, Tai Akera, Tadashi Murano, Tatsuo Furukawa and Sadao Miyata. All have had notable careers in pharmacology. Several students were awarded M.S. degrees and went on to careers in medicine, including Dr. Paul Quinn, who rose to the rank of Rear Admiral in the US Naval Reserve.

In addition to research activities and graduate training, I taught an evening course in Biochemical Pharmacology, presented the entire Pharmacy Pharmacology course over two semesters, gave medical school lectures, and spent approximately one hundred hours per year in medical school laboratory instruction. The usual "other" activities such as editorial boards, NIH study sections, attendance and presentations at scientific meetings, invited lectures, compiling data and writing papers for publications and preparing grants occupied other available time. Recreation included golf, participation in the department's bowling and softball teams, playing duplicate bridge with partner Hank Swain, and coaching Little League baseball. In retrospect, I fail to understand how my family tolerated my activities! There were other rewarding experiences. My wife and I were able to take advantage of my travels to scientific meetings around the world and to become acquainted with new and exciting people and cultures. One such event during my tenure at Michigan was participation in hosting the Tenth Annual Fall Meeting of ASPET in August of 1958. It was at this meeting that the Society decided to launch The Pharmacologist. These Fall meetings of the Society (actually held during the summer) were unforgettable events, and provided great opportunities to meet and interact with fellow pharmacologists and make life-long friendships. Their ill-advised termination has left a void that will probably never be replaced. Another highlight was an enjoyable visit and discussion with the author, Rachel Carson, then in the process of writing a book which would later be published as "Silent Spring".

The Michigan State University Days

A unique opportunity arose when a College of Medicine was established at Michigan State University in 1965. The University had a well-established College of Veterinary Medicine, but pharmacology had only a minor role in that program and was part of a combined Department of Physiology and Pharmacology. One of the two "veterinary pharmacologists" in that department was Dr. David Reinke, who had received his Ph.D. in Pharmacology at UM under Dr. Donald Bennett. The combined department was separated into two departments, and a national search was initiated for a department chair in pharmacology. I was selected, and assumed the Chair of the new Department of Pharmacology in July 1966. The department was to have the responsibility for teaching human medicine and veterinary medicine students. We subsequently were delegated the additional responsibility for osteopathic medicine and nursing students. In building a new department and meeting teaching duties, I needed faculty immediately and decided to seek out the possibility of recruiting recent Michigan graduates whom I knew well in Ann Arbor, and considered to be potentially good teachers and investigators. Two with UM backgrounds joined me in 1966. Dr. Kenneth Moore had been my graduate student in Ann Arbor and had been on the pharmacology faculty at Dartmouth. Dr. Gerard Gebber had been a student of Dr. Lloyd Beck's at UM, and had completed a postgraduate training at the University of Pennsylvania and at Tulane. That same year I recruited Dr. Jerry Hook from the University of Iowa on the recommendation of Dr. Lauren Woods, then Head of the Department of Pharmacology at Iowa.

Two of my UM graduate students joined me at Michigan State, Laurence Carr and John McNeill. Carr became the first MSU Pharmacology Ph.D. McNeill, completing his work at MSU, elected to receive his degree from UM and stayed on as Assistant Professor before heading to Canada and the University of British Columbia where he later became Head of Pharmacology and Dean. Dr. Tai Akera, who had been a postdoctoral fellow in my laboratory at UM from 1962-64, joined the MSU faculty in 1967 as a Visiting Assistant Professor and subsequently rose to the rank of Professor before returning to Japan in 1986.

In many respects the department at MSU took on many of the characteristics of the Seevers-led department at Michigan. Fundamental was that faculty as a group should have a wide breadth of research interests, rather than be restricted to a narrow focus or limited to a subdiscipline of pharmacology. This has and continues to serve both departments well since it provides the sources of information necessary for a first class teaching effort. A hallmark of both institutions was a policy of absolute freedom in the choice of research projects undertaken by an individual faculty member as long as they fell within University guidelines. Also advocated was the promotion of joint research and faculty from other biomedical units, particularly clinical departments. During my tenure as Chair, sixteen Japanese postdoctoral fellows trained at MSU.

In the ensuing eight years, a number of new faculty were added to the MSU department, including several with UM roots. Drs. Jay Goodman, Richard Rech, and Janice Stickney had received their doctorates at UM under Pharmacology Professors Tom Tephly, Edward Domino, and Ben Lucchesi, respectively. Dr. Gregory Fink had been a postdoctoral fellow at Iowa under Dr. Michael Brody, a UM pharmacology graduate. Also joining the department was Dr. Paul Sato, a graduate student under Dr. Bert LaDu, who succeeded Seevers as UM Chair. While MSU could attribute its early success to its UM ties, ten years after its founding, the Department of Pharmacology at MSU had achieved national recognition in both teaching and research.

One aspect that distinguished the two departments was the number and the relatively short tenure of the Chairs at UM after Seevers, which significantly impacted the department's effectiveness. Dr. Henry Swain served a number of terms as the "Interim Chair." In contrast, Michigan State's Department of Pharmacology has had three leaders since its inception. I served as Chair for twenty years until required to step down and Tai Akera was Chair for several months until Dr. Moore assumed that position. Moore held it until 2001 when Dr. Jay I. Goodman stepped in as Interim Chair. Another chair was appointed in the past year. During my tenure at MSU, the Department hosted the national Fall Meeting of ASPET in 1973, while I served as ASPET president. At that time, it was the largest meeting held at MSU with some eighteen hundred pharmacologists and guests.

An important and lasting product of collaboration between the two departments was the development of an Annual Graduate Student Colloquium. This was the brainchild of Drs. Lucchesi and Rech, which I enthusiastically supported. While initially only intended for UM and MSU graduate students and faculty, early on the departments at Wayne State University and the Medical College of Ohio at Toledo were included. The year 2003 marks the 31st birthday of that event. Students present their research in a friendly competition for recognition, and an opportunity to meet with their peers from the other institutions. A close relationship still exists between the UM and MSU departments after more than three decades, and both units continue to dedicate themselves to first-class professional teaching and graduate education and state-of-the-art research.

Extracurricular matters at MSU took up

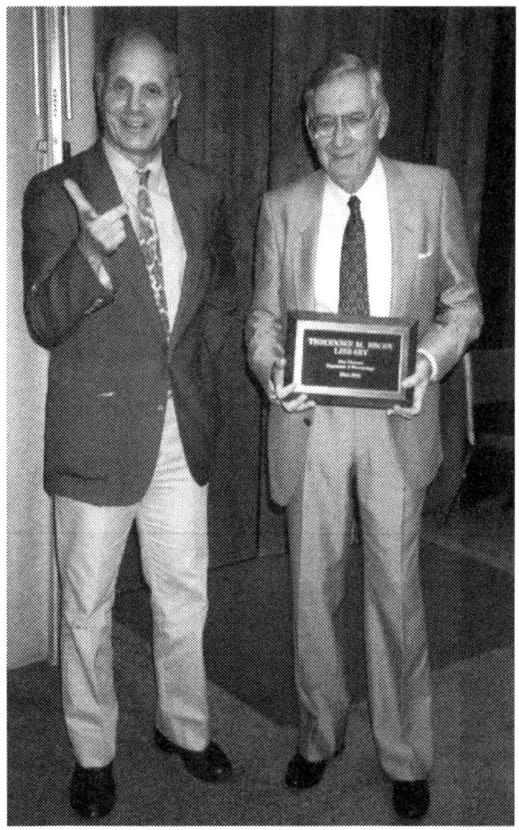

Drs. Kenneth Moore and Ted Brody held long tenures as Chairs at Michigan State University (at the dedication of the Pharmacology Library as the "Theodore M. Brody Library").

much of my time. Important were the daily adventures with my family. The usual committee work both local and national seemed to be endless, as were editorial board work, and manuscript and grant reviews. I served as a consultant to the Random House Dictionary of the English Language and also to the Pharmaceutical Manufacturers Association Foundation, both worthwhile endeavors. At the state level, I was a member of Michigan's Toxic Substance Control Commission. Among other highlights were my several trips to Japan, where I was able to visit again with former students and colleagues. Any available time was occupied by golf, not much different than in my days in Ann Arbor.

With faculty retirements and other losses over these many years there are only a few faculty remaining who can trace their roots back to UM; however, a close bond is still recognizable. I trust that I have instilled in and transferred to my students a part of that early heritage; teaching them to appreciate the uniqueness of pharmacology and the need to ensure its future. It is now critically important to maintain that same level of scientific curiosity and investigational ardor, dedicated teaching and willing service so characteristic of both departments. My greatest hope is that my students, and their students in turn, continue to pass on these traditions.

Recent Events

In 1995, I was honored by ASPET as the recipient of its most prestigious award, the Torald Sollmann Medal, presented for significant contributions over many years to the advancement and extension of knowledge in pharmacology. This was an unforgettable event. Equally as memorable are the many enduring friendships with colleagues and students fashioned over these many years.

In reflecting on the past half century, it has been my unqiue experience to have lived during what must be acknowledged as the "golden age of pharmacology," and to have participated in some small way in our achievements, all aimed toward the betterment of the human condition.

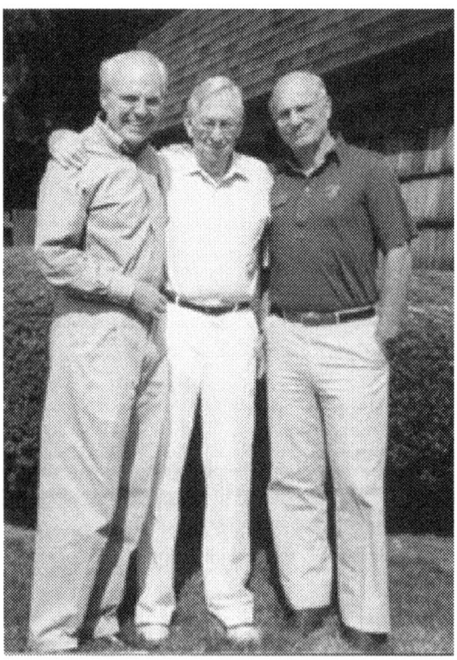

Dr. Brody with former students James Gibb (left) and Kenneth Moore (right).

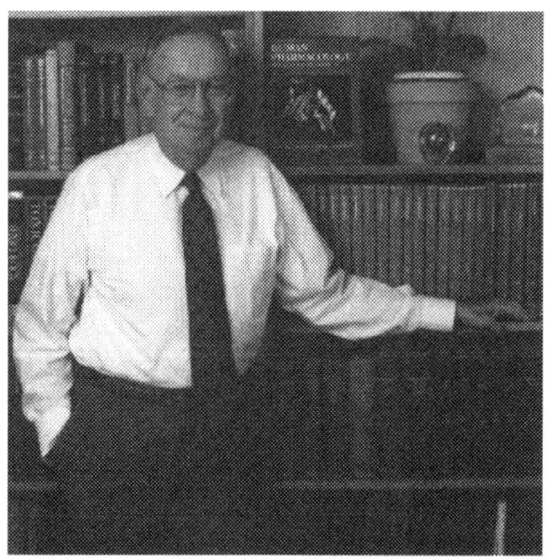

A distinguished Ted Brody, ca. 1992. Note the first edition of the pharmacology textbook he co-edited in 1991 on the shelf by his left shoulder. The upcoming 4th edition of the text will be entitled: "Human Pharmacology, Molecular to Clinical." It is scheduled for publication in 2005 by Elsevier.

Why I Came...and Why Did I Stay?

Edward F. Domino, M.D.

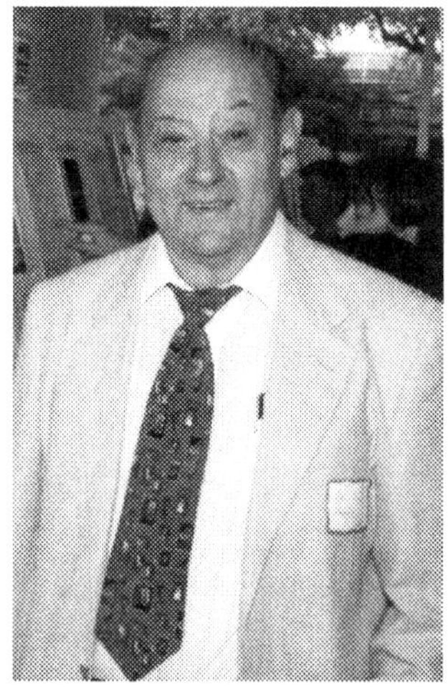

"Proximate cause" refers to a sequence of events in which, if the first did not occur, the subsequent events would not have resulted in the final one. It was a mouse running across the living room floor in a rented house in the Chicago Medical Center (507 S. Damen) while my wife, Toni, and daughter, Karen, were in the room that was the proximate cause of our move to Ann Arbor in September of 1953. There is nothing like a tearful, pregnant wife and a 16-month-old daughter concerned over a four-legged intruder to make you realize it is time for a lifestyle change.

In early 1953, I completed my rotating internship at Presbyterian Hospital, which was part of the old Rush Medical School. Eighteen months earlier, I had also completed the work for my master's degree in pharmacology. Then I worked as a part-time instructor in the Department of Pharmacology at the University of Illinois, Chicago. I spent a lot of time in the laboratory of Dr. Klaus Unna, a professor of pharmacology. He was trained in pharmacology in the German tradition of Schmiedeberg in Hamburg. When Hitler and the Nazis gained power, he had to leave Germany. He immigrated to the United States and took a job with the Merck Chemical Company in Rahway, New Jersey. It is there he described in detail for the first time the pharmacology of N-allyl-normorphine. Hart had reported its narcotic antagonistic effects in a brief abstract one year previously.

Dr. Unna was a classic German "geheimrat" M.D. professor who was extremely demanding of his students. He was especially interested in skeletal neuromuscular blocking agents. He and some of his students collaborated with Dr. Max Sadove in anesthesiology, studying the dose-paralyzing effects of a newly purified d-tubocurarine in man. He also used frogs and rabbits to study various neuromuscular blocking drugs before they were given to humans. In addition, he became interested in the compound benzimidazole as a centrally acting skeletal muscle relaxant first described by Goodman of Goodman and Gilman's textbook of pharmacology. The Smith, Kline and French pharmaceutical company gave Dr. Unna a grant to study a large series of chemical derivatives of benzimidazole called benzazoles. That project became the basis of my master's thesis in pharmacology.

As an instructor, I was helping teach the pharmacology laboratory course for sophomore medical students. My research involved work on many different benzazoles as centrally acting skeletal muscle relaxants. I even worked up chlorpromazine, then known to me as SKF-2601, in animals. To my chagrin, as a young man I was unimpressed with a drug that was an alpha-adrenergic blocking agent, induced hypothermia, enhanced barbiturate sedation, and antagonized apomorphine-induced vomiting in dogs.

Dr. Unna planned for me to continue research with him for at least another year or more. He was shocked when I told him I had

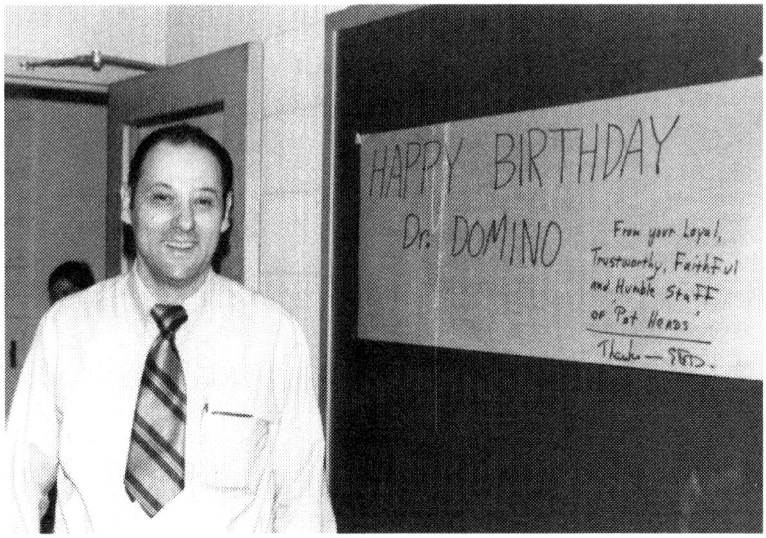
HAPPY BIRTHDAY
Dr. DOMINO
From your Loyal, Trustworthy, Faithful and Humble Staff of 'Pot Heads'

Pictured here in 1970, Dr. Domino receives a birthday card from his students and laboratory staff.

to look for a better job and intended to leave by September 1953. Finding a job was easier said than done. I later found out from Dr. Seevers that Dr. Unna actively discouraged potential employers from hiring me. That really hurt me because I didn't know why he would do that. Dr. Seevers said that Dr. Unna needed me to work in his laboratory, since most of his trainees were leaving.

Although obstetrics and gynecology or neurology had possibilities as career choices, I wasn't sure what field of clinical medicine most appealed to me. Clinical medicine would make too big a demand on my time and leave very little time for research, which I really enjoyed. In those days, the clinicians I knew worked as long and as hard as the house staff. I decided that I liked pharmacology a lot more.

I had a chance to go to the Federation Meetings in Atlantic City for job interviews the week of April 15, 1953. While attending the meetings, I met Sam Irwin, a young Ph.D. who had just graduated from the University of Michigan. He told me that a job had opened up in Michigan's Department of Pharmacology because Dr. Maynard Chenoweth, an associate professor, was leaving to go to Dow Chemical Company in Midland. I already knew that Harry Hardman and Ted Brody, both from Illinois, were at Michigan and were happy there. Sam was a gung ho, hypomanic fellow who took a liking to me. He immediately arranged for me to meet Dr. Seevers, who was interested but noncommittal. The only other solid contact was with Dr. James Dille, the chairman of the Department of Pharmacology at the University of Washington in Seattle. Both told me to write to them and they would consider my credentials. I left Atlantic City disappointed that job pickings were so slim. Sending my curriculum vitae to other departments of pharmacology was my only alternative but this did not payoff. By July 1953, I was getting desperate because I had had no job offers. I eventually got letters from both Ann Arbor and Seattle offering an instructorship beginning September 1st.

Toni and I decided in favor of Ann Arbor for several reasons. One was it was closer to Chicago where our families lived. The second was that we did not think we would like the rainy winter climate of Seattle. In addition, I had been stationed at the US Navy Base in Bremerton, Washington during World War II. While I was sitting in a movie theater in Seattle, an earthquake occurred. As I ran out of the theater in the dark the floor was moving up and down and cracking; it made a very unfavorable impression on me. I wrote to Dr. Seevers that I would like to come to Michigan, but would need a lot of equipment to start up a laboratory. He assured me that there would be no problem providing me with funds. So off I went to Ann Arbor to look for an apartment to rent for my growing family. Toni had to stay in Chicago to be close to her obstetrician who insisted that she should deliver the baby there and join me in Ann Arbor later. I found an apartment as part of a duplex at 1419 Morton Avenue. I was very happy with it at first, but we later discovered that the walls were very thin and we could hear the neighbors and vice versa. This soon became a major problem, causing us to move.

Dr. Seevers only offered me a nine-month appointment as an instructor of pharmacology at the University of Michigan. I tried to get a better deal than he was offering, but with Dr. Seevers it was take it or leave it. When I arrived at Dr. Seevers' office, I met Dotty Norton (later Overbeck), the whole of his departmental administrative staff. Dotty and I hit it off right away. I like her "tell it like it is" approach since it is mine as well. When she went into Dr. Seevers' office to tell him I was waiting, the door was left ajar. I could hear him say "Dr. Domino, who?" When she had to remind him that he had hired me, I realized I had a potential problem. He made it very clear to me that day what my duties would be as an instructor. He said that I was on a temporary status on the academic track. If I did well in teaching and research he would promote me to assistant professor the next year. I had to contribute to the Department as an active member so that he would look good. The only one in the entire University who would look after me was he, and, therefore, I had to do a good job. Any outside arrangements involving grants or money had to be cleared through him. My teaching duties came first with the comment, "I don't care if you are a great teacher, but you must be good enough to keep the students off my back." I later found out that Mark Nickerson had flunked about half of the sophomore medical students that spring and they all had to take pharmacology again in the summer term. That's how Nickerson got the title "Black Nick." Seevers was convinced that the problem was more Nickerson's teaching and unrealistically difficult exams rather than dumb medical students. The Dean's office was very disturbed over this issue and Dr. Seevers took the heat. He also emphasized that I must show independence in my research and not collaborate with others until he was convinced I was good. Inasmuch as I was on a nine-month appointment, he would cover my summer salary with his own research funds if I would contribute to his research effort.

Dr. Seevers decided I should take over an office and lab on the third floor of the old Pharmacology building. When I went with him to see the space he had assigned me, I was appalled. There were only a few cabinets, chairs and a desk and empty rooms. No research facilities. When I asked him for the research funds that he had promised me he explained that he had meant I could apply for grants. So began my years with Dr. Seevers!

A condition of employment at the University in 1953-'54 was that each person had to sign a special form indicating he or she swore allegiance to the United States of America and was not a communist. I've tried to obtain a copy of that form to include in this book, but I've been unsuccessful. Just nine months into my job as an Instructor, Michigan Congressman Kit Clardy held his Subcommittee hearings which involved Mark Nickerson. I was in the middle of a personal crisis of who to support. I chose to support both Seevers, my boss, and Nickerson my senior colleague and friend. Shortly after my arrival at Michigan, Nickerson asked me to join him in preparing a manuscript for a review of which was published in late 1954. Both Seevers and Nickerson accepted my middle of the road position and always supported me until they both died. My philosophy has always been that as human beings we all have good and bad qualities. To paraphrase the first Christian – let him without any bad qualities make the first disparaging remarks.

I wasn't involved in the secret US Army research conducted in our Department until

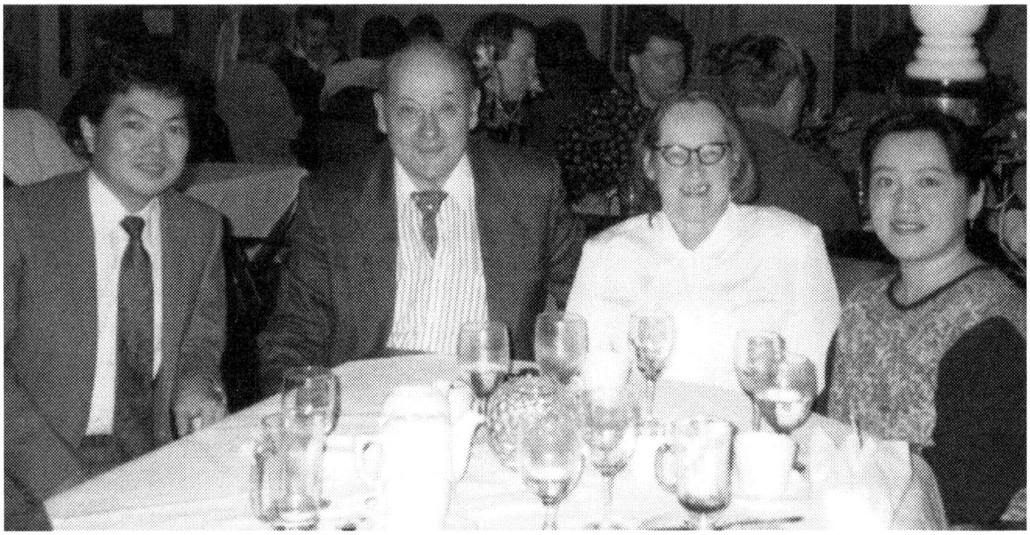

Chitoshi Kadoya, Ed and Toni Domino and Juri Kadoya.

1955 after Nickerson was dismissed. As the Principal Investigator with Secret clearance, Dr. Seevers needed a lot of people to work on his project; they were not informed of the chemical structures of the compounds they studied. Harry Hardman was first recruited and then me. Several years later Ben Lucchesi and Ed Alpert were recruited to help as well. In 1955 Harry was to study the cardiovascular effects, and I the central nervous system actions of a series of oily compounds with code names. A label on one of the containers indicated its molecular formula. It contained no nitrogen. Wow! Harry went to the library in the Chemistry Department for help in identifying its structure. Amazingly it was a synthetic red oil derivative of marijuana. It was similar to the Roger Adams compounds of the Department of Chemistry at the University of Illinois Urbana, where I learned my college chemistry. Harry and I told Dr. Seevers that we were studying marijuana derivatives. He promptly asked us to keep this a secret until we were cleared by the US Army. I already had a Confidential, then Secret security clearance from my years in the US Navy. In 1956 I was cleared for Secret by the US Army and later by the US Air Force, and again the US Army until 1986 for other classified research.

Harry Hardman's Memoirs describe some of the details of EA 1476, the best of the series of red oil derivatives we studied. This amazing compound produces artificial hibernation in dogs and monkeys for days, depending upon the dose administered. We felt then and still today the importance of a drug that can be used for temporarily treating thousands of survivors of atom bomb explosions before they can be treated definitively. Persons who claim this secret research was of minor significance should read our declassified publication (Hardman et al. and Domino et al. Pharmacology Review. 23: 295-316 and 317-336, 1976). Someday, somebody, somewhere, should pursue the amazing pharmacology of these chemicals especially EA 1476.

From the very beginning, I had a full time teaching load but promotions depended upon doing good research and the ability to obtain grants and publish. I could work in any field of pharmacology but the only one I knew well was centrally acting skeletal muscle relaxants and electroencephalography. Thus, I was a "budding" neuropharmacologist. The Rackham Graduate School provided me with my first grant, then the Cerebral Palsy Society, and subsequent pharmaceutical company funds through Dr. Seevers allowed me to establish a "first class" research facility, even better than what I had at the University of Illinois with Dr. Unna. I soon attracted (or was assigned by Dr. Seevers) graduate students and was on my way through promotions to a full professorship. Eventually, a number of postdoctoral fellows from all over the world came to work in my laboratory.

Each of my undergraduate, graduate, and postdoctoral fellows, and medical students made a major impact on me and on my research that would take too much space to describe. Their many degrees and publications provide the evidence of their contributions. I am proud of each of them, especially those who obtained their graduate degrees with me. John Kissel got me interested in brain neurotransmitters. Jane Heng Chin's work on morphine affecting tooth pulp evoked potentials in medial dorsal nucleus is still a classic. Dick Rech's studies on the effects of drugs, especially GABA, on isolated cerebral cortex again steered me toward neurotransmitters. Don Knapp's work on nicotine again got me back on the acetylcholine track. Roy Hudson's thesis on various drugs affecting central motor systems brought me back to extensions of my own Master's thesis research involving centrally acting skeletal muscle relaxants. Tony Dren's work with hemicholinium again stressed the cholinergic system. Joel Hoffman's work forced me to consider animal and human research on drugs and sleep as necessary compliments of each other. Ann Wilson Black's work again emphasized cholinergic mechanisms, which Jim Roppolo pursued further. Joe Pearl got me back into human marijuana research, and Maxine Stitzer into operant behavioral pharmacology in rats and humans. Mike Vasko, Gaston Labrecque, and Germaine Gwynn got me into narcotics and acetylcholine again, whereas with Lindsay Hough it was histamine. Ela Holsztynska renewed my long time interest in phencyclidine and showed important genetic differences in its biotransformation. Perhaps more than anything else, I can say I stayed at Michigan because of my students. I really had the best of two worlds, between my job as professor at Michigan and my part time work at the Lafayette Clinic in Detroit, which was arranged and approved by Dr. Seevers and the Medical School.

When Bert La Du became our chairman, he told me I was the last person in the Department to be on a nine-month appointment and insisted that I be put on a 12-month appointment. That arrangement was acceptable to me as long as I could continue to consult at the Lafayette Clinic.

As a member of the Department since September 1, 1953, I've seen, heard, and been a part of a number of disagreements among our faculty members. Some of these have involved legitimate differences of opinion, and others, insulted egos. As one looks back over the years it is clear that most of these squabbles do not deserve mention and are best forgotten by those involved.

Clearly the Nickerson Affair was the major newsworthy event, involving complex issues of communism, secret Army research, academic freedom, and the clash of some very strong personalities. Some of these issues have been described above and elsewhere in this volume.

In the past decade, there were three lawsuits initiated by members of our Department and subsequently settled by the University of Michigan. Tom Landefeld, an Associate Professor in our Department, initiated a lawsuit on January 10, 1997 against the Board of Regents, Dean Giles Bole, and Acting Chairman Ray Counsell. The suit addressed a perceived lack of diligence on the defendants' part in rooting out overt racism in the medical school faculty. About nine months earlier an article appeared in The University Record 51(24): 5, March 19, 1996 by J. Peterson "Medical School environment 'unwelcoming' to minorities and women, study shows." The study was commissioned by the Medical School and conducted by Nichols and Associates, Inc., a consulting firm based in Washington, DC. The Medical School was praised for its courage in doing this. Edwin J. Nichols, director of the team said: "I commend you for being willing to examine yourselves in this way." Dean Giles Bole responded, "Our consultants have identified some fairly sharp cultural issues about our environment that we need to deal with." For a period of time Dr. Tom Landefeld of our Department was an Assistant Dean in the Medical School involved in these issues. He filed suit on January 10, 1997. This case was resolved through a cash settlement on October 18, 1999.

In a second related lawsuit, Dr. Tad Smith, a Professor in the Department, filed a lawsuit against Jim Woods, Wendell Weber, Marshall Schlafer, Ben Lucchesi, Tom Landefeld, Jimmy Myers, Susan Rasmussen, and Joseph Smith on January 21, 1997. Tad stated that he had suffered injury to his reputation and good name, public disgrace, and indignity. The case involved a letter of support for Peggie Hollingsworth's promotion, which was alleged to contain forged and altered signatures, etc. The University hired a distinguished forensic expert who concluded that the signatures in the letter of support were neither forged nor altered. For good and valuable considerations, the case was settled on December 21, 1999.

In a third and related lawsuit, Peggie Hollingsworth, an Assistant Research Scientist in the Department was considered for a tenure track position. I had been on her doctorial thesis committee and knew of her research. I personally thought she was an excellent choice. She received her Ph.D. degree in toxicology.

I was not involved in the complex reasons why Peggie had been denied a tenured position but I thought she would be an excellent choice. Had she been promoted with tenure she would have been the first and only African American woman in the history of the Department or the Medical School to achieve that status. Roy Hudson, in his reflections in this book states "It is sad that to date no other African American has been hired as faculty in the Department." Peggie filed a lawsuit against the University of Michigan and Gilbert R. Whitaker, then Provost and Executive Vice President for Academic Affairs based upon the precedent setting irregularities in her review process. That case was settled for good and valuable consideration on December 21, 1999.

So who are the real "victims" of this second Shakespearean tragedy to affect our Department, Medical School, and University? I believe they are the plaintiffs, defendants, and each and every one of us associated with this Department. We humans must learn to solve our differences through compromises. Our Department's tarnished history is a lesson that must not be forgotten! That's why I've insisted these issues be part of this book.

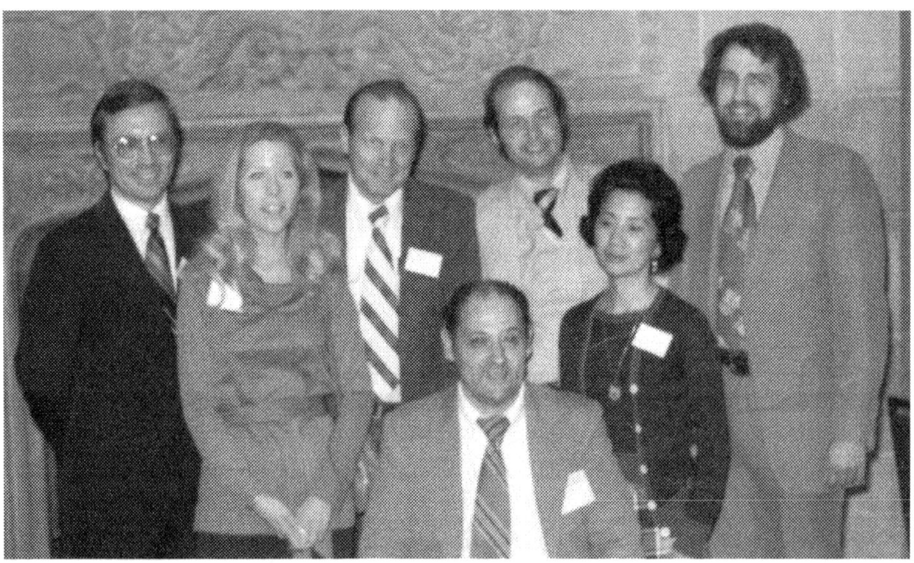

Ed Domino and former graduate students Tony Dren, Germaine Gwynn, Dick Rech, Mike Vasko, Jane Heng Chin, and Lindsay Hough, ca. 1970

I Remember...

Roy D. Hudson, Ph.D., LL.D.

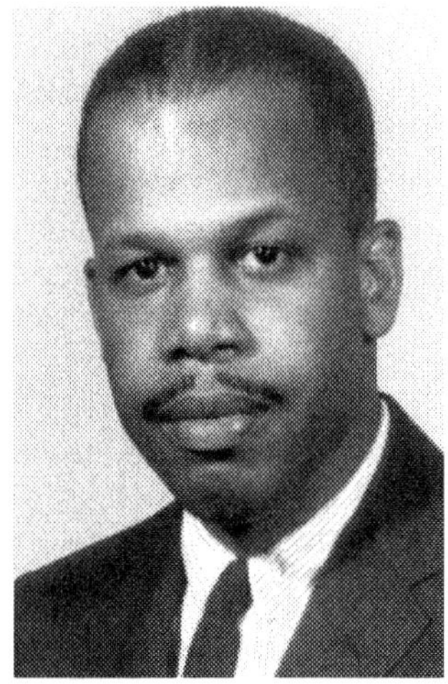

I came to The University of Michigan in 1955 after completing a B.S. degree in Biology at Livingstone College in Salisbury, NC. Having never heard of Pharmacology, I enrolled in the doctoral program in Zoology in the Division of Natural Sciences. During my initial year at Michigan, I was supported by the GI Bill (Korean Veteran) and The Danforth Graduate Fellowship. My appointment as one of 58 Danforth Fellows selected in 1955 from approximately 3000 applicants from the nation at large placed a special burden on my shoulders. Being the first recipient from my college, future appointments would greatly depend on my performance. Additionally, from a personal perspective, the renewal of the Fellowship was determined annually via an academic review process. My initial anxiety can be easily understood when one realizes that I came to the "Mighty" Michigan from a small, Black college with an enrollment of less than 500 students and a faculty having only two Ph.D.'s, one of which was in the Seminary and the other in Sociology. Although I graduated Summa Cum Laude, the question of coping at a place like The University of Michigan was yet to be answered.

The two high points of my first year at Michigan were my 4.0 GPA and the discovery of Pharmacology (not necessarily in that order). The latter would change my life forever and the former vindicated my preparation at Livingstone College for Graduate School.

Before proceeding I would like to say a few words about The Danforth Foundation. This Foundation was funded by the late Mr. & Mrs. William H. Danforth of the Ralston-Purina Fortune. The Foundation emphasized the theme of improving the quality of teaching and learning. The Danforths were dedicated to placing as many Christian teachers in the classrooms of the nation's colleges and universities as they possibly could. In this regard The Foundation endeavored to contribute annually to American education approximately 50 well-trained, academically able young men who had the vision of the high calling of the teacher. In facilitating the fulfillment of this goal, The Danforth Foundation brought all Danforth Fellows (old and newly elected) together each year for a week at a retreat setting in a conference with seasoned scholars to focus on the subject of "Teaching as a Christian Vocation." Many Fellows (myself included) were accompanied by their new brides, causing the Retreat to double as a "honeymoon" opportunity.

My association with the Danforth Foundation over the years has been an honor and a privilege. The 1955 class of Danforth Fellows (the fourth class) was the last to be greeted personally by Mr. Danforth prior to his death. Mr. Danforth was a strong influence in the lives of all Danforth Fellows. Among his many words to my class were, "I dare you—each one of you—to be a worthy example of the teacher you have the mind and heart to become." This statement lingered with me and continued to be a motivational force as I pursued my graduate studies at Michigan.

During the spring of my first year of graduate study a classmate mentioned her part-time work in the Department of Pharmacology. She said her employer was looking for a technician for the summer and invited me to meet him for an interview. I had never heard of Pharmacology but I did need a summer job so I agreed to talk with her employer. He turned out to be Dr. Ed Domino. We "hit it off" well and I was offered a job for the summer of 1956. It was here in Dr. Domino's laboratory that I got my first "taste" of research excitement and the utility of the scientific method. I was exhilarated and couldn't wait to discuss my new experiences with my colleagues in Zoology. As first year students in Zoology, we had not been introduced to the tools of research nor the analytical thought process so vital to its proper execution. In this respect I had an advantage over my peers in Zoology; Dr. Domino treated me more as a graduate student than a technician.

My first assignment as a "technician" was to work with John Kissel, one of Dr. Domino's graduate students. John exposed me to the "hows" and "whys" of the research methodology he was using. He was studying the effects of drugs on monosynaptic and polysynaptic neural pathways utilizing the patellar and linguo-mandibular reflexes. Added to this, John facilitated and inhibited these reflexes via electrical stimulation of specific areas in the brainstem.

My next experience came via a placement, along with Dick Rech, another of Dr. Domino's graduate students, in Dr. Donald ("Skip") Bennett's lab to learn the Heart-Lung Preparation. Dr. Bennett was a skilled teacher and brought the both of us along rapidly to the point where we could perform this procedure with minimal assistance. I was ecstatic! Not only did I continue to tell my Zoology colleagues, I wrote the Executive Director of The Danforth Foundation to let him know that I was already "into" research at Michigan before my second year had started. Dr. Domino observed that I was enjoying this research adventure and from time-to-time he would encourage me by passing along certain articles for me to read.

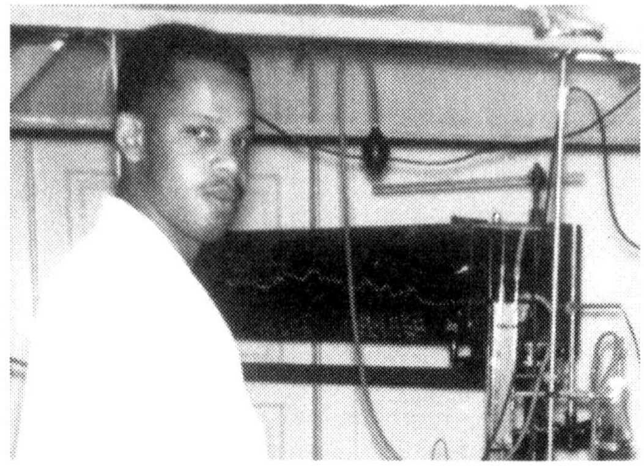

This was 1956 and Delay and Deniker (1952) and Courvoisier (1953) and several others were investigating the mechanisms of action(s) of psychotropic drugs, especially the Rauwolfia Alkaloids and the Phenothiazines. Dr. Domino launched a study using reserpine and analyzing changes in catecholamine levels in blood in conjunction with Glenn Kiplinger and Dr. Lloyd Beck. I participated by running the whole animal portion of the study and drawing the necessary blood samples. For a student never before exposed to research this was some "heavy stuff!" The above photograph shows me in the old Pharmacology Building on the Diag running an experiment on a dog using the now "retired" smoke kymograph. Learning to "smoke" a kymograph without smoking oneself and then preserve the data recorded thereon was a real art and one that I enjoyed, but that's another story.

The summer of 1956 had all too soon come to a close. I had gained a new perspective on scientific research and was now on my way to Massachusetts to "gain" a bride. Constance (Connie) and I were married on August 31, 1956 and following the annual Danforth Conference, we returned to The University of Michigan for her first year in The School of Social Work and my second year in Zoology. My experience in Pharmacology had really broadened my expectations regarding research in Zoology. However, my second year was also one of completing course work requirements thus intensifying my anticipation of the coming summer in Dr. Domino's lab. Despite my disappointment regarding research in Zoology during that second year there were two significant events that elevated my spirit greatly. In February, 1957 I received the Master's degree in Zoology and on June 13, 1957 Connie and I were blessed with a daughter, Hollye Lynne, who has continued to be a blessing to this very day.

During my second summer (1957), Dr. Domino gave me a project that ultimately produced my first publication with him and my first research seminars in Pharmacology and Zoology. We designed a study to observe the pharmacological actions of the isomers of atropine (i.e., d- and l- hyoscyamine). The results of our study appeared in the Journal of Pharmacology and Experimental Therapeutics, Vol. 127, No. 4, December 1959.

Duncan McCarthy, a graduate student in the Department, responsible for the student seminar program, noted my work and invited me to present it to the Pharmacology graduate students. You can imagine my trepidation! However, with a bit of encouragement from Dr. Domino and Duncan, I accepted the invitation. As a consequence of this commitment I "dug" deeper into the known physiology and pharmacology of atropine. The results of this seminar motivated me to repeat it in the Department of Zoology where it was favorably received.

Now the second summer was over and I was entering my third year of graduate study in Zoology. Included in this was the major hurdle of the Preliminary Examination qualifying one to continue in the program for the doctorate. This was a written examination given over a four-day period, three hours per day. I took this exam in April 1958. Of the several students taking the exam only three passed it at the level required for acceptance as a Candidate for the Doctorate in Zoology. I was one of the three. At this time I had invested three years in Zoology, selected a chairman for my doctoral committee, fulfilled one language requirement, completed all basic course work

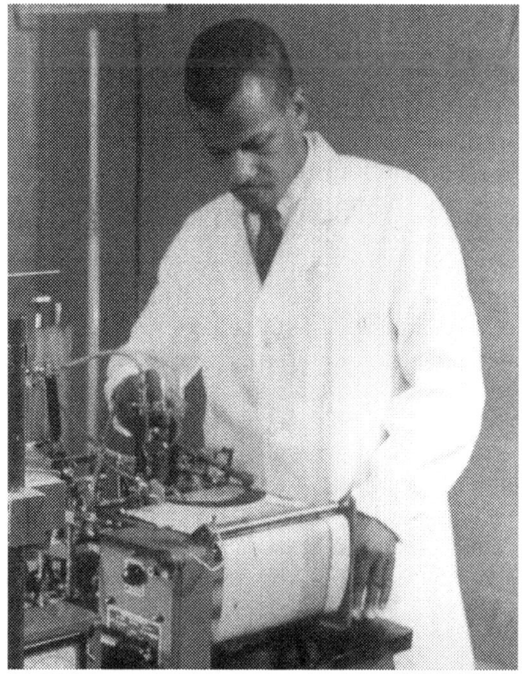

and the historical review for my dissertation in the concentration area of Endocrinology. Yet, when I should have been elated there was a feeling of discontent with the prospect of pursuing the doctorate in Zoology. After some serious "soul searching," I transferred into the graduate program in Pharmacology and started all over again! Although I was thrust back into the fray of basic science classes such as medical physiology (a nine hour credit course) with more than 200 medical and graduate students, I have never regretted this decision. In fact, it was one of the best decisions I have ever made.

As I had anticipated, my third summer was spent in Dr. Domino's lab but unlike previous years, I was no longer a technician but a bona fide "new" graduate student. The above photograph shows me using an ink kymograph during an experiment in the then "new" Medical Science Building I. This equipment was soon replaced by Grass and later, Offner polygraphs. Even so, I will always have a special attachment to the old "pulley and string" modes of collecting data.

I was now in Pharmacology! The atmosphere was electric with the desire to roll back the frontiers of research. Dr. Domino was enthusiastic, approachable and committed to pharmacology. He once even said that he would do pharmacological research even if he were not paid to do so. The students he gathered around him reflected his enthusiasm for learning and research. I considered myself to be in the midst of a living, learning, and teaching center that gave top priority to teaching excellence, and placed the learner at the apex of its planning. I felt that concern was exhibited for my own personal potential, my needs and learning experiences as well as for the advancement of pharmacology as a discipline.

I found the students in Pharmacology to be more friendly and less pretentious than most of those I had encountered in Zoology. Faculty members were supportive and responsive to inquiry— always more than happy to help. For example, Dr. Bennett ("Skip") worked with a number of us in the preparation for our oral preliminary examinations. Unlike Zoology, where the filter was the written preliminary examination, in Pharmacology it was the oral examination. I remember walking with my mentor, Dr. Domino, to the room where my preliminary evaluation was to take place. On the way there Dr. Domino said, "Roy, this is where they take your pants down and have a good look at you." Another professor observed that at the time of the Prelim one knows more on a broad basis than they will ever know again. But, I digress.

Although I was a first year graduate student in Pharmacology, I was in reality a fourth year graduate student. In this respect most of my "butterflies" were gone. I remember a few new Pharmacology grad students who came to Michigan with outstanding academic records expressing similar anxieties to those I had felt four years earlier, wondering just how they would perform given the requirement level and the competition at "Mighty" Michigan.

In 1961 I gave my first paper at the Federation meetings in Atlantic City, NJ. Following my presentation a very unusual thing happened. A well-known and respected scientist arose during the Q&A period but rather than asking a question he commended me on my presentation and the logic supporting my conclusions. Further, he complimented my mentor for preparing me for the occasion. I was overwhelmed!! It just so happened that Dr. Seevers, Chair of the Department of Pharmacology at Michigan, and Dr. Domino were in the audience. It was a good day for me and things were to get even better. After the session Dr. Seevers, Dr. Domino and I were standing together talking when Dr. Klaus Unna, Chair of Pharmacology at the University of Illinois, joined us. It is of interest to note that Dr. Unna was Dr. Domino's mentor, and that he himself had been trained by one of Dr. Oswald Schmiedeburg's students from Germany where Pharmacology (materia medica) began in the middle of the nineteenth century. Dr. Unna rather quickly made it clear that he was interested in my coming to "visit" with him in Pharmacology at the University of Illinois. Dr. Seevers was noticeably annoyed and said to Dr. Domino upon Dr. Unna's departure, "We've got plans for Roy." I did not know what this meant but shortly thereafter Dr. Seevers invited me to remain at Michigan as Instructor of Pharmacology. This was an offer I could not refuse!!

During the summer of 1961, I had the responsibility for the summer Pharmacology course. This was one of a few summer Medical School Pharmacology courses taught in the nation. Although I was appointed in the summer of 1961, my degree was not conferred until commencement of 1962. I was the first African American to receive the Ph.D. degree in Pharmacology at Michigan. Likewise, I was the first African American to be hired in a faculty position in the Department of Pharmacology. It is sad that to date no other African American has been hired as faculty in this department. As the first African American Assistant Professor of Pharmacology at the University everything I did was "history." I was one of three African American Professors in the Medical School. The others were the late Dr. Albert Wheeler of Public Health, who later became Mayor of Ann Arbor, and Dr. Ralph Gibson of the Department of Psychiatry/ Psychology.

It was in 1965 that Akira Tsujimoto,

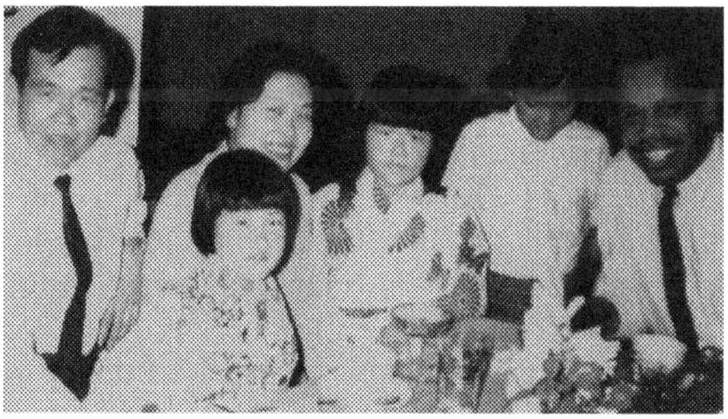

Dr. Tsujimoto and family pictured with Roy Hudson and his daughter.

M.D., Ph.D., a Japanese post-doctoral student, joined my laboratory. He was one of a long line of Japanese postdoctoral students who studied at Michigan dating back to the early 50s. When I arrived in the department as a student (1958), Dr. Seevers already had a demonstrated commitment to Japan and its quality of pharmacology instruction and research. In this regard he provided funding for many senior and junior Japanese scientists to tour (short term) or study for as long as one to two years at Michigan. The Japanese government recognized Dr. Seevers' contributions by decorating him with the Second Order of the Sacred Treasure of Japan and The Third Class of the Order of the Rising Sun Medal.

Shortly after Dr. Tsujimoto's placement in my laboratory I received an offer to move to Brown University in the Ivy League. This offer came at a very crucial time in my career— a time when I had been seriously considering administration as a means of making a broader impact on institutional resource availability for the researcher and a more inter-departmentally flexible research environment. Brown was offering a split appointment between its Graduate School as Assistant Dean and its newly formed "Medical School". Brown's medical program was interdisciplinary (without the usual compartmentalization). It was located in the Division of Biological and Medical Sciences and as such was a part of the graduate program of the University rather than being a separate professional school. This infrastructure would allow me to test my impressions of the impact that could be realized through administration while maintaining my position in medical research and teaching.

I distinctly remember the aura of sadness that filled my being the morning I approached Dr. Seevers' office to inform him of my planned move. I was and am grateful to Dr. Seevers for the opportunity he gave me to begin my professional career as a pharmacologist in the nation's top institution. I had had several good years at Michigan and a positive relationship with Dr. Seevers. It would not be easy to leave either. Just as I had been surprised five years earlier when Dr. Seevers invited me to remain at Michigan after my graduation, I was again surprised by his response to the news that I was planning a move. After listening to me struggle to get my "speech" out, he looked at me pensively and said, "You want to be a Dean? I'll talk to Dr. Hubbard." At the time Dr. William Hubbard was Dean of the Medical School (He was later to become President of The Upjohn Company where we would meet again). That very same day Dr. Seevers called me to his office and informed me that an Assistant Dean's position was available to me in the Medical School and told me to speak with Dean Hubbard. I was astounded by this unexpected turn of events. I thanked Dr. Seevers for his confidence in me and left his office torn between my gratefulness to him and my planned move. After some agonizing reflection and discussions with colleagues and Dean Hubbard, I decided to accept the invita-

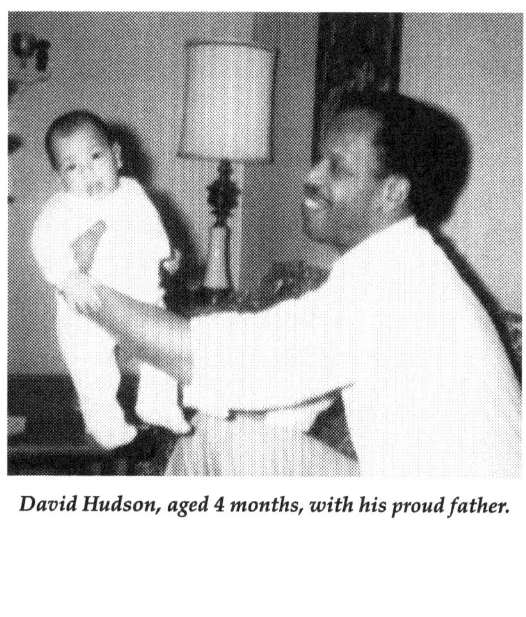

David Hudson, aged 4 months, with his proud father.

tion from Brown and left for Providence, RI, in July, 1966. Dr. Seevers permitted me to take all of my research equipment to Brown. This facilitated my research program in that I did not have to await the arrival of newly purchased research equipment. As soon as I acquired the necessary grants at Brown, I returned all of the loaned equipment. I served Brown as Associate Professor of Medical Science (tenured) and Associate Dean of the Graduate School. As a result of this move, Dr. Tsujimoto spent only one year in my laboratory working on evoked potentials in the brain. While in Rhode Island our family grew to four. Our son David Kendall was born on August 12, 1968. Like Hollye, he was a joyous addition to the family.

The '60s were years of Civil Rights unrest and activism in the Nation and in Ann Arbor. Al Wheeler (also President of the local NAACP Chapter in Ann Arbor) and I spent many days on the picket lines for various Civil Rights causes. The Department of Pharmacology never sought to curtail my Civil Rights involvement and seemed more interested (rightly so) in my research, lecturing, and committee responsibilities. For reference I list a few headlines from the Ann Arbor News citing some of my involvements; "High Level Anti-Bias Policy Must Hit All, Dr. Hudson Holds", by Larry Sullivan, February 26, 1964; "NAACP Backs Stand On 'U' Study Request", November 22, 1963; "Conference on Race-Religion Begins Tomorrow," May 24, 1963.

These were years when the country struggled, convulsively sometimes, to overcome deep and lingering injuries from times past and even present. Most of us at some point faced conditions that placed us in "awkward situations" having to deal with occurrences extraneous to our professional commitments but nonetheless an integral part of the fabric of our lives. Being the first African American student and faculty member in the Department presented me with some of those "awkward situations". These were more evident outside of the Department than they were inside. However, there were a few times when my colleagues were challenged by certain situations and with good intentions made what I considered "inappropriate" responses, comments, or inquiries. For example, one of my colleagues asked an entering pharmacology graduate student if the student would mind being placed with a "Black Professor". I don't need to explain the offensiveness of this inquiry since my appointment was one of equal faculty status. Another situation occurred as a result of a local pharmacology "tradition". It was "tradition" in those days that a professor would celebrate his grad student's passing of the prelim by taking them out to dinner. It just so happened that one of my grad students was a white female. When she passed her preliminary examination one of my colleagues asked, "protectively", if I would like to have him accompany us to the dinner celebration. Again, an act with good intentions but emphasizing the senseless "two world nature" of our existence in this country.

Racially-based incidents deriving from students aimed at faculty, from my experience, were rare. I can remember only one in the Medical School and one in the School of Pharmacy that happened to me personally. On the other hand, I did encounter one faculty faux pas unrelated to "good intentions." This occurred when a pharmacology graduate student requested a transfer into my lab from the lab where he had been assigned. In response to this, my colleague said (to me), that the male student's reason for wanting to transfer was so he could be with the female grad student in my lab. Apparently this faculty member could not conceive of the possibility that the transfer request just might be based on the usual academic reasons. Perhaps it never occurred to him that these two students had full access to each other without going through the trouble of initiating a laboratory transfer.

I recall my first faculty meeting as a young, impressionable member of the Pharmacology Faculty. This assembly emphasized that dimension of one's professionalism allowing the separation of issues from personal relationships. In that meeting there were intense differences of opinion— so much so that I wondered whether things might become physical at any moment. At the end of the session, I

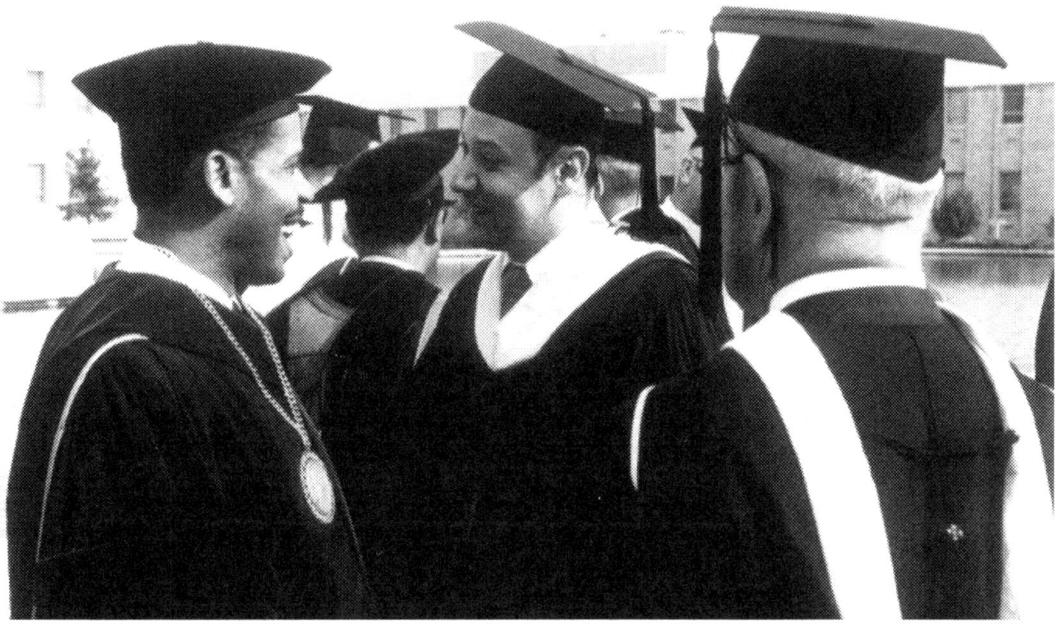

Ed Domino representing the University of Michigan at Roy's inauguration as President of Hampton University.

was amazed that persons on opposite sides of the debate paired up to go golfing, while other similar groups went bowling. There seemed to have been no carry-over from the heated discussion of a few moments earlier. I considered this a worthwhile faculty meeting for several reasons.

During the early '60s I remember two organizations issuing national rankings of pharmacology departments throughout the country. On one poll Michigan was listed as "number one" and Harvard was "second", while the other poll listed Harvard as "number one" and Michigan as "second." I recall the surge of pride we all felt, especially those of us recently added to the pharmacology staff. Our chests were fully expanded and sometimes "our feet did not touch the ground." It did not take the senior staff long to help us see that though the evaluation was just issued it was based on data accumulated over the past 20 years and as such had little or nothing to do with most of us presently on the faculty. While this was sobering, it remained an exhilarating, cutting edge experience to be in a department so highly rated nationally and to interact daily with scholars at Michigan and other universities. Also, it was a stimulus to us to make the next 20 years even better.

The personal bonds that were developed during the years at Michigan in the Department of Pharmacology have stood the test of time and continue to bring many of us together professionally and as friends. For example, in 1970 I was appointed President of Hampton Institute (name now changed to University) in Hampton, VA. Dr. Domino was at my Inauguration. Over the years he has remained interested in and supportive of my career. This is further demonstrated by his recommending me for the position of Adjunct Professor of Pharmacology in 1977 when I returned to Ann Arbor as a Divisional Vice President in the Pharmaceutical Research and Development Division of Warner Lambert/Parke-Davis. This recommendation was approved and I held the position until 1980, one year past the date that I joined The Upjohn Company and moved to Kalamazoo (May, 1979). Later I became Vice President for Pharmaceutical Research and Development, Europe at The Upjohn Company. During this

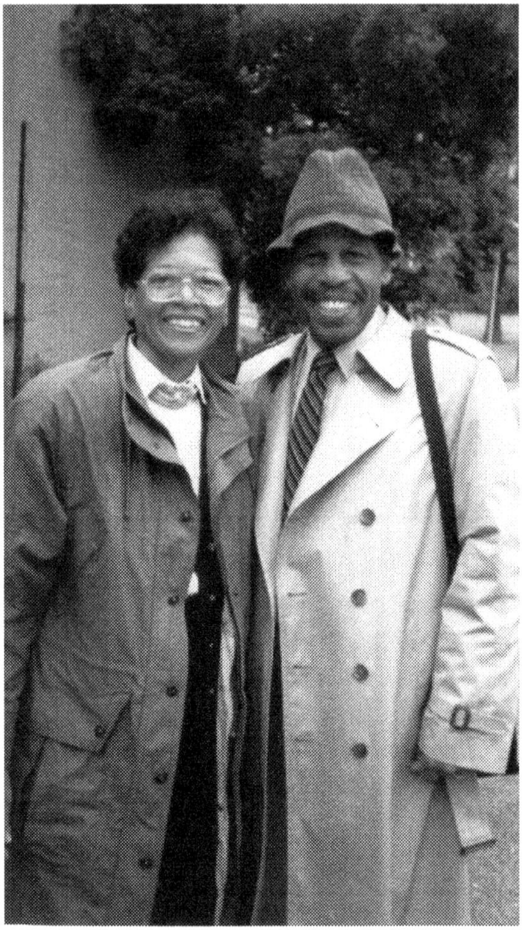

Roy Hudson with his wife Connie

time Connie and I lived in Overijse, Belgium. My office was in Brussels.

Again, in 1989 Dr. Domino recommended me for the King/Chavez/Parks Visiting Professorship at the University. His recommendation was approved and I returned to campus for a faculty lecture and a dialogue with University students. The Ann Arbor News covered the student session and issued a story in the Sunday paper (June 26, 1989) by Dov Cohen. The headline read, "Minority Students Encouraged To Form Own Agenda, Not To Be Used." In 1991 Dr. Domino encouraged me to present at the Centennial Celebration of Pharmacology at the University. I was very pleased to be a part of this historical celebration. The Department is truly a National Treasure and I consider myself blessed beyond measure to be a part of that history.

There are so many positive things I remember about my student days (1958-1961) and faculty days (1961-1966); (1977-1980); (1989) in the nation's first Pharmacology Department. These were vital and triumphant days, days of significant research discoveries, days of successes and failures, days of building lasting friendships, days of intellectual growth and development. I remember the summer softball games, Dottie Norton (now Overbeck), departmental dinners at the Seevers', gatherings at the homes of faculty and graduate students, interactions with international grad students and post docs, especially Dr. Showa Ueki (Japanese post doc) and his relentless pursuit of the elusive Renshaw Cell. I clearly remember one morning about 2:00 A.M. after another disappointing experiment, Dr. Ueki so aptly said, in his undaunted, spirit-filled manner, "That's what makes tomorrow so important!" For me this statement beautifully encapsulated the predominating force so evident in the lives of pharmacologists at Michigan (and perhaps everywhere). Finally, I say, in words similar to those used by the great poet, author and teacher, Margaret A. Walker in her signature poem, "For My People", so it was in Pharmacology at Michigan in those days, as we all looked to tomorrow for answers to, and people who, and days when, and places where, and reasons why, and discoveries of... scientific secrets providing for all of us a better way!

Reflections on the Past Forty-Six Years

Benedict R. Lucchesi, M.D., Ph.D.

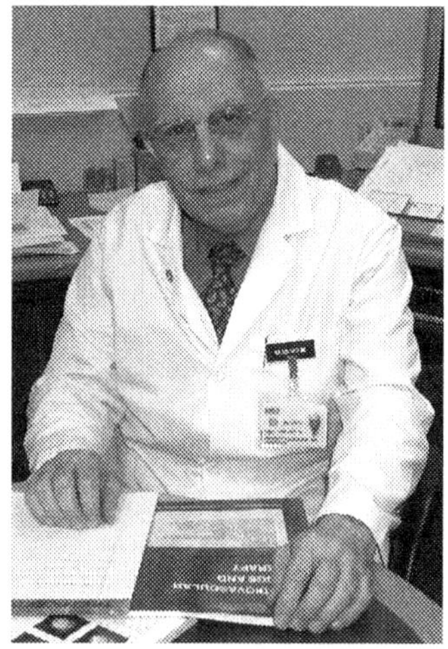

My fascination with science began to develop while in grade school, PS 127 located in Queens, New York, from which I graduated in 1948. It was the beginning of the atomic age and many schools became heavily invested in the teaching of science courses. My interest in subjects such as chemistry, physics, math and languages continued to grow throughout the time I attended Newtown High School, in Elmhurst, New York. During my years in high school I had the opportunity to work in a neighborhood pharmacy where I was tutored by one of the pharmacists in the compounding of prescriptions and learning about the action of drugs for the management of human diseases. My choice for a career was becoming clear and I made the decision to pursue a course of study leading to a bachelor's degree in Pharmacy. I applied to St. John's University and was accepted to begin my studies in September of 1951.

World War II ended in 1945 and the world had been relatively peaceful for almost five years. However, the era of relative peace was to end with the invasion of South Korea by its northern neighbors on June 25, 1950. The United States, under the leadership of President Harry S. Truman, joined with member countries of the United Nations to protect South Korea.

It was September of 1951 and I had completed my first week of college, when I received a notice from the President of the United States that I was to report for induction into military service. Along with many of my neighborhood friends I appeared as ordered for my health examination that consisted of a urine test for glucose, venous blood sample for hemoglobin and a complete blood count and a subsequent cursory chest and neurological examination. The physical examination was followed by a multiple-choice examination. The grades were tabulated and the new inductees were assigned to either the infantry or the marines. I was selected to become a marine and was ordered to obtain a crew cut and a toothbrush, and to report to Parris Island for training. It appeared that my college days were to come to an end. However, shortly before I was to leave, the orders to report for military training were canceled as I was given a college deferment that would remain in effect until I completed my studies, contingent upon maintaining a B+ or better average grade. The incentive to study and to do well was present very early in my college career. The next four years were to be an intensive period of study; at the same time I maintained a job in the neighborhood pharmacy in order to earn sufficient money for tuition and expenses.

Many students and faculty were called to join the military. One person in particular was a recently hired Ph.D. pharmacologist, Dr. Robert Bogner. Suddenly, the University was in need of an instructor to teach the lecture and laboratory course in pharmacology. St. John's University School of Pharmacy had the good fortune to hire Alfred E. Livingston, Ph.D. to replace Dr. Bogner. Dr. Livingston had retired from Temple University and was certainly a senior citizen. Despite his advancing years, he was a dynamic and dedicated teacher. His choice of textbook for the two-semester course was the Pharmacological Basis of Therapeutics, by Goodman and Gilman. His teaching style was to assign reading for each day of class and to call upon students to respond to specific questions. The classroom "discussions" were accompanied by a detailed laboratory emphasizing the use of classical methods for the study of pharmacologic agents. I was fortunate to have been given the opportunity to assist Dr. Livingston in setting up the laboratory. The pharmacology course and exposure to the laboratory solidified my decision to pursue graduate studies.

Dr. Livingston introduced me to the excitement associated with the study of drugs and the laboratory approach to research. He encouraged me to seek a graduate degree in pharmacology, but only after I had obtained a graduate degree in physiology. I followed his advice, and after completing my Bachelor of Science degree, I enrolled as a graduate student at St. John's University where I studied under Dr. Daniel Lilly, Chairman of the Biology Department. I was a teaching assistant in the mornings and a student in the evenings while conducting my thesis research during the afternoons. I completed my thesis "Purine Metabolism in Stylonichia pustulata" in May 1957. Throughout the six years of attending St. John's University I traveled each day from the borough of Queens to the borough of Brooklyn by bus and subway; a round trip requiring a minimum of 4.5 hours. During those long subway rides, I had the chance to read Goodman and Gilman's textbook from cover-to-cover three times.

In the early part of 1957, and nearing completion of my graduate studies in physiology, I took the examinations administered by the National Science Foundation (NSF) and placed number one in the country in pharmacology. Those long commutes and periods of reading yielded a benefit. I was certain that the fellowship would put me in a good position to gain acceptance at any of the major graduate programs in the country. Unfortunately, the NSF decided that pharmacology was not a top priority for funding and made the decision to use most of its money for the support of astronomy. At first I could not understand such a move on the part of NSF. Later the reason for this decision would become obvious to me and be recognized as one that would impact heavily on my career.

Once again, I approached Dr. Livingston for advice regarding the choice of a graduate school. He suggested that I apply to Georgetown University in Washington DC and to the University of Pennsylvania. I interviewed at the University of Pennsylvania and was subjected to a day long "interrogation" by Carl Schmidt, M.D., Chairman of Pharmacology and a number of distinguished persons including Seymour Kety, M.D. and Domingo M. Aviado, M.D. At the end of the interview, I was informed that despite my academic record and good showing during the interview, it was highly unlikely that I would be accepted into the graduate program at the University of Pennsylvania as they had never accepted anyone without an M.D. degree.

The visit to the University of Pennsylvania left me disappointed. I returned to Dr. Livingston for advice. I asked his opinion on the University of Michigan. I recall how he had often made reference in class about the work on narcotic analgesics being done by Dr. Maurice Seevers. Dr. Livingston seemed surprised by my question. After a brief moment of hesitation he implored me not to go to Michigan. When I asked for his reasons, he replied, "Once you go to Ann Arbor, you will never leave."

I had no difficulty making my decision and applied to the University of Michigan Horace H. Rackham School of Graduate Studies. My acceptance to the graduate program was received shortly thereafter. To my surprise, on the following day, I also received acceptance to the University of Pennsylvania as well as to Georgetown University. Dr. Livingston's premonition still rang clear in my memory and I accepted the opportunity to enroll at the University of Michigan. One thing is obvious, Dr. Livingston was correct. I can honestly say that I have never seriously contemplated leaving the University of Michigan and consider it an honor to have been permitted to be a student as well as a faculty member for the past 43 years.

It was a pleasant Sunday afternoon during the first week of September 1957. Family members had gathered at Grand Central Station in New York City to say farewell to Diana, my wife of three months, and me as we boarded the train that was to take us to Ann Arbor, Michigan. For our respective families this was an adventure as we were the first members of either family to leave the "Big Apple" and take the chance of crossing the Hudson River for the "western wilderness." Some 12 hours later the train arrived at the station in Ann Arbor, early on Monday morning.

As Diana and I left the train we gazed about in wonderment. The railroad station, a small stone building with many boxcars lining the tracks, was in marked contrast to New York's Grand Central Station. Somewhere inside the mass of freight cars were all of our worldly possessions. We were not to see our belongings for at least a week, as thousands of students were also arriving in Ann Arbor to begin a new life and it would require days locate and retrieve our possessions.

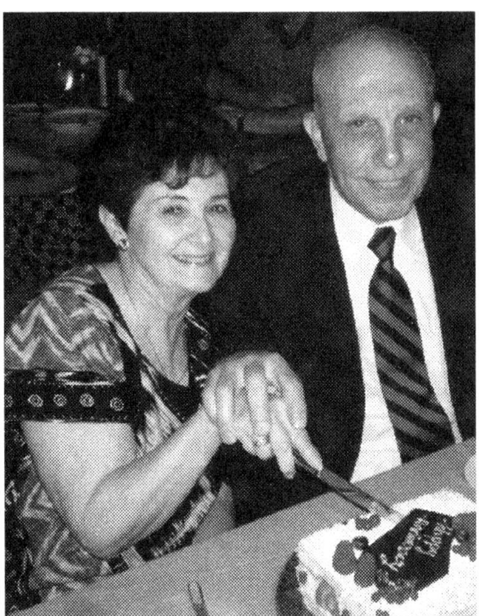

Ben and Diana Lucchesi's 40th anniversary.

We made our way from the station to what was then the original Bell Tower Hotel. That was to be our home for the next week since the University had informed us only a few days before leaving New York City that our apartment on North Campus would not be available. Thus, the Bell Tower became our "home" while looked for an apartment. We spent part of Monday searching, but without success.

On Tuesday morning, the ring of the telephone awakened us; my mother was calling from New York City. She informed me that I had received a letter from the draft board stating that I was to report for induction into the Armed Forces (US Marines). My deferment from military service had expired since having been deferred initially in 1951 and a second time during my graduate training at St. John's University. It appeared that my hopes of starting graduate school at Michigan were to come to an abrupt end. However, I had trust in the system and I immediately submitted an appeal to my draft board in New York City. In the meantime, we had to focus on finding an apartment. This too was not progressing well.

After almost five days of being refused by numerous landlords Diana and I were becoming discouraged. Suddenly a person unknown to us came to the hotel and said he had heard of our predicament and offered to rent us an apartment. The unexpected act of kindness was appreciated. And so Diana and I moved into our first Ann Arbor apartment, 537 North Main Street. Once more we visited the railroad station to find our possessions; this time we were successful. Our trunk had arrived safely. Now we could begin to set up our apartment and start our life in Ann Arbor. We rapidly grew fond of Ann Arbor despite having encountered a few obstacles and lingering uncertainties about our future. The fall term was about to begin and there was an air of excitement further enhanced by the fact that Diana obtained employment as a pharmacist at St. Joseph Mercy Hospital.

My appointment to meet with Dr. Seevers was scheduled for the afternoon. I arrived at the Pharmacology Department, located on the Diag on central campus; it was a magnificent fortress-like building built of solid stone and heavy timbers. I entered the departmental office and was greeted by Mrs. Dorothy Norton (later Mrs. Overbeck), who instructed me to wait until Dr. Seevers was ready to see me. In the meantime, Diana was waiting on one of the stone benches outside believing that my visit with Dr. Seevers would be short. This was not to be the case. I sat in the outer office along with another entering student, Edward Albert, who by coincidence had also just arrived from New York City. We became instant friends, with similar stories about life in the "big city." After what seemed like an eternity, I was asked to enter the chairman's office for my interview with Dr. Seevers.

He was an impressive figure seated behind the heavy wooden desk on which there sat a skull of a Rhesus monkey. I did not dare to ask the significance of this artifact. Dr. Seevers reviewed my academic record from St. John's University and noted that I had an advanced degree in Physiology along with a strong background in Biochemistry. He outlined a course of instruction, which included the medical school courses in Histology, Embryology, Neuroanatomy, Statistics, Pharmacology, and Pathology. I was also advised to audit the courses in Biochemistry and Physiology. It was the custom in the 1950s for graduate students in Pharmacology to take the same courses offered to medical students in the first two years with the exception of Gross Anatomy and Psychiatry. In addition, graduate students were required to take at least one graduate course each term outside of the Department of Pharmacology as well as graduate courses offered by the members of the Pharmacology Department. Along with the course requirements, graduate students were required to rotate among the laboratories in the Department and to participate in the teaching of medical students. In the third and fourth graduate years, the teaching assignments consisted of assisting in the medical student laboratories twice a week. As for my laboratory rotation, I was assigned to work under the supervision of Harold F. Hardman, M.D., Ph.D.

Thus I began my study of pharmacology at the University of Michigan Medical School. The academic environment was challenging and exciting. The Dean of the Medical School was Albert C. Furstenberg, M.D., an impressive figure who maintained an active clinical practice in Otolaryngology. Dean Furstenberg supported efforts to promote a research environment in the medical school and the recruitment of most outstanding educators in the basic medical sciences. The opportunity to study under such distinguished figures as Russell Woodburne in Histology, Bradley Patton in Embryology, Elizabeth Crosby in Neuroanatomy, Horace Davenport, Walter Wilde, David Bohr and others in Physiology, and Halvor Christiansen in Biochemistry, along with the faculty in the Department of Pharmacology, is by today's standards of graduate education incomprehensible. To be involved in such a heavy course load while at the same time participating in laboratory research required a total dedication that, for some reason, does not seem possible today. I should not forget to mention the fact that in addition to the courses mentioned, there was the requirement to pass examinations in two foreign languages. Having studied both French and German while in high school, I completed my language requirements during my first year. However, for many prospective students, the foreign language requirements proved to be a major hurdle and in some cases, their downfall. In later years, the Graduate School made the decision to eliminate the foreign language requirements for the Ph.D. degree, thus easing the pressure for many prospective students.

It was now October 1957 and the graduate program, while challenging, was exciting. Working with Dr. Hardman was rewarding although the classified nature of the project kept me from knowing exactly why we were studying a compound referred to only as EA 1476. This oily, viscous substance was essentially insoluble in water and it was my task to formulate the substance so that it could be

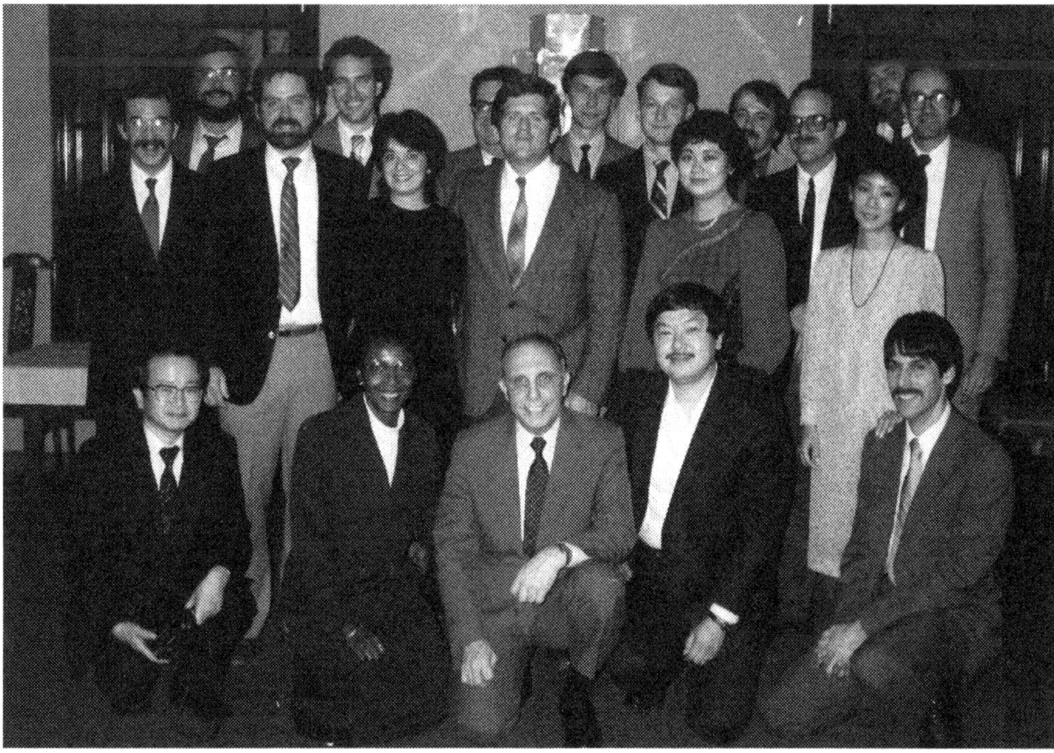

Former Lucchesi laboratory graduate students and postdoctoral fellows reunion in Washington DC, ca. 1970.

administered by intravenous injection. The task was relatively simple as I had a good background in preparing emulsions. Having accomplished this, we were well on our way to dosing animals with EA 1476 and observing a dramatic pharmacological event in which the animal (dog) essentially was put into a state of "suspended animation". The task given to the investigative team was to find the antidote that would restore the animal to its normal state. The reason why the United States Government and the military wanted this information remained a mystery for many years until the project was declassified. In addition, it was noted that EA 1476 had analgesic properties. Therefore, as a side project, Ed Alpert and I were assigned the task of evaluating EA1476 for its analgesic potential as assessed with the use of the rat tail-flick and the mouse hot-plate methods.

On October 4, 1957, the Soviet Union stunned the world when Sputnik rode into orbit on a ballistic missile. The first artificial satellite had been launched. Its two radio transmitters sent "beeping" signals to the world as it orbited the earth. By US standards, Sputnik was huge; at 184.3 pounds it was 20 times larger than the satellite the US was attempting to launch. Dwight D. Eisenhower was President of the United States and in a radio address to the nation he stressed the need to increase US investment in education and scientific research. A month later, the Soviet Union compounded U.S. discomfort by launching Sputnik II with a live dog named Laika as a passenger. The US failure to launch its small satellite in December 1957 further emphasized the magnitude of the Soviet accomplishment.

In the early days of the space race, the goal was to go to Mars. However, the United States lacked rockets of sufficient power to carry astronauts and the necessary life support equipment to such great distances. Therefore to reduce the necessary life-support payload, it was considered desirable to place the occupants into a state of suspended animation that could be reversed upon command by the administration of an antidote. EA 1476 was such an agent, if only an antidote could be found. This was the goal of our highly classified project.

In early December 1957 I received notice that my appeal for deferment had been denied and I was to report for induction into the US Marine Corps the first week of January 1958. Remembering the radio message from President Eisenhower and the urgent need to win the race into space, I exercised my last option, a direct Presidential Appeal.

I wrote a letter to President Eisenhower in which I indicated that my space related project would be interrupted if I were to be drafted into the military at this time. Dr. Seevers prepared a letter addressed to the Division of Manpower for the State of New York. I was instructed by Dr. Seevers not to open the envelope that had been sealed with wax and to deliver it to Colonel Dwyer in New York City. On December 23, 1957 I arrived at LaGuardia Airport shortly after the noon hour and took a taxi into the city where I met with Colonel Dwyer. I handed him the sealed envelope. He opened the envelope and carefully read the brief, but apparently impressive message. He made an immediate telephone call from one of two telephones on his desk, the red one. I could hear him asking the person on the opposite end to check a specific contract number. Upon receiving what was apparently a verification of the fact that I indeed was associated with the government research contract mentioned in the letter, Colonel Dwyer turned to me and wished me a Merry Christmas and a Happy New Year. I never found out what was in the letter crafted by Dr. Seevers. Whatever was written must have been important.

Upon my return to Ann Arbor that same evening, I found a letter bearing the return address of the Office of the President of the United States, The White House, Washington DC. The letter instructed me to disregard all future orders from my draft board. Sherman Adams, Secretary to the President of the United States, had signed the letter. I finally understood why NSF had allocated all of its fellowship funds to the study of astronomy. Charting the stars in our skies and beyond was of major importance if the United States was to maintain its superiority in the early days of the Cold War. I recognized that I had been granted an opportunity to continue my studies and was determined to make the most of this experience.

We continued with the study of EA 1476. Dr. Edward Domino and Dr. Hardman determined that the catatonic state induced by EA 1476 was reversible by the intravenous administration of dextroamphetamine. The response was dramatic and one that was certain to make a lasting impression upon a new graduate student. There was no better example of a drug-induced response. My fascination with drug actions and mechanisms was reinforced. In 1958, Powell and Slater reported the pharmacology of the first beta-adrenoceptor blocking agent (J. Pharmacol. Exp. Therap. 122:480, 1958) followed shortly thereafter by the classic publication of Moran and Perkins describing the cardiovascular effects associated with beta-receptor blockade (J. Pharmacol. Exp. Therap.124: 223, 1958). This event provided an opportunity to engage in a new and rapidly developing area of cardiovascular pharmacology.

At the time, I was working in Dr. Hardman's laboratory on a project involving the effects of ionization on drug actions. The study made use of the isolated turtle heart exposed to drugs under varying conditions of pH while monitoring the altered inotropic

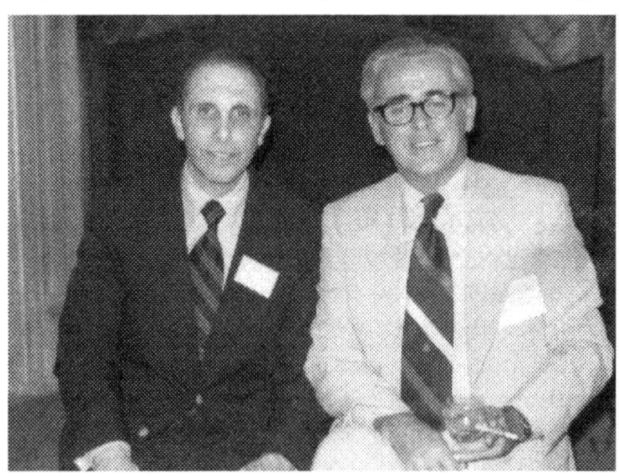

A young Ben and Harry

actions of specific pharmacological interventions. Therefore, it was possible to determine whether the ionized or unionized form of the drug was most active. Although interesting, my attention was being drawn to the study of beta-adrenergic receptor blocking agents.

I expressed my interests to Dr. Hardman. He was understanding and agreed that I could pursue my own interests in the evening while I assisted in conducting the studies on drug ionization in the daytime. He also allotted a budget ($800) to support my studies. I became totally absorbed in my research and soon determined that the drug, dichloroisoproterenol (DCI) possessed antiarrhythmic properties independent of its ability to block the cardiac beta-adrenergic receptor. My desire to continue the studies with DCI required that I obtain an additional research supply of the drug. A letter requesting an additional amount of DCI was sent to Dr. Irwin Slater, Director of Pharmacology at the Eli Lilly Company. Dr. Slater's response indicated that Eli Lilly had decided to discontinue the project on beta-adrenergic blocking agents because, "there did not appear to be a potential clinical application for this class of compound." Some many years later, upon a visit to Eli Lilly, Dr. Slater showed me an entry in his personal diary in which he recorded having sent such a letter (which I still retain in my files) and acknowledged that discontinuing the development of beta-adrenergic blocking drugs was the greatest mistake of his career.

Fortunately, Imperial Chemical Industries had undertaken efforts to develop beta-adrenoceptor blocking agents. It was a fortuitous happening that Dr. James Black presented a seminar in the Department of Pharmacology in which he described the basic pharmacological properties of pronethalol and propranolol. I had the opportunity to show Dr. Black my data on DCI and he agreed to provide me with pronethalol as well as propranolol. In order to demonstrate that the antiarrhythmic action of this class of compounds was independent of receptor blockade, I requested that the dextro- and levo-optical isomers be provided. Dr. Black was gracious and made available to me the dextro- and levo-rotatory isomers of propranolol. The data supported the concept that propranolol possessed antiarrhythmic properties that were separate from its ability to inhibit cardiac beta-adrenoceptors. Submission of our findings to the American Heart Journal was received with a total lack of enthusiasm. The response from the editor was as follows, "The drug you describe (propranolol) is of little interest to clinicians and your paper would be better suited for a specialty journal". Ultimately, the Journal of Pharmacology and Experimental Therapeutics accepted the manuscript despite the fact that one of the reviewers had recommended rejection of the paper. Dr. Neil Moran (Chairman, Department of Pharmacology, Emory University) instructed me to disregard the major objections since he had conducted similar studies and confirmed my results.

Propranolol was the first beta-adrenergic receptor blocking agent approved by the United States Food and Drug Administration, with the primary indication being that of an antiarrhythmic agent. My studies with this class of compounds formed the basis of my doctoral dissertation that I completed in December 1960; I graduated in May 1961.

The opportunity to engage in the study of beta-adrenoceptor blocking agents would not have been possible had it not been for Dr. Hardman who allowed me to pursue my "dream." I learned early in my career that when one comes upon a new finding, the excitement of discovery is the driving force. To this day, I try to emulate Dr. Hardman's approach in the training of graduate students and postdoctoral fellows. The pursuit of one's own findings is the most effective way of encouraging excitement and determination to seek new knowledge. Towards this end, each new student coming to my laboratory is provided with a key to the laboratory on the first day. I explain to each student the reason for having the key: for those times when an idea that comes in the mid-morning (e.g. 2A.M.), one need not wait for a later hour to explore it.

In the fall of 1959, Dr. Hardman announced that he would be leaving the University of Michigan to assume the chairmanship in pharmacology at Marquette University Medical School in Milwaukee, Wisconsin. Thus, I was left to complete my doctoral studies by correspondence.

Following Dr. Hardman's departure from the University of Michigan and at a time when I was completing my dissertation studies, I was summoned to meet with Dr. Seevers. To my surprise I was offered the half-time position of Instructor in Pharmacology with the understanding that I would apply to medical school, a totally unanticipated sequence of events, but an opportunity that I could not resist. So it was that I began my medical school studies in September of 1960. However, having taken essentially the first two years of medical school courses as part of the Ph.D. curriculum, I was given credit for those courses and was required only to take Gross Anatomy and Psychiatry over the next two years.

Thus, there was ample time to complete the writing of my dissertation and my first NIH grant submission. The grant, entitled "Analysis of Antiarrhythmic Agents," was approved for funding with a start date of January 1, 1961, and was funded continuously for the next 38 years, the last 10 of which were a Merit Award. Those final 10 years of the grant were among my most productive. The concept of the Merit Award should not be underestimated. The ability to conduct research with the guarantee of a period of uninterrupted funding provided an opportunity to follow "the science" as opposed to following the latest trends and fads in basic research. During this phase of my career, a number of animal models were developed that have become the "gold standards" in cardiovascular pharmacology. The most prominent model was the canine model of sudden cardiac death that is used by many to detect the antifibrillatory and profibrillatory actions of new pharmacological agents. The second model was that of spontaneous arterial thrombosis that provided the first clinically relevant model for the assessment of antithrombotic and fibrinolytic agents. Many graduate students, postdoctoral fellows and undergraduates were the beneficiaries of the NIH support as well as other foundation grants and industry contracts. Once again, none of this would have occurred had it not been for the fact that Dr. Seevers and faculty colleagues had not been willing to support me in the development of my career.

I specifically recall the day Dr. Seevers offered me the opportunity to be appointed as an instructor in the Department of Pharmacology, an offer I accepted readily. As I left the office along with Dr. Seevers, we encountered the young and successful Dr. Edward Domino. Dr. Seevers, in his usual and very direct manner, "asked" (ordered) Dr. Domino to transfer $5,000 of his research monies to an account in my name. Without hesitation, Dr. Domino complied with the "request". This was to be my first source of funds. This act of generosity was not to be forgotten and the debt was repaid (in principle) some many years later when there was a need to help a colleague. I believe I still have a responsibility to pay the interest, if the need should arise. Under Dr. Seevers' leadership we were trained to function as members of a family who cared for each other! Much of this behavior has been lost over the years, but I do see signs of its return. The measure of success goes beyond the number of publications or dollar value in grant support in a department. The measure of success in an academic setting should not exclude the human factor as determined by the training of future academicians and scientists in the discipline of pharmacology. More than ever before, the training of young scientists will require careful nurturing and guidance in the formative years and perhaps beyond. Leadership requires that those in charge be willing to set aside personal pursuits of scientific achievements and devote part or all of their efforts toward developing the next generation of scholars. Being a leader (chairman) should be viewed as a full-time occupation in which the major goal is to ensure the success of the discipline and the appropriate training of those who will inherit the responsibility for the development of new therapeutic advances in medicine.

In June of 1962 I began my third year of Medical School. The next two years were to be the most taxing in terms of the workload. In addition, my wife had given birth to Thomas, our first son, in November 1959, and our daughter Mary in September 1961, and was expecting our third child, Richard, who was born 12:45 A.M., January 1, 1963 (first born in Washtenaw County). The clinical years, along with the responsibility of conducting my research and tending to my teaching duties, were demanding. I learned to exist on a maximum of four hours of sleep a night. However, the excitement of the laboratory and acquisition of new knowledge related to the care of patients and clinical use of pharmacological interventions kept me infused with a desire to continue.

It was during my third year in medical school that I had the good fortune to be under the guidance of Dr. Richard Judge and Dr. Thomas Preston. Both were cardiologists who had degrees in electrical engineering. It was a time when there was a growing interest in developing implantable devices for pacing the human heart. Having a research laboratory at my disposal was an opportunity to work with my "teachers" in developing the first pacemaker produced by the General Electric Company along with an external device use to interrogate the implanted unit. This was an example of translational research in which basic animal laboratory studies evolved to the point of applying the knowledge to patients. This was to be my first clinical research experience and one that produced personal satisfaction in knowing that the lives of many patients benefited from our efforts. Also important is the fact that "student" and "teacher" worked together with each contributing their respective talents toward achieving a common goal.

In another incident, I recall the day in the operating room when a patient was under-

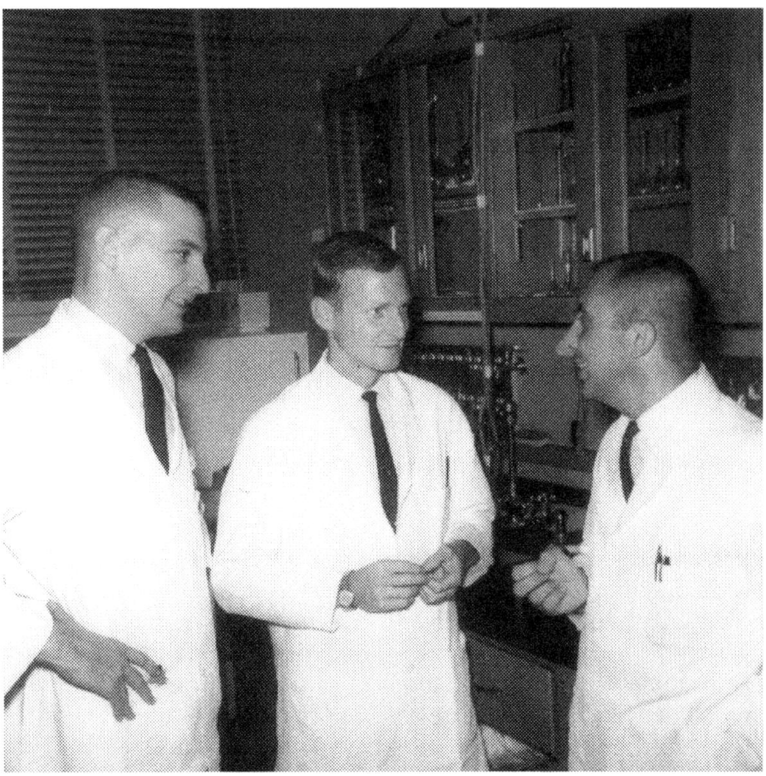

Leighton Whitsitt (far left) was a graduate student in Dr. Lucchesi's lab when they observed the "stone heart phenomenon".

going repair of an aortic valve. The procedure was done while the heart was in arrest and globally ischemic thus requiring the surgeon to proceed with the utmost of speed. All went well until the heart was reperfused upon restoring the coronary blood supply. To my surprise the heart went into contracture and did not recover its contractile function. This event had been described in the literature and was referred to as the "stone heart phenomenon." This experience was remembered and a short time later was recalled to my attention as a result of a laboratory observation.

Leighton Whitsitt, a graduate student was working in my laboratory and we were able to reproduce the "stone heart phenomenon" in the canine heart. Subsequently a grant proposal was submitted to the NIH in which I hypothesized that the reintroduction of oxygenated blood to the previously ischemic heart would lead to injury and cell death. I referred to this phenomenon as "reperfusion injury" and attributed the tissue injury to formation of oxygen free radicals. The NIH "Pink Sheet" summary statement began as follows: "This is a naïve concept and the investigator should return to medical school and take a course in pathology." The rest of the review and the ultimate decision should be self-evident. My rebuttal resulted in a site visit that failed to convince the reviewers that the concept of oxygen free radical-induced reperfusion injury was deserving of study. My own graduate students and some of my faculty colleagues voiced skepticism and refused to engage in or collaborate on the project.

As a last resort, I placed a telephone call to a colleague, Dr. Walter Freyburger, at the Upjohn Company in Kalamazoo, Michigan. Dr. Freyburger arranged for me to obtain the necessary research funding ($25,000) to develop my concept. At the time I was joined by Stanley Jolly, Ph.D., who had recently completed his doctoral studies under the guidance of Dr. Hardman in Milwaukee. Stan was given the charge of testing the free radical hypothesis. His masterful experimental protocol proved the correctness of the hypothesis. The paper was published in Circulation Research and the observations were soon confirmed by independent studies from investigators at Johns Hopkins University. Resubmission to the NIH to study myocardial reperfusion injury resulted in funding for 17 consecutive years.

The opportunities to take basic research to the bedside continued through my medical school years. In my senior year, I did an elective in cardiology and worked with Dr. Ernest Reynolds. We became good friends and engaged in joint research projects. I had the chance to show Dr. Reynolds the positive inotropic actions of glucagon upon the heart in the presence of beta-adrenoceptor blockade. This was of interest to me since beta-adrenoceptor antagonists have the potential to depress the heart and induce cardiac decompensation. At the time, an effective antidote for the reversal of cardiac depression secondary to beta-adrenoceptor blockade was not available. An earlier publication had mistakenly interpreted the data to suggest that beta-adrenoceptor blockade would block glucagon's positive inotropic action. However, my own study results were not in agreement with this and we were able to show that glucagon was an effective antidote capable of restoring cardiac contractility in the heart subjected to beta-adrenoceptor blockade. Additional studies conducted with the assistance of an undergraduate student, Peter Winokor, demonstrated that glucagon was an effective positive inotropic agent in an experimental model of chronic heart failure. Peter went on to medical school and subsequently entered private practice in the Detroit suburbs.

Dr. Reynolds remained unimpressed with my findings and did not see a potential application for the use of glucagon despite my repeated suggestions that it would be an effective means of augmenting cardiac output in both the failed heart as well as in the presence of cardiac depression associated with beta-adrenoceptor blockade. I was losing the argument with my "teacher" and ceased to pursue the subject.

A short time later, I was awakened by a telephone call. A husky and tired voice, but clearly that of Dr. Reynolds, said, "glucagon works," after which the caller hung up. I knew immediately that I had to go to University Hospital, where I found Dr. Reynolds and a cardiology fellow at the bedside of an elderly patient who had congestive heart failure and was being treated with digoxin. The patient had developed a rapid heart rate and inadvertently was administered intravenous propranolol for the purpose of slowing the heart rate. Unfortunately, the combined actions of digoxin and propranolol succeeded in inducing complete atrioventricular block and a low cardiac output state. The fellow contacted Dr. Reynolds, who upon recalling my "informal lectures," advised the fellow to administer intravenous glucagon. The patient, who was comatose and in a state of cardiogenic shock, gradually regained consciousness as her cardiac function and heart rate improved. For some time thereafter, glucagon was used at University Hospital for supporting cardiac function in patients with low cardiac output states, especially those awaiting heart transplantation. Another example of a basic laboratory observation applied to a clinical situation. To my knowledge, this was the first use of glucagon for the reversal of cardiac depression secondary to beta-adrenoceptor blockade. Unfortunately, the pharmaceutical company (Eli Lilly) did not consider developing glucagon for use as an inotropic agent.

On yet another occasion during my cardiology rotation I encountered a situation in which a patient developed ventricular fibrillation upon the intraventricular administration of a radio-contrast agent, Angio-Conray. Dr. William Weber rapidly resuscitated the patient and expressed his frustration with the new contrast agent that had induced potentially lethal arrhythmias in other patients. I invited Dr. Weber to come to my laboratory where we could examine Angio-Conray along with other available radio-contrast agents. At the time, Richard Dean was my graduate student and along with Dr. Weber and myself embarked upon a study to examine the effects of several radio-contrast agents when injected into the coronary circulation. It became apparent to us that the high osmolarity of the solutions (~1400 mOsmoles) was contributing to the problem and was responsible for severe disruption of the coronary vascular endothelium. We enlisted the technical support of Mallinckrodt, Inc., a major supplier of radio-contrast agents. We suggested that the osmolarity of the solution could be reduced significantly by combining two molecules into one while at the same time maintaining the degree of iodination required to achieve opacification (X-ray contrast) of the vessels. Our suggestions proved to be correct. The new low osmolarity contrast agents proved to be less damaging to the coronary vasculature and did not induce disturbances in cardiac rhythm. Subsequently Mallinckrodt marketed the new and more acceptable formulation that remains in use to this day.

Having the Ph.D. in Pharmacology along with a faculty position and laboratory space while going to medical school provided me with opportunities not available to most medical students or faculty. My situation was not unique as several members of the Department of Pharmacology had similar arrangements under Dr. Seevers. A number of my peers, Robert Reynolds, Edward Alpert, Carl Hug, and Raymond Ruddon, had similar opportunities provided to them. There were many others who came before (Dr. Hardman, Dr. Edward Cafruny, Dr. Donald Bennett), as well as others who followed. In the 1950s pursuit of both the Ph.D. and M.D. degrees was uncommon. Dr. Seevers was among the first to recognize the value of a broad training in pharmacology that required extensive classroom learning while in graduate school as well as the subsequent completion of a medical school curriculum. Equally important, he recognized the need to support the effort and to make an investment in the training and development of future pharmacologists.

I completed my medical school training in June 1964 and began full-time employment as an Instructor in the Department of Pharmacology. It was about this time when the Surgeon General of the United States was expressing concern over the health hazards associated with the use of tobacco and tobacco products. Dr. Seevers was appointed to chair the committee on Tobacco and Health. The American Medical Association-Education Research Foundation (AMA-ERF) agreed to fund studies to examine the potential adverse effects of tobacco on health.

Dr. Seevers, himself a smoker (of cigars) immediately issued "orders" that smoking would not be permitted in the Department. Furthermore, he was instrumental in removing cigarette vending machines from the student study areas (formerly located on the third level of Medical Science Building I) as well as prohibiting the sale of tobacco products at University Hospital. For many years Galen's Newspaper Stand, a medical student-operated venture situated in the main lobby of the hospital, had been the primary source of tobacco products. Dr. Seevers, with little support from faculty colleagues, led a "one-man crusade" against what he came to realize was a major public health hazard.

As a result of his long time interest in drug-related physical dependence, Dr. Seevers came to my office and suggested that I prepare a grant proposal to the AMA-ERF. The primary focus of the proposal was to examine the hypothesis that nicotine was "addictive" or could lead to the development of physical dependence. The study was to be done in human volunteers.

I found it interesting that Dr. Seevers had sufficient confidence in me to suggest that I prepare a grant proposal and engage in a clinical study involving a potentially dangerous substance that was to be administered to humans. As I contemplated the approach, I came to realize that the only way the study could be done was to conduct the investigation in a double-blind manner and to engage the subjects in an activity unrelated to smoking. Thus I called upon a faculty colleague, Charles (Bob) Schuster, Ph.D. Bob was a new faculty member and a trained behavioral psychologist. His research assistant, Ms. Grace Emly also was asked to join in developing the grant proposal that was completed in relatively short time and, to our extreme pleasure, was funded for a period of three years beginning in 1965.

The study involved the recruitment of healthy male and female volunteers over 18 years of age. During the screening interview we observed whether or not the applicant possessed a packet of cigarettes or spontaneously engaged in smoking during the interview. Once it was observed that the person was a tobacco user, he/she was sent forward for a complete medical examination and if found to be in good health was offered an opportunity to participate in the study.

The subjects were asked to come to the laboratory at 7A.M. They were to have abstained from food, caffeine, alcohol, and tobacco from 7P.M. of the preceding day. All personal belongings were removed and the subjects were dressed in surgical "scrub suits" and placed in a sound proof chamber with a one-way window so that they could be observed from the outside. An intravenous line was placed in a hand vein, electrocardiographic leads were attached and blood pressure cuff was placed on the forearm. After obtaining preliminary recordings of vitals, the subjects were given a standardized breakfast, reading material of their choice and of course, upon their request, we permitted them to smoke if they so desired. However, we provided the brand of cigarettes.

The door to the sound-proof chamber was closed and for the next eight hours, the subjects were engaged in carrying out a battery of psychological tests devised by Bob Schuster. At the appropriate time in the protocol, the subjects received either a placebo intravenous infusion of 0.9% sodium chloride solution for Injection or an intravenous infusion of nicotine in a dose equal to that obtained by smoking one cigarette. The intravenous infusions were administered in a pulsed fashion to mimic the manner in which nicotine would be absorbed during smoking a cigarette. The placebo or nicotine infusions were repeated every 30 minutes with each administration lasting 15 minutes. The question to be answered was simple. Would the exogenous administration of nicotine reduce the smoking frequency in a totally naïve subject who otherwise had no intent in discontinuing the use of tobacco? The result of the study was a total surprise. We were able to demonstrate for the first time that nicotine administered systemically would reduce the frequency of smoking thereby providing strong evidence to support the belief that the alkaloid produced a state of physical dependence. The study was published in the Journal of Clinical Pharmacology and Therapeutics and formed the basis for the subsequent use of nicotine patches and chewing gum for persons who desired to discontinue smoking.

I felt indebted to Dr. Seevers for having provided me with this opportunity. At the time I entered the study I was unaware that this would be the first time anyone had administered intravenous nicotine over an extended period to human subjects. Had I known that nicotine had never been administered in this manner, I certainly would have given more consideration to withdrawing from the idea. However, Dr. Seevers mentored us along the way. He always remained in the background, letting Bob and me share the credit for having conducted the first study of its kind and providing data that years later would be used against the tobacco industry in the government's effort to curtail the use of tobacco products based upon the fact that nicotine is "addicting." The three years of funding by the AMA-ERF were most exciting and served to heighten my desire to remain in an academic setting conducting research and teaching, especially at the University of Michigan.

As I look back over the years that I served as a faculty member, I can recall many pleasant experiences and events that hold significance to me. Among the most important is the number of predoctoral and postdoctoral students who have trained in my laboratory. I am proud of what each of them has accomplished, not because of me, but because they were able to take advantage of what the Department and the University was able to offer. I considered myself to be the catalyst that made the process move forward.

Shortly after Dr. Seevers retired in 1971, I contacted Dr. Theodore Brody who was Chairman of the Department of Pharmacology at Michigan State University and proposed that we establish an annual colloquium for graduate students. Ted was enthusiastic about the idea. The first colloquium was held in Ann Arbor on June 11, 1973, and was a resounding success. Graduate students from Michigan State University and the University of Michigan Departments of Pharmacology participated in a daylong series of scientific presentations with the entire program being managed by the students from both schools. News of the colloquium spread rapidly and the next year, graduate students from Wayne State University and the Medical College of Ohio joined in the annual event. The colloquium has been presented annually for the past 30 years. The participation of postdoctoral fellows has added to the importance of the event. The annual event provides an opportunity for over 100 trainees in pharmacology as well as faculty from four departments of pharmacology to come together and share their respective research findings.

As for my professional career, there are several events that stand out. In 1983 I received an unexpected invitation to give the opening talk at the International Society for Heart Research being held in London, England. The original keynote speaker, Dr. F.Z. Meerson from the former Soviet Union, was not permitted to leave his country. I accepted the invitation to travel to London with less than 96 hours notice and gave my first public presentation on the role of oxygen free radicals and neutrophils as contributors to myocardial reperfusion injury. I will forever remember my first visit to London in the month of July when the temperature soared above 100 degree F, or 38 degrees C. I soon discovered that air conditioning was not widely known in England and I also learned to have my cold drinks without ice. Despite having to endure these "hardships," I was happy to have had the opportunity to present my research to a learned audience. I would be forever indebted to Dr. Meerson, who was among the first to recognize the potentially toxic role of oxygen and its reactive metabolites. The debt would be subsequently repaid.

In 1988, I was in the process of organizing the XIII Congress of the International Society for Heart Research, to be held in May 1989. In need of a keynote speaker, I recalled my unpaid debt to Dr. Meerson and decided to invite him to the Congress. At the time, Mikhail Gorbachev was General Secretary of the Central Committee of the Communist Party of the Soviet Union. Mr. Gorbachev had announced sweeping changes in the Soviet Union. Therefore, I co-authored a letter to Mr. Gorbachev, dated June 9, 1988 (my 55th birthday) asking that Soviet scientists be permitted to travel to the United States to attend the XIII Congress of the International Society for Heart Research. On July 11, 1988 a reply came from the Kremlin stating that the Soviet scientists were free to travel to the United States. Dr. Meerson was the keynote speaker, and he, with many visitors from countries behind the Iron Curtain, added to the success of the meeting. The XIII Congress was attended by more than 900 registrants from 35 countries, all enjoying the perfect week of springtime weather in Ann Arbor. The meeting was so successful that I was asked to organize another meeting in 1998.

Another memorable event occurred in 1985 when I was selected to be the recipient of the Gustav Nylin Award presented by the Karolinska Institute in Stockholm, Sweden. The award was given in recognition for my studies related to the role of free radicals as a mediator of myocardial reperfusion injury. The award was significant as it happened at a time when our work was being refuted by many investigators in North America as well as by NIH Study Sections. To my pleasant surprise, my presentation at the Academy of Medicine in Stockholm was well attended and understood by scientists in Sweden. It was obvious to me that others shared my excitement about reperfusion injury as being more than a laboratory curiosity. At the conclusion of my talk I was approached by a medical graduate from Linkoping University, Dr. Hakan Walfridsson, who presented me with a copy of his doctoral thesis entitled, "Myocardial Oxygen Pressure of the Border Zone: Studies of Acute Coronary Occlusion in the Pig." It was apparent that others were beginning to focus on the role of oxygen as a contributor to myocardial injury. The attention given to my research findings by Swedish scientists provided me with the encouragement to continue my studies despite the resistance I was experiencing at home by colleagues and reviewers who found it difficult to accept the concept that the delivery of molecular oxygen could be detrimental to previously ischemic tissue.

I am most appreciative of the honor bestowed upon me in 1989 when I received the Award for Experimental Therapeutics from the American Society for Pharmacology and Experimental Therapeutics. The event was doubly exciting when I discovered that my entire family unexpectedly appeared at the award ceremony held in New Orleans. In 1990 my faculty colleagues in the Medical School bestowed upon me the honor of being selected for the Distinguished Faculty Lectureship in Biomedical Research. The lecture was presented in the Rackham Auditorium and attended by family and friends.

My friend and colleague, Dr. Charles Ross, received his Ph.D. in Pharmacology and went on to be a highly respected faculty member at the Medical College in Syracuse, New York. Dr. Ross, an African American, died prematurely as a result of cancer. Despite his long illness, he continued to serve his department and graduate school and to maintain an active roll in teaching and research. He was an accomplished renal pharmacologist who made significant contributions to understanding the mechanism of action of diuretic drugs. His enthusiasm for pharmacology, and life in general, was contagious. He was a role model for many and a friend to all who knew him. In recognition for his friendship and contributions to education, I established the Charles Ross Fellowship in his honor in 1991. For the last 10 years the Department of Pharmacology has awarded Summer Research Fellowships to underrepresented minorities who are selected to participate in research in the Department of Pharmacology. The program was one of the firsts of its kind in the Medical School and continues to flourish with the aid of contributions from alumni and grant support from the

Dean's Diversity and Career Development Committee. The Charles Ross Fellows are joined by other Summer Research Students supported by a competitive award from the Zannoni-Dalton Fund administered by the American Society for Pharmacology and Experimental Therapeutics.

The summer program began as a modest effort to introduce undergraduate students to the discipline of pharmacology and has grown to include high school and medical students who engage in a 12-week research experience with faculty in the Department of Pharmacology. The opportunity to work with the young, enthusiastic, and inquisitive students is both challenging and rewarding. Efforts devoted to the summer research program yield dividends in terms of shaping careers and making lasting contributions that give more personal satisfaction and a feeling of fulfillment far exceeding the pleasure derived from yet another publication or funded research proposal. Perhaps this is the reason why many decide to remain in an academic career despite the options to seek other means of employment.

I consider myself to be most fortunate to have been both a student and a faculty member at the University of Michigan Medical School. I enjoyed my days as a student in graduate school as well as in the medical school. During the course of obtaining my Ph.D. and M.D. degrees, I was fortunate to have been instructed by outstanding teachers and to make many long lasting friendships.

I would be remiss if I failed to express my appreciation to the late Dr. John Gronvall, who served as Dean of the Medical School. Dean Gronvall offered me the opportunity to serve as Interim Director of the Upjohn Center for Clinical Pharmacology. The experience was invaluable and gave me the opportunity to engage in clinical investigations leading to the development of several cardiovascular drugs, which include the topical nitroglycerin patch, intravenous nitroglycerin, bretylium and anagrelide.

Working with Dr. Gronvall on the Medical School Executive Committee offered another opportunity for growth and development. I gained a deep sense of appreciation for the enormity of the job of dean of the medical school, a position that also had the responsibility of managing the Medical Center. To this day I consider the Medical School Executive Committee and the Advisory Committee for Appointments, Promotions and Titles to be the most important committees in the Medical School. The decisions made in these committees have an important influence upon the lives of the faculty. Member participation on the committees is not to be taken lightly. The learning experience and the sense of contributing to the operation of the medical school make the effort worthwhile.

I express a deep sense of gratitude to Dr. Stefan Fajans who entrusted to me the position of Director of Research in the Michigan Diabetes Research and Training Center. The involvement in the Diabetes Center provided many important lessons, not the least of which was the preparation of two Center Proposals that were funded. It was also an opportunity to engage in an area of basic and clinical investigation that departed significantly from my primary interests in cardiovascular pharmacology. Dr. Fajans was an excellent mentor and remains a good friend.

My schooling and the performance of my faculty duties over the past 46 years would not have been possible had it not been for my wife Diana and my children, Thomas, Mary, Richard, Steven and John. They supported me during the years that I was in school and seldom at home. In the early days before our first-born son, Diana provided the support by working as a pharmacist at St. Joseph Mercy Hospital. In addition she served as a constant source of encouragement, especially during the third and fourth-clinical years of medical school that often clashed with my departmental teaching responsibilities and preparation of NIH grant applications. Diana had the major burden of raising the children, not an easy task when one must do it alone. My family was patient during the years when I was often away. We struggled to remain financially stable. There were few luxuries during those early days. The last year of medical school became extremely worrisome. We exhausted all of our savings and had only 90 dollars in the bank, with a mortgage, property taxes, tuition payments and children to support. The lowest point came when I was denied financial assistance from the medical school. The family held matters together; we continued to function and it all turned out well.

Part of the success was due to the caring attitude in the Department of Pharmacology. Mrs. Dorothy (Norton) Overbeck would be sent out to make periodic "scouting visits" to the faculty offices. Seemingly we would engage in idle conversation, most often focusing on family matters. Dotty was a keen observer who could sense when financial concerns were a problem and when there was a need for financial support. Somehow, the salary raises were always there when they were needed most. Together, both Dr. Seevers and Dotty were able to work miracles. We were indeed a family, both at home and at work, which cared for and supported one another.

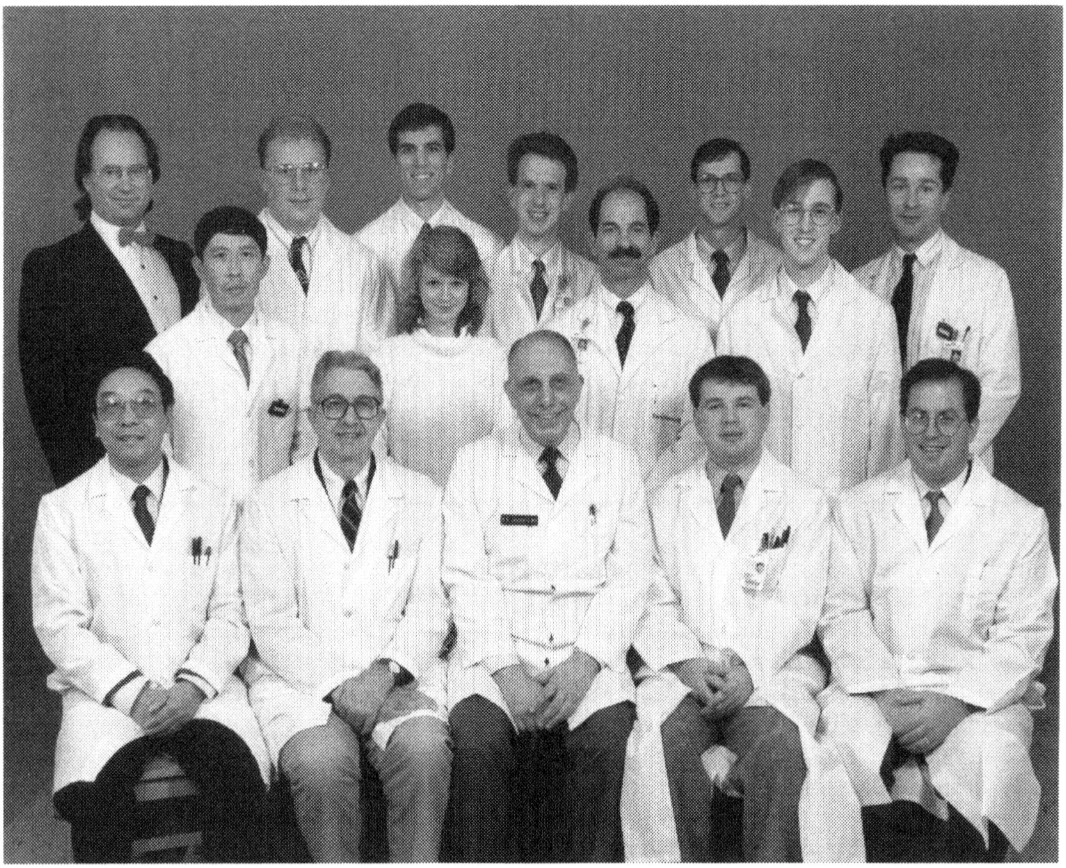

Front row: Dun-Xue Mu, James Davis, Benedict R. Lucchesi, Michael Ranier, William Rote Midde row: Liguo Chi, Laura Sell, Steven Werns, Peter Manly Back row: Edward Driscoll, Michael Gralinski, Gregory Friedrichs, Kenneth Kilgore, Jonathon Homeister, Shawn Black, ca. 1991.

Memoirs: 1957-1960

Anand L. Misra, Ph.D.

I arrived in New York in July 1957 on a Smith-Mundt Fulbright scholarship to pursue studies on the use of radioisotopes in biological research. The program was managed by the Institute of International Education in New York; the Institute made all the arrangements for my short stay in New York, and my travel to Syracuse, NY, for a six-week orientation program. This involved short stays with American families and in University dormitories; visits to supermarkets (which were quite novel to me at that time), beaches, and industrial factories (such as the IBM research center in Yorktown Heights, NY); and familiarity with American sports, the US Constitution, and the educational system at Syracuse University. This was indeed a pleasant educational experience for someone who had not seen skyscrapers before, and gave me a feel for the American way of life.

After the orientation program, I arrived in Ann Arbor, a beautiful, neat, clean, and crime-free University town, and reported to Mrs. Dorothy (Norton) Overbeck, the Administrative Head of the Pharmacology Department, situated in the historic old building on the left side of the Diag directly opposite the University library. Dotty, as everyone affectionately called her, informed Dr. Maurice Seevers of my arrival. Dr. Seevers greeted me warmly in his office and made me feel welcome instantly, describing in detail his pleasant trip to Jaipur and Udaipur (India) some years earlier. He then introduced me to Dr. Lauren Woods in his first floor office. After a preliminary chat about the orientation program, Dr. Woods gave me an idea of the scientific program I was to pursue with him. He also introduced me to his assistant, Dr. Lawrence Bruce Mellett, and to Dr. Salah El-Dareer from Egypt, who had been working in the department for a few years and with the other members of the staff.

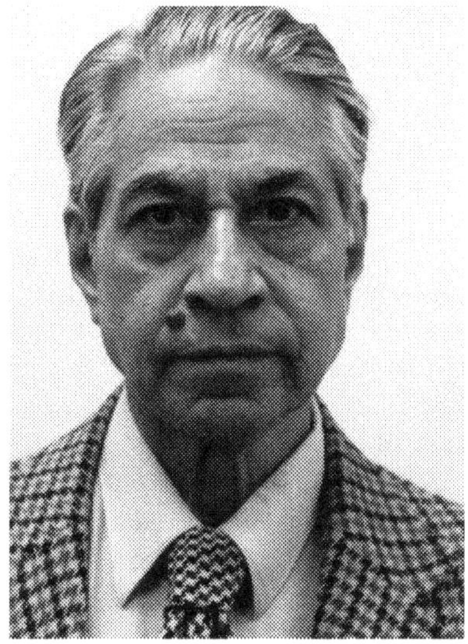

Bruce, being a senior member of Dr. Woods' group, was, with his usual sense of humor, very helpful on a day-to-day basis to all newcomers in our group, with all kinds of general information, scientific procedures and techniques, etc. He was also actively pursuing his own research on disposition and metabolism of opiates and cancer chemotherapeutic agents supported by Dr. Woods' grants from the National Institutes of Health.

Dr. Woods and I then moved to the basement laboratory, where the work with drugs labeled with ^{14}C-radioisotope was being carried out. The method of counting radioactivity with a Geiger-Muller counter using a thin layer of radioactive material spread on metal planchetts was laborious and time-consuming. Dr. Katherine Anderson, an organic chemist who was shortly going to leave the department to join Dupont Company in Delaware, had developed a facile synthesis of morphine-N-methyl-^{14}C using "cold" normorphine and paraformaldehyde-^{14}C. This preparation was widely adopted by commercial firms supplying ^{14}C-labeled morphine to investigators around the country.

Dr. Woods, however, was already thinking of switching to the newly developed technique of liquid scintillation counting of weak beta emitters (^{14}C and ^{3}H) and had already purchased the first manually operated model of the Packard liquid scintillation counter on which I gained experience initially. We encountered frequent problems with the blowout of electronic vacuum tubes used in the counter and Dr. Woods and I would get down on our knees to check the circuits in the back of the counter to replace the defective tubes. However, very soon we replaced the machine with a Packard transistorized counter, which was a great improvement over the previous model.

At about this time a short note on tritiation of organic compounds by exposure to tritium gas appeared in the Journal of the American Chemical Society by Dr. K. Wilzbach. We got our micronised morphine (prepared according to the tips offered by Dr. Anthony Glazko of Parke-Davis Company to Dr. Woods) tritiated at a commercial house offering such a service. Because of enormous decomposition and browning of morphine due to high tritium radiation flux, the final product had to be thoroughly purified to remove labile tritium and colored impurities to obtain the colorless morphine-^{3}H. On checking its purity, however, on buffered paper chromatography, we found a very large portion of radioactivity resided in a trace contaminant (later shown to be dihydromorphine. ^{3}H along with the bulk of morphine-^{3}H having comparatively lower radioactivity. Using large sheets of buffered cellulose paper, we were able to chromatographically separate morphine-^{3}H from its contaminant and use it for biological studies in the rat.

These studies using radiochemically pure tritium nuclear-labeled morphine reported in Nature (1960 and 1961) established the formation of normorphine-^{3}H as an in-vivo metabolite of morphine in the rat for the first time. These results were confirmed within a year by Dr. Kristen Milthers from Denmark and were interesting in the light of the mechanistic hypothesis of N-dealkylation of opiates advanced at that time by Dr. Arnold Beckett in London, England.

In collaboration with Henry Jacoby, a graduate student, I also carried out studies on the disposition and metabolism of Normorphine-^{3}H, which along with our morphine studies found their way into two publications in the Journal of Pharmacology and Experimental Therapeutics (1961). Our present tritiation technique and ^{14}C-labeling did not provide us with labeled morphine of very high specific activity, which was one of the objectives of Dr. Woods for the study of its regional distribution in different anatomic areas of the dog brain. However, studies with the ^{14}C-labeled morphine and ^{3}H-dihydromorphine were successfully completed by Sal Mulé and Carl Hug, Jr., two graduate students in our group. Dr. Hiroshi Kaneto, a visitor from Japan who joined us in 1958, was actively pursuing morphine receptor binding studies. The commercial availability of morphine-^{3}H of very high specific activity in 1972-73 enabled Dr. Solomon Snyder of Johns Hopkins University in Baltimore, MD to successfully demonstrate the presence of opiate receptors in the rat brain. Similar techniques had earlier been used to demonstrate the presence of steroid receptors in the rat brain using steroids of very high specific activity to obviate non-specific binding of these steroids.

During 1958, we made the move to the new Medical Science Building. Dr. Woods provided us with tote boxes and transport and assigned us the responsibility for moving our respective laboratory equipment and other materials to the new laboratory. The move was undertaken in a very smooth manner without any breakage or loss of material in the shortest possible time. It was indeed a pleasure to work in the spacious new laboratory.

Because of its research, teaching, and Dr. Seevers' international reputation as an expert authority on problems of drug dependence, our pharmacology department had well-deserved recognition as a top-notch institution. The reputed faculty of the department acted as a magnet to attract visiting scientists from all over the world to spend some time in the department, learning techniques and having scientific discourses with friendly and helpful staff members.

Dr. Seevers had initiated and developed a program for the training of Japanese pharmacologists in the Department in 1951, so we witnessed the arrival of a large contingent of Japanese students and staff members for training in various sections of the Department for varying periods of time. I recall the short visit of Dr. R.B. Arora, Head of Pharmacology at the All India Institute of Medical Sciences in New Delhi (an institution supported by the Ford Foundation) to our Department, and spending some pleasant evenings with him. Dr. Frank Fraser of Addiction Research Center in Lexington, KY, also spent some time with us discussing narcotics research problems over evening dinners in downtown Ann Arbor. Dr. P.B. Saxena and Dr. A. Maiti came to work for a short time in the neuropharmacology laboratory of Dr. Domino.

There were memorable saki parties in the Department, particularly one on the arrival of Dr. Hiroshi Kumagai, Head of Pharmacology at the Tokyo University. We also used to have several parties a year at Dr. and Mrs. Seevers' home.

The regular seminar schedule in the Department, as well as the tea and cookie parties arranged by Dotty, brought us in contact with several distinguished scientists from the country for fruitful exchange of ideas. Dr. Donald Bennett and Dr. Duncan McCarthy kindly organized trips to Dow Chemical Company (in Midland, MI) and Parke-Davis in Detroit, which were an invaluable experience for me. Professional associations at Ann Arbor were very informal. The thoughtfulness of Dr. Woods made me feel at home in every possible way. Because of my interest in soccer, he provided me with football tickets several times and also funds for attending the Federation meetings in Atlantic City and Chicago. These meetings stimulated my scientific interest and provided an opportunity to meet other scientists and exchange scientific information. There were several invitations at Dr. and Mrs. Woods' Barton Hills home in Ann Arbor, where, along with their children David, Douglas, and Judy, the Woods were very gracious hosts. Dr. Woods made my stay in Ann Arbor really pleasurable and productive and the valuable period of my training was a rewarding experience that contributed significantly to my professional advancement. It was indeed a privilege for me to have the opportunity to work with Dr. Woods, and he has my sincere gratitude for his many acts of kindness. My pleasant association and friendship with him that started in 1957 continues to this day with my deep regards and admiration.

One memory of which I am not so fond is that Ann Arbor, which is such a beautiful place in summer and spring, takes on a different appearance in winter. This is not a pleasant one, especially for a person coming from a tropical climate. The winter wonderland, snowy, windy, and cold, may be a treat for photographers of all shades, but was a bit of a damper on my spirits during the severe winter months. However, it did not affect the tempo and tenor of our scientific activities.

I am appreciative of all the help that members of the department rendered to me during my sojourn to Ann Arbor. Other than Dr. Seevers and Dr. Woods, Dotty Overbeck paid special attention and consideration to all visiting scientists, as did Bill Sheldon (the store manager) and Bob Shepherd (the workshop manager).

Reflections on My Years in the Department: 1957-1960

Ken Moore, Ph.D.

Arrival

Although it was in early June 1957, I remember my first full day in Ann Arbor as if it were yesterday. My wife, Barry, 2-year old son, Grant, and I had arrived the previous evening and had found lodging in a rooming house on Longman's Lane, located on what was then the western edge of Ann Arbor. The owner, Mrs. Longman, was a gaudily dressed elderly woman with flaming red hair. She was very kind and showed us to the basement of her house that was filled with small cubicles, two of which were to be our bedrooms for a couple of nights until we could get into a university apartment on North Campus. It was only later that we were to learn that Mrs. Longman's rooming establishment had been a well-known house of ill repute years before we arrived.

The next morning with a map in hand I proceeded to walk toward The University of Michigan campus in search of the Department of Pharmacology. A light rain was falling and as I passed a bank, the large thermometer on the outside indicated the temperature was 92°F! How could it be raining and be so hot? Hoping to make a good first impression I had dressed in my only suit (made of warm wool) and it was not long before I was sweating profusely. How could people live in such heat? I located the old pharmacology building on the original university quad next to the library. I introduced myself to the lone woman in the small departmental office who turned out to be Dottie Norton (subsequently Dottie Overbeck). She greeted me warmly and made me feel comfortable, but then proceeded to make me feel uncomfortable by telling me details of her recent surgical procedure to correct a "female problem." Wow— Americans were certainly open!

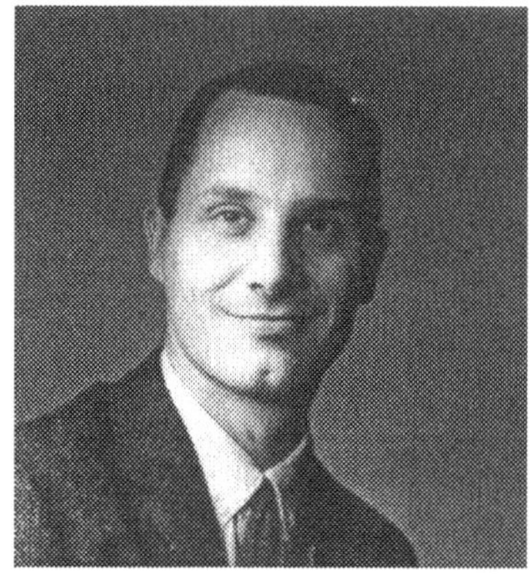

After getting the "low down" on the Department from Dottie, she ushered me in to meet the Chairman (not Chairperson in those days), Dr. Maurice Seevers. Accustomed to the formal interactions with faculty at the University of Alberta, I stood at attention to be greeted by a powerfully built man with a large bald head and enormously strong hands. He greeted me with a vigorous handshake saying, "Ken, how the hell are you? I've been waiting to meet you." Wow again! One of the most prestigious men in American pharmacology was waiting to meet me?! Americans were not only open, but relaxed and extremely friendly. So began the first day of what was to be one of the most exciting years of my life. A year in which faculty and graduate students in the Department introduced me to the thrill of pharmacological research and started me on my career as a pharmacologist.

How did I chance to come 2,500 miles from my home to the Department of Pharmacology at the University of Michigan? I had grown up in a railroad community in northern Alberta, Canada, and my early ambition had been to work on the railroad with my dad. But, through a series of circumstances, I ended up receiving a B.S. degree in pharmacy from the University of Alberta. After working for less than a year in a dispensary (which I hated), I was encouraged to return to the university by Deane Calvert, a friend who had been in the class a year ahead of me in pharmacy school and was then in a M.S. degree program in pharmacology. Although I was married and had a newborn son, my wife, knowing I was not going to be happy working as a pharmacist, encouraged me to return to graduate school. I worked with Deane during the second year of his program and we became close friends. Barry typed his M.S. thesis and then the letters of application to the Ph.D. programs in departments of pharmacology throughout the US Despite sending out about 50 letters, the only positive response was from the Department of Pharmacology at The University of Michigan. Deane was to be the first of five graduates of the Faculty of Pharmacy at the University of Alberta to earn Ph.D. degrees in pharmacology from The University of Michigan in the space of 10 years (Jim Gibb, Jack Diamond, John McNeill, and I were others).

As I continued to work on my M.S. degree at the University of Alberta, I received letters almost weekly from Deane filled with exciting details of the research that he and others were doing in Ann Arbor. Near the end of my second year of study I had tentatively accepted a "real job" working on nerve gas research in a Canadian government lab in a desolate region of southern Alberta. Deane was very persuasive in having me apply to the graduate program in the Department of Pharmacology at The University of Michigan. I received a generous offer from Dr. Seevers to enter the Ph.D. program (only later did I learn there was a great difference in the cost of living in Edmonton, Alberta, and Ann Arbor, Michigan!). I am certain that my acceptance into the graduate program was based on the recommendation of Deane, who also arranged to have his parents drive my family and me to Ann Arbor.

Life in Ann Arbor

My first summer in Ann Arbor was filled with new adventures; in the laboratory, classroom and in married housing on the North Campus where we were surrounded by families from different regions, backgrounds, and cultures. We were all "in the same boat"—trying to complete our educations while living on a tight budget. I had come to the US on a student visa in order to avoid serving with the military in Korea. The only way Barry could accompany me was on a Visitor's permit that required that she travel to Windsor, Canada every six months and reenter the US. Her Visitor's permit prevented her from working, so she became a full-time mother.

In 1958 my oldest daughter, Sandra, was born at St. Joseph Hospital and although it meant additional expenses, it did make us eligible to rent a 2-bedroom apartment. This gave me somewhere to study. Up until the time we moved, I had to spend the evenings studying in the bathroom of our two room apartment with the fan on to drown out the noise of Barry entertaining our friendly neighbors. We had a TV!

Living on the edge of poverty for three years was not fun, and although people would tell me, "You'll look back on these years and laugh," I never have. It was difficult having to "purchase" Christmas and birthday gifts for my children and family with Gold Bell stamps, and eat tuna fish casserole every week (but not once since leaving Ann Arbor!). What I do remember with fondness are the friendships with people who gave us encouragement and assistance during a very difficult period in our lives. Ted and Ethel Brody were tremendously supportive as were the many graduate students (including Dunc and Maggie McCarthy, Glenn and Marti Kiplinger, Tom and Isabel Baum, Mike and Natalie Brody, Ben and Diana Lucchesi) who helped us in hard times and provided much of our entertainment. Except during our last month in Ann Arbor we were unable to afford a car, but kindly neighbors frequently transported Barry to do shopping. People we hardly knew would take us on picnics and help during medical emergencies. Many friendships made in Ann Arbor more than 40 years ago have endured to this day.

Graduate Program

The various activities in the Department offered new experiences every day. I had initially hoped to study with Ted Brody, but as his lab was full, I was assigned to work with Hank Swain. I spent several months using the dog heart-lung preparation to study cardiac electrical conduction. Although the research was not what I had hoped to pursue, it afforded me the opportunity to learn a lot of techniques to which I would not otherwise have been exposed. My experiments were conducted in a large communal room on the second floor that was shared by Lloyd Beck and Hank. People were physically and intellectually involved with each other's experiments. I learned a lot of autonomic pharmacology from Lloyd Beck as I was "pressured into service." After numerous unsuccessful attempts, I finally learned how to smoke the perfect kymograph paper. Not the best surgeon, I often had bleeding emergencies as I opened dogs' chests; these emergencies were often resolved in a relaxed manner by Glenn Kiplinger who occupied an adjacent lab bench. Glenn also lightened the days with numerous stories. A tiny lady from South America (Dr. Ibarra?) also worked next to my bench. Her small stature required that she stand on a box to do surgery. She never wore a lab coat and unlike me she was never covered in blood. Others in the room included Ben Zimmerman, studying hemorrhagic shock with Lloyd, and Joanne Moore working with Hank on the effects of a mysterious compound ("sheep dip") in isolated hearts. Joanne was generous in providing both emotional and technical support. These experiences in cardiovascular research prepared me for subsequent years when while on the faculty at Dartmouth Medical School. Dick Rech (another contemporary graduate student in Ann Arbor) and I developed medical student labs employing isolated guinea pig hearts and demonstrations of autonomic drug actions using Lloyd Beck's hindlimb perfusion technique.

Working in the large communal laboratory with a number of other individuals afforded me the tremendous learning opportunity that would not have been possible if everyone had worked in separate laboratories. Indeed, when the Department moved to the Medical Science Building I the following year, people tended to remain in their own modern labs, and some of the community spirit was lost— a casualty of progress I suppose.

Eventually, I was able to work with Ted Brody studying the effects of toxic organotin compounds on mitochondrial function (oxidative phosphorylation, ATPase activity, swelling properties) and subsequently on tissue levels of catecholamines. The latter studies started me on a 40-year career of exploring the effects of pharmacological/endocrinological manipulations on the dynamics of aminergic neuronal systems in the mammalian brain.

With a few exceptions, most of my fellow graduate students focused on their research projects, although the formal didactic part of the program was fairly rigorous. During the day we attended lectures and laboratories in histology, embryology, physiology, pharmacology, pathology, etc., with medical students and then attended specialized graduate courses in pharmacology in the evenings. I remember some of the medical school lectures as being superb, especially those by Elizabeth Crosby in neuroanatomy and Horace Davenport in physiology. The formal courses were meant to prepare us for oral comprehensive exams and I believe I knew more about general basic biomedical sciences the night before my comprehensive exam than at any other time either before or after my examination. Unfortunately, during my oral exam I forgot 90% of what I had learned. Indeed, even though I somehow passed the exam, the experience was so stressful that as a faculty member at Dartmouth Medical School and Michigan State University, I lobbied successfully against the oral comprehensive exam and for the written exam. At Michigan State University students are subjected to rigorous questioning after their formal seminar presentations that are made at the end of their first and third years of study and at the time of their thesis defense. In this way the questioning is less freewheeling and directed more to the area of the individual's research emphasis.

Graduate students today, as they did in my time, gripe about formal coursework but after all is said and done, I believe the courses prepared me for subsequent teaching duties and research endeavors. For example, I never fully appreciated the value of the course in pathology until several years after joining the faculty at Dartmouth Medical School when I needed the assistance of a pathologist to help me understand the toxicity of alpha-methyltyrosine. I am perhaps a dying breed in that I have resisted efforts to reduce required graduate coursework to the "bare bones." It is interesting that many former MSU graduate students have informed me that after having been on their own for several years their general knowledge of basic biomedical sciences learned from their coursework increased their confidence when shifting their research focus to new areas.

Faculty

I was very fortunate in having Ted Brody as my graduate mentor. He provided me the resources and freedom to follow my own research ideas (often jointly with Deane Calvert) and then was appropriately critical of my results. At times when I became discouraged with lack of progress and road blocks provided by unexpected data, Ed Domino, whose lab was adjacent to Ted's, was usually able to identify something positive in my results and encouraged me to pursue leads. From Ted and Ed I learned that when dealing with students and fellow faculty members, it was important to evaluate results critically but always accompany criticism with supportive enthusiasm. One of the joys of research is making new discoveries and then sharing these with colleagues. With this in mind I have always tried to counsel students who are considering positions/jobs to avoid situations where they would be isolated scientifically.

Senior graduate students were assigned to work with a faculty member supervising pharmacology laboratories for medical students. I was fortunate in being paired with Don Bennett who was an excellent one-on-one teacher. He was very helpful in showing me how to teach medical students in a laboratory session, often through the Socratic approach, and how to demonstrate the actions of drugs in experimental animals. These experiences benefited me when, as a young faculty member at Dartmouth Medical School, I had to develop and supervise medical student laboratories in pharmacology.

Dr. Seevers was very supportive during my stay in Ann Arbor. Although I was much in awe of this man for his many accomplishments and stature in the field of pharmacology, his "down to earth" nature made it relatively easy to talk to him. An unusual aspect of our discussions was that they were often held in the men's washroom; he didn't want to waste time and I was eager to speak with him at any time or place. In contrast to Dr. Seevers' "earthy manner," Dr. Lauren Woods, second in command of the Department, was more formal and as a student I was a little intimidated in his presence. It was not until years later, frequently through my association with the American Society for Pharmacology and Experimental Therapeutics that I got to know Dr. Woods better and to appreciate the sincerity and warmth of this gentleman-scholar.

Harry Hardman was a junior faculty member while I was in Ann Arbor but I didn't get to know him well as he was in medical school much of the time. In 1960 I completed all requirements for the Ph.D. degree and left to accept a faculty position at Dartmouth Medical School. At the same time, Harry joined the faculty in the Department of Pharmacology at Marquette University School of Medicine (now the Medical College of Wisconsin). My associations with Harry were strengthened when he was appointed Chair of his department in 1962 and recruited Deane Calvert to join his faculty. Get-togethers in Milwaukee between Deane's and my families were often facilitated by Harry's kind invitations to present seminars/lectures in his department. Our visits increased when Deane was found to be suffering from colon cancer that subsequently caused his death. Deane's death was a great personal loss as well as a loss to our discipline for I believe had he lived, he would have been a major contributor to pharmacology in the USA. My relationships with Harry and his family have continued and I was honored in 1999, along with a former fellow graduate student Ben Lucchesi (Harry's first graduate student), to speak at a celebration of Harry's contributions to the Medical College of Wisconsin.

Reflections

On reflecting back on my career, I realize how fortunate I was to have become associated with the Department of Pharmacology at The University of Michigan. By chance Deane Calvert applied to and was accepted into the graduate program and through his guidance and efforts, I too was afforded the opportunity to develop my teaching and research skills in this great department of pharmacology. I was able to learn from a distinguished group of faculty, many of whom subsequently became chairs of departments of pharmacology throughout the USA. These included Drs. Beck, Brody, Cafruny, Carr, Hardman, and Woods. Many of the graduate students who were my contemporaries at The University of Michigan influenced my learning during the time I was in Ann Arbor, and subsequently during the development of my career. Tragically, some of the top students had their careers cut short by untimely deaths (Deane Calvert, Tom Baum, Mike Brody), but others have remained friends for over the 40 years that have passed since we worked and studied together; these included Joanne Moore, Ben Zimmerman, Ben Lucchesi, and Dick Rech.

In 1966, Ted Brody was recruited to chair a new department of pharmacology at Michigan State University; the nucleus of his faculty was composed of graduates of the Department of Pharmacology at The University of Michigan. In addition to me, these included David Reinke, Dick Rech, Jerry Gebber, and Jay Goodman. Over the past several years, Jerry, Jay, and I have been recognized as Outstanding Alumni of the Department of Pharmacology at The University of Michigan; we share a proud heritage. In my former position as Chair of the Department of Pharmacology and Toxicology at Michigan State University, I had to be loyal to the green and white, particularly when it came to competition against the hockey, football and basketball teams wearing the maize and blue, but I will always appreciate the important influence that the Department of Pharmacology at The University of Michigan played in providing me with a strong base in the discipline that I love.

Editor's note: Dr. Ken Moore stepped down from Chairperson on September 1, 2001 to Emeritus Professor status on January 1, 2003.

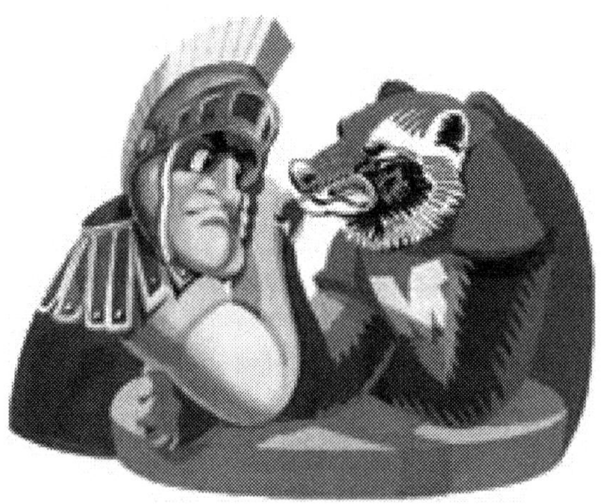

Memoirs: 1958-1963

K. Roger Hornbrook, Ph.D.

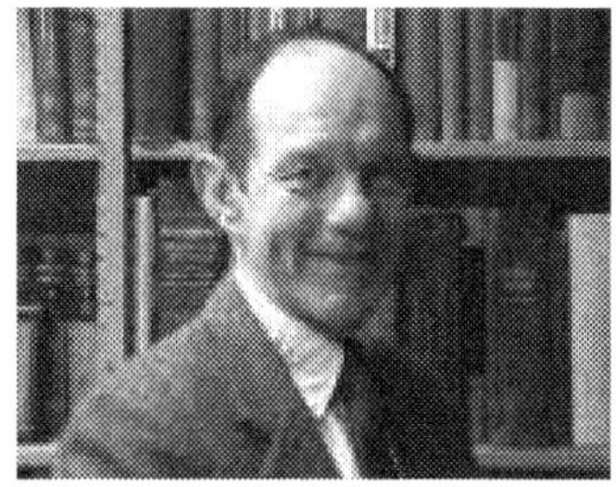

I arrived in Ann Arbor in 1958, freshly married and having no concept, in what I was about to become involved. Initially, I worked with Skip Bennett for two years. I do not think that there was an in vitro or in vivo preparation with which I did not have some experience. That experience included being sentenced to the basement to chase, and sometimes catch, rhesus monkeys. That time in the monkey colony afforded me the opportunity to observe Dr. Yanagita's initial experiments on self-administration. The experiments he did with cocaine and morphine left a long-lasting impression. The set up at that time was large and not as refined as later years; nevertheless, the responses of the monkeys to inject as much of the drug as they wanted got imprinted indelibly in my mind.

In Skip's laboratory, we did enough dog heart-lung preparations and cat papillary muscle preparations that there is probably a special torture chamber in dog/cat heaven for the lot of us in that environment. Probably, I am one of the last folk to be trained to do smoked drum kymographs and fix them with shellac. Lots of procedures have changed markedly. Doing statistics and a sum of squares on the Marchand calculators was the greatest advance in the world. Now, I am not certain that students understand that calculating a standard deviation requires the calculation of a sum of squares. Another great advance was not having to do carbon copies for the dissertation.

In 1960, I got a hankering to work more in the biochemical area and went to work for Ted Brody. I was the token US citizen in Ted's space–at least for a while, until Paula Stern arrived–sandwiched in between those bloody Canadians, savages from the north. Deane Calvert and Ken Moore left the laboratory just before I went there and Jim Gibb, Jack Diamond and John McNeill came while I was measuring my 11,322nd phosphate determination. Paula Stern and I held the fort against the northern invaders, but there was also the Japanese invasion of post-doctoral fellows, including Dr. Furukawa, Dr. Akera and Dr. Murano. Some days I was the only person around who did not speak Japanese and felt totally out of the loop, especially when they whispered in Japanese.

Another major change has been the loss of student laboratories from the medical school curricula. They were time consuming but it was a great opportunity to talk with students and to find out what was really bugging them. The opportunity presented to me as a graduate student to work with monkeys and all the other species of animals which pharmacologists use from time to time has been of great value to me as I have wandered along through the academic world. In many ways, I regret the demise of the student laboratories as this was one opportunity to establish some relationship with the medical students.

I am proud to have been associated with the Department of Pharmacology at Michigan and realize now what a strong, dynamic department it was at that time. When you are a student fighting for survival, such thoughts never seem to occur to you.

Reminiscences of Pharmacology at Michigan

Carl C. Hug, Jr., M.D., Ph.D.

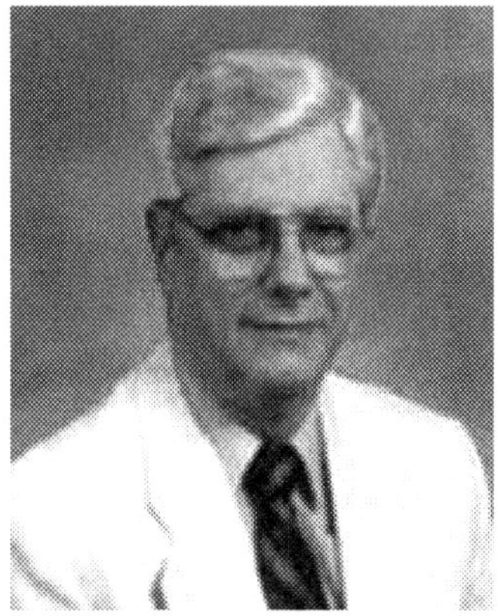

My interests in a teaching career began during my very first lecture in college while Dr. Hugh C. Muldon, Dean of the School of Pharmacy at Duquesne University, was presenting an introduction to inorganic chemistry. I thought: "Now that's a job; you stand up and tell people what you know." My interest in pharmacology stemmed from the influence of Dr. John Adams and my work as an assistant in the pharmacy research laboratories. As a pharmacologist, Dr. Adams advised me to obtain a Ph.D. degree in one of the following five university departments of pharmacology: Emory, Illinois, Iowa, Michigan, or Tulane. Applications were made, visits were scheduled, and our first stop was in Ann Arbor. My wife Marilyn and I met Dr. Maurice Seevers in his office in the old pharmacology building on the Central Campus. He came in from a golf game to meet us. We left his office with Marilyn saying, "He reminds me of a sugar daddy!" I said "We don't have to look any further," and I canceled the visits to the other four departments.

Back at Duquesne, Dr. Adams warned, "If you go to Michigan you will go to medical school." I said , "No way," thinking of my wife and two children to feed. Fortunately, NIH fellowships were sufficiently generous ($173.00 monthly) to meet our basic expenses.

Drs. Bob Gussin and Tony Dren also attended Duquesne University School of Pharmacy. They stopped by to see me as they were on their way back to Pittsburgh, having visited several other Big 10 departments of pharmacology. They had the same reaction to Michigan as I did. Once they met Dr. Seevers, they signed on the dotted line.

One day Dr. Seevers called me into his office and said, "What are you going to do with your life?" I responded, "Teach and do research." He said, "Where?" I said, "In a pharmacy school or a medical school." He offered, "If you are going to teach in a medical school you need a union card. You have to go to medical school." Through the efforts of Dr. Fred Shideman and Dr. Seevers, American Cancer Society Postdoctoral Research Scholarship awards were obtained for Dr. Ray Ruddon and me. These awards paid the equivalent of an instructor's salary as well as tuition costs in return for alternating six-month periods as a medical student and as a faculty member investigator. Dr. Ruddon and I alternated our six-month rotations, lectured to our own classmates, and finally graduated together in 1967. I learned many lessons while at Michigan. Following is a sample of a few.

From Maurice H. Seevers, M.D., Ph.D.:

1. Cut the crap. Get to the point. Keep the big picture in mind.
2. If you want the uninterrupted attention of the listener, talk to him in the men's room.
3. Lecture outlines don't need to be any more than four lines; one can only transmit four main points to a class in a 50-minute lecture.
4. A handshake agreement accompanied by a smile is very much better than any-

thing that can be written on paper.

5. [On training people for only a brief period.] Actual experience in pharmacology and interactions with pharmacologists provide the individual with an understanding and appreciation of pharmacology that is impossible to attain by any other means, and creates a life-long supporter of the discipline.

From Lauren A. Woods, M.D., Ph.D. (my first research advisor):

1. Organization leads to productivity and productivity leads to satisfaction.
2. Always keep a clean shirt in your office.
3. Knowledge trumps a loud voice.

From Edward F. Domino, M.D.:

1. Never take "no" for an answer. Determination and persistence eventually succeed.
2. Enthusiasm attracts good people and spurs them on to success.
3. You get a lot more accomplished if you let others help and give them credit for their work.

From Edward J. Cafruny, M.D., Ph.D.:

1. Strunk and White's textbook is invaluable when you have to rewrite your thesis.
2. It is not what you say, but how you say it that makes a good impression.

From Anand L. Misra, Ph.D.:

1. Safe handling of radioisotopes is excellent training for maintaining sterile technique.

From Edward J. Carr, M.D.:

1. If you want to pique the interest of medical students, use practical examples of how knowledge of pharmacology improves clinical practice.

From Henry H. Swain, M.D.:

1. If you are considerate of others, including medical students, you will be rewarded.

From Theodore M. Brody, Ph.D.:

1. If you can't keep up with the rumor mill, befriend someone who can. It sure helps in interpreting formal communications of all types.

Since leaving Ann Arbor to move to the Department of Anesthesiology of Emory University School of Medicine in Atlanta in November of 1971, I have continued to draw on the experiences and to recall the advice of faculty members, fellows and graduate students from way back then. In many ways, the practice of anesthesiology is applied pharmacology, and the basic principles of pharmacokinetics and pharmacodynamics are just as important today as they ever were. Despite the dramatic advances of molecular biology and genetics, the everyday practice of medicine requires good understanding of dose vs. response relationships and their variability in order to achieve safe and effective use of drugs. I continue to teach these principles every day in the operating rooms and intensive care units, and actually get some kudos for my efforts.

The training, experience and advice I received from the relatively young but very good pharmacology faculty that I met in 1958 have stood me in good stead throughout the past 30 years in the specialty of anesthesiology. They have allowed me to enjoy a rewarding career as a teacher, investigator, physician, and administrator. And even more importantly, there is a continuing legacy of the Michigan influence in the hundreds of medical students, residents, fellows and faculty members with whom I have worked at Emory University School of Medicine and its affiliated hospitals in Atlanta, Georgia.

Memoirs: 1959-1980

Roger Lininger, B.S.

My friend, Ron Chipps, informed me about a possible summer position in the Department of Pharmacology. Ed Domino interviewed me and hired me right away. I performed electronics technician tasks from 1959 until 1963. In those days, Dr. Domino's laboratory had all kinds of electronic equipment, so I fit well because of my background in electrical engineering. I enjoyed organizing things which was good because there were many people working in the lab and they had a tendency to not put things back where they belonged.

There were many technicians, undergraduate and graduate students, as well as, postgraduate fellows working in the laboratory. I recall postgraduates: Dr. Irene Gierasinski from Poland, Dr. Ken-ichi Yamamoto from Shionogi Pharmaceutical Company in Osaka, Japan, and Dr. Katsuda from Kyushu University in Fukuoka, Japan. Some of the graduate students included: Don Knapp, Roy Hudson, and Tony Dren. Roy left for Brown University and later became president of Hampton University. Ray Riciputi worked with Irene concentrating on rat behavioral pharmacology. Earl Morris was an undergraduate electronics whiz who spent his summers in the Domino laboratory as a rat-trainer. I kept in touch with Earl over the years and still consider him a friend. Mary Corcoran was a key person who handled paper work and scheduling of experiments.

Dr. Seevers occasionally came to the lab and watched me work. He never said anything, but just watched me doing electronic chores and repairs. He smiled and then went on his way. I remember Dotty Norton Overbeck well. She had a Masters degree in speech which was handy because every so often she dealt with problems requiring use of her unique talents in letting people know where they stood.

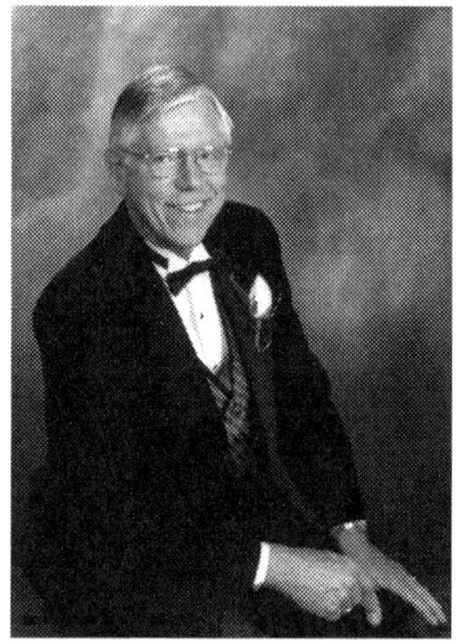

Dr. Domino obtained two special computers of average transients which were called CAT computers. They were used for quantifying animal brain electrical evoked potentials and later in humans, especially in the anesthesia induction room of the old University Hospital. Mary did a lot of the patient recordings when Doctors Guenter Corssen and Robert Sweet were involved. Dr. Corssen had been a German tank commander on the Russian front during World War II and had received an Iron Cross for bravery. He prided himself on fighting communists. On one memorable day, I was helping Dr. Corssen with a drug study. He was called out of the room and I was left alone with a sedated patient who had been given droperidol and fentanyl that scared me. So I quickly got help from one of the residents.

One of the most memorable experiences I had was setting up the electronic equipment at St. Barnabas Hospital in the Bronx, New York, as part of an evoked potential study Dr. Domino did with Dr. Irving Cooper, a famous neurosurgeon. We filled a station wagon with electronic equipment and drove to New York through Canada. I had all the equipment well packed and organized. Then we went through Canadian customs and they insisted that we unpack everything so they could inspect it, before they would let us into Canada. This experience convinced us that we should make our return trip through the US. One day during our stay we went out to lunch at an Italian restaurant with all of the people from Dr. Cooper's laboratory. The waiter went around the table taking orders and everybody ordered Italian sausage. When they came to Dr. Domino, he wanted Polish sausage. The restaurant did not have any, but Dr. Cooper insisted that they find some. Shortly after, the grinning waiter served Dr. Domino the Polish sausage. It might have been sweet Italian sausage doctored up with a lot of garlic, but Dr. Domino accepted it as Polish sausage.

We set up our electronic equipment in the surgical operating room at St. Barnabus Hospital. We had administrative and sterility problems, but we solved them all. This was my first introduction to working with Parkinsonian patients being operated on under local anesthesia while their brain evoked potentials were being recorded. Sixty cycle alternating current was a big problem interfering with our recordings, but I learned to solve that problem by using a very logical approach, i.e., pulling out everything and inserting one a.c. plug at a time to find the offending equipment.

Bill Sheldon worked for the Department for many years. He was in charge of the stockroom and told Dr. Seevers that he was planning to retire and that somebody would have to be found to take his place. The new person would have to train with him for a while, but Bill was pretty hard to get along with. In fact, someone else had worked with him for a while, but had given up and quit. The Department needed somebody who was good at organizing things because, in addition to managing the stockroom, they would be in charge of eight large student laboratories on the seventh floor of Medical Science Building I. I was offered this position in 1963. Although Ed Domino wanted me to stay on in his lab and offered me a salary increase, Dr.

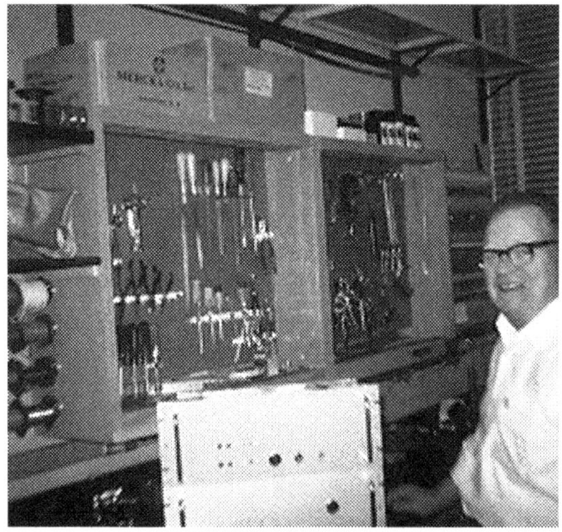

Bill Sheldon ca. 1967 in his work area in the stockroom. Bill just finished a job— two power supplies for rat and monkey avoidance experiments. Bill did neat work and put everything away in its proper place.

Seevers offered me a far better deal. Since I was planning to start a family, I needed the extra money. I could also continue to do some electrical/electronic repairs. It turned out to be very interesting.

When I started working under Bill, I volunteered to answer the stockroom phone in order to impress him. However, I soon found out that I needed to spend several weeks on the job before I learned the ropes well enough to answer the many questions that I was asked. Bill ran the stockroom with an iron hand. He shouted and swore fiercely whenever someone did something behind his back. He smoked pint-sized cigars which hung out of the corner of his mouth when he talked. One day, he invited me to his house to see his bird feeders. I asked him what he particularly liked about the feeders and if he was looking for any special birds. He said, "No I just like to see who is going to rule the roost." When I heard that I knew what his own behavior was like when it came to running the stockroom.

I liked working with Dr. Seevers. I referred all of the complaints about the stockroom to him and he always backed me up. If we needed more supplies there would always be money to buy them. I quickly learned to let Dotty Overbeck know where I was and what I was doing. She handled the day-to-day problems of the Department with the same backing of Dr. Seevers. As a result, things usually went very smoothly, and this was his method of running the Department.

One of my tasks was organizing the eight student laboratories. We had enough equipment for four complete laboratories. It was necessary to lay out all of the equipment for the four laboratories which were held on Tuesday and then switch to the other four laboratories for Thursday. We did this for the entire winter/spring semesters. Each laboratory had four medical students at each of six tables. Naturally, there was a lot of setting up and cleaning after each lab session. I decided to set up a gold star system for the cleanest lab. This system worked because I made up a chart that everybody could see. This included all the labs and the doctors' names who were involved. Since I awarded gold stars for the cleanest laboratory; it was possible to check the progress of a certain lab from week to week. Everybody helped clean up because none of the doctors wanted to have their names look bad. At the end of the term, I invited the students from the winning lab to go to the Pretzel Bell for beer which I bought with my own money. I didn't drink much myself, but it was fun to treat them because they had saved me a lot of work.

The smoked paper kymographs were probably the most unusual pieces of laboratory equipment at that time. A piece of heavy paper was removed from a roll. One side was glossy and smooth. Two ends of the paper were glued, after it was cut to fit onto a rotating drum and extension arm of the kymograph. Benzene was burned to create carbon soot to coat the paper. The paper had to be cranked at a steady speed to obtain a uniform coating of carbon. If the drum was cranked too slowly the paper would burn. After smoking the paper, I carried the paper to the appropriate lab, and put it on the kymograph drum, and then adjusted its roller to tighten the paper. In addition, I had to set up all of the mercury manometers for recording blood pressure which was done by a one little pen floating on the mercury and another scratching the carbon coated paper. When the autonomic drug experiments were run it was a big responsibility because there were all the drugs and six kymographs for each of the four laboratories that needed to be set up on any given Tuesday or Thursday. There were also 24 dogs each Tuesday or Thursday that had to be anesthetized for measuring their arterial blood pressure. After the experiments, the smoked paper had to be removed, and passed through an ethyl alcohol solution of shellac, and hung up to dry. At the end of an experimental day, after shellacking 24 of the records, I was intoxicated from breathing all that alcohol. Later, I found out that the benzene was carcinogenic and between the alcohol and the benzene, I'm amazed that I never got sick. Electronic polygraphs eventually replaced these antique methods.

Another of my tasks was assembly of the student laboratory manuals. Each of the professors in the department was responsible for writing up at least one of the student laboratory experiments. Getting them to meet a deadline was one of my biggest problems, but somehow we got it done. I also kept track of the money that was collected from the medical students for their laboratory fees. There was a small safe, in room M6413 of Medical Science I, where Dr. Seevers kept some drugs of abuse, as well as, the money I collected from the students. I was concerned that someone would be waiting for me when I came in early in the morning with a gun, or a knife and want me to open the safe, but that never happened.

There was also a small safe in Jim Woods' office on the sixth floor of Medical Science I, in which the morphine, etc., for the monkey colony was kept. Some scoundrels came in during one Thanksgiving vacation and loaded the very heavy safe onto a dolly. They were trying to take it out through the steam tunnel when it slipped off the dolly and severed one of the steam pipes. The thieves took off leaving the safe for the steam maintenance people to find. Dr. Woods appeared on the 11:00 o'clock TV news trying to explain what happened. I don't think he said very much about the contents of the safe, for a very good reason.

During my time in the stockroom, I also became acquainted with Bob Shepherd who was in charge of the machine shop. Much of our research apparatus was constructed in this shop. Bill Sheldon and Bob Shepherd never got along with each other. One day the two of them traded insults and went after each other. Bob had two hammers and was angrily trying to hit Bill's head between them. Dr. Seevers quickly stepped in and settled the argument. He told them, "If anything like this happens again you are both out of a job." After that incidence Bob and Bill never spoke to each other. If Bill wanted anything from the machine shop he sent me down to get it.

Toward the end of Dr. Seevers' career he wasn't well. He came to work, but we knew things weren't right with him. I offered to get him anything he wanted, but on some occasions he would be in tears. It was something to see a man of such great status brought to his knees. After Dr. Seevers retired, Dr. Henry Swain took over as Interim Chairman. Soon Bob Shepherd became ill and died rather quickly. His widow came to the Department to pick up his tools. We didn't know which ones were Bob's so Dr. Swain and I just collected a bunch of tools and gave them to her. Shortly after, Bob Austin took over in the machine shop with Tom Laramee assisting.

The curriculum of the sophomore medical students changed many times over the years. The student laboratories eventually were no longer needed for teaching. After that, my position was strictly running the stockroom. I missed Dr. Seevers, Dotty Overbeck, and the old guard. I realized that it was time for me to look for a new job. The Division of Nuclear Medicine's Cyclotron Project was just beginning in 1982. Someone was needed to run a new medical cyclotron. They offered me the operator position which I accepted. The move from the Pharmacology Department changed my life at the University, but that's another story.

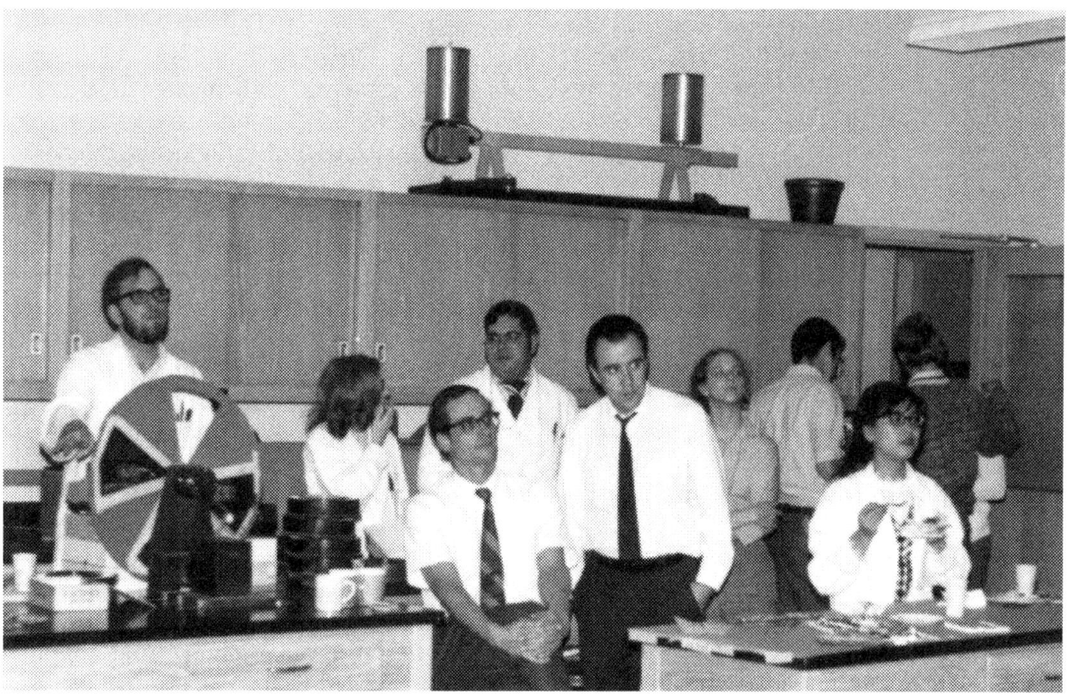

Listening to a summary of an experiment during a medical student laboratory session. Note the kymograph and ice bucket on top of the cabinets, ca. 1975.

Memories of Michigan

Paula H. Stern, Ph.D.

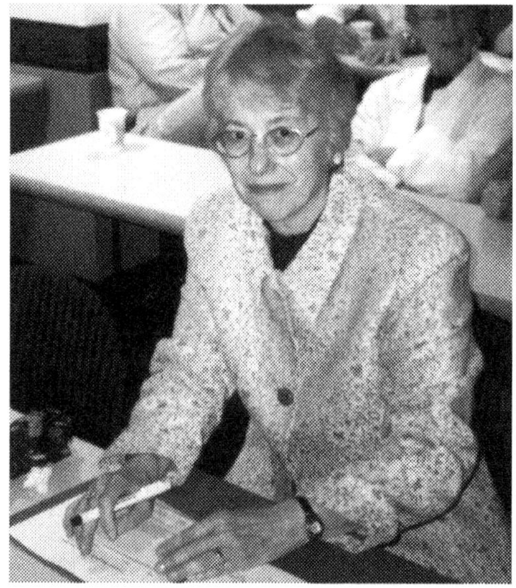

How did I happen to come to Michigan? I came to Pharmacology serendipitously. As an undergraduate, I was a biology major at the University of Rochester, and, inspired by one of my teachers, the eminent Johannes Holtfreter, I decided to become an embryologist. Robert Stern, my fiance, was studying in Cincinnati, so I planned to go to graduate school there. I spent a summer in Woods Hole taking a Comparative Embryology course, and while there I happened to meet a faculty member from the Department of Pharmacology at the University of Cincinnati. Shirley Bryant, an electrophysiologist, worked on squid in the summer and myotonic goats in the winter.

I had no idea what a pharmacologist was, and Shirley explained it to me in very simple terms, "you can do practically anything and call yourself a pharmacologist." When I arrived in Cincinnati to interview for graduate school, I learned that the embryologist on the faculty had, unfortunately, recently passed away. I remembered Shirley's words and went to visit him and interview in the pharmacology department.

I became a graduate student in pharmacology at Cincinnati as a student of Julius B. Kahn, Jr., working on cardiac glycosides and ion transport. At some point in my research I wanted a method to look at cardiac muscle metabolism, and tried to measure oxidative phosphorylation. Under ideal circumstances, healthy tissue should give a P/O ratio of 3.0, but I never got any values better than 2.0.

Julius suggested that we visit his good friend Ted Brody at Michigan, who was a pioneer in the application of oxidative phosphorylation. I was very excited when Julius showed me a letter he had received from Ted a few days later saying that his lab regularly assayed oxidative phosphorylation in many different tissues, and we were welcome to come to the lab and learn how to do it.

We drove up to Michigan and spent the day in Ted's lab. Of course, everything went wrong. Ted himself did the experiment with us, and as I recall, we obtained a ratio of 1.9! I felt terrible, thinking that my presence had been a distraction, that explaining things to me and answering my questions had prevented him from doing the steps as quickly as necessary, causing the tissue to deteriorate. Naive as I was at that time, I did not realize that directors of large lab groups did not spend their time doing those types of assays, and I did not even consider that Ted, the guru of the field, might have been a bit rusty. I did have a great day there, and recall meeting Roger Hornbrook, Ken Moore and the late Deane Calvert. I thought it was a superb group.

As fate would have it, my husband decided to transfer to Michigan, and I applied and was accepted to the Department of Pharmacology and to Ted's lab. The project that Ted proposed was to follow up on Deane's studies on the hepatotoxicity of carbon tetrachloride. I spent many hours in the cold room, decapitating rats and homogenizing livers. I got quite adept at measuring oxidative phosphorylation as well as in methods such as administering carbon tetrachloride by stomach tube and setting up cross-circulation models.

The lab continued to attract good people. We had two core groups: the New Jerseyites (Ted, Paul Quinn, and myself), and those who came down the pipeline from Alberta (Deane, Ken, then Jack Diamond, Jim Gibb, and John McNeill). The latter group had a sign by their desks, which read something like, "You are now entering the Canadian Sector." There was also the inimitable Dick Bird, Ted's technician, who would willingly entertain us with tales of his exploits, including his "noonies" with Rosie.

The lab also hosted several visiting faculty members from Japan, including Tatsuo Furukawa, who was a collaborator and co-author on one of my first papers, and who became a good friend. My husband, Robert, and I would visit with Tatsuo and Tatsuko, and they introduced us to Japanese food and customs. Robert had read a lot of Japanese literature in translation, and we had some good literary discussions. In recent years, we have visited Tatsuo and Tatsuko in Fukuoka, where they were unbelievably gracious hosts. Several years ago, Tatsuo invited me to speak at a Japan/China pharmacology meeting. Participating in that meeting, at which I was the only non-Asian, was one of the most memorable experiences of my career.

One of the significant national events that occurred during the years I was in the lab was Alan Shepard's space flight. Someone brought in a TV. Roger got pretty excited over it and picked up a rat and lifted it up in the air and then back down. I guess it was the first *rat*stronaut. Once, I helped Jack Diamond prepare a prop for one of his seminars. He was working on the rat uterus, and one of his slides was of a rat in a round wire cage. To stimulate interest, we made a cardboard cutout of a model from Playboy and put it in a similar cage. I believe his seminar line was, "Because we couldn't use this species." My assistance with that project didn't help my feminist credentials very much!

The lab windows faced the river and the golf course. Sometimes we thought we could spot our esteemed advisor, along with Ed Cafruny and Lloyd Beck, having small 'scientific workshops' on the golf course. The hallways in the Medical Science Building were wide and clear enough for recreation. The faculty would practice their golf swings with yardsticks from the lab. The Canadians would play hockey using large rubber stoppers from Bill Sheldon's stockroom as hockey pucks. We would also play ice bucket-top frisbee. There were labs from the biochemistry department across the hall, and Bill Lands would occasionally take a break from his lipid research to join in the pseudo-athletic activities.

We worked hard too. I remember that there were many late nights, starting with the evening graduate courses, and then continuing with experiments, which often ended in the wee hours. Some of the students lived in U Terrace, so it was just a short walk over the hill. I often walked home with Gerry Gebber after long experiments. The graduate courses, in addition to being bonding experiences for us, were very solid, introducing us to classical and current pharmacology. In fact, I could not bear to discard my notebooks, and still have them. There were lots of seminars, and although I can't remember any specific speakers, I can still recall my awe at how Ben Lucchesi, who was still a student when I first came to the Department, would always ask penetrating questions. There were a number of excellent teachers in the Department. They must have been good role models, because I know that several of us have received teaching awards during our subsequent academic careers. My antibiotics lectures were especially well-received, and I must give credit to Hank Swain for both the format and some corny jokes (e.g., the "three deaf mycins").

One of the most agonizing experiences was typing my Ph.D. thesis. In those pre-computer days, the theses had to be typed on special plastic sheets, which were then used for reproduction and microfilming. Erasing smudged the sheet, so you usually had to start the page over if you made a mistake. Most of the students had the sense to hire professional typists, but I felt that I could type well enough to do it myself and save money.

I decided to rent an IBM Executive electric typewriter, which was supposed to give a more professional, finished appearance to the document, since different letters had different numbers of spaces, e.g., "i" was one space, "s" was two spaces, "m" was three spaces. It was fine, unless you needed to center or align things, which of course you had to do a lot for making tables. The whole process was agony, and it was not made any better by the fact that I was doing it in the summer and our apartment at U Terrace was not air-conditioned. I lost about 10 pounds while typing my thesis. Along with my notes from the graduate courses, the plastic version of my thesis is another memento I have kept.

Looking back on my experiences in the Department of Pharmacology at the University of Michigan, one of the most valuable aspects of training there was being exposed to the range of questions and the diversity of techniques. It exemplified and confirmed for me Shirley Bryant's statement that you could do almost anything and be a pharmacologist. It also made me feel personally confident that I could apply any technique or move in any direction. Allowing myself to do this has led to a very fulfilling career.

The other rewarding aspect was the permanence of many of the friendships I made. In addition to my colleagues from the Brody lab, Janice Stickney and Bob Gussin have remained good friends. I tell my own students that even though they will go in many different career directions, they will retain their connections with their fellow graduate students and enjoy reliving their experiences and keeping up with their lives when they meet at scientific meetings and elsewhere.

Where is the field of pharmacology going? During my career, I have heard murmurs that pharmacology is dying as a discipline, that it could be merged with biochemistry, or with physiology, and that some departments had done this already. But now we see that pharmacology is stronger than ever. New techniques, crystallographic, genomic, proteomic, electrophysiological, cyber networks, rapidly become part of the methodologic armamentarium of pharmacology. New concepts in membrane structure, signaling, cell communication and behavior, become viable new targets for development of therapeutic agents. Research interactions and collaborations between academia and industry have become stronger and well accepted. Pharmacology is as exciting as ever, and in the future it should be even more so.

Thanks for the opportunity to reflect.

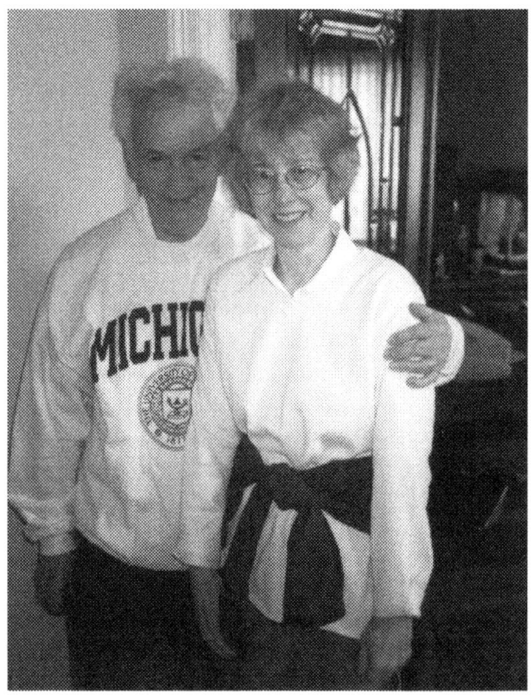

Paula and her man

Vignettes: "I Remember When..."

Staff and Students of the 1950s and Beyond

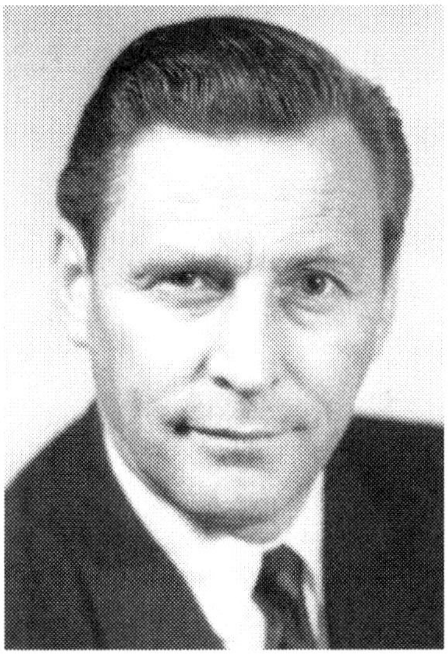

Lloyd Beck, Ph.D., 1953-1969

As far as memories of the Department go, my most treasured memories are of that group of talented young men who came into my laboratory as Ph.D. graduate students. One of them went on to attend Medical School after he graduated. The others went on to produce an astounding body of important research while at the same time being excellent teachers and administrators. The major universities and drug companies that benefited from their expertise were indeed fortunate institutions.

John W. Kissel, Ph.D., 1953-1958

I came to the Department in 1953, registering for school on my honeymoon. Those were hectic days — breaking into a new department, beginning married life, expecting a baby, the Mark Nickerson "problem" swirling around me, my requesting a transfer from Dr. Seevers' opiate addiction project so that I could work under Dr. Domino, etc. At this point, I don't trust my memory sufficiently to contribute to any history book.

There are a couple of memories that did pop into my mind. I remember the maze of cages in the basement of the old building that was dedicated to the opiate addiction project. Residing in these cages were monkeys that were physically dependent on heavy doses of opiates. They had to be injected repeatedly on a strict schedule without interruption.

Both grad students and technicians made up the injection crew, but only one person needed to be there at a time. The injection procedure required the injector to be in the cage with a free-moving monkey. The technique involved pushing the animal up against the side of the cage with one hand and injecting with the other. It usually went pretty smoothly, but one time the monkey snatched the loaded syringe out of my hand. This was a red alert situation! If he injected me, they would have found me unconscious on the floor of the cage the next morning — if I were lucky.

I don't recall how the incident described above was resolved, but I know that monkey

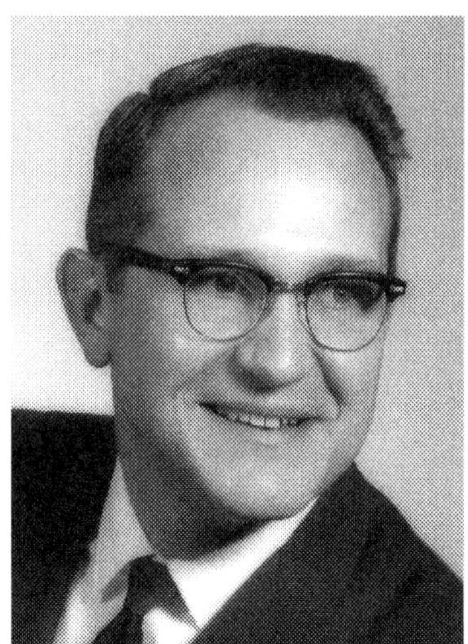

did not inject me. Going up to the deserted Pharmacology building in the middle of the night was always adventuresome.

The other incident involved a graduate course being taught by a member of the Pharmacology faculty, possibly Lloyd Beck or Ed Cafruny, who incorporated a great deal of anatomical detail in his lectures. One of my fellow grad students thought he would heckle the teacher. He brought a box of colored pencils and during the lecture "accidentally" dropped them all over the floor. Everyone got a big kick out of it. You can see that it didn't take much to amuse us in those days.

Glenn F. Kiplinger, Ph.D., 1954-1959

I started at the U of M in 1954 working in Ted M. Brody's laboratory. At that time, Dr. Hosoya was a visiting fellow. I met Dr. Kumagai, Dr. Tanabe, and Dr. Watanabe also, but the real influx of Japanese postdocs started after I left.

This became most obvious with the number and exceedingly high quality of papers presented at the Seevers Symposium in May of 1970— many from the Japanese. That symposium was just prior to Dr. Seevers' retirement and it was my great pleasure to have initiated the Symposium and to have aided in its organization.

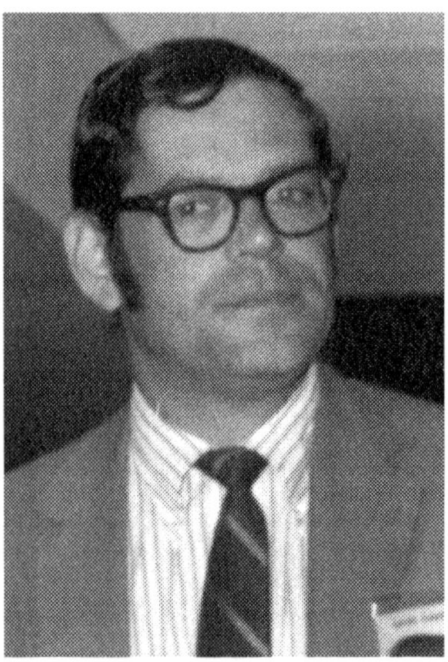

My memories of my husband Ed Cafruny, M.D., Ph.D.
Marilyn Cafruny, 1955-1965

Capturing the Michigan years of Pharmacology and especially locating and biographing that faculty that has endowed Michigan Pharmacology with its international renown, is a remarkable venture. Half a year ago I could have included pictures of those past wonder years when my husband Ed

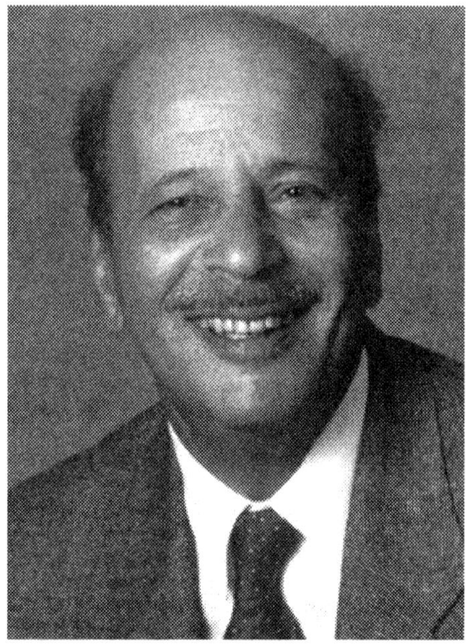

worked in the Department — the handsome, young, lab-coated faculty, dedicated workers, and competitive friends. I am still in the throws of unpacking from my recent move to Vermillion, South Dakota. The past three years have been spent trying not to think of tackling over a half-century of possessions accumulated in the menacing attic of a large house, and the discarding, saving, discarding again, retrieving, and then finally discarding that has had to happen.

Ed always referred to his Michigan training as "classic" — he was proud of that training. Those who may remember Ed from "the old building" especially will empathize with his comments. This is a sweet and sad journey for me down "memory lane."

Richard H. Rech, Ph.D., 1956-1959

Though I started my Ph.D. program in 1956, I took a seminar course earlier, taught by Dr. Edward Domino, as an elective for my M.S. program in hospital pharmacy. The course dealt with CNS drugs— neurotransmitters. I remember being terrified to present my topic in front of such an august group of scholars. During the 1958-59 year, Dr. Showa Ueki and I shared a laboratory. He had learned little verbal English and I even less Japanese, but somehow we managed to communicate. One reflection on his character is that he was saddened for some weeks after one of his EEG subjects, a favorite beagle, finally had to be sacrificed.

The students in my era were a closely-knit group. I remember Glenn Kiplinger always brightened Mondays with a slew of new jokes. Where he got his supply was always a mystery to me. I often collaborated with my classmates— Don Bennett and I worked on reserpine effects in the heart and lung, and Duncan McCarthy and I combined our labor on several older monkeys who were subjected to surgery to prepare neuronally-isolated cortical islands. This latter effort ended unpleasantly; the last monkey was an aggressive female that broke free and bit Duncan severely on the shoulder. I believe he spent about a week in the hospital. The episode cured me of any aspirations to work with rhesus monkeys.

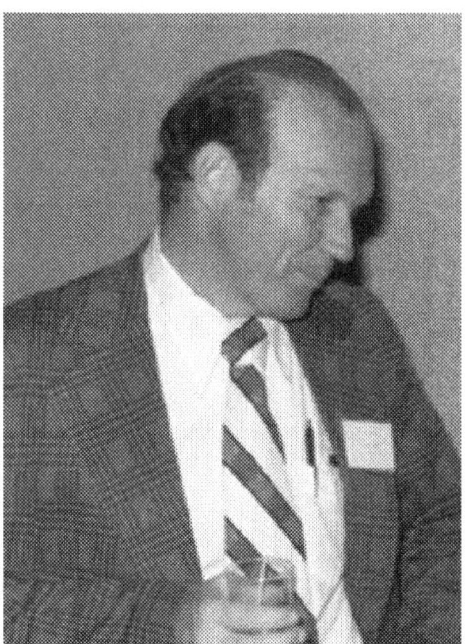

When I had a particularly difficult set of data to analyze, I often sought out Lloyd Beck. He would review the data over five to 10 minutes and give me an answer that seemed to come from left field. It would then take two to four hours to tease out of Lloyd the mental leaps of insight that he utilized to arrive at this profound solution.

Ben G. Zimmerman, Ph.D., 1956-1960

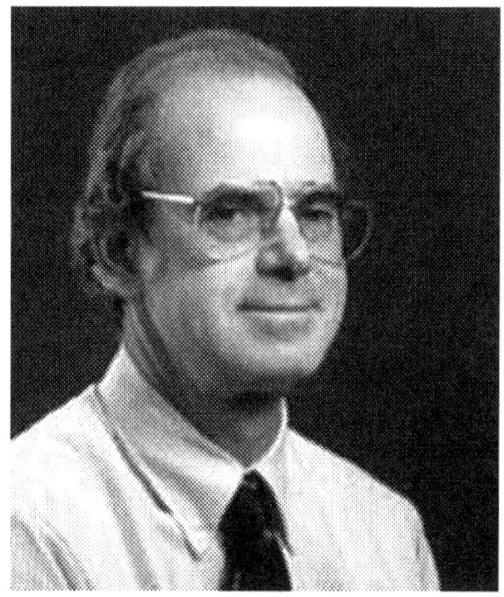

As I look back, I must say that I treasure many of the experiences that I had while a graduate student at the U of M. One which stands out is the friendship that I had with Akira Sakuma who was a postdoc working in Lloyd Beck's lab at that time.

Sakuma was not only a very personable and communicative individual, he was also very helpful when it came to statistics and experimental design. He spent many hours teaching statistics, particularly analysis of variance, to me, Mike Brody, and others in the Department. Sakuma was and probably still is very knowledgeable in mathematics and especially statistics. He even designed a short course on the subject that he presented to the graduate students. The material that he gave us was very well thought out, and the handouts he prepared as well as the statistical analyses that he performed on my thesis data are still intact and kept in my filing cabinet. Every now and then I actually refer to them in order to carry out analysis of variance on my experimental data. Just recently I took out the material and showed the people in the lab these 40-year-old handwritten analyses. They could hardly believe that Sakuma's analyses were that old, let alone that someone would have saved them for that long.

His impact on me and undoubtedly on others was certainly long-lasting, and I feel very fortunate that I was a student at the time that he joined the lab. For a time we kept in touch, and I did bump into Sakuma at the 1965 International Physiology Congress in Tokyo. However, I regret to say that I have lost contact with Sakuma; every so often I think about him and wonder what he is doing now.

Certainly Lloyd Beck had the greatest influence on my scientific training. He was a tremendous influence on me and other graduate students and postdocs. Lloyd was able to train us in his own unique style. He had a way of getting even raw recruits (such as I was at the time) to think and be enthralled about cardiovascular pharmacology. I owe a lot to him.

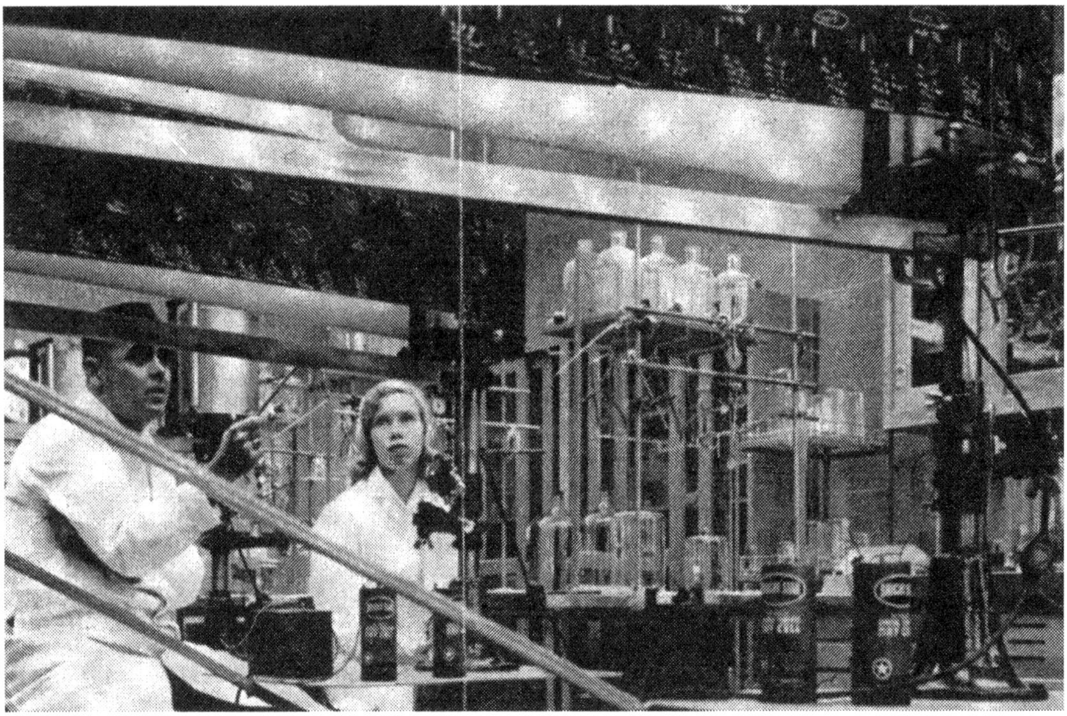

A photograph of three smoked-paper drum kymographs (try to find them) used for recording cardiac contractility of the isolated turtle heart. Pictured is Dr. Harold Hardman (left) and his research assistant examining the results of an ongoing experiment. The studies focused on the inotropic action of theophylline under different conditions of pH, which altered the ionized state of the drug in solution. Dr. Hardman was among the first to demonstrate that the ionized state of a given drug could modify its pharmacodynamic response, ca. 1958.

1957

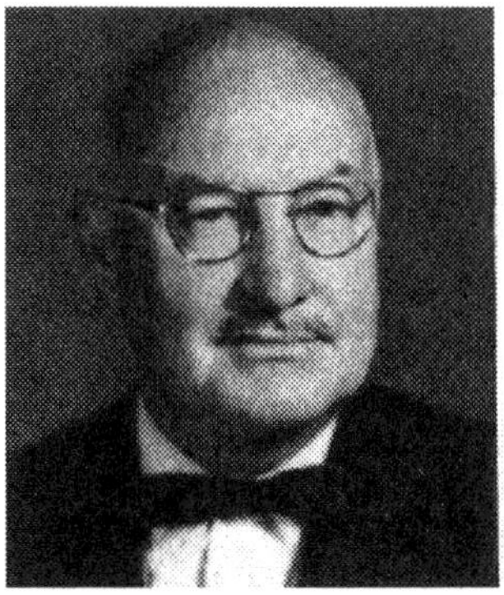

Maurice Seevers

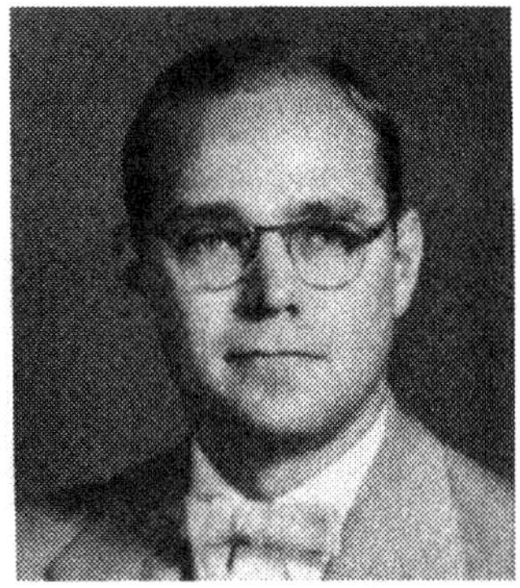

Lauren Woods

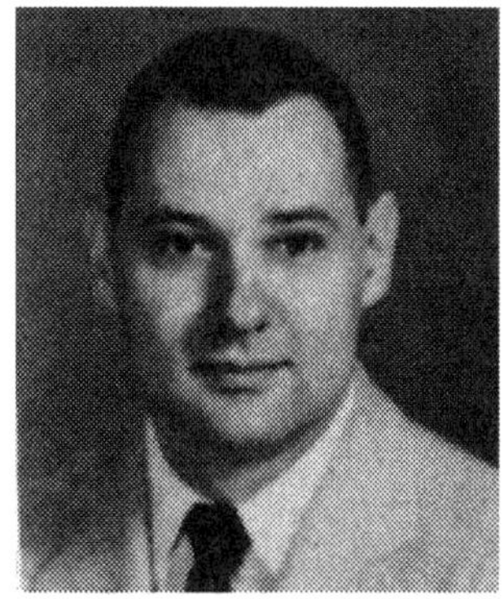

Edward Domino

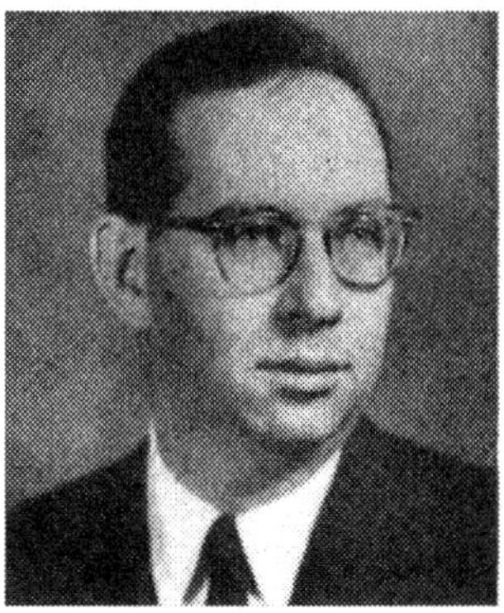

Ted M. Brody

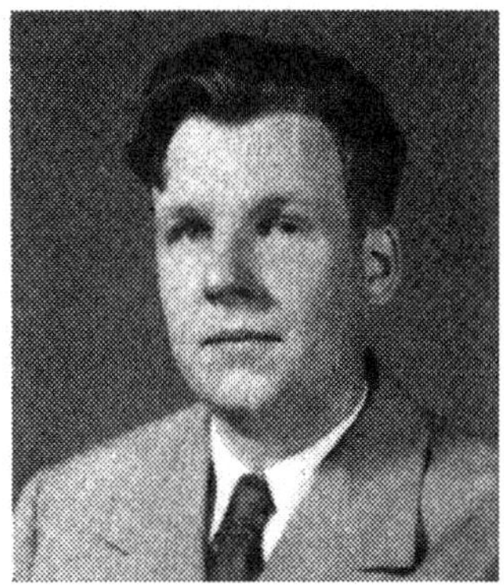

Edward Carr

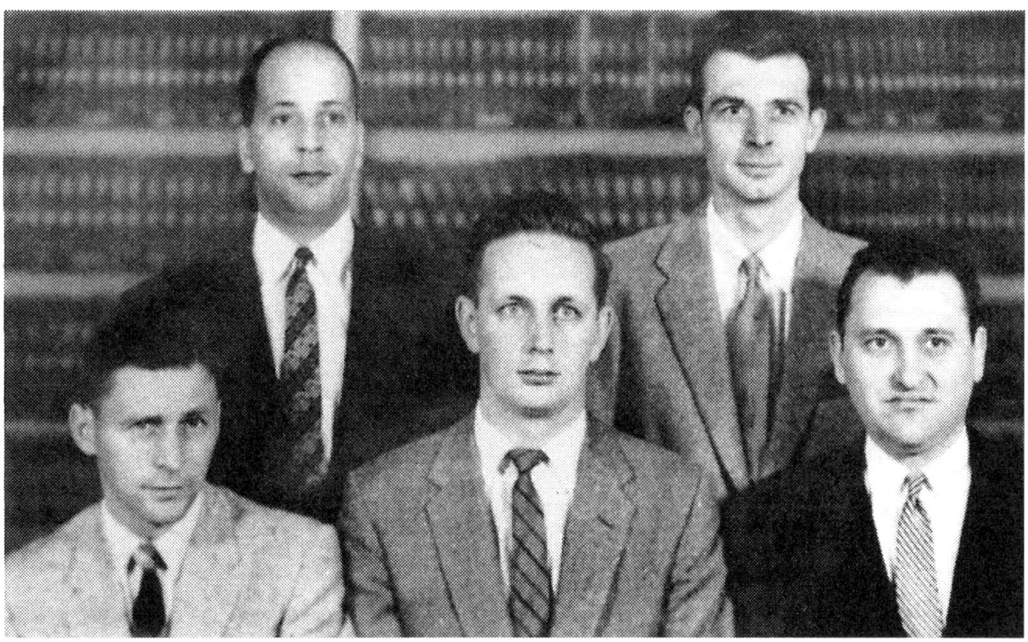

Front row: Lloyd Beck, Henry Swain, Lawrence Mellett   Back row: Ed Cafruny, Gerry Deneau

1958

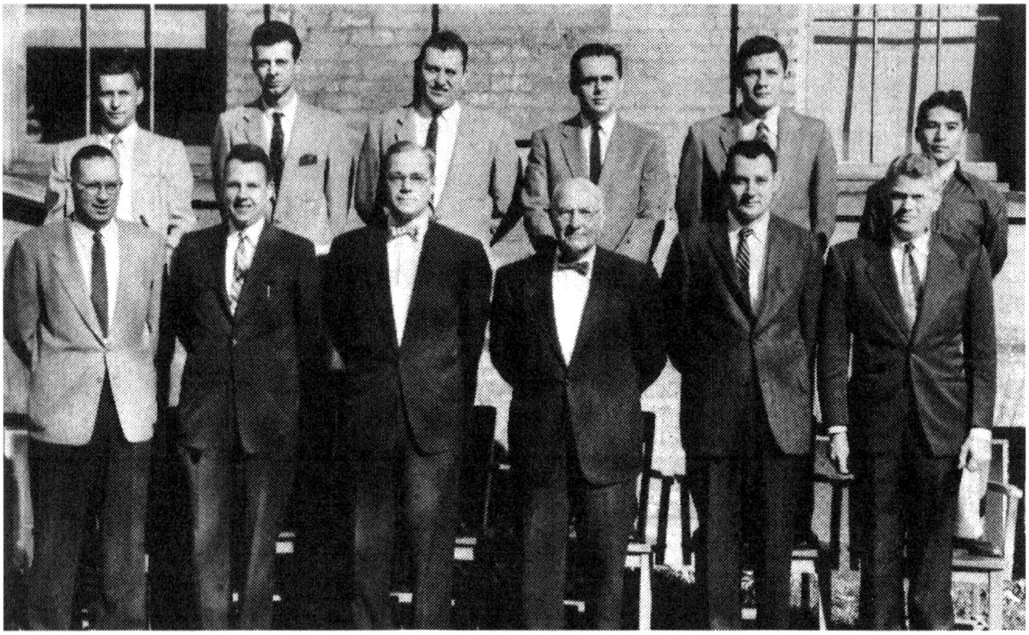

Front row: T. Brody, E. Carr, L. Woods, M. Seevers, E. Domino, R. Laird
Back row: L. Beck, G. Deneau, L. Mellett, H. Hardman, D. Bennett, S. Ueki

1959

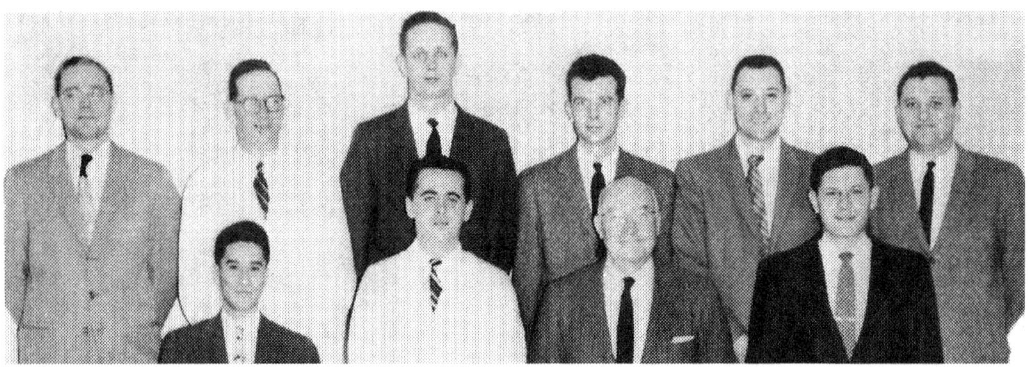

Front row: S. Ueki, H. Hardman, M. Seevers, D. Bennett
Back row: L. Woods, T. Brody, H. Swain, G. Deneau, E. Domino, L. Mellett

17

Memoirs: 1960-1965

*Ronald S. Chipps, M.D.**

I spent three years in the Department of Pharmacology. From 1960 to 1961, I obtained a postdoctoral fellowship and worked in the lab of Hank Swain. Then, from 1963 to 1965 I served a fellowship in clinical pharmacology, receiving my Masters of Science in Pharmacology in 1965. Most of my memories of the Pharmacology Department date back to the year I spent in Hank Swain's lab. It was an extremely pleasant year despite the fact that it taught me that I had very little aptitude for basic science research. I was very impressed by the quantity and quality of the pharmacology faculty at that time. I found all of the faculty members to be easily accessible, friendly, and helpful. I particularly enjoyed my contact with Ben Lucchesi, and have been able to maintain some contact with him over the years. I continue to value his friendship.

I still remember many of the extracurricular activities that were carried out while I was in the Department. One such activity was partridge hunting in Northern Michigan with Lloyd Beck. I still remember Lloyd's highly technical descriptions of the shots he missed. I also remember the parties held mainly at Alex Heingartner's house, and Dr. Kiro Shimamoto trying to teach us some Japanese songs after we had had quite a bit to drink. I know everybody had a good time at those parties.

My main contribution to the Department of Pharmacology was talking Roger Lininger into taking a position in Dr. Domino's lab. Roger was a grade school and high school classmate of mine from Kalamazoo. Roger worked in the Department for several years, taking over the stock room when Bill Sheldon retired. Roger later finished off his career at the University by working with the PET scanner at the University Hospital.

I had completed my internship prior to my year of working in Hank Swain's lab. I then completed my internal medicine residency at the University Hospital before returning for the clinical pharmacology fellowship. The clinical pharmacology fellowship was served in the Hypertension Unit and I had very little contact with the Department of Pharmacology during that time. When I completed my fellowship, I served for two years as an instructor in Internal Medicine in the Medical School and continued to work in the Hypertension Unit. I then worked for the Upjohn Company for five years, setting up their employee health surveillance program and also doing some clinical medicine.

I worked in clinical research for six months but quickly realized that was not where I wanted to spend my career. I went into the private practice of internal medicine in Kalamazoo and have served as chief of our hospital internal medicine department and medical director of our local peer review organization. In 1993 the hospital purchased my practice and I have been able to practice medicine with no administrative responsibility since.

My experience in pharmacology has been very helpful to me over the years. My training in hypertension occurred just at the time the importance of hypertension was being realized and effective drug therapy was first appearing. Over the years one-third to one-half of my practice has continued to involve the management of hypertension.

* Deceased

Memoirs: The Years 1960-1964

Gerard L. Gebber, Ph.D.

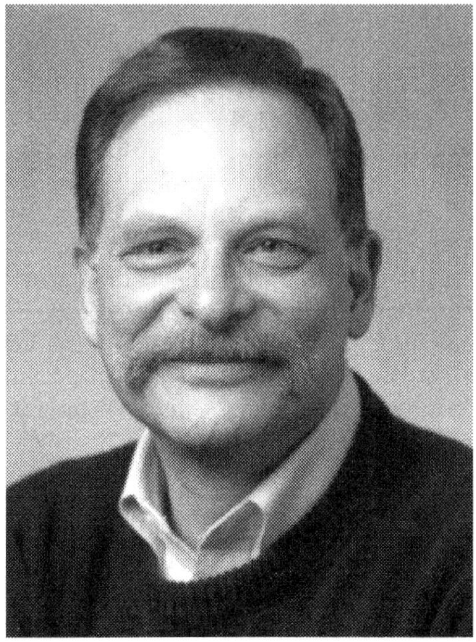

I arrived in Ann Arbor to begin my first year of graduate school in September 1960, two years after the Department moved to Medical Science Building I. I was young, brash, and my ego far outshone my accomplishments, a problem that I have not quite outgrown in the ensuing years. On our first day as enrolled students, Dotty Norton ushered Jack Davitt, Joe Luciano and me (the entering class along with Dave Reinke) into Dr. Seevers' office. After a brief welcome by Dr. Seevers, I promptly asked him where and how large my laboratory was going to be. Jack and Joe were quite taken aback but Dr. Seevers simply gave me a long look, turned to the window facing north, pointed to the VA hospital and said something like: We will have to watch you for awhile, but I'm sure that you will end up there. It took almost a full semester before I realized that he was referring to the psychiatric ward. Dotty quickly scooted us out of Dr. Seevers' office and introduced us to Skip Bennett.

Skip was in charge of first year student "rotations." This incident is germane to the theme of my memoir which is to compare how things were done in the early 1960s with present day practices. Skip indicated that we had a day to choose between the laboratories of Lloyd Beck, Ted Brody, and Ed Cafruny, all of whom had openings. I went off for the first time to visit the men's room on the sixth floor of Med Sci I and when I returned, Skip informed me that Joe was joining Ted's laboratory and Jack would train with Ed. Whether I liked it or not, I was assigned to Lloyd's laboratory. As it turned out, I liked it a lot.

Lloyd was part of the second generation of faculty carefully chosen by Dr. Seevers whose nose for talent had vaulted Michigan into the forefront of Pharmacology in the 1950s. By the time I entered graduate school, Maynard Chenoweth, Harry Hardman, Mark Nickerson, Lauren Woods, and Fred Shideman had already left the department to assume chairs and directorships elsewhere. They were replaced by an equally talented and even larger group including Ed Carr, Ed Domino, Gerry Deneau, Bruce Mellett, and Hank Swain. Ben Lucchesi, who had just completed his Ph.D. and was taking an M.D. degree, held an instructorship. Ben was rapidly developing into the superb and productive scientist he is today. Moreover, he was making great progress in bouncing verbal insults and erasers off of the heads of medical students. Over the years, he has perfected the former talent. By necessity rather than inclination, he has dispensed with the latter practice.

Not only was the faculty comprised of accomplished scientists who were excellent mentors, but many of them were uniquely unconventional. Lloyd Beck's imagination was far ranging and all dogma was suspect in his eyes. He insisted upon the same for his students. Can any of the graduate students of the 1960s forget Ed Domino's unbridled enthusiasm for his research, Ed Cafruny's perfect lectures always delivered without a note in front of him, and Ed Carr's conversations with himself held daily while eating lunch in the old hospital cafeteria? How about Hank Swain's electronic circuit of the heart whose blinking lights brought us, but hardly ever the circuit, to the threshold of ventricular fibrillation? Was this the intended purpose of the demonstration?

The graduate students of my day were well matched to the faculty. I am reticent to single out individual accomplishments in fear of further distorting the record. Nevertheless, imitation is a sincere form of flattery and it is true that many of us quickly took on the characteristics of our mentors. Bob Gussin was in charge of Ed Cafruny's laboratory by his second year of graduate school. Ed went on to a Deanship and Bob is currently perhaps the longest serving Vice President of Research of any of the large pharmaceutical firms in the USA. Both Paula Stern and Ken Moore followed Ted Brody as President of ASPET. Mike Brody and Ben Zimmerman who preceded me as students in Lloyd Beck's laboratory emulated Lloyd's innovative and competitive approach in their research careers as I have tried to do.

On a more personal note, after serving for a short time as Lloyd's hunting dog (Lloyd's real dog had died just before the beginning of the pheasant season) I was promoted to the status of full-fledged hunter. In the fall of 1960, Lloyd took me hunting for the first time. Being fresh out of New York City, this was a new and exciting experience for me. Lloyd said that I didn't need a gun and asked me to walk about twenty yards in front of him. Later he complained that I wasn't kicking the bushes hard enough. Suddenly, I flushed a hen pheasant and Lloyd brought the bird down with a shot aimed directly over my head. I exacted my revenge in 1964 when I finally won our annual "buck a bird" contest. Of course, we ate everything we shot after I picked the shotgun pellets out of his birds and mine. Is there a graduate student currently in the Department who has served as a hunting dog? I suspect not. More seriously, my greatest pleasure in graduate school occurred on those rare occasions when I was able to catch Lloyd in error. Believe me, that was hard to do.

Whereas the Department today is primarily cellular and molecular in its orientation, the 1960s represented the heyday of integrative, whole animal studies at Michigan. Integrative biology is currently in resurgence, especially in the neurosciences which is my research area. My experience in Pharmacology started forty years ago with the kymograph. This "primitive" instrument did not present an obstacle to good research and new ideas in Lloyd's laboratory. When I remark upon this to my current students, they think me to be a bit strange. After all, they have written software allowing them to delve into the principles of nonlinear dynamics and self-organization within large-scale neural networks. Nevertheless, they may be partially correct about my strangeness but for the wrong reasons. Back in the 1960s, we smoked our kymograph paper over a benzene flame, a well-established carcinogen today. Also, our recordings of blood and perfusion pressures were etched into the smoked paper to create a white-on-black record by a hand-cut plastic "flag" attached to a wooden stick bobbing up and down on a column of mercury. Naturally, mercury was always spilling out of the manometer onto the floor. From there, it rolled across the laboratory to collect in the corners or we collected it and dumped it down the sink where over the years it accumulated by the pound. Finally, in 1961, Michigan's Chemical Safety unit told us clean up the mess. Someone who will remain unnamed had the bright idea that we should vacuum the laboratory and sink traps (thus vaporizing the mercury).

By this time, both Lloyd and Hank Swain who shared the laboratory were, in my opinion, acting strangely ("mad hatter" syndrome). Chemical Safety ordered urine to be collected from all of us for a month's time. I remember lugging a five gallon jug back and forth from the laboratory to the apartment I shared with Jack Davitt and Joe Luciano.

Luckily, everyone survived.

I also lost high frequency hearing and developed tinnitus in my left ear during the course of my four years at Michigan. By this time, Ben Lucchesi was finishing medical school. So I asked him whether I might be developing an acoustic neuroma. Ben looked at me, smiled and remarked something like: I doubt it, its probably the grinding of the Sigmamotor pumps that you use to perfuse the dog's hindquarters. Lloyd's laboratory had four set-ups, each with two or three pumps that were grinding incessantly throughout the day. The sound of my pumps resonated off of a wall two feet from my left ear. Despite these trials and tribulations, no one complained and no one sued. We were Kamikazes in the truest sense of the word.

We solved problems by improvisation rather than equipment upgrade. Lloyd had the idea that baroreceptor-induced reflex vasodilatation in hindlimb skeletal muscle had both an active and passive component. He and Mike Brody proposed that the passive component was due to inhibition of vasoconstrictor outflow while the active component reflected activation of a second set of sympathetic fibers that released histamine. Lloyd further postulated that the time constant of passive vasodilitation (due to decreased norepinephrine release) should be slower than that of the active component. My first job in the laboratory was to test this hypothesis. Since we didn't have a differentiator or a method to export kymographic records to such an instrument, I decided to run the kymograph drum at an astounding rate of one foot per minute to obtain records from which I could easily calculate dp/dt before and after the injection of an antihistamine. Thus, data collection was limited to about 8 minutes per roll of paper. I would then run to the "smoking" room to fix the record in shellac, smoke a new paper, run back to the laboratory and load it on the kymograph. The sequence was repeated ad infinitum under Lloyd' s watchful eye. I went from 165 to 138 lbs in my first year of graduate school, but it was great because the experiment worked.

Lloyd was forever changing his ideas, interpretations and experimental approaches for the better, an important lesson for me. On the other hand, he resisted changes in instrumentation. When some new Grass Model 5 ink-writing polygraphs were delivered to Ed Domino's laboratory, I was fascinated by these "electronic marvels." I suggested to Lloyd that we might get rid of our kymographs and replace them with polygraphs. Lloyd agreed to consider my proposal but after visiting Ed's laboratory decided against it. He said that it would be a real come down to go from beautiful white-on-black records that were ten inches in height to swiggles written on green-lined paper that was only five cm in height. There was no photocopy machine in the department in the early 1960s. Neither was there a mechanism for digitizing data for exportation to a graphics program. So we cut and pasted our "typically best" kymograph records on poster board. If we made a mistake, the data were lost and it was back to the laboratory to repeat the experiments. On numerous occasions, I lost the fruits of a hard day in the laboratory by brushing against the kymograph paper which was shoulder high when mounted on the drum. My rank in the Department was denoted by the perpetually present black smudge on my white laboratory coat.

In 1997, I was honored to receive an Outstanding Alumnus Award from the Department. It was an especially rewarding experience for me. As I stepped to the podium to deliver my lecture, I realized that the seminar room in Med Sci. I once had been the laboratory in which my thesis work was performed. The tradition and excellence in Pharmacology at Michigan today can be traced back, in good part, to Dr. Seevers' tenure as chairman in the 1950s and 1960s. I played a small part in that story and am forever grateful to those who guided my formative years as a graduate student.

Memoirs of the Early 1960s: The Magnificent Years

Anthony T. Dren, Ph.D., Robert Z. Gussin, Ph.D., Jack Diamond, Ph.D., Donald W. DuCharme, Ph.D., James W. Gibb, Ph.D., Jerome A. Levin, Ph.D., and Morris S. Zedeck, Ph.D.

For the Department of Pharmacology at the University of Michigan, the early 1960s were notable in that the largest single group of students was admitted to the Ph.D. program. In 1961, 12 students were admitted, seven of whom graduated and thereafter modestly referred to themselves as "The Magnificent Seven." We, the seven graduates, were Jack Diamond, Tony Dren, Don DuCharme, Jim Gibb, Bob Gussin, Jerry Levin, and Morris Zedeck. Because of our diverse backgrounds (American/Canadian, east coast/west coast, Masters degree/ undergraduate degrees, pharmacists/non-pharmacists, some married/ some single, children/no children, pharmaceutical industry experience/academic experience) and our varied therapeutic interests, the interactions and friendships that developed within the group were academically stimulating as well as highly rewarding, exciting and long-lasting.

Several influences helped us, as new arrivals, get connected to the Department and to the faculty. When we arrived, Dorothy Norton Overbeck was a superb resource, helping us get oriented to the campus and being a particularly good friend to the married students. Dr. Seevers provided the NIH funding, albeit modest, for us to pursue our goals. Bill Sheldon let it be known that he was the boss of the storeroom and that we'd need his cooperation if we had plans to graduate.

The Seven matured and developed a sense of worth from their mingling and interactions with the cast of characters that made up the faculty, the postdoctoral fellows, the advanced students, and the new arrivals of the early 1960s. Each of us was required to interview with, and rather quickly select, the mentor with whom we were to spend the remainder of our time in the Department. Departmental research activities didn't permit much down time.

Diamond and Gibb trained with Ted Brody and shared lab space with Paula Stern, Roger Hornbrook, and Paul Quinn, and subsequently mentored Bill George and John McNeill. Tony Dren trained under Ed Domino and followed in the footsteps of Don Knapp and Roy Hudson while sharing lab space with Julian Villarreal, Bart Meyers, John Rosecrans, Elliot Piperno, and Kenichi Yamamoto. Jerry Levin spent two years with Don Bennett and interacted with Ed Alpert, Dave Reinke, Hank Jacoby and Al Rosenbaum. Jerry then joined with Don DuCharme, who had already started his dissertation research in Lloyd Beck's lab, and the two finished under Lloyd while closely interacting with Gerry Gebber, Jerry Carlson, Al Pollard and Suleyman Kayaalp. Bob Gussin teamed with Ed Cafruny for his training and shared the seventh floor lab with Charlie Ross. Morris Zedeck trained with Bruce Mellett and shared lab space with Carl Hug, Ray Ruddon, Paul Davis and Jim Johnson.

The maturing and professional growth of The Seven did not develop solely from the expertise and mentoring of their faculty preceptors. Didactic training included hallway debates with Ben Lucchesi involving the never-ending questions, "Who are dumber and which are lazier, medical students or graduate students?" Hands-on training included witnessing and participating in the "Golf Olympics" and the hallway "Virtual Bowling" conducted by Cafruny, Beck, Brody, Swain, and Mellett. Another maturing influence, since we were a 100% male group, was the privilege we

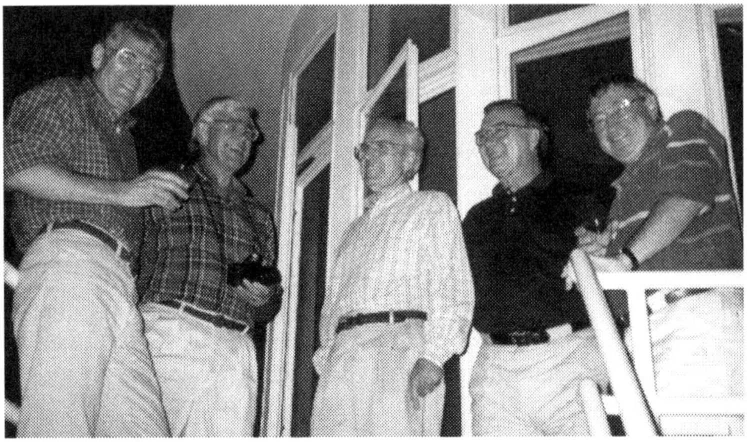

Five of the "Magnificent Seven" gathered in Long Island, NY, in 1999. From left to right: Jack Diamond, Donald W. DuCharme, James W. Gibb, Anthony T. Dren, and Robert Z. Gussin

had of standing shoulder to shoulder alongside Dr. Seevers in the men's room, as recipients of his "Urinal Philosophy."

A high point in the mutual support and cooperation among the Seven came when we were scheduled to take the oral Preliminary Exams. Each candidate was required to take the exam individually. The exam was administered by the full faculty in a closed room; each faculty member had the opportunity to ask one question. Even though all of us had already passed the written prelims, we were intimidated by the importance of this exam because of the potential impact on our careers and personal lives. We were told that Dr. Seevers would ask the first question and that it would be broad and general and in his area of expertise.

The group decided that to adequately prepare for the exam, we should get together at frequent intervals to study and practice presentation skills. The shared thought was that we wanted to help pull each other through this ponderous gauntlet. Each of The Seven made up a few broad, general questions and wrote them on a slip of paper. The questions were placed in a brown paper bag and, one at a time, each candidate would draw out a question and answer it in front of the group. This routine improved our confidence for this milestone exam and enhanced our bond with one another. However, even with this preparation, Dr. Seevers joked as each of us concluded our exam, "Boy, would I like to measure your adrenaline levels today." Needless to say, despite the high anxiety, all of The Seven passed. Once the oral "prelims" were passed, an external sign of acceptance within the Department, and a highly gratifying experience, was to have Dr. Seevers greet you by your last name rather than by "How Ya Doin', Boy." Bill Sheldon provided the second sign of acceptance by distributing lab coats without large acid holes once the prelim exam milestone was achieved. Laboratory research in the era of the early 60s was markedly different from approaches prevalent in the '70s and thereafter. CNS, cardiovascular, autonomic nervous system and renal research was conducted in live, whole animals. Even the biochemists in Ted Brody's lab started their research activities with whole animals. Laboratory instrumentation and techniques of the day ranged from eight-foot smoked-drum kymographs for hind-limb perfusions and frog rectus abdominus muscle bioassays to scintillation counters, sophisticated Grass and Offner (Beckman) polygraphs, microelectrode techniques for recording single cell discharges in central nervous system neurons and Computers of Average Transients for recording cerebral evoked potentials.

Campus activities also influenced and

fused the ties between The Seven. Medical classes in Physiology, Histology, and Neuroanatomy were conducted in the hot, non-air-conditioned, old East Medical School building. Thus, summer lectures and labs took extraordinary perseverance to stay awake after the walk down the hill to the main campus. However, waking up for the initial physiology lecture was unavoidable. Who can forget the impact and classical "rude awakening" by Horace Davenport starting off his lecture with a blast from his "Big Bang" cannon? All in the group took evening classes on the main campus to pass the requirement for reading proficiency in two foreign languages; late night studying together as a group was commonplace. Instructors of influence who molded the scientific scope of our group included Horace Davenport for Physiology, Elizabeth "Ma" Crosby and Ed Lauer for Neuroanatomy, David Bohr for Cardiovascular Physiology, Walter Wild for Renal Physiology, Jim Rank for Neurophysiology, and Jim Olds for Experimental Psychology. Biochemistry was the province of Bill Lands. But where was there a better Pharmacology faculty than: Maurice Seevers, Ed Domino, Lloyd Beck, Don (Skip) Bennett, Ted Brody, Ed Carr, Ed Cafruny, Gerry Deneau, Roy Hudson, Ben Lucchesi, Bruce Mellett, Bob Shuster, Hank Swain, Julian Villarreal, and Tomoji Yanagita?

The Seven acquired football tickets and attended games as a group, often followed by after-game parties at the Maiden Lane apartment complex or in the University Terrace and North Campus married-student housing areas. On Saturday mornings, the group often met at the Department to write up and finalize the week's research activities and then departed before noon for the stadium. The all-day pre- and post-game activities served to enhance camaraderie within the group and provided a release from the day/night rigors of laboratory research.

Several notable scientific endeavors initiated by the Department coincided with our tenure. The Department achieved international renown with drug dependency research, including nicotine research, and provided groundbreaking scientific data on the capacity of nicotine to reinforce self-administration behavior and affect human physiologic parameters. The Upjohn Center for Clinical Pharmacology was funded to initiate training in clinical drug development research. Dr. Seevers participated on the Surgeon General's Advisory Committee on Smoking and Health and helped co-author the first Surgeon General's report on the hazards of cigarette smoking. Other areas of international interest included sleep/dream research, the discovery of active vasodilatation phenomena, dissociative anesthesia, the self-administration monkey colony, renal stop-flow analysis for determinations of diuretic and cardiovascular drug mechanisms and sites of action, drug effects on oxidative phosphorylation, and the metabolism of cancer chemotherapeutic agents and narcotic analgesics.

Following their Michigan years, five of The Seven pursued additional training and obtained postdoctoral fellowships. Those five departed to work with renowned investigators and research institutions. Jim Gibb left for additional NIH training with Sidney Udenfriend as the first NIH Pharmacology Research Associate Trainee Fellow. Jerry Levin entered Bob Furchgott's lab at the SUNY Downstate Medical Center. Bob Gussin departed to Alfred Farah's lab at the SUNY Upstate Medical Center in Syracuse. Jack Diamond continued at the University of Michigan and then joined Jean Marshall's laboratory at Brown University. Morris Zedeck left for Arnold Welch's laboratory at Yale and continued with Alan Sartorelli. The two others, Tony Dren and Don DuCharme, bypassed academic postdoctoral training and opted to enter the pharmaceutical industry directly; Dren to Abbott Laboratories, DuCharme to the Upjohn Company.

Publications, promotions, and accolades followed. All are elected members of professional scientific societies and have contributed as committee members, chairpersons and members of editorial boards, particularly for the American Society for Pharmacology and Experimental Therapeutics, The American Society for Clinical Pharmacology and Therapeutics and the American Heart Association.

Gussin, Gibb, and Dren served on the Pharmacology Centennial Advisory Committee that helped to organize the memorable centennial celebration for our Department; Don DuCharme was an invited speaker at the celebration. Professional levels of achievement and influence include: numerous scientific discoveries accompanied by the issue of more than 30 US and international patents, two pharmacology department chairmanships, four full professorships, eleven adjunct academic appointments, several distinguished alumnus and professional society awards, three industry Senior Scientist appointments and therapeutic area Directorships, one International Clinical Research Directorship, one Corporate Vice Presidency and one Honorary Doctorate.

With 38 years of contributions, The Seven have begun to reduce our workload of professional activities. However, even though retirement has been an option, all are still active professionally. Gibb is Pharmacology Chairman Emeritus at the University of Utah and is a consultant within the Corporate Office of Science and Technology at Johnson & Johnson. Diamond is Professor Emeritus at the University of British Columbia and continues to run an active pharmacology laboratory. Dren is a Consulting Professor in a newly initiated Clinical Research Management Program at the Duke University Medical Center. Gussin continues as a consultant to the firm of Johnson & Johnson. Levin has developed his own private entrepreneurial business in alternative medical treatments. DuCharme has continued his extensive volunteer involvement with the American Heart Association and has also initiated and maintained his own private entrepreneurial business. Zedeck continues as a consultant in forensic pharmacology and has an academic affiliation with the John Jay College of Criminal Justice.

The Department of Pharmacology and the University of Michigan were good to us. In turn, the Seven have rendered credit, honor and fame to the Department and to the University. We are widely published on a myriad of topics and have maintained the commitment to excellence in our personal and professional lives that was fostered by The Department and the University. We the Seven are proud to have received our scientific training and professional start from our mentors and colleagues in the Department of Pharmacology at the University of Michigan.

An Addendum to the Magnificent Years

Morris S. Zedeck, Ph.D.

My time spent in the Department of Pharmacology at the University of Michigan was very special. I know this because 38 years after leaving Ann Arbor, I still have very warm feelings for my classmates (the "magnificents," Jack Diamond, Anthony T. Dren, Donald W. DuCharme, James W. Gibb, Robert Z. Gussin and Jerome A. Levin), my labmates (Carl C. Hug and Raymond W. Ruddon), my mentors, the Department and the University. That these feelings still exist is even more significant given the fact that, after leaving Michigan, I ventured into an area of pharmacology one might term non-classical, i.e., cancer research. While the classical pharmacologists attended ASPET meetings each year and maintained relationships, I attended conferences related to cancer research and did not see my classmates and labmates for many years. In spite of this, I always felt close to each of them and part of the family. Whenever our paths did cross, even after a long hiatus, it was as though we had seen each other only the day before. I take this opportunity to thank each of them for the feelings of warmth and friendship.

It is difficult to find a specific reason for the closeness that developed over a four-year period. We came from diverse backgrounds. Some of us were married, some with children, some had advanced degrees and some were older than others. We had one trait in common though, and that was to work hard and make the best of what we considered a wonderful opportunity to study, with financial backing, in what was the best department of pharmacology in the United States, if not the world. When we were not attending class, you would find each of us working in his respective laboratory, days, nights and weekends. We were

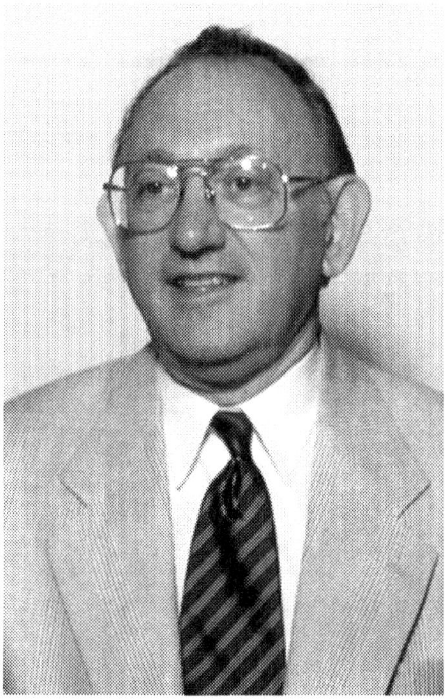

always ready to help each other. I cannot recall a single incident of non-cooperation between any of us. This common focus of diligence, exemplified by the Department members, may be one reason for our close bond. We felt special as individuals and as a group. Perhaps it was the camaraderie we witnessed among our six different mentors that made us feel united as a family. Perhaps it was the funny stories we shared about our daily experiences that made us a clique. This sense of cooperation was evident throughout the Department. In my laboratory, headed by Bruce Mellett, I could always count on Carl Hug and Ray Ruddon for assistance, lively discussions and friendship. When my research led to the merger of cancer chemotherapy and renal pharmacology, my intrusion in Ed Cafruny's laboratory was welcomed by Bob Gussin and Charlie Ross, who were not only cooperative and instructive but whose friendly presence made long nights pass quickly. I can still see myself sitting in front of the Fiske osmometer. Other memories include listening to the funny stories of events which took place in Lloyd Beck's laboratory as told by Don DuCharme and Gerry Gebber. These tales were told outside in the hallway and not in their laboratory, as everyone wished to reduce the risk of being exposed to mercury vapor. I fondly recall the times Jerry Levin and I got together at the Jewish holidays and when he tried to teach me how to smoke a pipe, being in awe when Jim Gibb and Jack Diamond would describe the cold winters in Edmonton, Canada, and being impressed when Tony Dren would manipulate the needle of his stereotaxic instrument. I will always be indebted to Paula Stern who risked her life to teach me how to drive my stick shift VW Beetle. These are but a few of the hundreds of memories I have of my brief stay in Ann Arbor.

To this day, though I have not seen some of "the magnificent seven" or other members of the Department for several years, I still feel part of a family, part of the Department of Pharmacology and part of the University. Corny as it sounds, I occasionally don University hats or sweatshirts, I still root for the Wolverines and I feel proud when I meet other University alumni in my travels and listen as they also speak highly of their days in Ann Arbor. I have fond memories of my four years in Ann Arbor and I am proud of my affiliation with the Department and the University. I know that I will always be accepted as a member of our group of "the magnificent seven," of the Department and of the University.

The Journey from Michigan to Virginia

John A. Rosecrans, Ph.D.

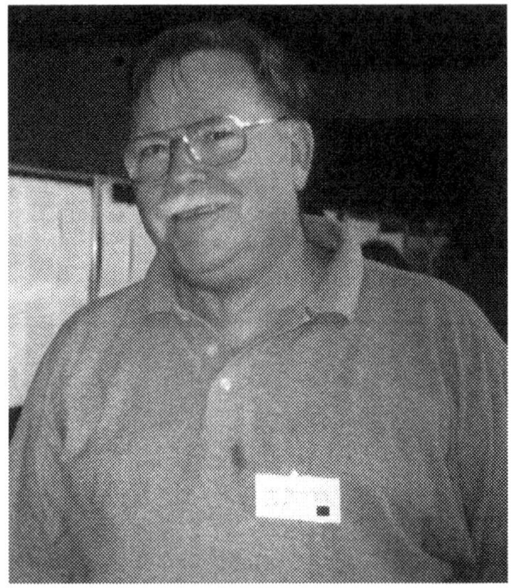

When I was first asked by Ed Domino to write this treatise on my time at the University of Michigan I had some doubts as to whether I could really come up with a worthwhile story. However, as I began to look back into why I chose to become a postdoctoral student at the UM, and what the long-term outcome was, a very interesting scenario emerged. My stay at the UM was extremely important to my growth at the time, and was also central to my development as a scientist in later years. The story has covered many years and has involved many people, especially Ed Domino.

I should begin this story as a recent Ph.D. graduate from a small Department of Pharmacology of a new School of Pharmacy at the University of Rhode Island (URI), in Kingston, Rhode Island. Coming to Kingston itself was an earth-shattering experience for me, having been born and having attended college in New York City, then arriving in a town that appeared to be in the 18th century. Those years, however, were important, as I realized that what I really wanted to do was research.

As I was writing my Ph.D. dissertation I was exploring several postdoctoral sites and realized that I needed additional training in a broad-based pharmacology program. Michigan was it. My interests in CNS pharmacology also led me to Ed Domino, and I moved to Ann Arbor in January 1963. I arrived as an NIMH Postdoctoral Fellow with a salary of $7,500. The fellowship was to explore CNS histamine arousal mechanisms. I was married with two children and found a house in Ypsilanti, MI; driving to and from Ann Arbor was an endearing experience. Just getting on the expressway was enough to make me long for the East Coast. I never saw such speed, especially in the snow; these people appeared crazy. My first trip seemed to be never-ending, as I passed cars and trucks overturned along the side the road. Of course, I am exaggerating, but please realize that I didn't learn to drive until I arrived in RI in 1958. Why would anyone own a car in New York City?

The Years in Ann Arbor

I was overwhelmed by the Pharmacology Department at the University of Michigan; I felt like I had been cast into an oasis of knowledge and research experience, one that I couldn't possibly maneuver. The first thing I noted was the enormous amounts of equipment, especially in the Domino lab. Much of it was neurophysiological, with one or two behavioral set-ups. The Domino lab was bustling with technicians, postdocs, and graduate students, and I really felt lost for a time. I couldn't possibly fit in! One thing that helped me, though, was the fact that most of the graduate students were pharmacy graduates. That did make me feel somewhat at ease, since I had also graduated with a B.S. in Pharmacy. Thus, I had to somehow fit in. Over the 18 months I was in the Department of Pharmacology I did realize that I knew as much as anyone at my level coming from a small department, and felt more comfortable each day.

Ed Domino was very helpful in trying to help me get settled, as did others in the lab; Tony Dren and Julian Villarreal, both graduate students, were especially helpful. Julian had received a M.D. from the University of Mexico and was a postdoctoral fellow working on a Ph.D. Roger Lininger, who was a senior technician, was interesting and had a great sense of humor, but enjoyed ice fishing; I could never understand why anyone would fish through a hole in the ice.

My first assignment was to help Ed Domino and Bart Meyers, a postdoc in the lab, put together an instructional videotape of the behavioral phenomena of spontaneous alternation. That is, we had to demonstrate that if a rat was placed in a T-maze, it should turn alternately left or right in the arms of the maze when placed in maze on successive trails. The idea was that certain drugs, mainly CNS-acting anticholinergic drugs, would block this effect and the rat would go to one side only. The first part of the tape was to get the rats to demonstrate alternation, which they wouldn't. After several hours, and after many different rats, the phenomena were finally demonstrated, and there was also enough footage to demonstrate the effects of the drugs, and we all went home. The interesting part of this demonstration was to see Ed Domino exhibit frustration and laughter at the same time; it was a wonder and really showed how human everyone was. It was a delightful experience, one that helped me begin to let down my guard and take in the fullness of the Michigan experience.

I had several other such experiences that proved to me that I had made the correct choice in coming to Michigan. Working in the same lab with other postdocs such as Don Knapp and a Japanese scientist, Dr. Yamamoto, was also quite interesting and informative. One Monday I came into the lab to conduct some cholinesterase assays on brain tissue and I found that the tissue was destroyed due to thawing of the frozen tissue. This was frustrating, but after talking with Dr. Yamamoto the reason was discovered; researchers in Japan would turn off all electrical equipment on weekends because of power surges that were prevalent at that period of time. Thus, the freezer plug had been pulled on the Friday before I was to do my assay.

The next task was for me to conduct my first experiments in cats to show that there were histaminic receptors that were involved in arousal. In this study I needed to anesthetize a cat, but I was too impatient to get the study going and was subsequently scratched by a very angry animal. This was indeed demoralizing. Needless to say I never did another such experiment and very quickly changed projects at Dr. Domino's insistence. My first task was to prove myself and I failed immediately. The Domino laboratory was internationally known for its work with cholinergic agents and one project of interest involved the enzymes that metabolized acetylcholine, the cholinesterases. I thought, this is something I could certainly do, as I had developed several assays to measure brain amines while a graduate student. Consequently, I was assigned to develop an assay to measure cholinesterases. The lab however, was a neurophysiological lab not a neurochemical lab, and it was obviously my job to put together such a lab station.

The first thing I did was to research the current methodology; I found that there were several ways of doing the assay, for example colorimetric assays. However, the best and most accurate method was to measure the change in pH of acetylcholine via its hydrolysis by acetylcholinesterase, a method that employs a pH-Stat apparatus, available by a company RadiometerR that was also quite expensive. I proposed purchasing such an apparatus to Dr. Domino, and his reply was, "Build one!" I had never built anything in my life except model airplanes, and even they rarely flew. So here I was, at one of the most prestigious departments of pharmacology in the world and I had to develop a procedure with equipment I had to build myself, or be considered a failure.

To make a long story short I was able to diagram what equipment was needed to do the job, but the overall cost would be equal to or greater than the cost of the pH-Stat. I even visited Dr. F. Foldes' laboratory at Montifefiore Medical Center at the Albert Einstein College of Medicine in New York, and worked for a couple of days with one of his research associates who was proficient in cholinesterase research using the pH-Stat. I was convinced that we needed to use the pH-Stat.

Ed Domino did finally come through but not in way I thought. He remembered that there was such an instrument at the University of Michigan Mental Health Center and we trudged over there. Ed persuaded them to loan us the equipment. How he did it I will never know but we did get the equipment and I was saved the embarrassment of not being able to build the instrument. I developed the assay and we conducted several studies that were published showing the relationship between behavioral disruption and the inhibition of acetylcholinesterase. This approach was also used to show that the consequent decrease in acetylcholinesterase was correlated with an increase in brain acetylcholine that was evaluated by Tony Dren. This study was extremely important at the time, but even more important in later years as several of my own students at the Medical College of Virginia used similar approaches to evaluate nicotine's mechanism of exerting discriminative stimulus control of behavior.

Having completed my first year of postdoctoral research, I ventured on to another project studying the relationship between the catecholamines and the cholinergic system. This involved learning how to measure tissue catecholamines, and was directed by Dr. Ted Brody, who was also supportive of my research needs. In fact, I set up an assay procedure using his equipment with the help of one of his students, Jim Gibb.

I might add that I got to know most of the graduate students in the department, especially on our long drives to FASEB meetings in Atlantic City, NJ. These were very memorable trips. The research experience was invaluable to my development as a scientist and was facilitated by the discussions with faculty and students and the many seminars. I also attended the department evening course sequence, which were very inventive, short courses in different areas of pharmacology, CNS, drug metabolism, etc. I later tried to persuade our faculty in Virginia to develop a similar series, but it never did take.

The faculty was a very hard-working group (and still is) of scientist-teachers well known in their respective fields. They became immediate role models as to how to what a professor should be. One faculty member, Dr. Roy Hudson, who was an instructor in pharmacology, also impressed me. He was personable and one of the best teachers in the department. I came across Roy again after moving to Virginia. He had been elected to be the President of Hampton University in Norfolk, VA and needed a copy of Goodman & Gilman's textbook of pharmacology. There were no medical schools in Norfolk so I bought him a book and got to chat about our mutual time at UM.

While in Ann Arbor, my wife and I had a third child, Laura, who was born at St. Joseph Hospital on the day before President Kennedy was assassinated. What a memory to come away with!

After the University of Michigan

During my second year of postdoctoral training, Ted Brody came to me with a job possibility at the University of Pittsburgh. Dr. Joseph Buckley, who was chairman of the Department of Pharmacology in the School of Pharmacy at Pittsburgh contacted him about a faculty position that Ted felt was perfect for me. I visited Pittsburgh and consequently become a research assistant professor in the summer of 1965. My research at Pittsburgh involved the "Effects of Chronic Stress on the Development of Experimental Hypertension." I was able to use much of what I had learned at UM to continue this work and we published a very interesting paper describing the chronic effects of stress on tissue and urine catecholamines. I also worked with a colleague, Dr. Herbert Barry III, who was a renowned behavioral pharmacologist and had a great influence on my major research over the last 34 years, the discriminative stimulus effects of nicotine. I also co-taught with Dr. Dan Abraham who is now chair of Medicinal Chemistry at the Medical College of Virginia (MCV).

For a variety of reasons, among them that the University of Pittsburgh was having financial problems, I moved on to the Yale University Department of Psychiatry and worked with Drs. Danny Freedman and Nick Giarman. During that period my research was focused on hallucinogenic drugs such as LSD. I developed procedures to evaluate this chemical's effects on brain neurochemistry (brain serotonin) and adapted some of the procedures developed at the University of Michigan in Dr. Brody's laboratory. So everything was coming together. The last piece of the puzzle involved Ed Domino again. After finishing a long study on LSD, Nick Giarman invited me into his office to pass on the word that Paul Larson, chairman of the Department of Pharmacology of the Medical College of Virginia, was looking for a person to fill the role of psychopharmacologist in his department. This was communicated via Ed Domino who was good friends with Paul Larson. In fact this relationship becomes more interrelated, as Paul was also a good friend of Dr. Maurice Seevers, who was then chair of Pharmacology at the University of Michigan.

The Michigan-Virginia Connection

The major reason I am writing about Virginia and my time there is because of the intimate connection between Michigan and me. I arrived in Richmond on July 1, 1967; I had been hired as assistant professor at MCV, which later became part of Virginia Commonwealth University (VCU). MCV was one of the oldest colleges in Virginia, aside from the University of Virginia and William and Mary. Virginia is the State of Presidents and I should also point out that MCV was to be the major medical school of the Confederacy. My building, McGuire Hall (named after Hunter McGuire who was in essence the surgeon general of the Confederate States), was located diagonally from the Confederate White House. I might also add that when we became VCU, Dr. Lauren Woods, who was on the faculty of the University of Michigan when he did most of his research involving the narcotic antagonists, became the first vice president of the health sciences division of VCU.

The Department of Pharmacology at that point had only six faculty members when I arrived and Paul Larson was insistent that I apply for a nicotine grant from the American Medical Association Research and Education Foundation (AMAERF). The AMAERF had a grant program with the goal of learning more about nicotine and smoking and health; it was funded by American tobacco companies, which became a problem later to some universities. The government had never considered nicotine a drug and there were no funds for such research at the NIH. In fact NIH support of nicotine as a psychoactive drug didn't occur until the mid-1980s; nicotine grants usually ended up in the Cancer Institute.

Important to my research was the fact that Dr. Seevers was chair of the committee that awarded AMAERF funds, and Paul Larson was a member of the committee. The time spent at the University of Michigan was important in that I had learned much about cholinergic drugs, especially how to approach studying the mechanisms of action of nicotine. Needless to say, I was awarded funds to start up a CNS nicotine research laboratory within six months of arriving in Richmond and was funded via these funds for almost 10 years. I had always felt that I received the funds for nicotine only because I was on the faculty of MCV until Paul Larson retired in 1975 and mentioned to me that the committee and outside reviewers were very impressed by my first grant.

I was able to conduct research on nicotine in a systematic and logical manner with no concerns about competition, since few researchers (except for Ed Domino) were interested in this most fascinating of chemicals, nicotine. In fact, one of my colleagues from Yale suggested that I spend more time on a "real drug" such as LSD.

Ed Domino's influence has been central

to my approach to sorting out how nicotine is working in the brain, at least at the basic science level. The approach was very simple and partly evolved from Julian Villarreal's research project. The approach used simple pharmacological interaction studies that involved the central-acting nicotine antagonist mecamylamine and the muscarinic antagonist atropine. Mecamylamine would antagonize nicotine but not a muscarinic agonist such as arecoline, and atropine would antagonize arecoline but not nicotine. We could also use select antagonists that would not enter the brain to show that nicotine was acting in the brain. In this way we were able to sort out where and how nicotine was acting in the brain. This approach was especially useful in our studies that involved studying nicotine as a discriminative stimulus (DS) that has led to our understanding of where nicotine has its primary site of action. Every graduate and postdoctoral student who works in my laboratory is required to read Domino's early work involving cholinergic drug interaction studies before they begin their own studies involving nicotine.

In the spring of 1970 Dr. Seevers visited Richmond and Paul Larson persuaded those of us with AMAERF grants (we had four grants) to present our research findings during an informal seminar session attended by Drs. Larson and Seevers. Dr. Seevers' understanding of our research involving the nicotine DS was especially gratifying to me. Dr. Seevers was a pioneer in encouraging the development of laboratories with the goal of evaluating the ability of psychoactive drugs (such as cocaine and morphine) to be self-administered by laboratory animals, especially primates. The University of Michigan had one of the first such laboratories and has been a model for other such laboratories.

Thus, I was a little wary of Dr. Seevers' thoughts and comments about what we were doing. Our research model was based on the ability of rats to elicit DS control of behavior which was a relatively new approach developed in only a couple of laboratories, and was especially new to us. Much to my delight, Dr. Seevers astutely observed that what we were measuring in our DS studies was the subjective effect of a drug, nicotine, that could induce an organism to self-administer it. He was able to immediately understand what we were doing, i.e. that we were evaluating the ability of a rat to detect nicotine's subjective effects in a manner similar to that perceived in the smoker. This was important to me, and may have even surprised Paul Larson as to the significance of our research. I attribute this observation to our success in continued funding from the AMAERF. These observations have also been important to my research over the last 34 years. We have further shown that smokers can detect nicotine much like our rats, supporting Dr. Seevers comments in 1970.

My last important direct encounter with Michigan was a visit in 1987. I was invited to present a paper at a nicotine symposium organized by Dr. Ovide Pomerleau who is a professor in psychiatry, and the behavioral medicine program at the University of Michigan. It was great going back to Michigan, 20 years later, to see the growth of the University. Most of the people I had known were no longer at the University. I also never did check to inquire if the RadiometerR pH-Stat was still in the laboratory.

Final Remarks

My time at Michigan was one involving both learning new methods and ideas and dealing with my own shortcomings. The postdoctoral years are important as you are only beginning to learn your craft. The Ph.D. is only a starting point for the long, hard road of continuing study. At the time I was frustrated by not being able to accomplish enough each day. However, as the years have accumulated I have realized that going to Michigan was an extremely important decision as to my own development as a scientist. The hypotheses I developed had their roots in my work in the Domino laboratory and the University of Michigan Department of Pharmacology. It was indeed a worthwhile journey.

The Michigan Days: 1965 to 1969

Stephen G. Holtzman, Ph.D.

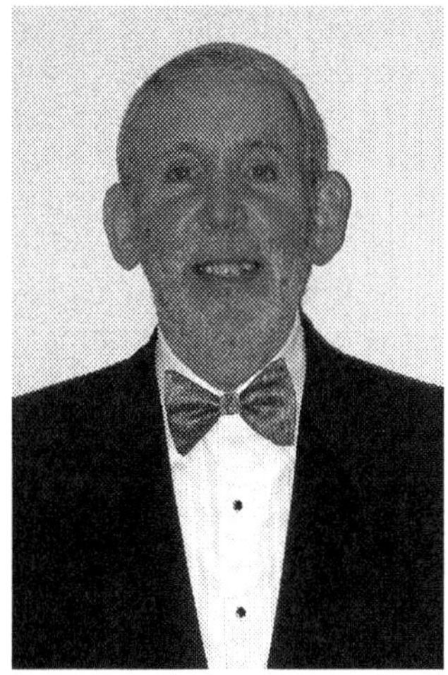

I went to The University of Michigan because I did not go to Tulane University. I had applied to five or six graduate programs in pharmacology. I was accepted by the program at Tulane, with a fellowship, and I sent a thank you letter saying that I would come. The acceptance letter from Michigan came later, in April, I think, suggesting that I was not at the top of the list of their candidates. Nevertheless, I was interested. I had read about the program at Michigan and was impressed by the number of prominent faculty in the pharmacology department. In addition, a former faculty member of my undergraduate program in pharmacy, Dr. George Zografi, had joined the faculty of the pharmacy school at Michigan a year or so earlier and expressed considerable enthusiasm for his new institution during return visits. I was convinced. I accepted the offer by Michigan of a position and fellowship, and I withdrew my acceptance of the position in the Tulane program. It was a fortunate decision. I entered the Michigan graduate program in July 1965, and left four years later with both a Ph.D. and a wife. That's what I call a great program.

Nine of us started in the pharmacology graduate program that year, and seven of us eventually completed it. All seven ended up on the faculty of an academic institution, which must be a record of some sort.

After arriving in Ann Arbor, I learned to my dismay that several of the eminent members of the pharmacology department, a major reason that I was attracted to the Michigan program in the first place, had recently left. I made the rounds of laboratories, looking for a faculty advisor, and chose Dr. Julian E. Villarreal. Julian, as he was known to everyone, had just been appointed an Instructor in the Department so that he could take over a program of drug screening in morphine-dependent rhesus monkey. That program had been directed by Dr. Gerald Deneau, one of the recently departed faculty members.

Julian had a medical degree from the University of Mexico and had just completed a research project with Dr. Ed Domino and then another for the Ph.D. degree under the auspices of Dr. Maurice Seevers. He needed only to write and defend his doctoral dissertation in order to be promoted to assistant professor. However, as was characteristic of Julian, he never did today what he could put off until next month. He finally defended his dissertation about six months before I defended mine. Julian's procrastination meant that he remained an Instructor during the entire time that I was in the program. Because an instructor could not chair a doctoral advisory committee, the chair of my advisory committee was the department chairman, Dr. Seevers.

The selection of such a junior person—one who, technically, was still a graduate student—as an advisor was, in retrospect, an incredibly naïve decision. But it was the right decision. Julian was a brilliant and innovative scientist and a compassionate and supportive mentor. He was also a friend.

Julian won me over by enthusiastically extolling the joys of using behavioral approaches in drug research. [It should be obvious by now that I have a weakness for enthusiasm.] So, I was destined to become a behavioral pharmacologist. I could not have been in a better milieu. Dr. Charles "Bob" Schuster, one of the pioneers of behavioral pharmacology, was conducting research on rhesus monkeys one floor below ours, using the recently developed technique of intravenous drug self-administration. His research assistant was Jim Woods, who had not yet added the title of "Dr." to his name. Down the hall from us Dr. John Falk, the discoverer of "schedule-induced polydypsia" and another notable behavioral pharmacologist, had his laboratory in the Department of Pathology (for reasons that were never clear to me). Dr. William Stebbins, a behavioral physiologist, had his laboratory across the street in the Kresge Building. Across another street was an old house that looked like it might have once belonged to the Addams Family, which was the home of the Brain Research Institute and the laboratory of Dr. James Olds, the father of intracranial self-stimulation. It was an enriched and stimulating environment in which to discover behavioral pharmacology.

During the summer of 1966 I began to date Yung-Fong Sung, a rising second-year medical student, who at the time was a summer research fellow in Dr. Ben Lucchesi's laboratory. We married two years later.

Snatches I remember:

*Being bitten on the hand by a rhesus monkey at 1:00 am while trying to measure its rectal temperature.

*Julian's desk and office floor became piled high with documents that he never quite got to. His solution: he moved to another office, a small one on the sixth floor of the Medical Science Building (there was only one Med Sci building then). It took us days to find him.

*Dr. Hans Kosterlitz, the person who discovered endogenous opioids in 1975, visited our laboratory, accompanied by Dr. Seevers. He got too close to the cage of "Joe," a stump-tail macaque, who promptly grabbed Kosterlitz' tie. While Joe pulled the tie into the cage, Julian and Seevers tried to pull Kosterlitz away. By the time they succeeded, the knot on Kosterlitz' tie had been reduced to the size of an acorn. Another minute or two and the enkephalins might have remained undiscovered for years longer.

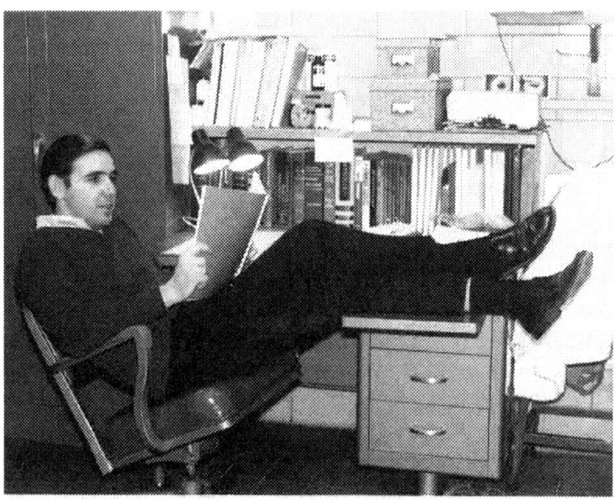

A young Holtzman studying pharmacology.

Memories of the Michigan Pharmacology Department Odyssey in and Beyond

Maxine L. Stitzer, Ph.D.

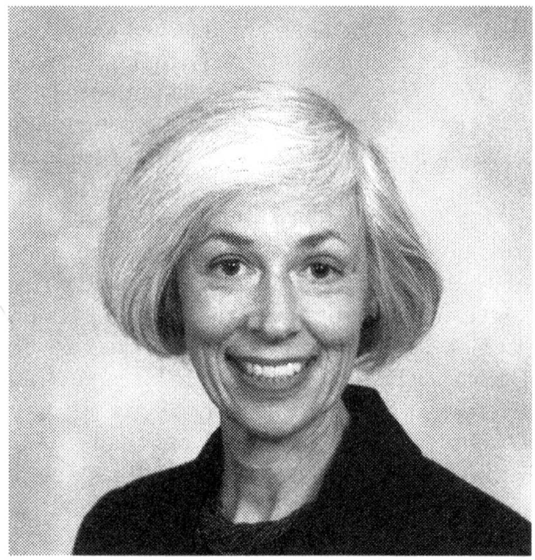

I felt like a lost soul when I first came to the University of Michigan in 1964. The campus was so big! And coming from California, the winters seem very chilly! Where were the other psychologists? And what exactly was I supposed to do? James Olds, the famous neurophysiologist with who I had aspired to work, said he had no room in his lab. So I landed at the Mental Health Research Institute, where a lipid biochemist was looking for help to run rats through a water maze. (Those little guys can really swim!) I read the Worm Runner Digest, edited by James O'Connell and learned about what happens when planaria eats another planaria. Meanwhile, I heard rumors of interesting work going on at the Pharmacology Department across the street, and went to investigate. Indeed, I found people there who were using new methods of operant conditioning as a tool to systematically investigate how drugs affect behavior. Dr. Edward Domino gave me my first break – the chance to study the effects of nicotine on the operantly controlled behavior of rats. We did a nice little dose-effect study and published a paper in a much respected pharmacology journal (Stitzer, Morrison & Domino, 1970). Meanwhile, I was wandering down to the basement to see what was going on in the monkey lab. Julian Villarreal and Bob Schuster were studying opiate dependence in a colony of addicted monkeys. Bob Schuster was implementing the revolutionary concept of using catheterized monkeys to study the reinforcing effects of drugs – designing what turned out to be a powerful self-administration model of drug abuse. Steve Goldberg was finishing his dissertation work on body temperature effects of opiates and Steve Holtzman was showing that long-lasting conditioned withdrawal responses could be elicited and using classical conditioning techniques. This all seemed very interesting.

Meanwhile, the then president of the U.S., Richard Nixon, had launched the first "war on drugs." As part of a new training initiative, Ed Domino applied and the Department received funds to train "Psycho-pharmacologists." I was one of the first to sign up for the opportunity. It meant some financial support during graduate training and the chance to take some very interesting classes with medical students while working on our psychology requirements. This early training in pharmacology and scientific methods was critical for success later in my career, as well as the careers of the other psychology graduate students.

The chance to move downstairs to the behavioral pharmacology laboratory came after Bob Schuster left for the University of Chicago. Jim Woods, a fledgling faculty member himself, was thrown into the foray of mentoring an unruly bunch of graduate students that included myself, Gail Winger, John Carney, and Carol Iglauer. We had technical problems in those days – the rhesus monkeys' intravenous catheters would become infected and the animals often died before their useful laboratory life had run its course – and right in the middle of our experiments! Gail Winger and I managed to pull off a study of sedative self-administration (Winger, Stitzer & Woods, 1971). Gail had infinite patience with the monkeys and a real knack for handling them. I, however, was ready to quit graduate school out of sheer frustration. Jim Woods, in his best mentoring style, convinced me to change my dissertation project to a more manageable study involving pigeons. This suggestion saved my career and I am grateful to this day. My gratitude also goes to Ed Domino, who took me back into his laboratory after I had finally earned my degree in 1971. During this brief sojourn, I began dabbling with a new interest that was taking shape in the field – the translation of animal behavioral pharmacology research into research with humans (Stitzer & Domino, 1974).

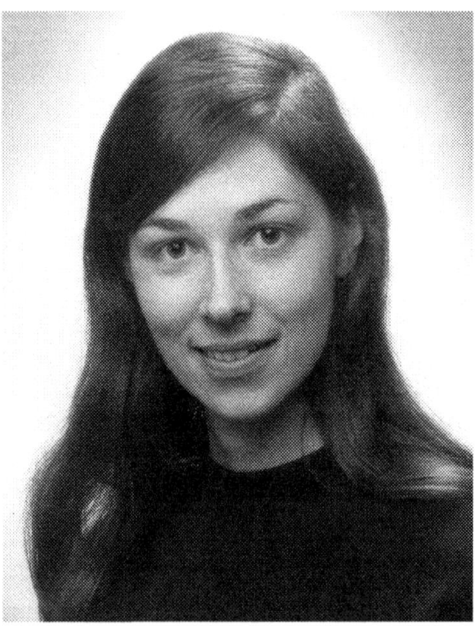

A younger Maxine

The idea of working with humans had not yet coalesced as a clear goal for me when I left Ann Arbor to take a post-doctoral position in another animal behavioral pharmacology laboratory in Boston. However, it soon became apparent that I was drawn to the human work that was just beginning to get established in a few laboratories. I was extremely fortunate to find George Bigelow and Roland Griffiths who had established a nascent human behavioral pharmacology laboratory at Johns Hopkins University School of Medicine in Baltimore, MD, where I started working in 1974. We named our laboratory the Behavioral Pharmacology Research Unit, and we were off and running with a vision of excellence and innovation that has served us well for 30 years.

During the time at Johns Hopkins, I have had the opportunity to conduct or direct a wide range of human behavioral pharmacology and drug abuse treatment research studies. Working in collaboration with a wonderful group of colleagues and postdoctoral students, and with a level of sophisticated research support that is unsurpassed in the nation, a large body of research has been produced whose main themes include: 1) studies of acute opioid physical dependence in humans, 2) systematic research on the pharmacology of methadone's treatment efficacy, 3) studies of buprenorphine's clinical pharmacology and its development as a new opioid dependence treatment medication, 4) studies of physical dependence, craving and relapse in nicotine dependence and 5) development of contingency management interventions for use in drug abusers. This research has advanced the field of drug abuse in a number of important ways and has led directly to some of the new treatments that are being used today.

Over the years, I have had the honor to receive several research career awards that have recognized the contribution made by myself and my colleagues at BPRU. These have included a research contribution award from the Maryland Psychological Association (1998), the Nyswander-Dole award from the Association for Treatment of Opioid Dependence (2000), the Brady-Schuster award from Division 28 of the American Psychological Association (2000) and the Marian Fischman award from the College on Problems of Drug Dependence (2003).

Looking back on graduate school at the University of Michigan, I am grateful for the high quality and stimulation education that was available. The graduate program to which I and my fellow psychology graduate students were exposed was unique in its combination of psychology and pharmacology training. In retrospect, this program could serve in part as a model for the training that psychologists will need in order to gain prescribing authority, a movement that is about to become a reality in this country. For us, the training that we received opened up fascinating career options in academia and prepared us extremely well to succeed in them. More importantly, we made lasting friends and supportive connection among fellow students and U of M faculty that have been a source of joy through the years.

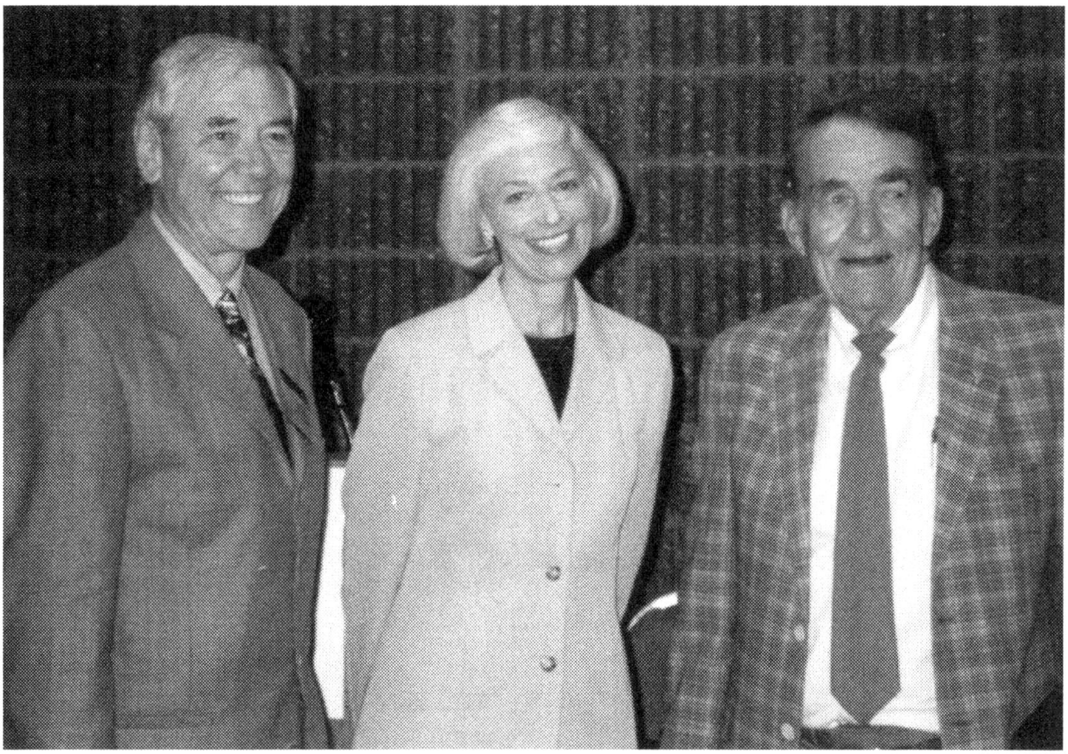

Three intellectual pillars of behavioral pharmacology, from left to right: Drs. Charles Schuster, Maxine Stitzer and Joseph Brady.

Memories: 1965-1971

Thomas Tephly, M.D., Ph.D.

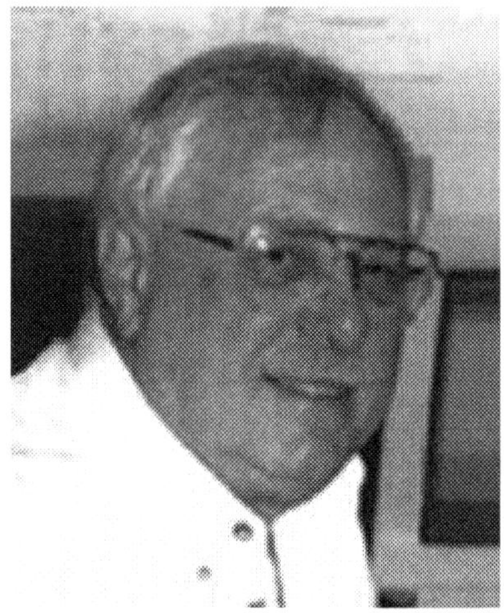

In 1965, Dr. Ed Cafruny moved from the Department of Pharmacology at the University of Michigan to the Department of Pharmacology at the University of Minnesota. I was in Gil Mannering's lab and finishing my medical school program in 1965. I was working on both drug metabolism and methanol toxicity in the lab and starting to explore further professional opportunities. Ed mentioned that I should contact Dr. Seevers, the chair of pharmacology at Michigan, to see if there was a possible opportunity there. I did, I was invited to give a seminar, and I was offered a job as an assistant professor. I was very happy to have the chance to pursue research at Michigan and, interestingly, I moved to Ann Arbor with my family in the same moving boxes that Ed Cafruny used to move to Minnesota. Then, when we got to Ann Arbor I learned that we inherited the same phone number that Ed had had in Ann Arbor!

When I arrived in Michigan I immediately got three graduate students and a lab which was completely empty except for a Mettler balance, courtesy of Ed Domino. How were we to begin doing any research? No start-up funds existed in those days. I was also told that I had to develop my own course, teach part of the medical school course and continue the summer course in medical pharmacology. I started writing an NIH grant the day I arrived (which was funded), I wrote for small grants on campus (also funded), and we had a lot of help from Dr. Ted Brody who really was a savior for chemicals and advice. I will never forget that initiation and I will never forget Ted Brody for his help. Over the next five years our research went well. We worked hard and the graduate students who began with me were extremely bright and enthusiastic. I might point out that each of them, Bill George, Jay Goodman, and Jeff Baron, are professors of pharmacology today.

In 1971, I was offered a position at the University of Iowa as Director of the Toxicology Center and Professor of Pharmacology. I accepted this position and my family and I moved to Iowa City. We have been here ever since. This marked the fourth Big Ten University that I had been at: I got my Ph.D. at the University of Wisconsin, M.D. at Minnesota, first job at Michigan, and present job at Iowa. I love the Big Ten and in each of the departments I have had great experiences. Specifically at Michigan, who could ever forget Dr. Seevers? I remember, with respect and joy, the interactions with Carl Hug, Ray Ruddon, Ben Lucchesi, Tad Smith, Hank Swain, Lloyd Beck, Ed Domino, and Ted Brody. Too bad we can never go back in time; I have such happy memories of Michigan.

Memoirs: 1966-1970

Paul Bass, Ph.D.

The people in the University of Michigan Department of Pharmacology made a strong impact on the research at Parke-Davis. The company research facilities moved to North Campus in 1959. At least two of us, Duncan McCarthy and I, had very close ties to Pharmacology at the University. In addition, Dr. Seevers was a personal friend of Cal Bratton, the Head of Pharmacology at Parke-Davis. In 1966, while working at Parke-Davis, I received a lecturer appointment in Pharmacology.

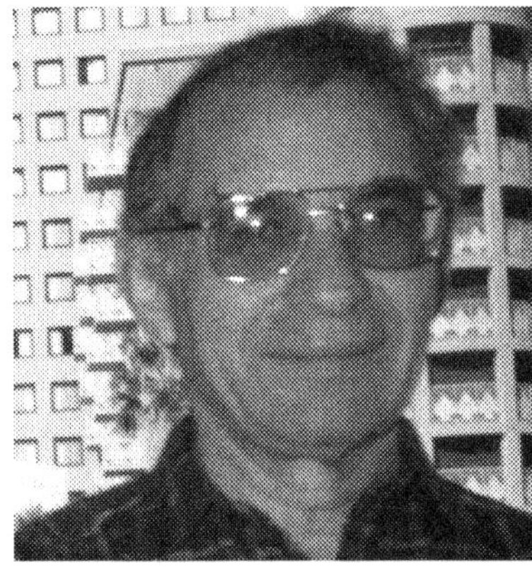

Parke-Davis sponsored my postdoctoral education. I joined the company at their new facilities in Ann Arbor in January, 1960. Between 1962 and 1970, the students and faculty from the Department of Pharmacology and other departments from the Medical School with whom I worked had free access to the laboratories at Parke-Davis. Much of the collaborative research that led to various publications was conducted at the Parke-Davis facility. The company benefited greatly because these bright people from the University facilitated research for understanding the mechanisms of drugs acting on the gut smooth muscle in the unanesthetized animal.

Dr. Donald (Skip) Bennett and I had excellent scientific interactions, developing several methods for monitoring gastrointestinal motor activity. After Skip went to Dow Corning, Drs. Carl Hug and Ray Ruddon, as well as several graduate students, continued to interact with me. Henry Jacoby was the first graduate student to study and develop a muscle transducer for chronic recording of gut motor activity. After many failures, Hank built the first force transducer that lasted approximately seven days. David Reinke as a graduate student in collaboration with Skip and I extended the life of the muscle transducer to approximately six months. Norman Weisbrodt and Jerry Carlson, for their Ph.D. dissertations, studied the actions of various drugs on the small intestine and colon. I also recall interacting with the late Julian Villareal. He helped characterize CI 750, a non-narcotic antidiarrheal agent that was synthesized and patented by Parke-Davis.

In addition, I interacted closely with several faculty and residents in the Departments of Medicine and Surgery. These were Dr. Bob Bolt, a professor in the Gastroenterology division of the Department of Medicine; Gene Overholt, a resident in Medicine; and Jack Ludwick, a surgical resident. Ludwick, who stayed on as an assistant professor, worked closely with Skip and me on several aspects of biliary tract pharmacology.

The gastrointestinal force transducers developed at Parke-Davis and the University have a continuing story. After coming to the University of Wisconsin at Madison, my wife Ruth learned to construct them and set up a cottage industry. There is still a demand for these transducers and she supplies the world—Japan, many European countries, and even Turkey. We have generated several sizes so that gut motility can be recorded from animals as small as the rat to larger domestic animals.

Memoirs: 1968-1970

Marcus V. Gomez, D.V.M., Ph.D.

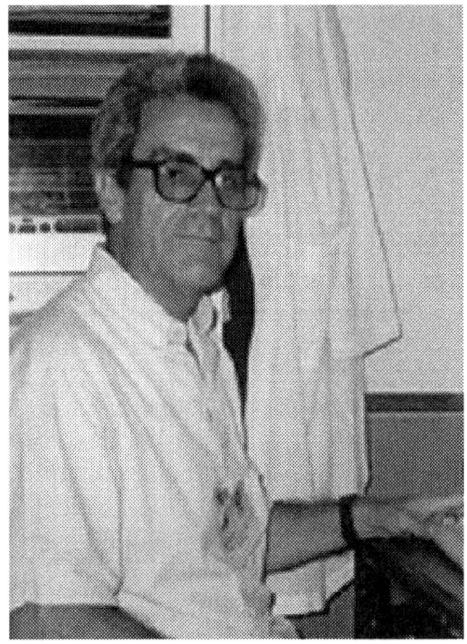

For two and half years (1968-1970) I had the pleasure of working in the Pharmacology Department at the University of Michigan with Dr. Edward F. Domino. At that time Dr. Domino was working on a research project with Dr. Otto Z. Sellinger of the Mental Health Research Institute at the University of Michigan. The research project was related to the effects of hemicholinium-3 (HC-3) on choline metabolism and acetylcholine (ACh) synthesis. During the development of the research we obtained data showing that HC-3 not only inhibited the ACh synthesis but also stimulated the incorporation of radioactive choline into phospholipids, specifically lecithin. This new data was shown to Dr. Brian Ansell in one of his visits to the Pharmacology Department. I believe Dr. Ansell, at that time, did not believe in our data and even criticized it. A few years later, in 1973, I was present at one of Dr. Ansell's conferences at the meeting of the International Society for Neurochemistry in Tokyo. Dr. Ansell initiated his presentation by mentioning that he was going to talk about the new and relevant aspects of the effect of HC-3 on phospholipid synthesis as described by Gomez, Domino and Sellinger three years earlier.

My postdoctoral position at the Pharmacology Department caused a profound change in my area of research interest. Before I was a biochemist only devoted to protein purification, specifically scorpion neurotoxins. After my postdoc, I was also interested in aspects related to the effects of these neurotoxins in synaptic transmission. Thus after my return to Brazil in July 1970, I used the tityustoxin that I had purified in 1967 to initiate studies with the effect of this neurotoxin in the release of ACh in brain cortical slices. We showed for the first time that this toxin binds to the Na^+ channel and has antagonism with tetrodotoxin. As far as we know this was the first demonstration of neurotoxins antagonism.

Neurotoxins were our main research field, and later we began studies with toxins purified from the venom of the spider Phoneutria nigriventer. One of these toxins is a potent blocker of calcium channel, blocks glutamate release, and may have potential use in neuronal ischemia. Another toxin from the venom only acts in insects and has no effect in mammalian tissues, having potential use as biologic insecticide.

In 1975 I returned for a short visit to the Pharmacology Department. At that time, Dr. Domino asked me to help one of his Ph.D. students, Lindsay Boardman Hough. Dr. Hough got his Ph.D. degree in 1978, and he sent me a copy of his thesis. I have kept it for more than 20 years. In his thesis, on page ii, Dr. Hough dedicated to me some words that may give an idea of my feeling toward research: "To Dr. Marcus Gomez, who made research more fun than work."

How the University of Michigan Department of Pharmacology Changed My Life

Joe Graedon, M.S.

When Ed Domino asked me to contribute a chapter to a book he was planning about the history of the University of Michigan Department of Pharmacology, I agreed reluctantly. The more I thought about it, though, the more uncomfortable I became. My short time in the Department was one of the most difficult periods in my life, and some of the memories remain painful even 30 years later. Nevertheless, I owe Ed and the "boys" a huge debt of gratitude. Without my trial by fire and the knowledge I gained, I wouldn't have been able to create the unusual career and satisfying life I now enjoy. So, here's the unusual story of Joe Graedon's amazing pharmacological adventure.

I guess it all started as a result of one of those bizarre moments that happen when someone accidentally triggers extraordinary excitement. For me it was during a guest lecture at Penn State University when I was an undergraduate. Bill Dement was giving a talk about sleep research. It must have been 1966 or 1967. I was totally captivated. He discussed various sleep stages from REM (rapid eye movement sleep) to stage IV (slow wave, "deep" sleep) and provided a glimpse into the brand new world of sleep research. I was immediately hooked and started reading as much as I could. But there wasn't much research opportunity for a psychology undergraduate at Penn State in this burgeoning new field, so I was left to my own devices.

When I graduated in 1967, I was unsure what direction to take with my life. The Vietnam War was heating up, and as a Quaker I had decided to seek conscientious objector (CO) status. A friend told me that her pharmacologist father knew of a lab where I might be able to serve my obligation and also do sleep research. Although I was clueless about pharmacology as a discipline, the idea of sleep research was intriguing.

I met with Carl Pfeiffer, M.D., Ph.D., head of the neuropharmacology laboratory at the New Jersey Neuro-Psychiatric Institute in Princeton, and he was quite open to my proposal for CO status. My local draft board saw that I would be working in a "mental institution" and sanctioned my request without delay. I initially did bioassays on monoamines such as spermine, spermidine, and histidine in Dr. Pfeiffer's lab, and then worked for Dr. Leonide Goldstein, an amazing mentor. I participated in several sleep studies involving methaqualone (Quaalude) and also was involved in fascinating research on LSD and other hallucinogens. (And no, despite ready access to dozens of vials of pure Sandoz LSD, I was never tempted to try it or any of the other hallucinogens we kept in the refrigerator.)

We hooked up with a creative biochemist, Bernard Polis, Ph.D., who wanted us to test free radical compounds on brain physiology in rats and rabbits. This was around the time that the Russians were beaming microwaves into the US Embassy, and Dr. Polis had been encouraged to try to find out what those microwaves might be doing to animal neurophysiology.

Working in this environment was an incredibly heady experience. Every day was exciting and challenging. I loved this stuff and couldn't wait to pursue the dream that began to grow there, a career in neuropharmacology that would focus on mental illness and sleep neurophysiology. Leo said the place to go would be the University of Michigan and the man to work with would be Dr. Ed Domino. So, that was the next stop in my adventure.

I remember rolling into Ann Arbor in

the early summer of 1969. What a time! The Vietnam War was now going full blast. The protest movement was also ramping up with huge marches on Washington. The "summer of love" was changing the cultural landscape. And a field in Woodstock, New York, would make headlines, along with that now unforgettable phrase, "That's one small step for man, one giant leap for mankind."

For me, life was now study-study-study! I remember being totally captivated by microanatomy. It was hard but fun, and getting my first "A" in grad school was rewarding. I will also never forget meeting Maurice Seevers. The chairman of pharmacology was short, fat, and incredibly kind to newbies. His lecture on drug abuse was amazing. Here we were in the middle of this drug culture with so much emotional nonsense in the media about marijuana and such. I seem to recall Dr. Seevers sharing with us that he had tried just about everything there was to take, from heroin and barbiturates to amphetamines and cocaine. We sat there in stunned silence. He hadn't much liked the barbiturate experience, but he admitted that cocaine was incredibly seductive.

Fall semester was trial by fire: heavy-duty coursework, intense pharmacology with the med students, and intimate interaction with faculty. What a crew they were! These folks were generally arrogant, demanding and unforgiving. They thought their little research niche was the most important place in the universe, and whatever the other guys were doing was less significant. Tad Smith took the cake. We were frequently reminded that, when he was at Harvard, things were different, presumably better, tougher and more rigorous, as if we were coasting at U of M. He shared how he would read up on some arcane area of research as a student and lie in wait for an unsuspecting professor with an impossibly difficult question, suggesting that if we were real scholars we would follow in his footsteps.

In general, the graduate student experience was awful. The faculty seemed unsupportive and divided. There was an awful lot of backbiting and general criticism of each other's work. There were exceptions, of course, faculty members who did not try to set traps to humiliate insecure grad students. A few seemed to genuinely care about our well being, but the overall atmosphere was incredibly intimidating.

I remember Ed Domino telling me early on to forget the arcane and antiquated EEG. Think cellular, he said. I needed to be focusing on neurons, not on the whole brain. Ouch. That hurt. Ed seemed genuinely sorry to see the old world of intact animals replaced with brain slices, but it was the new reality. My rotation in Ed's lab was at a time when course work was so intense that I didn't have much time to absorb anything else.

A rotation with Tad Smith made my time with Ed seem like a picnic. I remember the big scissors to cut off the heads of the rats so we could "harvest" the brains faster and get the brain slices quicker. I must not have been very good at it. The most memorable time with Dr. Smith was the "man to man" lecture he administered when he told me that some people were cut out to be pharmacologists and others weren't. The clear message: Joe Graedon, you ain't one of us. I beseechingly suggested that some of us might be able to provide something of value, albeit in nontraditional ways, but there wasn't much sympathy for that argument.

Hank Swain seemed like my last hope for a mentor. I was about as interested in cardiovascular pharmacology as in being a dogcatcher, which is sort of what I became. I remember collecting dogs in the basement, injecting an anesthetic and then praying they'd survive until I got them into the slowest elevator in the world and unloaded them into Hank's lab.

For some reason the anesthetic always seemed to precipitate bronchospasm, so I had to perform an emergency tracheotomy the moment I got them into the lab. Then there was the chest opening, threading the catheter into the heart and a series of electric shocks designed to induce ventricular fibrillation. I remember one of the more valuable lessons that Hank taught me was that so-called anti-arrhythmic drugs could actually have a pro-arrhythmic effect.

Now that was an eye opener, and it started me asking heretical questions, like how many other drugs may be harming more than helping?

My time with Dr. Swain was also problematic. I was no surgeon. Cutting up dogs was not my forte, and using those antiquated smoked papers on revolving drums to measure blood pressure was pretty bizarre. Hank was the best damn lecturer I ever encountered at U of M, but he did have his emotional ups and downs, maybe leftover in part from the residual mercury poisoning he had experienced. I am sure I disappointed him on more than one occasion. He did force me to think critically, however. His disdain for some of his colleagues intrigued me. I remember him asking me impossible questions about the cause of SIDS (sudden infant death syndrome) and CHF. I tried to bullshit my way through these difficult questions, to his obvious disdain. Ultimately, I learned that if what I was hearing in lectures or reading in textbooks didn't make much sense, maybe it wasn't that I was stupid; maybe the answers just weren't there. That was one of the greatest gifts I took away from my U of M experience, and Hank was largely responsible.

Oh yes, there was one other huge gift, this time from Ed Domino. I remember sitting in on a lecture he was giving to some medical students about drug interactions. He talked about MAO inhibitors and tyramine—the "cheese" effect. I seem to recall other interaction issues during that lecture as well. It truly intrigued me. When I first appeared on "Good Morning America" in 1976 to talk about the original edition of The People's Pharmacy, my discussion of food and drug interactions was the focus. In particular, my brief discussion of the dangers of mixing MAO inhibitors with cheddar cheese, salami or pickled herring really captivated the American public and helped propel the book to number one status on the New York Times bestseller list.

But I am getting ahead of myself. Despite my decent grades and positive attitude, my esteemed professors did not see fit to give me a chance to pursue a Ph.D. I was given a master's degree instead and sent on my way. As I recall, there were quite a few "casualties" in our group. It had been a rough two years for all sorts of reasons, and I was glad to be done. The trial by fire had left lots of scars.

I had learned an enormous amount of information about the human body. My physiology class with the grand old man, Dr. Davenport, was worth the price of admission. And I truly did develop a love for pharmacology. I discovered that this "bastard" field, a quicksand between biochemistry and physiology, really is where the action is. I learned to love the multi-disciplinary nature of this profession. To this day I love the practical meeting of basic science and clinical application. I still believe that the way the system is set up to teach medical students is nonsensical. Asking researchers who get their jollies from focusing on minutiae instead of the big picture lends itself to irrelevance. That most physicians seem to rely on drug sales reps for their continuing pharmacological education has always seemed like an indictment of the entire process.

After receiving my terminal master's degree, I followed my wife Terry to Oaxaca, Mexico, where she was planning to do field research in medical anthropology. During a preliminary trip I met the director of the local medical school, Dr. Fernando Galindo. We hit it off immediately and he asked me to help him set up a pharmacology laboratory program for his second year medical students. I was probably one of the last graduate students at U of M to have served as an assistant in the pharmacology laboratory program for med students. I still had all my notes and handbook materials. I managed to scrounge some drugs from Hank Swain and Leo Goldstein, and with great trepidation brought them into Mexico. I feared I might be one of the rare individuals jailed for smuggling drugs into Mexico rather than the other way around.

Terry helped me translate my notes (and some other text material) into Spanish. And so this "farmacologo" commenced a career teaching enthusiastic Mexican medical students in Spanish some of the same material I had learned at U of M. The class was a roaring suc-

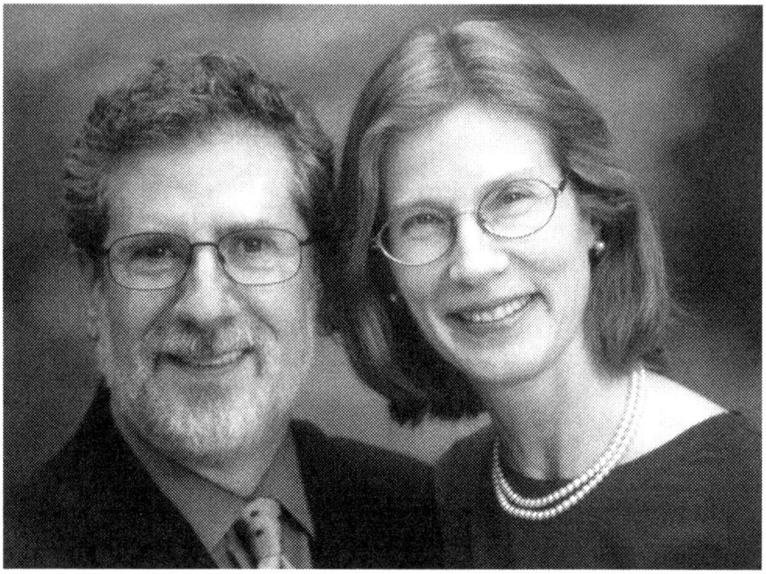

Joe Graedon and his wife Terry have collaborated on "People's Pharmacy" books for over 25 years. They also host a public radio program heard all over the country.

cess, both to my ego and for my students. We used the same ridiculous smoked paper we had used in Hank Swain's lab to record blood pressure in dogs. The only difference was that my students had to capture their dogs on the street with great fear and trepidation, since there was always the risk of rabies.

The lab class was taught each morning five days a week (repeated to five successive classes of roughly 25 students). By the end of each week my Spanish had improved enough so that the Thursday and Friday classes really could understand what I was talking about. I rotated the classes so that each group could benefit from this learning curve.

Since my afternoons were free, I started thinking about writing a book that had been floating around in my head ever since I left U of M. It would be an effort to translate my love of pharmacology into laymen's terms with lots of practical information. So, in 1973 I started on The People's Pharmacy. We spent one more year in Oaxaca, during which time I was promoted to teaching a regular pharmacology class in addition to the laboratory program. I loved it and the students seemed to appreciate the material as well.

During a recent visit, my old students, many of whom are now leaders in the medical community, reflected fondly on their pharmacology classes so long ago. My favorite assistant, Hector, now a formidable pediatrician, was heading up the pharmacology program himself.

When we returned to the US, Terry commenced her thesis and I worked diligently on the manuscript that would eventually be published as The People's Pharmacy. We moved to Durham, NC, where Terry got her first job as a medical anthropologist at the Duke School of Nursing. My book was published in 1976, and eventually became number one on the New York Times bestseller list.

Since then, many other books have been published, including a novel—a medical mystery co-authored with my friend Tom Ferguson, M.D., called "No Deadly Drug." Terry and I have been collaborating on "People's Pharmacy" books for over 20 years. Over three million copies of various works have been printed. We also write three newspaper columns together each week that are syndicated to papers all around the world. Some of our client newspapers include The Los Angeles Times, The Houston Chronicle, the Cleveland Plain Dealer, the Baltimore Sun and the Seattle Times. Circulation of our client papers is over six million weekly. We also co-host an award-winning radio show heard on over 500 stations, including public radio, the In-Touch Radio Reading Service, and Armed Forces Radio.

We lecture all over the country on drug-drug, drug-food, drug-nutrient and drug-herb interactions. We interact with FDA folks, especially those who approve new drugs and those concerned about drug surveillance. We have a wonderful working relationship with clinical pharmacologists like Ray Woosley. Television appearances have included "Dateline NBC", "20/20", "Oprah Winfrey", "Live with Regis and Kathie Lee", "Today", "Good Morning America", "CBS Morning News", and "NBC Evening News" with Tom Brokaw.

None of this would have been possible without my experience in the Department of Pharmacology at the University of Michigan. So, I owe a huge debt of gratitude to Ed, Hank and Tad, and all the others who made my life miserable so it could become wonderful. Thank you, guys, from the bottom of my heart.

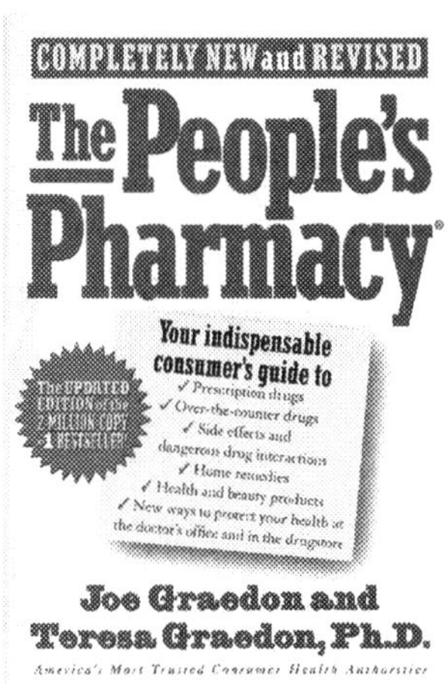

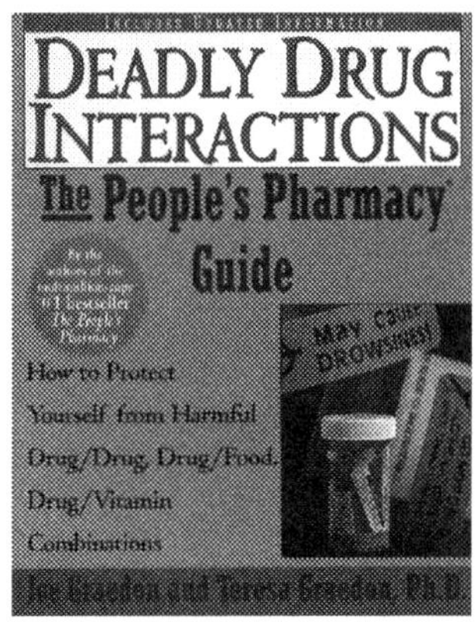

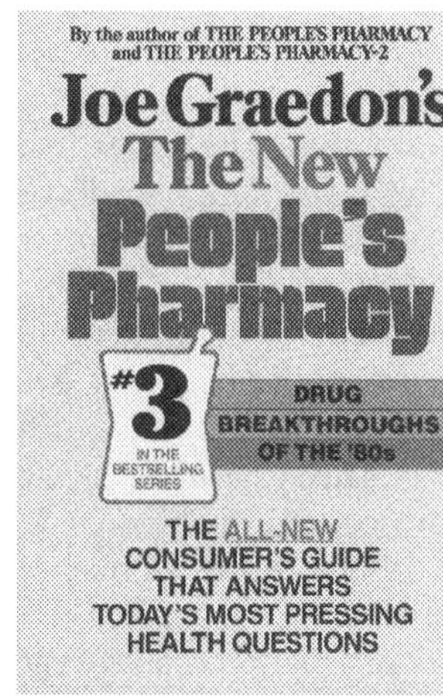

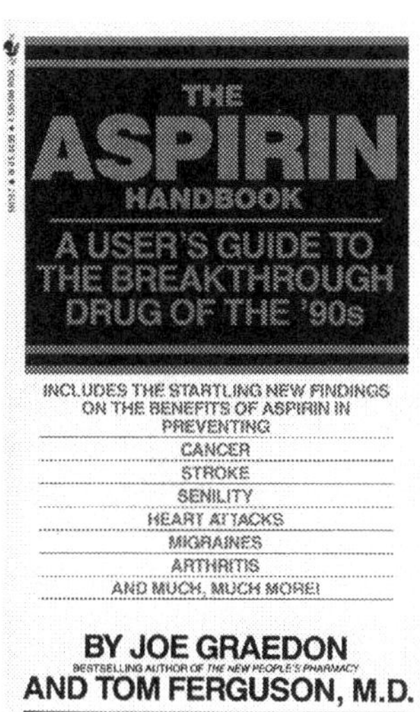

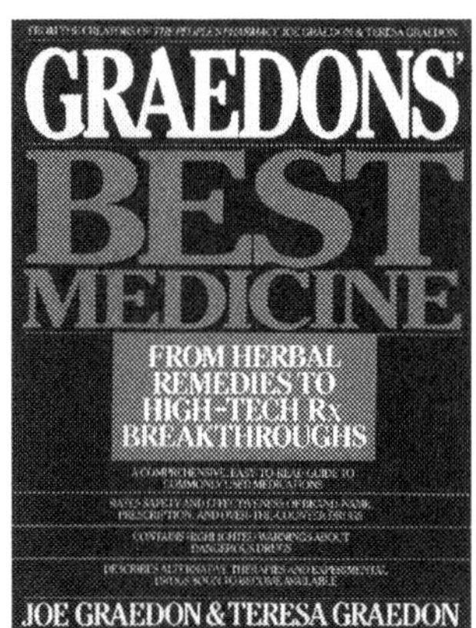

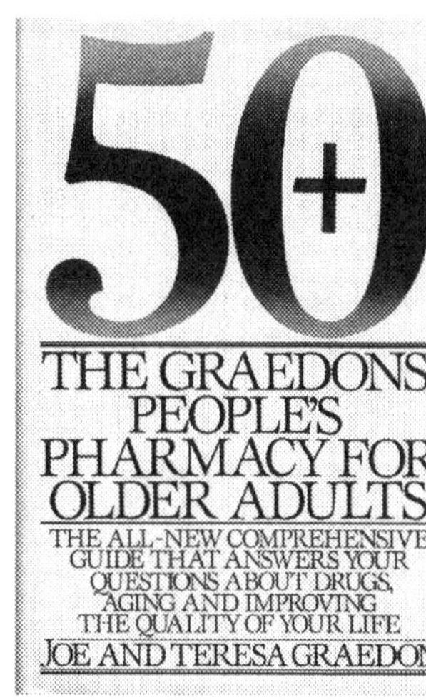

From Classical Pharmacology to Chronopharmacology

Gaston Labrecque, Ph.D.

I had the privilege of getting my graduate training in the laboratory of Dr. Edward F. Domino at the beginning of the 1970s. Dr. Maurice Seevers was the chairman of the Department of Pharmacology and many laboratories were studying on the effects of narcotic analgesics.

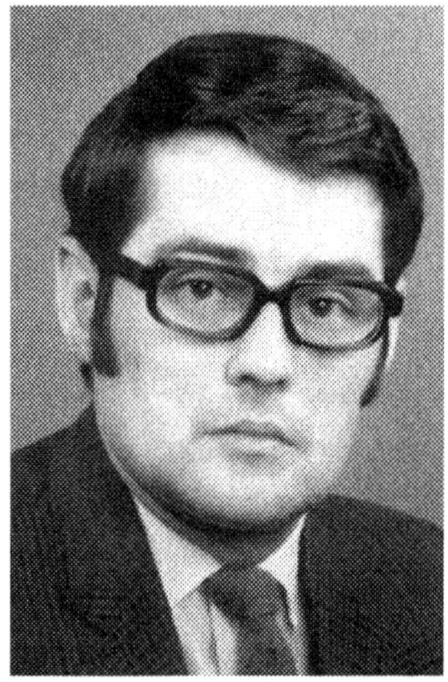

In these days, the "classical" pharmacologists of the department were looking at the effects of narcotic agonists and antagonists either on animal behavior (monkeys, mice, rats) or on the different neurotransmitter systems of the brain. In Dr. Domino's laboratory, most of us were looking at the effect of morphine and related agonists on the central cholinergic system, mainly on the brain levels or the release of acetylcholine from the neocortex.

The graduate students were taking many courses in biology and pharmacology, in addition to the regular seminars of the Department and the usual laboratory meetings. The graduate courses and meetings were scheduled at different hours of the day and the research activity of the graduate students was realized around them. Some students began their experiments either very early in the morning (6:30A.M.) to be able to attend the afternoon meetings or after lunch (1:30P.M.) when our business activities were scheduled in the morning. This working schedule allowed the students to get data quickly and to graduate as soon as possible.

When reviewing our data, Dr. Domino and I were astonished to find that the doses of morphine needed to raise brain acetylcholine content varied by a factor of 30-fold from one experiment to the next. Many working hypotheses were suggested to explain this extremely large variability in drug effect and we tried to answer the following questions: Can technical problems (including the student himself) explain the data? Does cigarette smoking around the acetylcholine bioassay equipment be responsible for the data? Can an "unknown" factor interfere with the bioassay or the effect of the drug and if so, which one?

It turned out that neither technical problems nor cigarette smoking were responsible for the large variations found in the effect of morphine. However, we observed that the results obtained in the early morning experiments were always similar, but they were completely different from the afternoon data. Our later studies showed that the brain levels of acetylcholine varied by more than 50%, depending on the hour of sacrifice: acetylcholine was maximal in early morning hours and minimal late in the afternoon. When brain content of the cholinergic neurotransmitter was highest, a very large dose of morphine was needed to significantly raise its cortical levels and vice versa. We concluded that the hour of morphine administration was the "unknown" factor explaining the variation in morphine effect.

This was one of the first studies showing the importance of the hour of drug ad-

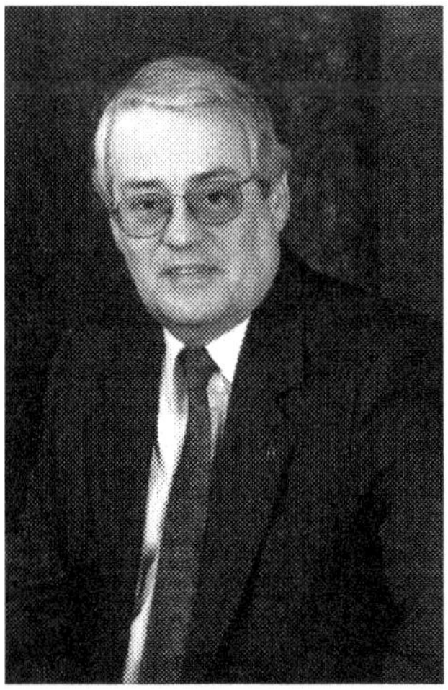

Professor Gaston

ministration on the effects of medications. The subject of chronopharmacology, time-dependent variations in the effects and the pharmacokinetics of drugs are now phenomena more easily recognized by the scientific and clinical communities. The hour of drug administration is now being accepted as a factor modifying the effects of medications. For instance, clinicans are aware that serious cardiovascular problems are occurring mainly in the early morning hours, and drug delivery systems are designed to take the time-dependent variations into account in patients. Drugs designed to use the body rhythms are now available in the United States and Canadian markets.

The outstanding training received in Ann Arbor and the objective but critical approach learned during my training years were very useful in developing the new field of chronopharmacology. Chronopharmacology may become the "classical" pharmacology of the 21st century and the Department of Pharmacology of the University of Michigan was directly involved in its development.

Editor's note: Gaston must unequivocally credit his wife, Marcelle, for providing the proximate cause for his life-long career in chronopharmacology. She did not believe in the bioassay used to quantify ACh and she put aside samples collected on the brain and gave him blanks to run the assay. When she found out that he was not making up the data, she told him that she now believed in the bioassay methodology and that she was ready to spend as many hours as needed in the laboratory.

Male Holtzman rats usually were maintained on a 12 hour light— dark cycle. Morphine effects were quantitatively different on total rat brain acetylcholine levels. At 0800 Gaston had shown that 10 mg/kg of morphine i.p. did not significantly change brain acetylcholine levels. This negative data did not fit with my preconceived ideas.

However, when Gaston repeated this experiment at night the effects were dramatic. The same dose of morphine at 1900 hours produced a 45% increase in acetylcholine levels that were highly significant ($p < .001$). Even one-tenth the dose of morphine (1mg/kg) was effective when administered during the first hour of the dark period ($p < .01$). At first I suspected this young French Canadian graduate student could not calculate and administer the correct dose of morphine to a rat when left alone at night. I confirmed that he knew exactly what he was doing. He now found his Ph.D. thesis topic and eventually a future career in a fundable and important area of research.

Of Mice and Men

Teresa Sagalés, M.D.

Perhaps I should apologize for borrowing John Steinbeck's title, but reminiscing on my days at the Department of Pharmacology in Ann Arbor brings mostly memories— of mice and men. Let me make it clear, I am referring to real mice (Mus musculus) and real men (you will easily realize that I could avoid repeating the qualification) so, do not expect any drama and please do not imagine that I am comparing myself with that extraordinary writer.

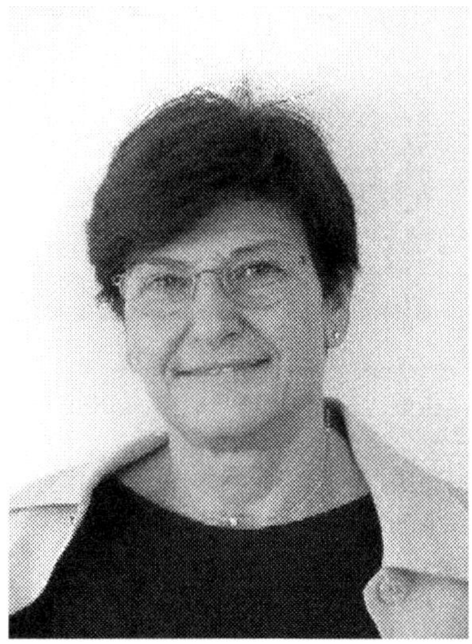

What about mice? After all, there are mice in practically all departments of pharmacology, but I remember mine for a series of reasons. When I came to Ann Arbor I had had very little contact with laboratory mice. I knew that they were nice creatures and also rather clever. What I did not suspect is that before long I was going to consider them quite intelligent. During my time in Ann Arbor I was involved in research on the interactions among cholinergic mechanisms, sleep and memory. That means that I had to evaluate the process of learning, and in mice this usually means resorting to mazes or to the shuttle box. The first strain of mice that I worked with were an absolute failure as far as learning was concerned and I soon had to switch to another. The new ones were lovely, with bright dark fur and easy to handle, and they seemed to do well in the first experiments. Soon, however, the counters started to pick up an incredible number of failures. They were not so. It was not as if the animals had become dumb enough as to accept whatever shock was delivered; they simply had discovered that staying on a single rod they did not endure any shock whatever color light was turned on.

Many will claim that this is an experience not uncommon in this type of situation. Possibly, but this was not to be the only show of intelligence on the part of the little animals. At one time of my research, it seemed appropriate to measure the effects of sleep deprivation on brain acetylcholine concentrations and on memory. That task was not easy, but quite interesting. I remember building my own stereotaxic apparatus for mice, implanting permanent EEG, EMG and EOG electrodes and having some fun at devising a procedure to achieve the goal of sleep deprivation in mice. Finally, I settled for an island-like arrangement. Washing basins at the laboratory were filled with water and a rod large enough to allow a mouse to stand on top of it (but definitely not to fall asleep) was erected at the center. Of course, I needed objective proof of the deprivation of sleep, and this was achieved by means of continuous polygraphic recording through the implanted electrodes, connected to a suitable apparatus. Simple, isn't it? Well simple it was, but it took quite a while for the experiments to run smoothly. The reason: many mice discovered that if they kept turning around, the twist of the cables connecting them to the EEG machine facilitated a jump to the border of the basin and to limited liberty and unlimited sleep.

And men. My memories of men in Ann Arbor center mostly about my boss, Dr. Edward Domino, and I know that Sergio Erill, my husband, who was also at the Department, will not be offended if I say so. Actually, I got in touch with the Department of Pharmacology in Ann Arbor through Sergio, who was there on a postdoctoral fellowship to train in clinical pharmacology with Dr. Ted Carr. My job in our country, Spain, was in clinical neurophysiology and I wanted to take advantage of the stay in the US to do some research in a field not far from that. Dr. Domino had been recommended to me as a very good scientist and I wanted very much to work with him. So, I was not taken aback when he said to me that his custom was to push his students as hard as it was needed to obtain high quality results, that is, using his own words, to squeeze them like a lemon. I am glad of this opportunity to clarify that I never felt squeezed, just the opposite. What I got from Dr. Domino was support, coaching, help and friendliness. If this is the fate of his lemons, it is worth being one.

I probably gave Dr. Domino more than one headache, and I particularly remember his bewilderment when we discussed the authorship of my first research article there. As I said above, I came to Ann Arbor as the wife of a postdoctoral trainee, Sergio Erill, and everybody naturally referred to me as Teresa Erill. This was quite OK to me, after all everybody addressed me as simply Teresa and I had no second thoughts at being Mrs. Erill. So far so good, but women in Spain keep their maiden names in every official document (passport, driving license, diploma, etc.) and it was quite clear to me that I should be Teresa Sagalés, M.D., in any research paper. Sergio, whose English was far better than mine, did his best to explain this, at that time, very strange state of affairs to Dr. Domino, who probably thought that this Spanish rigmarole was just an excuse to hide the fact that I was a secret member of woman's lib.

I have written about Dr. Domino, my boss, and Sergio, my husband, and you may wonder if they did ever get in touch. They did,

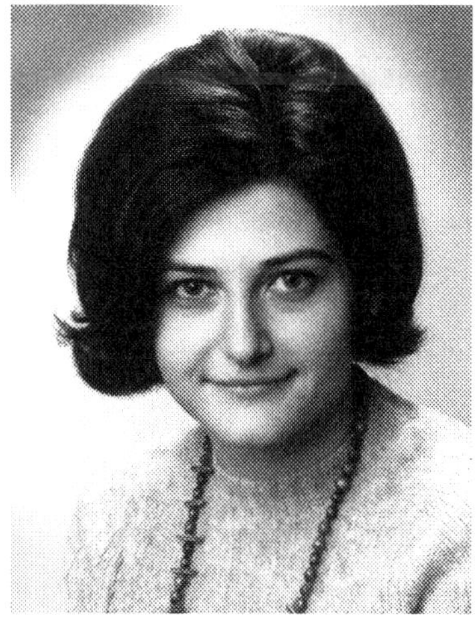

A younger Teresa

indeed. We three co-authored two research articles dealing— no surprise— with cholinergic mechanisms, sleep and clinical pharmacology, and 30 years after our time in Ann Arbor they are now involved in a psychopharmacology project. Nevertheless, there is an anecdote that even now always brings a smile to our faces. One morning Sergio got a request from Dr. Domino to see him at his office sometime in the afternoon. The poor soul did not say anything to me but, knowing how wild (that is what people say) I could be, he feared that I had done something quite unspeakable and was frightened to death. When the time of the meeting came, he was confronted with Dr. Domino's anxiety about my wellbeing. At this time I was six months pregnant, and he just wanted to enlist Sergio's help in convincing me that running in the corridors and descending stairs at full speed, as I had done all my life, comported a serious risk of miscarriage. Perhaps I complied with their united admonitions, because in due time I gave birth to a lovely girl.

Once, someone at the Department asked me if there was ever any competition between my husband and me, both being physicians and working quite close and sometimes even together. The answer was the same that I would give today, an emphatic no. However, I have to confess that there was something that sometimes interposed between Sergio and me in Ann Arbor: mice. I remember how funny he looked once when he found me attempting mouth to mouth resuscitation of a mouse. It had stopped breathing just when I had completed a rather complicated placement of electrodes in its brain and I hated the idea of my work going into thin air. Anyway, this was an isolated instance and what I remember now is something different. In my shuttle box experiments it was not uncommon that when I picked up a mouse out of the box at the end of them the little animal would walk along my arm (often under the sleeve of my coat) and end at my neck— to pee. The poor little things were probably scared but I assure you that whatever summary cleansing I tried before reaching home and the shower, something was interfering between Sergio and I on our way home (but just then!).

Writing all this, the richness of our life in Ann Arbor and the happiness that we experienced there comes back to my mind with a strong hint of homesickness. We left Ann Arbor just three weeks after the birth of our daughter, and I never came back to work at the Department after the delivery. I remember that the labor contractions started one afternoon while I was working there and I delayed my return home as much as possible to complete what I was doing. I felt like leaving something unfinished. Is it perhaps because of that feeling that I have always longed to return to the Department?

Editor's note: Dr. Teresa Sagales received her M.D. in 1966 from the University of Barcelona. Teresa worked as a Postdoctoral Fellow in my laboratory from 1968-69. Following her work at U of M Teresa went on to obtain her Ph.D. from the University of Granada in 1986. Currently Teresa is Director of Postgraduate Courses of Clinical Neurophysiology at the University of Barcelona and also the head of the Department of Clinical Neurophysiology at Hospital Universitari Vall d'Hebron.

She is a member of various international societies including: American Sleep Disorders Association, Catalonian Society of Clinical Neurophysiology, European Sleep Society, Iberian Association for the Study of Sleep Pathology and the Spanish Society of Neurology.

Dr. Sergio Erill received his M.D. in 1963 from University of Barcelona, and obtained his Ph.D. from the same institution in 1967. Subsequently, he was a postdoctoral trainee in Clinical Pharmacology in the Department of Pharmacology and the Upjohn Clinical Pharmacology Center. From 1967-1971 Dr. Erill was Associate Professor at Autonomous University of Barcelona. He was Chairman and Professor for three years at University of Bilboa of the Department of Pharmacology starting in 1976. Shortly after that he became Chairman and Professor of the Department of Pharmacology at University of Granada Medical School until 1983. In 1983, the Esteve Foundation was established in order to honor the late Dr. Antonio Esteve. The Esteve Foundation's main goal is to promote pharmacotherapy through ways of scientific communication and discussion. In 1983 Dr. Erill became Director of the Esteve Foundation in Barcelona. In 1989, he became Senior Director of Research and Development of Esteve.

In 1967, Dr. Erill received the Merck International Fellow in Clinical Pharmacology award. In 1970, he was given the Spanish Board of Internal Medicine Certificate. From 1978-1980, he was Chairman of the Spanish Board of Clinical Pharmacology. From 1982-1986, he was President of the Spanish Society for Pharmacology. Starting in 1983 and for the next nine years, he was a member of the WHO Expert Panel on Drug Evaluation. From 1987-1988, he was Chairman of the Spanish National Drug Surveillance Board. From 1991-1995, he was a member of the Selection Committee of the Merck International Fellowships in Clinical Pharmacology.

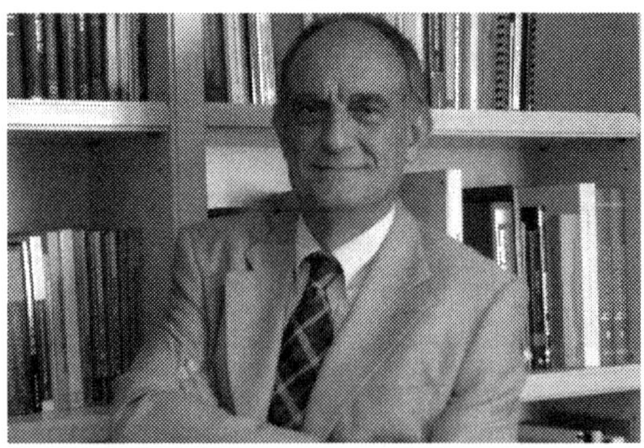

Dr. Sergio Erill

My Impressions of the Department of Pharmacology in the '60s and '70s

Ann Wilson Black, M.S.

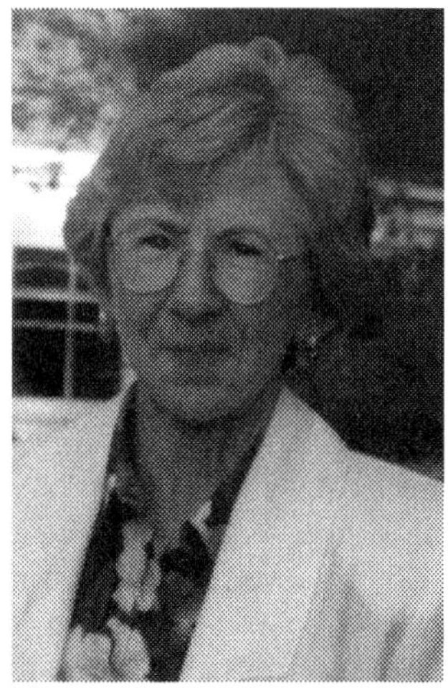

The 1960s and 1970s were exciting times for everyone on college campuses in America. There was student unrest, rock and roll music was at its peak, and love flourished everywhere. However thrilling it was to be out of school, the blunt reality of living meant finding a job. With a B.S. in Science from the University of Michigan, the field of opportunity appeared to be research. My first job interview was with Dr. Edward Domino in the Department of Pharmacology, who hired me on the spot. I had never worked in a research laboratory and thought it would be similar to the chemistry labs I had taken in school. The 10-plus years I was there proved that research involves not only bench work, but reading current literature in the field, writing reports, and presenting the results. I stayed for so many years because I had the opportunity to work with many other groups and departments, and Dr. Domino had endless new projects for us. I also learned that my paycheck came from grant money; this provided an additional incentive to be in the forefront of research.

I had the privilege of knowing Dr. Seevers and his administrative assistant, Dorothy Overbeck, who really ran the daily operations of the Department. While they often appeared formidable and stern, they were very accomplished, caring and wonderful people. Dr. Seevers often invited the whole department to his home to view his wonderful greenhouse full of bonsai trees. Dr. Domino's labs were somewhat unique because of the variety of people there, including postdoctoral people, lab workers, graduate students, and visiting scholars. The graduate students were always interesting. They entered pharmacological research as green and naive students but left as competent and inquiring scientists. We enjoyed their wild ideas and friendships as they progressed through their research. Their new ideas and questions always kept us on our toes.

Passing prelims and the oral exam was always a time of great tension. Finally, when word came the student had passed, all retired to the Pretzel Bell for an afternoon of celebration. Since we always had new students every year, it was an annual event we greatly enjoyed. Now, the majority are scattered all over the United States but still manage to keep in touch.

I had many opportunities in the Department of Pharmacology under the guidance of Dr. Domino. All researchers were encouraged to publish their work and give visual and/or oral presentations at meetings. I gave my first oral presentation to a large lecture hall full of scientists. I am sure everyone who has done this remembers his or her first oral presentation. Your heart rate accelerates to unknown levels, your mouth is as dry as the Gobi desert, and you wonder if the words will come.

After a few years in the Department, I had reached a plateau in knowledge and advancement. I decided to return to school and earn a master's degree in pharmacology. At that time in our Department, a master's degree was given when a person failed their oral exams for a doctorate degree. I did not want to do that so I entered the Medicinal Chemistry program and transferred to the Department of Pharmacology a year later. The Department, after several meetings, decided I could give an oral presentation of my work or write a small thesis. Of course, I wrote the thesis and received the Master's degree with the encouragement and guidance provided by Dr. Domino.

There were few women in the field of research when I started; however by the 1970s we saw at least one new female student enter the program almost every year. It was so unusual to find women in research at that time, I was often asked at national meetings if I was the wife of so and so enjoying the sights. However, women from all nationalities started to enter research at this time, especially from Japan, and have found rewarding careers.

Some of the highlights from my years with Dr. Domino should be mentioned. We learned all sorts of techniques since his interests were varied. Dr. Domino's curiosity even extended to his vacations since he always brought back exotic plants or other specimens. He collaborated with Dr. Wagner, the pharmacokineticist who could cover a blackboard with equations nonstop for hours. I remember keypunching hundreds of cards containing all the information for producing equations describing first order kinetics of the plasma concentrations of drugs. It took the computer days to produce the results and all those cards were later recycled into large Christmas wreaths.

Dr. Domino had the first quadrapole mass spectrometer on campus. While it appears crude now, it opened windows of opportunity in research just as technical breakthroughs have today. We were able to detect, identify, and measure compounds at concentrations that had been unattainable in prior years. We investigated the pharmacology of many different drugs of abuse. There was no trouble finding volunteers for marijuana research since the United States government supplied very potent stuff.

Other controlled substances were tested in animals to determine plasma concentrations and to find ways to quickly eliminate the drugs to reduce toxic events. At that time, all animals were housed in one large room, even monkeys. From a health standpoint monkeys can be dangerous to work with despite precautions. Once we had a group that became positive for tuberculosis after being in the facility for a couple of weeks, but this did not stop Dr. Domino's planned research. Under quarantine he did the experiments himself and samples came out the door in a gloved hand.

The number of labs that Dr. Domino was in charge of increased over the years and so did the staff and visiting scholars from all over the world. They came from Japan, South America, Spain, Russia, and Italy and each left an impression that coming to America to do research was a great honor for them. The Japanese soon introduced us to sake on Friday afternoons— a wonderful wine that helps close the week. Even at that time, the Japanese were some of the most intense and thorough scholars I have ever met.

Dr. Bartolini and his wife from Italy worked with leeches. The muscles of the leech are very sensitive to acetylcholine and the degree of contraction was used to assay acetylcholine content in samples. The leeches were kept in large glass container with a tight lid and small opening for air. No one ever volunteered to pick them up. One morning a graduate student had to take the leeches up to the next floor. He had forgotten to make sure the lid was secure. As he was walking down the hall we heard his voice rising in intensity and finally the sound of breaking glass. The leeches had found an escape route and decided the student's arm was the next meal.

Dr. Gomez from South America left us with many stories. The visiting Russian scientist, Dr. Yuri Burov, did not trust us at first. His eyes of cold blue steel finally softened after a year when he realized how valuable friend-

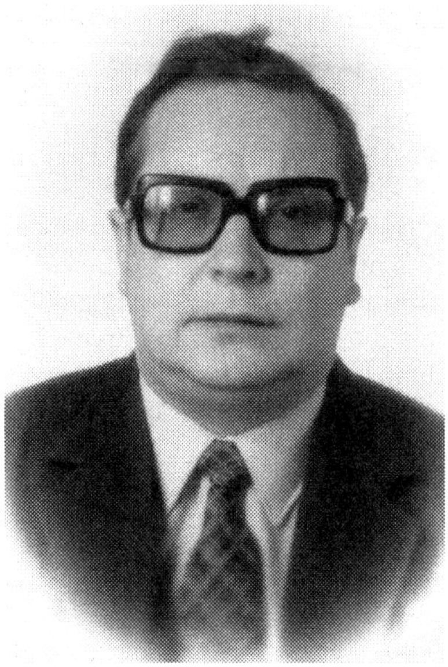

Dr. Yuri Burov was a USSR / USA Cultural Exchange Fellow.

ship can be between people.

Looking back, I find the years I spent in the Department of Pharmacology went very rapidly. They were times of intense learning as well as fun. I had the privilege of working with some unique scientists whose ideas and skills have guided me in my work. Dr. Domino is a great teacher and I am grateful to have had the time to be in his laboratories. I think being an excellent teacher is as important as making some important discoveries, since through teaching ideas are spread everywhere.

I think in the future at the university level, pharmacology still has the challenge to educate the physician about drugs better than it has in the past, and to continue to be the place to try new ideas. It may be worthwhile thinking about the department as becoming a center of excellence in some specific field. These are just my thoughts on things.

Editor's note: Ann Wilson Black worked with me for eleven years. She began as a laboratory technician in the Department from 1966-1972, and then as research assitant after she received her M.S. degree in pharmacology. In 1974 she was a medical technician in my psychopharmacolgy laboratory at the Lafayette Clinic. She then came back to my laboratory in the Department until 1977. She graduated with a B.S. in zoology and chemistry in 1965. After a year in medical school at Wayne State University she decided she would rather pursue a research career. Her initial research with me involved the bioassay of brain acetylcholine in both frog rectus and leech muscle preparations. She ended up using sophisticated gas chromatographic-mass spectrometric (GC-MS) selective ion techniques with our first GC-MS equipment in the laboratory M6414 Medical Science Building I. The GC-MS equiptment filled an entire roon. Bob Austin and Tom Larmee had to install two massive window air conditioners to keep the entire room cool. The water cooling system for the GC-MS required an equally impressive circulating system where the pump would leak periodically. The water would accummulate on the floor and dribble down to the fifth floor office of the Chair of Biochemistry. After several such accidents in which water dripped down on the desk of both Minor Coon and later Jack Dixon, I got to know both of them very well indeed!

In 1977 Ann got an offer from Warner Lambert to work across the Huron River at the former Parke-Davis facility. She started as an associate and soon was promoted to a scientist status in their Department of Pharmacokinetics and Drug Metabolism. She is especially proud of her seminal study on the pharmacokinetics and biotransformation of atorvastatin (Lipitor).

I owe Ann a lot for the many years of excellent work she did with me.

Vignettes: "I Remember When..."

Staff and Students of the 1960s and Beyond

James W. Gibb, Ph.D., 1960-1965

My training in the Department of Pharmacology at the University of Michigan had a major positive impact on my career. I am particularly indebted to the Department for the general broad-based curriculum that was offered during the time I was a graduate student. We were required to take most of the courses required of medical students in the first two years of medical school, which provided an excellent foundation on which to build my pharmacology career. This has, indeed, been a valuable asset as my research interests have developed and diversified.

I was particularly fortunate in having Dr. Theodore M. Brody as my mentor and research advisor. He provided the opportunity to learn state-of-the-art techniques and concepts in the area of biochemical pharmacology. He was a considerate, kind individual who provided the environment to develop scientific skills; he has continuously been a strong advocate of each of us who had the opportunity of working in his laboratory. I forged close friendships and associations at Michigan, particularly as part of a group we call the "Magnificent Seven." There was an esprit de corps that developed during my time as a graduate student at the University of Michigan that persists even to this day.

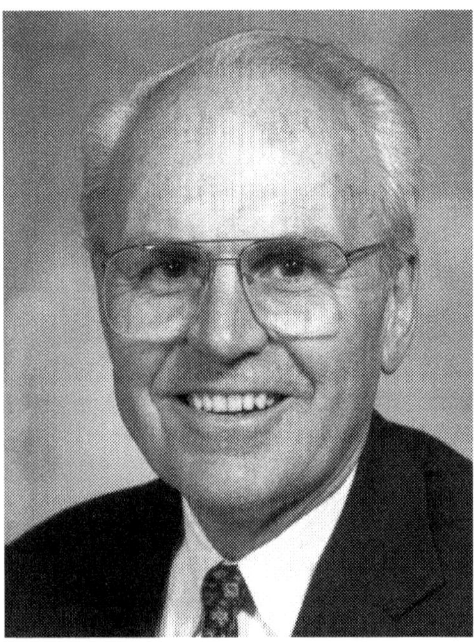

The Pharmacology Department at the University of Michigan has a strong tradition of excellence of which all graduates are proud. I am indebted to faculty, fellow graduate students, postdoctoral students and to the institution for an outstanding education and experience which sets graduate students apart in the academic and scientific community and prepares us well for careers in pharmacology.

Prem N. Saxena, M.D., 1960-1961

Under the Rockefeller Foundation Fellowship, I worked with Dr. Edward F. Domino in the Department of Pharmacology at U of M from January 1960 through January 1961; it was my first visit abroad. I chose to work on electro-pharmacology, with Dr. Seevers' permission. Dr. Domino taught me techniques of unipolar and bipolar stimulation and recording from various brain structures, including isolated cortex preparations.

We found that electrocortical recruiting as well as arousal responses could be obtained, the former by bipolar slow frequency stimulation and the latter by high frequency stimulation of neurons located in the midbrain, thalamus, and caudate. Sedatives like phenobarbital, chlordiazepoxide, thioridazine, etc., enhanced the recruiting response and suppressed the activating response. The two systems— the recruiting and activating— are closely located. Because of the time limit, I

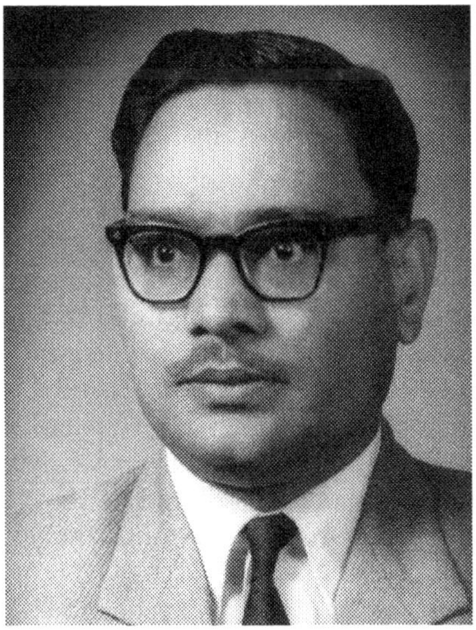

could not finish the work at Michigan and continued it in Lucknow on my return. The work became my Ph.D. thesis and it was then published.

I found the people very sympathetic in Ann Arbor. I was encouraged to learn the techniques of isolated heart-lung preparation under Dr. Swain, limb-perfusion under Dr. Beck, and EEG recording in humans under Dr. Bagchi, in addition to the techniques taught by Dr. Domino, whom I consider my esteemed teacher. I was also able to attend lectures on statistics by Dr. Sakuma and on cardiovascular pharmacology by Dr. Swain.

I maintained correspondence with Dr. Domino for a number of years, periodically requesting reprints of his work. It has been 42 years since my departure from Ann Arbor, and I continue cherishing the memories of my association with Dr. Domino and others of the Department.

Janice Stickney, Ph.D., 1962-1967

I accepted the opportunity to begin the Ph.D. program in the Department during the summer of 1962, immediately following graduation from Oberlin College. Although this was not my plan initially, I think that having the summer to transition from the small liberal arts college environment to that of a large multi-faceted university was a wise beginning for my graduate program. I will always appreciate the decision of the Department faculty to offer me this choice.

There were many aspects of the graduate program that contributed significantly to my scientific and personal growth. Two of the more important were the breadth of scientific exposure (including Department seminars, university seminars, and continuous discussions with fellow students and faculty) and training in the scientific method; and friendships with faculty and students, many of which continue these 30 years later. In fact, for a period of nine years (1972-1981) when I was a faculty member in the Department of Pharmacology and Toxicology at Michigan State University, I had an opportunity to work with several University of Michigan Pharmacology Department alumni, including Ted Brody (MSU chair), Gerry Gebber, and Jay Goodman. I was especially fortunate to have been able to work closely on several occasions with Tai Akera. Tai is very knowledgeable and was always very willing to discuss practically any aspect of cardiac pharmacology and toxicology. He was also a good friend.

In 1989, Ray Ruddon invited me to participate in a panel discussing minorities in science, which was held at the Rackham Auditorium as an activity during Martin Luther King, Jr. Day. Over the years I have been invited by the University of Michigan Pharma-

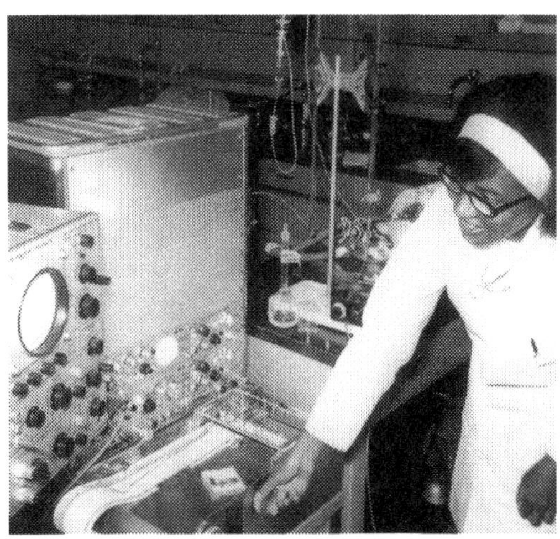

cology Department graduates to give seminars at their respective institutions. Also, at various times, my service on national committees was concurrent with that of other University of Michigan alumni. I continue to keep in touch with many graduates and past fellows of the Department.

John H. McNeill, Ph.D., 1963-1967

I look back very fondly to my years as a graduate student at the University of Michigan. Fixed in my mind are the lifelong friendships that I made plus the excellent training and education along with the deep sense of pride that I have in being a member of such a historical and strong Department. Remembered also is the awe that we held for Maurice Seevers as well as the terror that Skip Bennett, Lloyd Beck, Gerry Deneau, and Ben Lucchesi could instill during the evening graduate courses. My mentor, Ted Brody, certainly had a lot to do with the success of my career, and I owe him a great deal. The excellent lectures presented by Roy Hudson, Hank Swain, Ed Cafruny, Ben Lucchesi, and the rest of the Departmental faculty really impressed me.

Remembered from other departments are: the awesome sight of Horace Davenport striding into a classroom, the patience of David Bohr, Judd Coon playing the piano to make a point during a biochem lecture, the Socratic teaching of Gerry Abrams in pathology and evening "hall hockey" tournaments played with rubber stoppers against Bill Lands and the biochemists on the sixth floor.

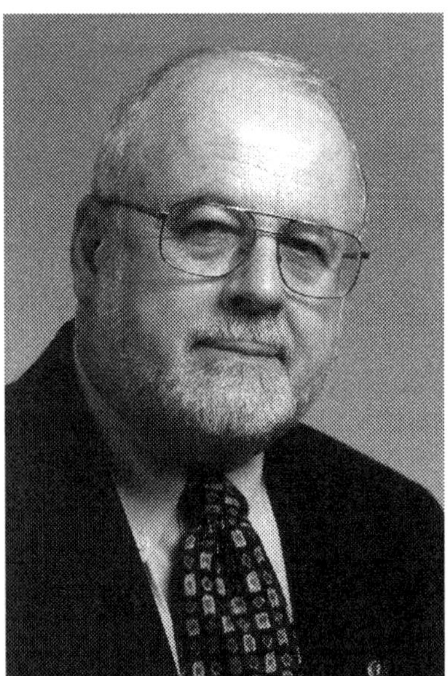

During the '60s there was no greater thrill than packing 10-12 graduate students chaperoned by some unfortunate junior faculty member (e.g., Roy Hudson) into a U of M station wagon and driving to Atlantic City for FASEB. Days were spent in sessions and in walking the boardwalk and (at least some) nights were spent at the infamous Hialeah Club.

Ted's lab at that time had the "Three Canadians," Jack Diamond, Jim Gibb, and me. We had followed in the footsteps of Deane Calvert and Ken Moore from the western prairies of Canada. Our accents were laughed at and we retaliated by putting a sign on the door of the lab stating, "You are now leaving the American sector" in about 12 languages including Finnish, which Gibb happened to speak.

Another fond memory is of Bill Sheldon, who ran the storeroom. Bill seemed to take great delight in taking 20 minutes to select the absolutely worst lab coat from the back of the laundry to give to a graduate student. The secret, we soon found, was to always ask a question about fishing before making a request to Bill. It always put Bill in a good mood and you got a decent lab coat!

George E. Bacon, M.D., 1964-1967

Following my Pediatric Residency, I was taking postgraduate training in Pediatric Endocrinology at the University of Michigan. The clinical experience was excellent, but the laboratory facilities at that time (1964) were limited. The Clinical Pharmacology program, under the leadership of Dr. Ted Carr, offered the research and basic science availability which I felt I needed for a career in academic medicine. I was able to pursue my interest in steroid metabolism and dose-response curves

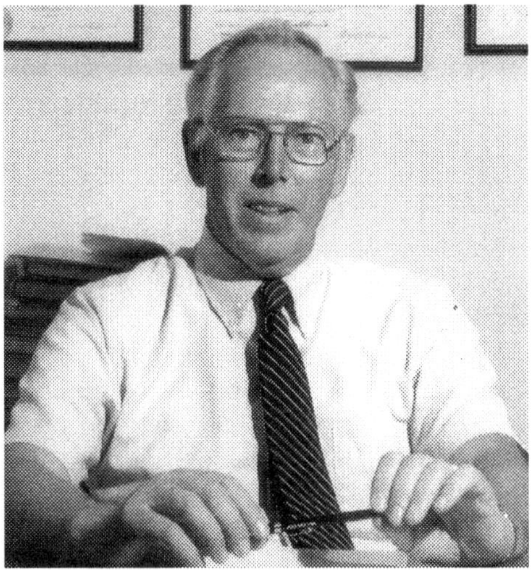

to administered glucocorticoids in particular. A Master's degree in Pharmacology was a nice bonus!

With this background, I was able to have a fulfilling career in pediatrics (which, incidentally, included two "terms" as acting director of the Upjohn Center for Clinical Pharmacology).

Norman Weisbrodt, Ph.D., 1965-1970

For me, the late '60s at Michigan were filled with memorable events, both professional and personal. Quite a few of us rookies began the program in 1965, seven if I remember correctly. It really was great having fellow students like Steve Holtzman, Jay Goodman, Jeff Baron, and others for support as we all got started. I also appreciated being assisted by the more senior students. In particular, I remember Leighton Whitsitt, Jerry Carlson, Jan Stickney, Guy Curtis, Larry Carr, and Mary Kay Wolpert more or less taking me by the hand.

Of course, the faculty members during that time were very supportive. My first contact was with Ben Lucchesi, who with patient explanation and sharp humor gave me my first introduction to the high quality of research being conducted in the Department. Shortly thereafter, Roy Hudson took me into his lab where I first helped Jerry and Mary Kay with their experiments. With their help, I got started on experiments of my own, but

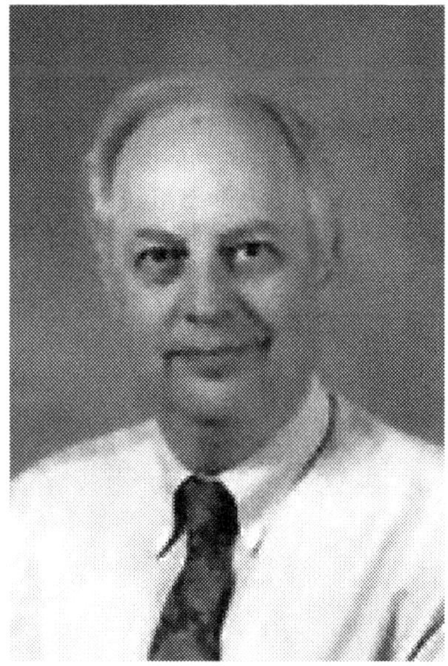

Dr. Hudson left in the very early stages. Fortunately, by that time Paul Bass, Ray Ruddon, Carl Hug, and Jerry Carlson had started some very interesting studies on the effects of nicotine on intestinal motility. I soon was hooked and began my thesis work under the guidance of Drs. Bass and Hug.

During that time, I was fortunate to work with many wonderful people both in the Department and in the very active labs Paul Bass ran at Parke-Davis. I particularly remember Gene Overholt who was a resident in Medicine; Jack Ludwick, a resident in Surgery (whose house I rented while he was in the military); and Jim Wiley, who in addition to taking me fishing a few times, taught me to make gagges. I also was able to seek advice from many knowledgeable people. Although I met with him only a few times during my studies, Dr. Seevers was immensely supportive. Indeed, I think he saved me from certain disaster during my oral preliminary exams. I also recall David Bohr patiently explaining smooth muscle electrophysiology to me. In addition to this personal attention and the constant supervision of my mentors, Drs. Bass and Hug, I also received the benefit of many great teachers. In particular, I remember the lectures, both in the classroom and in the hallways, of Drs. Swain, Beck, Tephly, Lucchesi, and Smith.

During the time I spent at Michigan I also got married, Cathy and I had two children, I played in many softball games, and we saw some great football. Although my work and travels since leaving Ann Arbor have taken me closer to the discipline of physiology, I have always maintained my initial interest in pharmacology. And as it turns out, two years ago our departments here at the University of Texas at Houston were merged so that I once again find myself a card-carrying pharmacologist.

Arthur M. Cohen, Ph.D., 1966-1970

I was a graduate student in the Department from 1966 through 1970, and did my thesis research under the direction of Dr. Raymond W. Ruddon. Although my specific project was concerned with the mechanisms underlying the induction of hepatic drug metabolizing activity by phenobarbital, the strength of the overall program at Michigan provided me with in-depth knowledge and appreciation for all aspects of pharmacology. These included the molecular and physiological properties of the central and autonomic nervous systems as taught by Dr. Ed Domino, Dr. Charles B. Smith, and Dr. Lloyd Beck. I was also fortunate to be a lab assistant for Dr. Ben Lucchessi when the Department was still conducting in vivo cardiovascular demonstrations for the medical students. As has often been said, the best way to learn a subject is to involve yourself in teaching it to others.

Perhaps more than anything else, the rigorous scientific atmosphere in the Department provided me with the tools to become an independent investigator and to properly evaluate the published literature. Having worked with colleagues from a wide spectrum of university backgrounds, I have come to appreciate even more the strength of the program at Michigan. The Department has truly earned its long-standing reputation as a leader in graduate pharmacology education. I am fully confident that it will continue to successfully meet the changes and challenges that face the discipline of pharmacology as we move into the era of genomic biology.

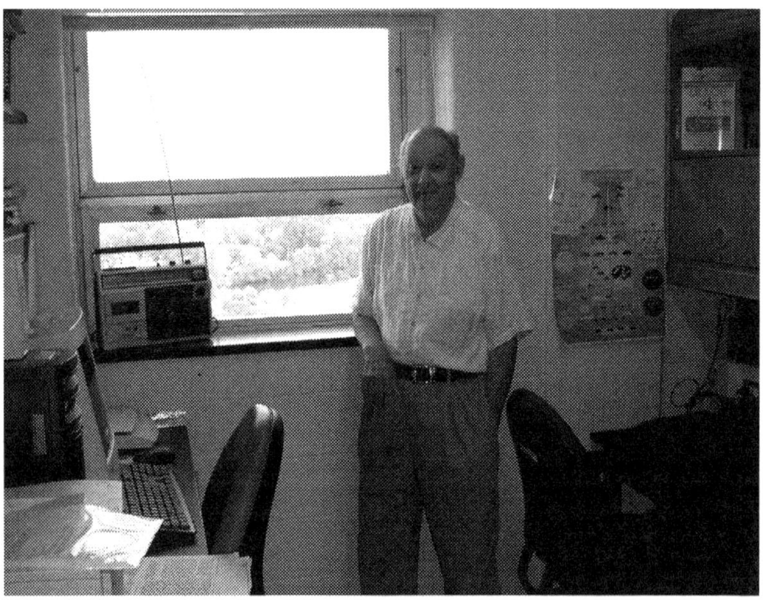

Ed Domino standing in his old lab, M6412-14 in Medical Science Building I, which was previously occupied by Drs. L. Woods, B. Mellett, C. Hug and R. Ruddon. Guess who occupies it today.

1961

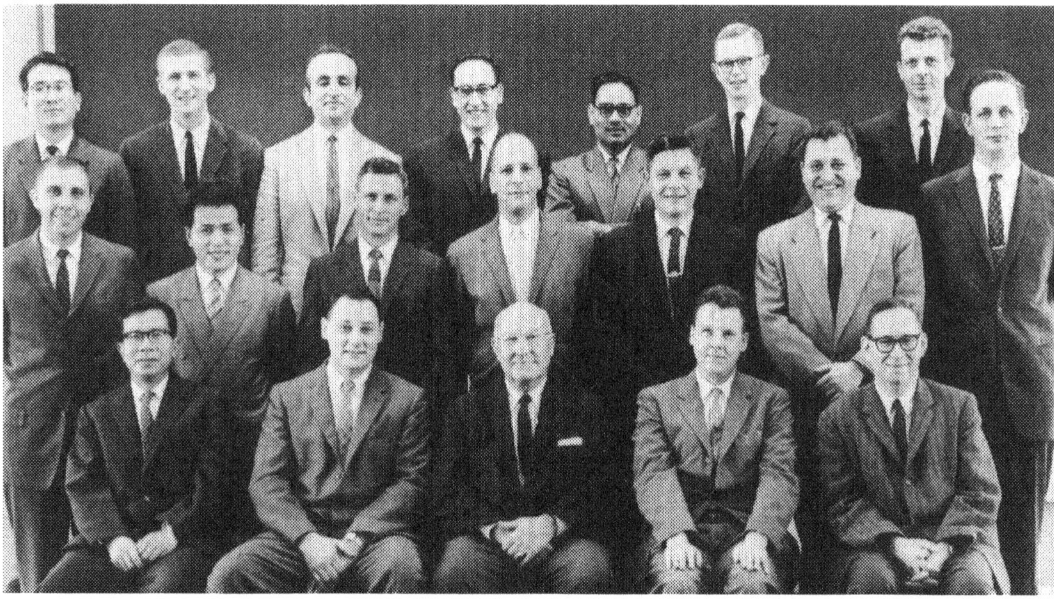

Front row: K. Shimamoto, E. Domino, M. Seevers, E. Carr, T. Brody
Second row: B. Lucchesi, T. Yanagita, L. Beck, E. Cafruny, D. Bennett, L. Mellett, H. Swain
Third row: S. Takaori, R. Renolds, S.O. Kayaalp, J.L. Magana-Garcia, P. N. Saxena, R. Chipps, G. Deneau

1962

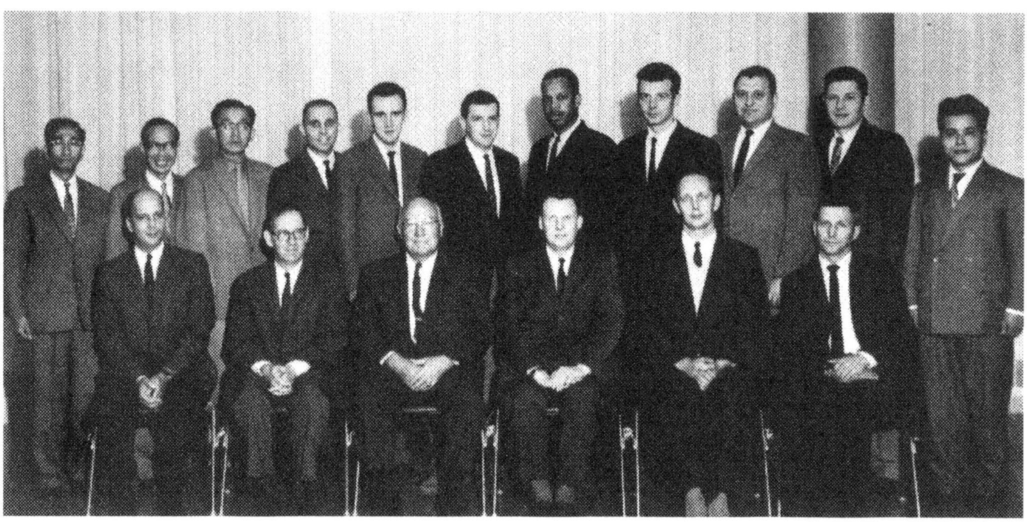

Front row: E. Cafruny, T. Brody, M. Seevers, E. Carr, H. Swain, L. Beck
Second row: S. Hisada, S. Iida, T. Furukawa, B. Lucchesi, J. Villarreal,
M. Segal, R. Hudson, G. Deneau, L. Mellett, D. Bennett, T. Yanagita

1965

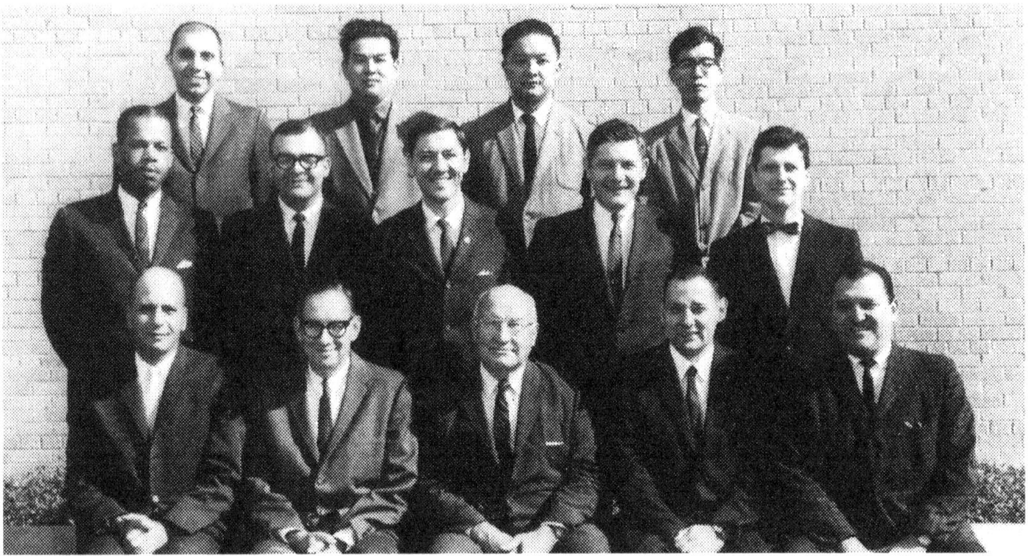

Front row: E. Cafruny, T. Brody, M. Seevers, E.Domino, L. Mellett
Second row: R. Hudson, E. Alpert, C. Schuster, D. Bennett, C. Hug
Third row: B. Lucchesi, K. Yamamoto, S. Matsuoka, N. Katsuda

1966

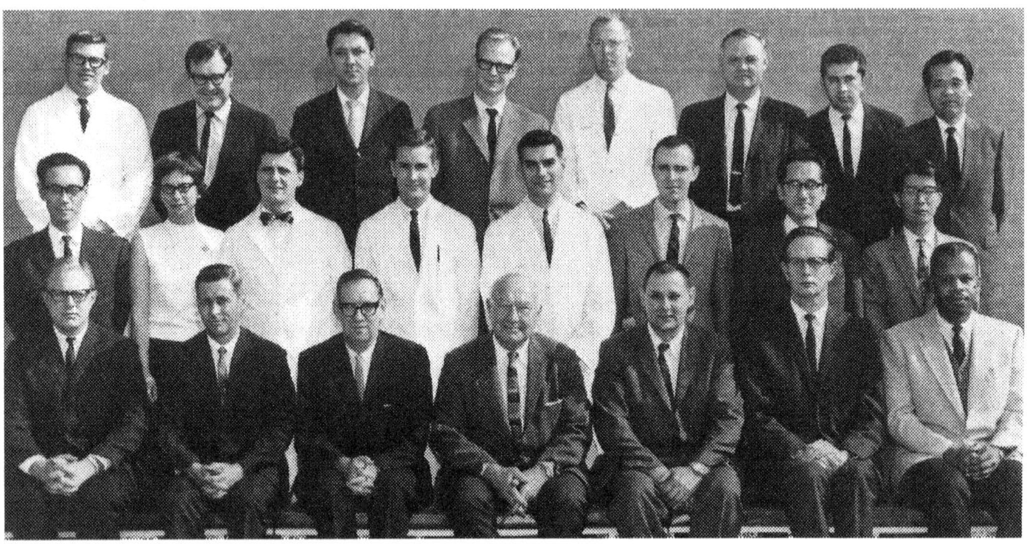

Front row: T. Tephly, L. Beck, T. Brody, M. Seevers, E. Domino, H. Swain, R. Hudson
Second row: S. Tadokoro, P. Stern, C. Hug, M.K. Shellenberger, R. P. Carson, J. Villarreal, H. Itoh, N. Katsuda
Third row: J. Diamond, A. Morrison, C. Schuster, H. Kampffmeyer, G. Bacon, B. Tilton, U. Estrada-Robles, A. Tsujimoto

1967

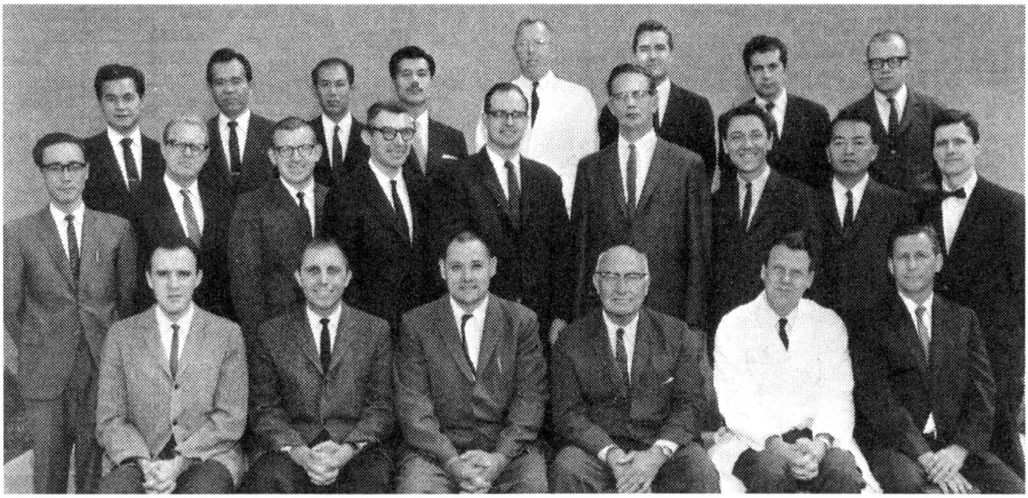

Front row: J.Villarreal, B. Lucchesi, E. Domino, M. Seevers, E. Carr, L. Beck
Second row: S. Tadokoro, T. Tephly, R. Ruddon, W. Baird, C. Smith, H. Swain, C. Schuster, H. Kawamura, C. Hug
Third row: M. Miyasaka, A. Tsujimoto, I. Iwami, Y. Nakai, G. Bacon, M. Shellenberger, U. Estrada, D. VanDyke

1968

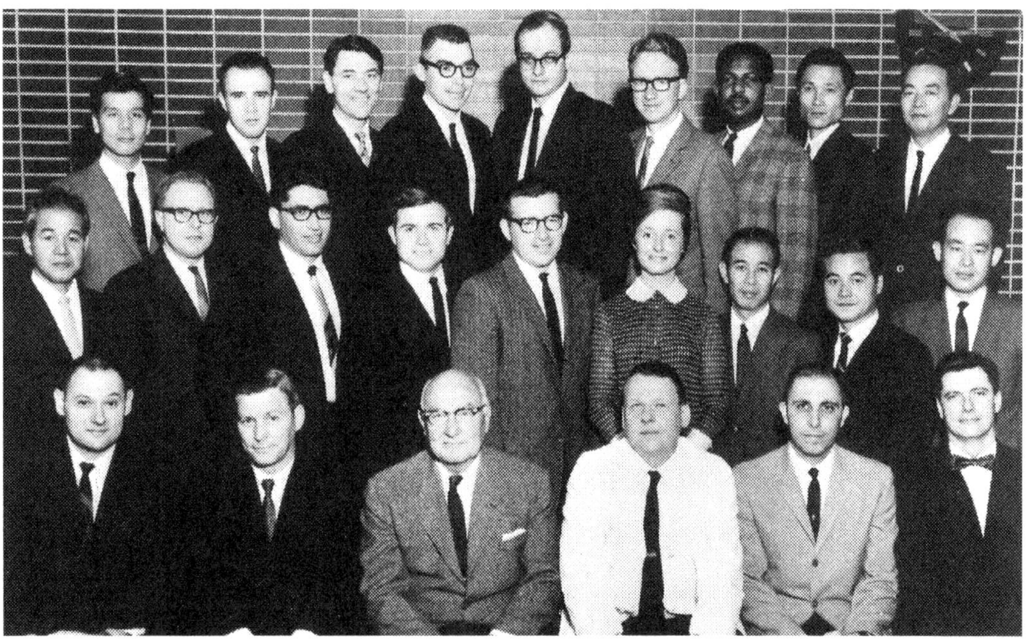

Front row: E. Domino, L. Beck, M. Seevers, E. Carr, B. Lucchesi, C. Hug
Second row: K. Matsusaki, T. Tephly, M. Shaffi, J. Johnson, R. Ruddon, A. Von Baumgarten, T. Iwami, M. Miyasaka, T. Oka
Third row: Y. Nakai, J. Villarreal, C. Schuster,W. Baird, C. Smith, E. Hvidberg, C. Inniss, M. Hitomi, H. Kawamura

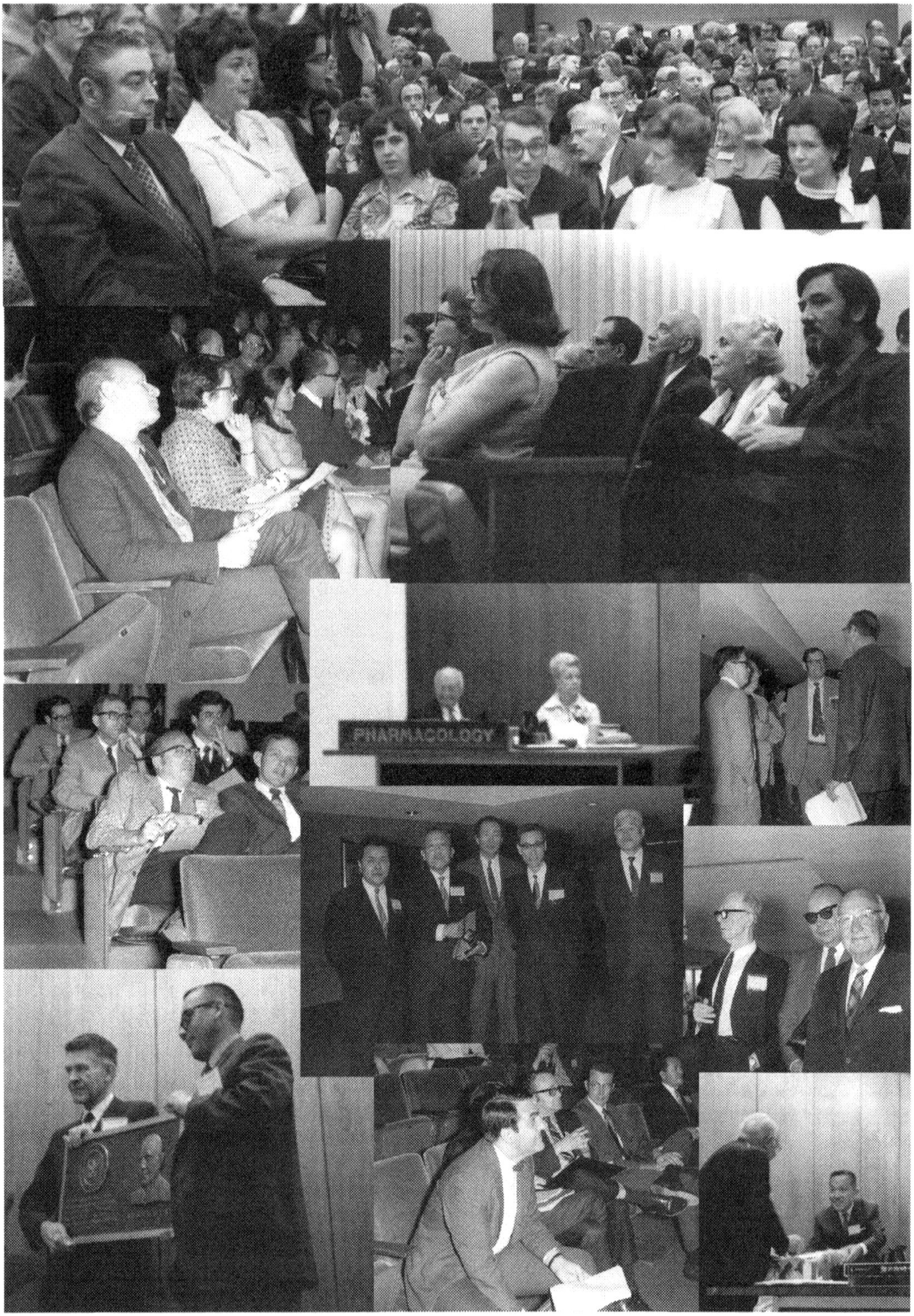
PHARMACOLOGY

18

Memoirs: 1970-71

Alessandro Bartolini, M.D.

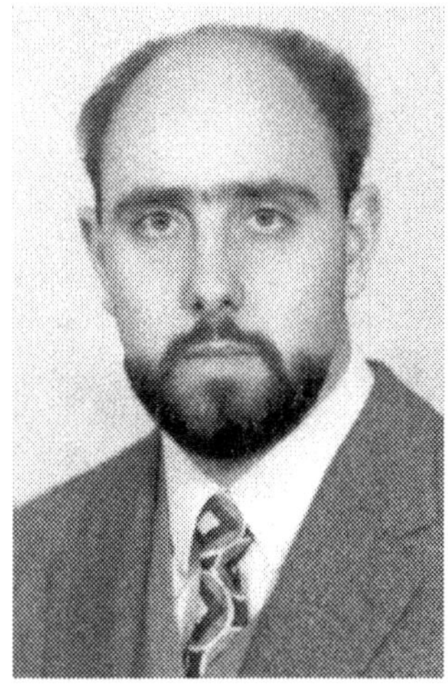

I spent 18 months in the laboratory of Professor Edward F. Domino at the University of Michigan, from January 1970 to July 1971. This period was very pleasant and undoubtedly one of the most useful for my education and university career.

First of all, my stay in Ann Arbor was of fundamental importance in learning how to understand and speak English. I wish to thank Dr. Domino for allowing me to attend the Intensive Course in English at the UM English Language Institute during the first two months.

In the UM Department of Pharmacology, I also learned novel research methods especially useful for studying neuropsychopharmacology. For example, I learned how to inject drugs into rodents intracerebroventricularly, how to dissect specific brain areas, how to collect samples of acetylcholine released by the cat hippocampus, how to induce degeneration of optic nerves in order to detect possible variations of neurotransmitters in both lateral geniculate bodies and superior colliculi, and so on. My way of thinking about research approaches was greatly influenced not only by Dr. Domino, my "American mentor," but also by other learned collaborators such as Hiroshi Kawamura, Ann Wilson, Margaret Mohrman, Gaston Labrecque, Michael Newman, Michael Antonaccio, Larry Weisenthal, and many others I had the opportunity to meet during my stay in Ann Arbor.

On my return from the University of Michigan I continued, at the University of Florence, research concerning the physiopharmacology of the central cholinergic system. Thus, together with my collaborators, I found interesting correlations between cholinergic and antinociceptive systems.

Certainly the time that I spent in Ann Arbor had a strong impact not only on me from a scientific point of view, but also on my family. We had the opportunity to visit some very fine places in the USA and to make friends with many lovely people. Among these I would like to mention Ernestina and Giuseppe Parravano (a Professor of Chemistry at UM) and Dorin and Robert Smith (a clinical pharmacologist at the Glaxo Pharmaceutical Company). My wife, Lia, and daughters, Olga, Paola and Valentina, and I have very fond memories of Ann Arbor and America, and all of us are extremely grateful to Dr. Domino and to the University of Michigan for the fantastic opportunity offered us. Lina, who was born in Florence after our return to Italy, is very sorry to have missed the opportunity. However, Lina, now a medical doctor, hopes to visit the University of Michigan as soon as she obtains her Radiology Specialization from the University of Florence.

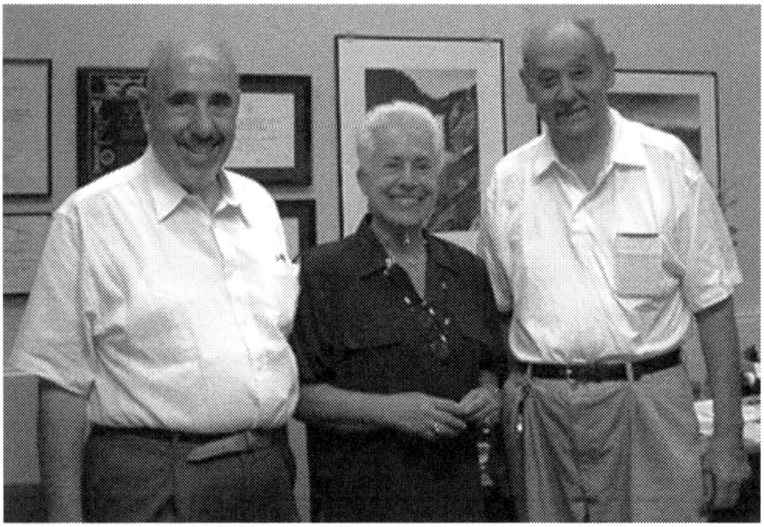

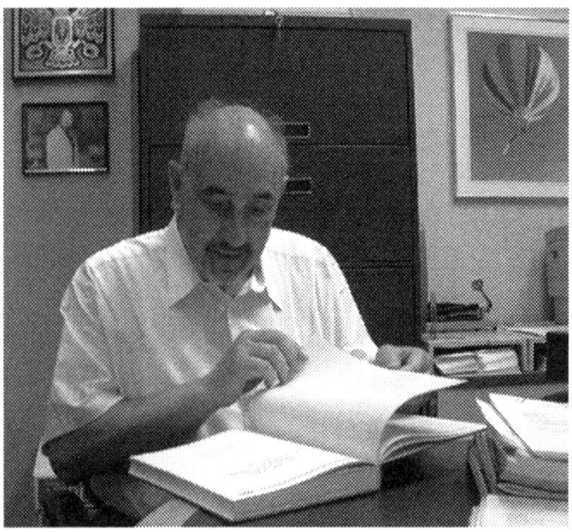

Above: Dr. and Mrs. Bartolini stopped in to the Department of Pharmacology in 2002 to visit Ed Domino.

Left: Dr. Bartolini

Below left: During their visit they met Marta, in Dr. Lucchesi's lab, who returned to Italy in late 2002.

Below right: Valentina Bartolini plays on the grass near Medical Science I.

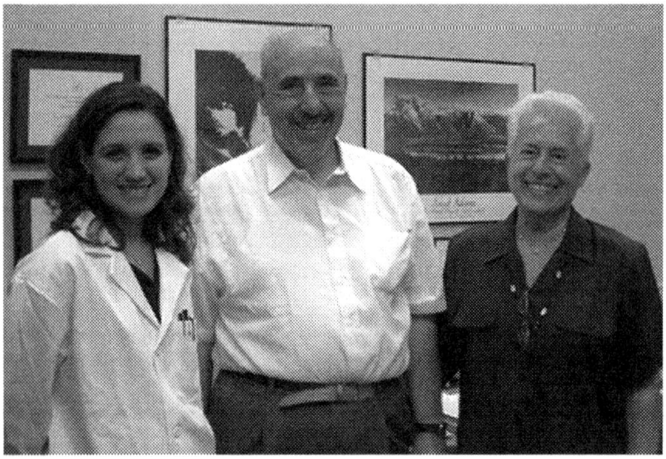

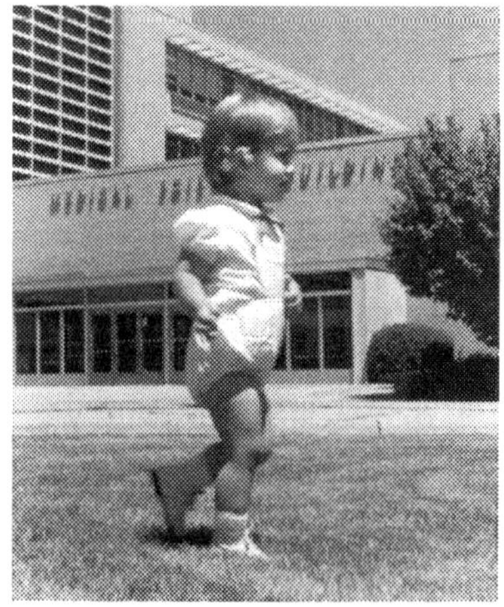

A Brief Reflection on My Years as a Graduate Student, 1970-1974

Richard E. Tessel, Ph.D.

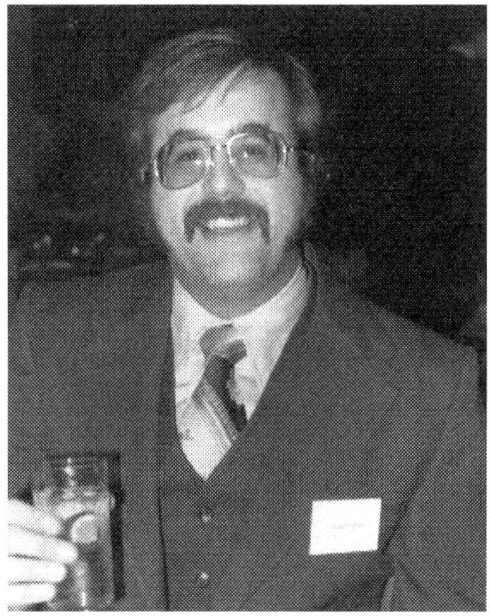

My story in the Department of Pharmacology at the University of Michigan began in 1970. The previous year, I had graduated with a master's degree in Experimental Psychology from the Department of Psychology at the University of Illinois at Chicago Circle (as it was then called), moved to Los Angeles with my wife, Pat, and our daughter Lauren, and found a job at Longview State Hospital for the Mentally Retarded. However, that same year I lost the job because the then-governor of California, Ronald Reagan, decided that such hospital facilities were not really necessary.

I somehow heard that a training program in psychopharmacology existed at the Department of Pharmacology at U of M, and Ed Domino was the contact person. I wrote to Ed and was informed that the training program had lost its funding, but he asked if I would like to become a graduate student in the Department. Having published a few papers involving the effects of drugs on behavior, I decided that, yes, it would probably be good for me to understand more about drugs, and getting a Ph.D. had always been one of my dreams.

I formally applied to the Department and was subsequently told that my acceptance in to the pharmacology program depended upon the acquiescence of a Dr. (C.B.)"Tad" Smith. I probably made Tad's life less than pleasant because I called him repeatedly, begging him to "please!!!" accept me. Unbeknownst to me, even though I eventually learned that Tad had done behavioral work at Harvard with some of the most important people in behavioral pharmacology. He was less than excited to have some unknown psychologist join the Department. Nevertheless, I was accepted and began life in the Department as a rotating NIH predoctoral student in the laboratory of (my nemesis?) Dr. Smith. At the same time, a young woman named Peggie Hollingsworth also joined Dr. Smith's lab as a new graduate student. However, unlike me, Peggie had been at the University working as an electron microscopist, and had heard a great deal about the intimidating Dr. Smith. One episode in the lab underlines her feelings about Dr. Smith at the time. Peggie was sitting at the lab's hood doing something with glassware when Dr. Smith, in a relatively mild voice, said "Peggie." Glassware went flying and she fell over backwards off her seat. Aghast, Dr. Smith said "Peggie, get a hold of yourself." Despite this, Peggie eventually decided that Tad really wasn't so bad and married him.

When my rotation in Tad's lab was over, I contacted Dr. Benedict Lucchesi and asked if I could do a rotation in his lab. At that time, Ben sported a crew cut and always wore a white shirt and a tie. In addition, I was admonished by him that in *his* lab, male students were required to also wear ties. However, I'd forgotten this requirement, and attempted to gain entrance to his lab without a tie. Of course, I was refused entrance and I went down to Dr. Carl Hug's lab to complain about this antediluvian requirement. He said, not to worry, and made a bow tie for me out of paper toweling spotted with black Magic Marker dots. I then nonchalantly returned to Ben; he took a second or two to inspect the tie but did allow me into the lab that day.

As I remember it, I enjoyed working with Ben until he thought that I was taking much too long to catheterize a dog's coronary and yanked the surgical instruments from me. I think that that was when Ben decided that cardiovascular pharmacology was not for me. I then entered Dr. James H. Woods' lab. After much hard work, frequent scientific discussions with Jim, John Carney (who helped me with the many electromechanical operant programming problems I seemed to always be having), Gail Winger, and others whose names currently escape me (I apologize!) and occasional gatherings at Howard Johnson's for all-you-can-eat fried fish-eating competitions (the winner received a free dessert), I earned my Ph.D. with Jim. Working with Jim and seeing how he handled research led me to believe that I also had the capacity to do science.

During my rotation with Jim, I talked to Tad about the possibility of comparing the atrial rate effects of cocaine and a quaternary of cocaine, cocaine methiodide, in his lab. He acquiesced, and with his explanations of mechanism, we got a nice paper out. In addition, with regard to Tad, early in my career at Michigan, Tad taught a section of the Experimental Pharmacology course we were required to take. Tad gave us an open-ended question about receptor theory to report on based on our own library research. This terrified me, but thanks to the support of other students, I was able to calm down enough to think. Anyway, I got the best grade of my career at Michigan from Tad, for which I continue to be very appreciative.

Lastly, I really appreciated Dr. Julian Villarreal because he asked the first question of me during my doctoral orals, a question he had gotten me to think about previously, in order to increase my confidence. I think I answered his question well enough but the orals seemed to go from bad to worse after that.

Looking back over the past quarter century since my graduating from the Department, I have many fond memories of the faculty and students of that long-ago time. These included Ed Domino's ever-present briefcase containing urine specimen cups for human research he was involved in, as well as the ASPET and FASEB meetings in Atlantic City I was encouraged to attend as a student. Perhaps more importantly, at Michigan, I learned what it meant to be a pharmacologist, a condition for which I have always been grateful.

Editor's note: Richard E. Tessel obtained his Ph.D. at the University of Michigan under the mentorship of Dr. James H. Woods. His primary research theme here at Michigan was the relationships between the structure and the locomotor stimulant and reinforcing actions of several fenfluramine analogs. From 1974-1975, he was Postdoctoral Fellow of the Department of Pharmacology at the University of Colorado School of Medicine. In 1975, he went to University of Kansas to become Assistant Professor, Associate Professor and then Professor in the Departments of Pharmacology and Toxicology.

He is a member of the American Society for Pharmacology and Experimental Therapeutics, American Association for the Advancement of Science, Behavioral Pharmacology Society and the American Society for Neuroscience. From 1981-1999 he was a member of the Memorial Advisory Board for the Journal of Pharmacology and Experimental Therapeutics. In 1999, he became a member of the Editorial Board of Experimental and Clinical Psychopharmacology.

His main area of interest is operant behavior and mechanism of recovery from brain damage.

UM Pharmacology in the Mid-1970s

Fulton T. Crews, Ph.D.

The UM Department of Pharmacology was a fantastic dynamic forum of scholarship for a broad range of pharmacology in the mid-1970s. Neuropharmacology remained a strength through the efforts of Drs. Jim Woods, Tad Smith and Ed Domino continuing the strong tradition that Moe Seevers had started long before. This faculty provided critical thinking from molecular to behavioral studies on Neuropharmacology as well as bridging between warm and fuzzy friendship and overly strict paternal guidance. New faculty neuropharmacologists who seemed almost peers to the graduate students and postdocs were Drs. Peggy Gnegy and Ron Holz, who further strengthened the advice and insight faculty could provide to students. Great discoveries were being made to understand the adaptive mechanisms by which drugs modified the brain and behavior. Pharmacogenetics was a major theme due to the arrival of Drs. Burt La Du, Wendell Weber and Vincent Zannoni. They were student-friendly faculty emphasizing the importance of genetics and unique drug response to medicine long before molecular biology made sequencing the genome a goal. Ben Lucchesi was always popular for his cutting edge cardiovascular studies and his entertaining way of pressuring students to work hard. The Department had a great sense of success and history. Cancer and cellular pharmacology included Drs. Ray Ruddon and Bill Pratt who spearheaded advances in cellular and molecular techniques, leading the Department into the emphasis on molecular pharmacology that was in the near future. All the graduate students knew and understood that as students from the first Department of Pharmacology in the United States we were expected to carry a tradition of excellence throughout our careers and exceed our own expectations.

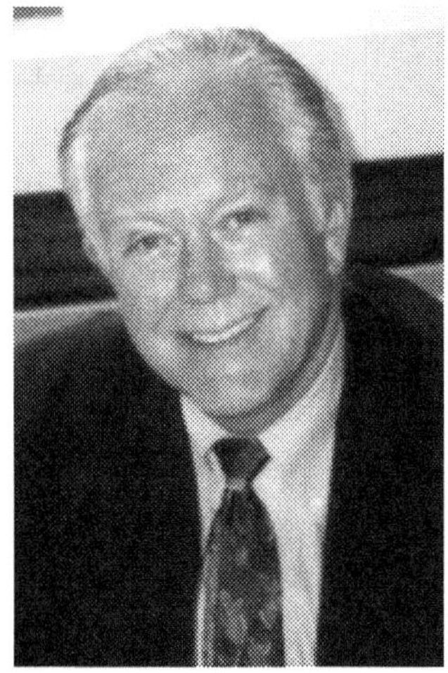

The environment was great in the 1970s. Most students and faculty interacted as a community. Me, John Lazo, Mike Vasko, Lindsey Hough, Bill Pratt, Ray Ruddon, and others regularly played competitive weekend basketball and football games. Bill Pratt regularly lost control to the great entertainment of the students and one year Ray Ruddon broke his achilles tendon causing much concern and taking him out for a season. These sporting-social events bonded faculty and students in wonderful ways.

Dr. Hank Swain always had some type of pharmacology history social. Drs. La Du and Weber would open their houses and orchid displays with lots of free food for socials. Dr. Lucchesi always provided an excellent Italian buffet when host. As scientists we all have scattered across the world, but those I have kept in touch with have grown great success from their foundations at UM and remain appreciative of the tradition of UM Pharmacology we shared and to which we now contribute.

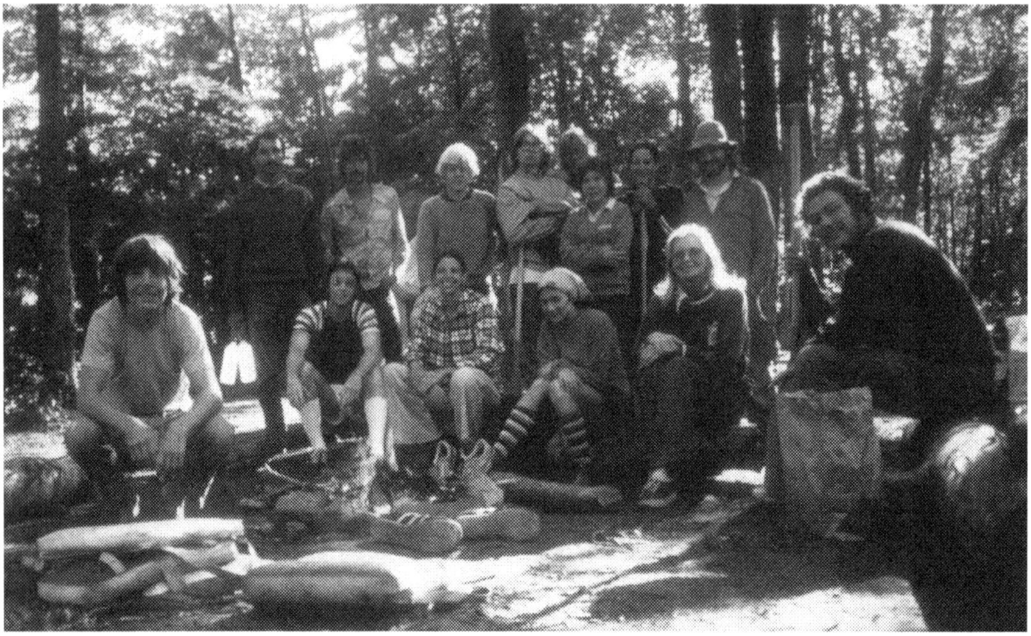

Pharmacology Canoe Trip, 1976. Front row: David Crews, Jeff Milliken, Barbara Waszczak, Rita Valentino, Virginia Crews, Fulton Crews. Back row: Arthur Ensroth, George of Jim Woods lab, Darryl Russ, Timothy Geary, Ellen Sheets, Irene Glowinski and Kenneth Ensroth

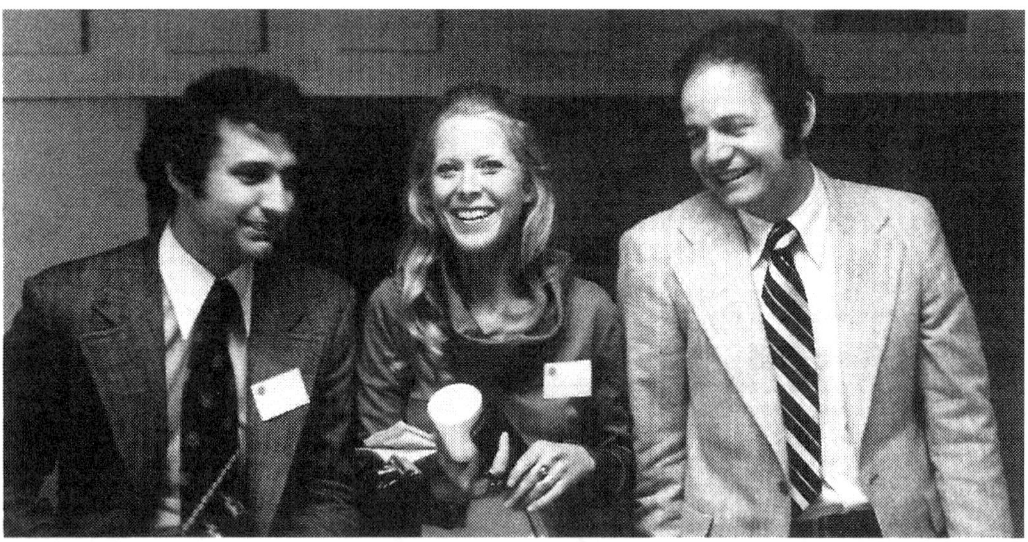

Lindsey Hough, Germaine J. Gwynn, and Mike Vasko in 1975; they all received their Ph.D.s working in Ed Domino's Lab.

Memoirs: 1974-1990

Oksana Lockridge, Ph.D.

I spent a total of 20 years at the University of Michigan Medical School before moving to the University of Nebraska Medical Center in 1990 where I am a full professor. Before joining the Pharmacology Department at the University of Michigan, I was in the Biochemistry Department for two years as a postdoc with Vincent Massey, and then in the Human Genetics Department for two years as a postdoc with Arthur Bloom.

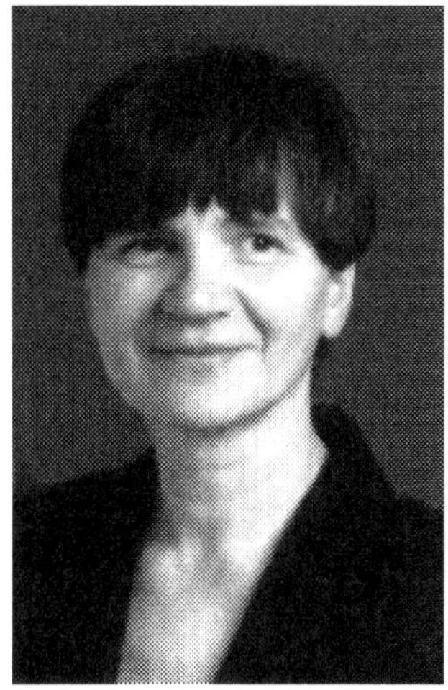

When Bert La Du was hired in 1974 as the new chairman of the Department of Pharmacology, he recruited me to join his laboratory. When Bert first arrived to assume his post as chairman he was invisible for several months because he was hospitalized with a detached retina. This period of unsupervised time allowed me to develop my research goals for serum butyrylcholinesterase. I decided to purify the enzyme and to titrate the number of active sites, using techniques I had learned in Vincent Massey's biochemistry laboratory.

In 1974 there was no simple purification method for serum cholinesterase. Once I had purified the enzyme by electroelution on a huge polyacrylamide gel, I started searching for a simpler procedure. Affinity chromatography was appealing. I made several affinity columns using different ligands, and, with the help of a pharmacy student named Karen Mesch, finally hit on one that is used worldwide today. The procainamide-sepharose 4B affinity column is extremely useful for purifying butyrylcholinesterase from human serum, as well as recombinant butyrylcholinesterase expressed by mammalian cells and acetylcholinesterase from fetal calf serum. This affinity matrix has become so useful that other people now make it in large quantities and I buy it from them rather than making it myself.

One of my favorite memories of the affinity column concerns the first time I tested it. I am not the cautious type and therefore loaded all of my partially purified enzyme on the column to see if it would stick and if I could elute it. Bert knew what I was doing but, though he was a little worried that I might lose the precious enzyme sample, he did not interfere. Bert liked to encourage people to take the initiative, so he stood back and let me commit all of my sample. He did say, however, that if it worked he would take us out to dinner. It worked beautifully. I expected a dinner in Ann Arbor, but Bert lavished us with a dinner in a place 3,000 miles away. We went to a meeting of the International Society of Human Genetics in Mexico City where Bert took me, Rita Valentino, and Harry Eckerson to dinner.

Having a method that allowed me to purify butyrylcholinesterase from large volumes of human serum led me to my next big project, the sequencing of the protein. I was lucky that in 1982 the Biochemistry Department had George Tarr working on sequencing cytochrome P450 for Jud Coon. George Tarr had developed methods for the manual sequencing of small quantities of peptides. I learned those techniques from him and from

Shawn Black, a graduate student with Dr. Coon. I needed only to buy a pump, a Speed-Vac, and a heating block to do the Edman degradation. I already had an HPLC for purifying the peptides and I purchased a second HPLC for analyzing the phenylthiohydantoin derivatized amino acids. I manually sequenced 1400 peptides and finished the entire sequence of 574 amino acids in three years. I am proud of this work because it was a big project and the sequence I published was correct down to the last amino acid. When I started the sequencing of this protein, no amino acid sequence for any cholinesterase from any organism was known. Knowledge of the sequence was important because it showed that the cholinesterases belonged to a new class of serine esterases.

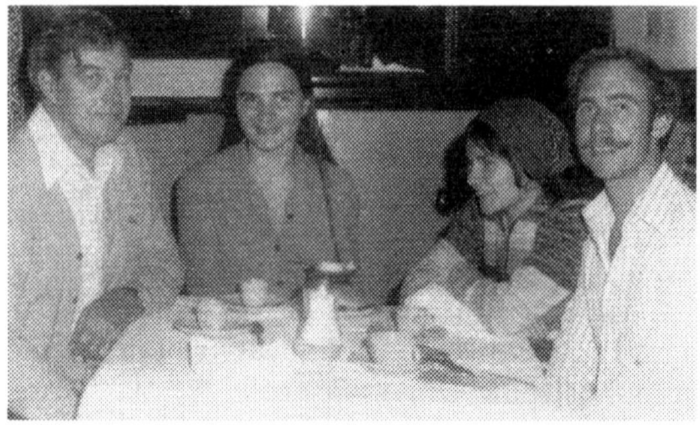

Bert LaDu, Oksana Lockridge, Rita Valentino, and Harry Eckerson share a dinner in Mexico City, Mexico while attending the International Society of Human Genetics Meeting.

The molecular biology revolution came along while I was manually sequencing peptides. It was clear that the amino acid sequences I was generating were useful for making probes for searching for the cDNA. After a lab meeting where I presented my amino acid sequences I went home and decided that I wanted to try looking for the cDNA. I planned to speak to Bert about it in the morning. When we got together the next day we found that we had been thinking the exact same thing and that we were in agreement about looking for the cDNA. We knew nothing about DNA in 1983. None of the people in the Pharmacology Department knew anything about DNA either. Up until that day we had been strictly protein chemists and enzymologists. Yet with a sense that this was the right direction for us and that it was a lot of fun we decided to jump into this new field. Our success in this new endeavor made me always unafraid to try radically new things, and has shaped my philosophy that I can use whatever techniques I need to answer a question. It does not matter whether or not I am an expert in a particular method; I can either figure out how to do it, or I can find someone willing to collaborate and do it for me.

We made some big blunders when we first got into the DNA business in 1983. I can laugh about them now because, despite our naivete, we achieved our goals. At that time a 17mer oligonucleotide cost $2,000. Bert and I designed and ordered a probe, using the genetic code we found in a biochemistry textbook. When the oligonucleotide was delivered to us, the paperwork that came with it showed thymidine where we had requested uracil. We were upset by this change, and Bert called to find out why the company had made the change. In this way we relearned a lesson from biochemistry: DNA uses T but RNA uses U nucleotides. Boldly Bert asked the company to make us a second probe for free, since they should have consulted with us before changing the nucleotides. The company did provide us with a second oligo for free, and, with two oligonucleotide probes in hand, we set about to screen a liver cDNA library. A competition started in the lab as to which project would succeed first: would the protein sequence get finished first or would we find the cDNA clone first? I was working on both projects. I set up the DNA sequencing that allowed us to check for positive clones. The lab searched for the cDNA clone for four years; the peptide sequence was completed in three years. Close to 30 people helped us with screening for the cDNA. Cheng Gao (now on the faculty at Indiana University) was an undergraduate student who introduced us to many DNA techniques. Antje Klem (now at Hoffmann La Roche in Basel) was beautiful, hardworking, and bright. She screened lambda phage libraries and exposed the filters overnight in cassettes to x-ray film. She would arrive at work at 9 a.m., one hour after Bert. Bert was so eager to know whether a positive clone was in a new set that he simply could not wait that hour. Instead, he learned to develop film himself. Theresa Vaughan (now an anthropologist in Oklahoma) and Arnaud Chatonnet (now a scientist in Montpellier, France) were part of the screening team. But the king of them all was Steve Adkins. He was the one who found the cDNA clone for butyrylcholinesterase.

The lab was in a fever to find the clone. Six to eight people were screening at all times. When I heard that there was a brain cDNA library in Cleveland in Terry Rosenberry's laboratory that might have the clone we wanted, I got permission from Terry to screen the library. At the time, Terry was in Paris on sabbatical so it took a while to get permission; those were, after all, the days before e-mail. As soon as we had permission, Matt Kott and Theresa Vaughan volunteered to make the 12 hour round trip drive to Cleveland to pick up the library. Steve Adkins set up agar plates so he could plate the new library the moment it arrived in Ann Arbor. Matt and Theresa arrived back in the lab late on a Monday evening in August. Steve was waiting; he plated the library that night. He made four sets of filters, hybridized with four different probes, and by Friday he knew he had it. One clone was positive with all four oligonucleotide probes. The joy in the lab was intense; after four years of searching we had a clone of human butyrylcholinesterase.

Though in our hearts we knew we had the clone we still had to prove it. Steve plaque-purified the lambda phage clone and subcloned it in preparation for DNA sequencing. We manually sequenced a number of the subclones and exposed the films overnight. In the lab, we set up bets as to how many of the subclones were butyrylcholinesterase, and the range of bets reflected a variety of optimistic and pessimistic personalities. It turned out that all six clones represented butyrylcholinesterase.

With these achievements we were finally in a position to fulfill Bert's lifelong goal: find an answer to the question, what is the basis for the atypical variant of butyrylcholinesterase? It was known that this was a genetic variant and that people who had the mutated enzyme were unable to breathe for two hours after they received a dose of succinylcholine that was intended to paralyze their muscles for only three to five minutes. Bert had saved all blood samples that had come into his lab for phenotype analysis. His 30-year collection included large pedigrees and every type of variant known. Bert contacted the physicians who had sent him the original samples to ask if they could get fresh samples, and Dr. Harold Lightstone in Pennsylvania visited patients in their homes to get the blood we needed. Another lucky break was that Mary McGuire wanted to work for a year before starting medical school. She was assigned the project of looking for the mutation in atypical butyrylcholinesterase and she succeeded. The method Mary used was the polymerase chain reaction. This was a new method in 1987-88. It came along at just the right time, when we most needed it. Mary found that the negatively-charged aspartic acid 70 was glycine in all persons who had the atypical phenotype.

Bert had achieved his lifelong goal and, despite pressure from the department to retire, was totally uninclined to give up research at such an exciting time. It was too much fun and everything was working. Bert remembered that, during his time as chairman, it was

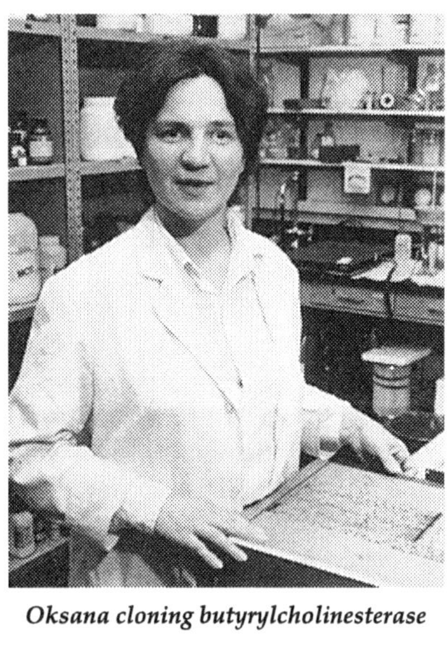

Oksana cloning butyrylcholinesterase

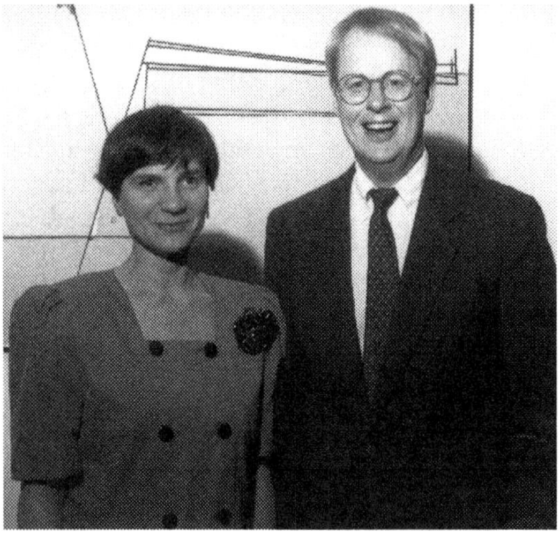

Oksana Lockridge in 1989 upon receiving the University Research Scientist Award from the President of the University of Michigan.

difficult to get people to give up lab space. He wanted to cooperate even though he and I together had huge amounts of grant money, and therefore needed lab space. The compromise he decided on was to retire officially but to take the title of emeritus professor. In 1990, Bert moved his laboratory to the anesthesiology department so pharmacology could assign his space to a young rising faculty member, Rick Neubig. That year, I moved to the University of Nebraska Medical Center in Omaha. I made the move with Ray Ruddon who was hired as Director of the Eppley Institute. In Nebraska, I have continued working on the cholinesterases. My proudest achievement since leaving Michigan is the making of the acetylcholinesterase knockout mouse. To our great surprise a mouse can live, breathe and move without acetylcholinesterase. Another surprise is that the mouse is very sensitive to the toxic effects of organophosphorus agents, even though the target of these poisons, acetylcholinesterase, is absent.

I loved living in Ann Arbor and I loved the University of Michigan. It was wonderful to be able to find expertise in new techniques and new areas of research just down the hall from me. I could usually borrow any equipment or any reagent I needed. The intellectual environment was great. People worked late into the night because they loved what they were doing. I remember Ben Lucchesi showing me Current Contents on a computer disk, which was still a novelty in the late '80s. Ben appreciated the power of the personal computer several years before the rest of us caught on. I also remember Ed Domino talking about his experiment to treat Alzheimer's disease with peanut butter. The idea was to increase the dietary intake of choline because Alzheimer's disease is characterized by a deficit of cholinergic neurons. A dietary increase of choline was intended to increase the amount of the cholinergic neurotransmitter acetylcholine. Ed Domino gave memorable talks. Another one that has stuck with me through the years is one in which he talked about the effects of phencyclidine. He mimed the feelings of limblessness, and emphasized that the hallucinogenic effects could recur days or weeks after a single dose.

Wendell Weber and Bert La Du were on a program project, so the two labs interacted together to discover the basis for individual differences in response to drugs. Wendell worked on N-acetyltransferase. His graduate student Karen Martell was the first person in his lab to find the NAT gene. We showed her how to use the polymerase chain reaction and she found the NAT gene on her first try. She was lucky because NAT contains no introns. Another person whom I remember fondly from the Pharmacology Department is Vincent Zannoni. He was a charming man who collected art and had a beautiful apartment. He designed and hand-made beautiful rugs at home. The patterns were often copies of famous paintings. Vincent Zannoni was also editor of Drug Metabolism and Disposition. He took a personal interest in the careers of his graduate students and helped them to achieve their goals. Peggy Gnegy was the only female faculty member of the Pharmacology Department during my time there. Peggy Gnegy, Wendell Weber, and Vincent Zannoni were all hired by Bert La Du, while he was Department chairman, between 1974 and 1979.

Memoirs: 1974 and Beyond

Wendell Weber, M.D., Ph.D.

I joined the Pharmacology faculty at the University of Michigan in the Spring of 1974, but the events that led there began at least a dozen years before that.

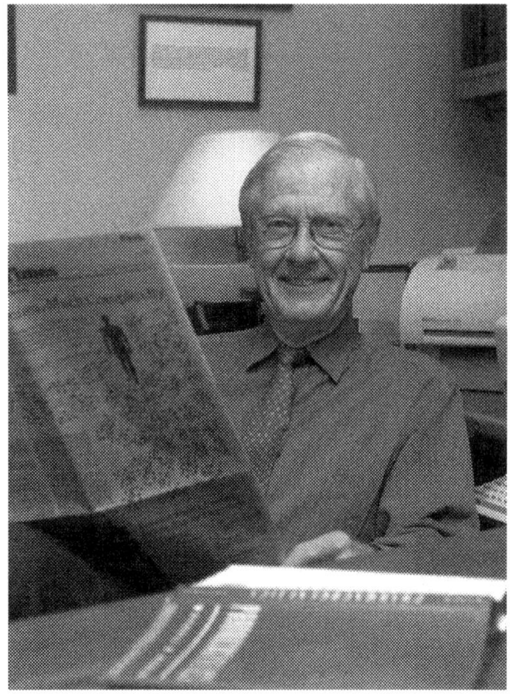

The Trek to Ann Arbor

After completing an internship and a pediatric residency at UCSF Moffitt Hospital/ San Francisco General Hospital in 1962, I spent the next year doing research and studying human genetics at the Galton Laboratory, University College, London, England, with Lionel Penrose as a Special fellow of the NIH. At University College, I shared a laboratory with Bert La Du on sabbatical from the NIH, and chanced to read Werner Kalow's book just published on pharmacogenetics. During that year, Bert was invited to the chair of the Department of Pharmacology at New York University Medical School where I joined him in 1963, continuing in his laboratory as a NIH Special Fellow. In 1965, I joined the pharmacology faculty at New York University. When La Du decided to leave for the University of Michigan in 1974, I joined him in Pharmacology there.

In 1961, while a pediatrician-in-training at San Francisco General Hospital, I encountered a patient — a 6 year-old African-American boy — with jaundice. He was admitted with a tentative diagnosis of hepatitis, but he appeared to be in good health with no signs of liver disease. I was aware by then that persons sometimes respond differently to drugs because of variations in their genes, especially among different ethnic groups. Tests revealed that the boy's jaundice was triggered by a reaction to an antibiotic he had taken. It turned out he was missing an enzyme that protects red blood cells from the drug, so his cells broke down converting the hemoglobin to bilirubin which caused the jaundice in his eyes. This experience combined with reading Kalow's book and my association with Bert La Du led me to a research and teaching career in pharmacogenetics — a nascent field concerned with the connection between drug effects and genes.

One of the first pharmacogenetic traits to be discovered involves acetylation, a process by which natural chemicals help the body excrete drugs and other chemicals to which people are exposed. From Kalow's book I first learned about this trait and that little was known about its cause. In the 1950s, dye factory workers in Germany who manufactured aniline dyes developed bladder cancer. At the same time, some patients who took the new anti-tuberculosis drugs, isoniazid, complained of numbness and tingling in their fingers and toes. Researchers showed that both groups had problems with acetylation. Affected persons were "slow acetylators." The dye factory workers could not convert the dye chemicals fast enough so the dyes became cancerous in their urine. In the tuberculosis patients, the problem was compounded because the isoniazid bound to vitamin B6 flushing it from their bodies and causing them to become B6 deficient, which further lead to the numbness and tingling in their extremities.

Genetic studies in tuberculosis patients in North America and Japan established the heritable nature of "slow acetylation," suggesting that a genetic polymorphism in isoniazid acetylation was responsible, but little else was known about the origin of the trait. When the opportunity arose at NYU in the 1960s to search for its cause, I jumped at it. Two other pharmacogenetic traits —"glucose-6-phosphate dehydrogenase (G6PD) deficiency" and "succinylcholine sensitivity" — were under investigation, but they both could be studied in peripheral blood. The hereditary difference in acetylation polymorphism for isoniazid and various other therapeutic drugs, on the other hand, is in the liver. Since liver biopsies were intrusive and impractical, and DNA technology to get the gene from blood cells would not be developed for about 25 years we had to resort to other study methods.

We set out to answer the question "What causes "slow acetylation?" We used New Zealand white rabbits for this purpose. To be on solid enzymoloigical grounds, we first examined the enzymatic mechanism of drug acetylation and found it behaved as a "ping-pong Bi-Bi" reaction. Put simply, this means that the enzyme swings back and forth between free and acetylated forms as it catalyzes the acetylation of drugs. As these studies progressed, we found we needed a stable, replenishable source of rabbits, and to this end we developed a colony of about 80 rapid and slow acetylator rabbits, breeding those with acetylating enzyme mutations to study their metabolism. But adequate space to house the colony at the NYU Medical Center in the 1970s was unavailable so we kept the colony in New Jersey and upstate New York. Maintaining adequate control of the colony located many miles away from the laboratory proved difficult and while we were struggling with this inconvenience, the possibility of moving to the University of Michigan came about. Jim Neel, who was then Chair of the U of M Department of Human Genetics, expressed a strong interest in pharmacogenetics and encouraged us to develop a pharmacogenetics program here. When Bert La Du decided to leave NYU for the Pharmacology Chair at Michigan in 1974, I decided to join him.

The Move to Ann Arbor

In Ann Arbor, we continued to concentrate on the rabbit acetylator trait with the aid of the rabbit colony, which we moved to the University from New York and maintained in the Department throughout much of the 1980s. But we also explored the acetylator trait in greater depth in humans, monkeys, chimpanzees and baboons, and in mice, hamsters, and rats. Eventually, we switched from rabbits to inbred mice as a lab animal model for pharmacogenetic studies of acetylation. During the next two decades, we gathered a great deal of fascinating information about the metabolic, genetic, toxicological, developmental, and molecular genetic aspects of acetylation polymorphism in these species. During that period we received generous NIH support, and maintained an NIH program project in pharmacogenetics which helped support pharmacogenetics research in our lab and that of several colleagues in Pharmacology and Human Genetics for 10 years.

The emergence of recombinant DNA technology during the 1980s brought genetic analysis of protein polymorphisms within reach of many investigators, including our laboratory. Since then, the pace of pharmacogenetics research at all levels has increased enormously. The genes for acetyltransferase, the enzyme responsible for acetylation, as well as for many other pharmacogenetic traits were cloned and sequenced, and the existence of variants of those genes was demonstrated. Whereas a connection between a susceptible

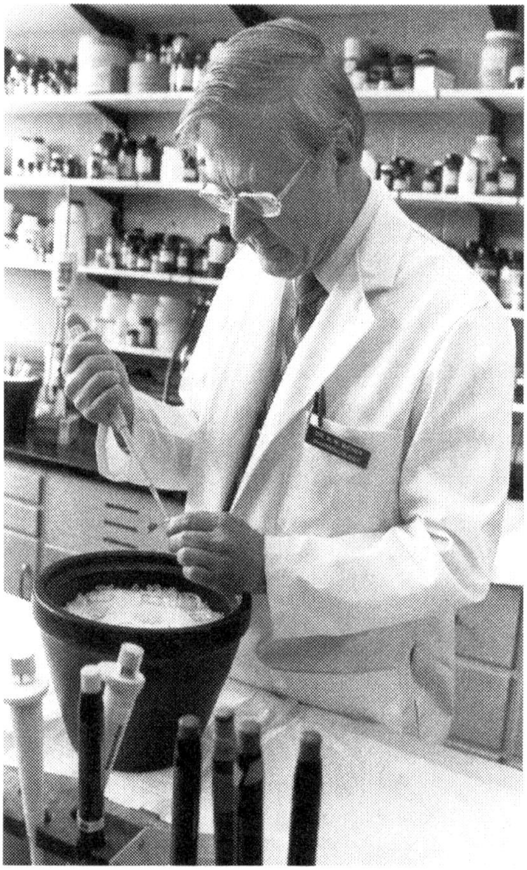

Wendell at work

phenotype and its genotype could, heretofore, only be inferred, it could, with the advent of DNA technology, be directly established. We were first to establish the molecular basis of the mouse acetylation polymorphism and its location on chromosome 8. In collaboration with investigators in the Department of Human Genetics, we constructed congenic acetylator lines of mice and hamsters that have greatly clarified the role of acetylation polymorphism in toxicology, particularly that involving carcinogenesis. The mouse and hamster congenic lines are both in use today in several laboratories here and abroad. In quick succession, after we reported sequences of hepatic N-acetyltransferase peptides of rabbit liver acetyltransferase in 1987, two functional human loci, NAT1 and NAT2, were identified, characterized, and mapped to human chromosome 8. Our laboratory was among the first to demonstrate the occurrence of diverse mutations in both of the human genes for acetylation, and to explain the essence of the phenomenon of "slow acetylation" of arylamine and hydrazine drugs and carcinogens.

The Years in Ann Arbor

The last 40 years has witnessed the transformation of pharmacogenetics from a young science that involved a handful of academic investigators to a worldwide phenomenon that has attracted the attention of clinical scientists, pharmaceutical investigators, and those on the front line of medical care. My laboratory has devoted most its research for some 35 years to studying the pharmacogenetics of acetylation. The field has been shaped mainly by the study of drug metabolizing enzyme polymorphisms like the acetylation polymorphism. I would like to acknowledge the 15 Ph.D. students and a like number of postdoctoral fellows and research associates that contributed to the progress we made.

As one of the first human hereditary traits affecting drug response to be discovered, the acetylation polymorphism occupies a singular position in the annals of pharmacogenetics. No better example exists to teach us how a broad spectrum of responses to exogenous chemicals, including drugs, can arise from a single, genetically determined, metabolic theme, and to demonstrate how we may achieve a better understanding of such traits in devising strategies to prevent human illness of environmental origin. During the last 10 years, the field has undergone a period of rapid growth and redefinition as pharmacogenomics. As a result of progress, improved patient care through customized drug treatment and new drug discovery are within the foreseeable future.

Memoirs: 1975-1979

Lindsay B. Hough, Ph.D.

The time I spent in Ann Arbor was truly special. I never worked harder in my life, and never learned more. Even the chance to go into this world famous program at Michigan to study was beyond any of my reasonable expectations. Ben Lucchesi will say to this day that my admission was an aberration – but I think I see him smile when he says it.

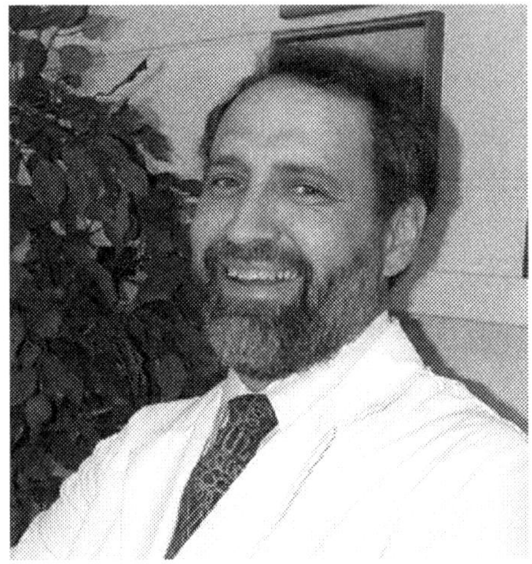

What made it so special? Many reasons. The first, of course, was the faculty. No one would ever turn away a student with a question. I can recall sitting with every one of them – one on one – day or night – sometimes for hours – working on a problem. I have several vivid recollections. I wonder if Fulton Crews and Ben Lucchesi remember the night that Fulton and I were in the lab studying well past 10 p.m. and we wandered into Ben's office. He had just finished his overheads for one of his famous nursing lectures. Despite the hour, and despite whatever all three of us were supposed to be doing, he gave us (right on the spot) a good piece of the lecture on Wolf-Parkinson-White syndrome. I still remember it, including those color overheads. I remember that on another Sunday afternoon, when I was in the middle of an experiment, Bert La Du wandered into the lab. I was all excited about microwave irradiation and histamine in the brain. We must have talked about it for most of the afternoon! I will never forget my first manuscript. Even before I gave a copy to Ed Domino, who was my mentor, I asked Vince Zannoni to take a look at it and we proceeded to argue about it for days. Vince, of course, had no reason to spend any time reading my manuscript except to help me, since he was not an author on the paper. I, of course, probably thought the paper was perfect, even though I had never written a manuscript before. There were many others who helped me in different ways— Bill Pratt and Hank Swain both wanted to "round me out"— admittedly a tall order. Then, of course, we can't forget those famous Domino lab meetings where none of us would have a clue as to what the research problem of the week was. Ed was so broadly trained, so knowledgeable about pharmacology, and so excited by it all, it was an amazing and humbling experience to spend so much time with him. Many of us will remember him telling us that "the train is pulling out," but trying to stay on that train was a tall order.

There is little doubt that the other students and postdocs who were in the Department at the time I was also contributed to the uniqueness of the place. It's no surprise that the people who were trained there are the leaders in pharmacology today. They were smart, motivated and spirited, and I learned from all of them. We studied and worked together and still found the time for some laughs. I recall the day that Rick Tessel told me he was giving reserpine to monkeys and I, just having had my first pharmacology course, asked him if he was making them depressed. He replied without hesitation, "I don't know Lindsay, why don't you ask them." I remember lots of trying times and fun times with my classmate Fulton Crews. One of my favorites was when I suggested to Tad Smith that he shouldn't be so hard on Fulton (his student). After all, I pointed out, Fulton was going to make him famous when their Nature paper was accepted and published (it was). As I recall, we both exited the hallway very quickly while Tad was still changing colors. I have lots of memories of times spent with Mark (Wally) Vogel. Even though he was a cardiovascular pharmacologist (the best "armchair pharmacologist around" according to Lucchesi), I remember the two of us spending lots of nights sitting up late on the front porch trying to figure out how the brain works. I had lots of good times with my lab mate Mike Vasko. I'll never forget the time that Mike was finishing up his thesis work and we had all signed up for round-the-clock morphine injections for tolerance/withdrawal studies. I bolted out of bed Sunday morning at 3 a.m. and realized I had missed the midnight injections. (I had a great excuse, but can't include it here.) Fortunately, it all worked out and Mike still speaks to me at meetings.

Ann Arbor itself is a special place. The excitement of football games, the incredible mass of talent, the amazing variety of intellectual pursuits, the beauty of the campus— all these combine to make it unlike anything anywhere else.

Most remarkable to me is that I have so many fond memories of my time in Ann Arbor when 14-16 hours of most days were spent doing experiments. Even that is a time to be cherished— a time when your obligations are limited and your purpose is clear. I'll close by recalling a late night when Ed Domino and I left the lab together. It was after 11 p.m. My experiment had started at 7 a.m. and Ed had worked a full day, gone home for dinner, and returned to work that evening. As we walked out, I told him I was so tired that I didn't think I could keep up the pace. He told me to enjoy it— that this was a special time in my life and that it would never be simpler. Of course, he was right.

Editor's note: Lindsay B. Hough was born on October 16, 1950 in Paris, Kentucky. He received his B.S. Chemistry degree in 1972 at the University of Kentucky in Lexington. He obtained his Ph.D. in Pharmacology here at University of Michigan in 1978 (I was privileged to be his Ph.D. thesis advisor). His primary research theme at Michigan was histamine metabolism in the brain. In 1979, he was postdoctoral at the Mount Sinai School of Medicine in New York. From 1980-1982, Dr. Hough became Assistant Professor at Mount Sinai School of Medicine. From 1983-1984 he became Associate Professor at the same institution. From 1984-1986 Dr. Hough became Associate Professor at Albany Medical College. In 1985 he became Vice-Chairman of the Department of Pharmacology and Toxicology, and in 1986 as Professor of the Department of Pharmacology and Toxicology at the same institution. Presently Dr. Hough is Professor and Associate Director at the Center for Neuropharmacology and Neuroscience at the Albany Medical College.

Dr. Hough is a member of the American Society for Pharmacology and Experimental Therapeutics, American Association for the Advancement of Science, Society for Neuroscience, and the American Pain Society.

In 1971, Dr. Hough was the recipient of the Advanced Undergraduate Achievement Award from the University of Kentucky. In 1972 he was the Sullivan Scholar at University of Kentucky. From 1973-1977 he was an NIH Pre-doctoral Fellow at University of Michigan. In 1976 he was given the Duncan A. McCarthy Jr. Memorial Award from University of Michigan. He was a NINCDS Postdoctoral Fellow from 1978-1980. From 1980-1982, he was the recipient of the Pharmaceutical Manufacturer's Association Faculty Development Award.

His areas of interest since graduate school days have been the neuropharmacology and neurochemistry of histamine in the brain.

Memoirs: 1977 - Present

Margaret E. Gnegy, Ph.D.

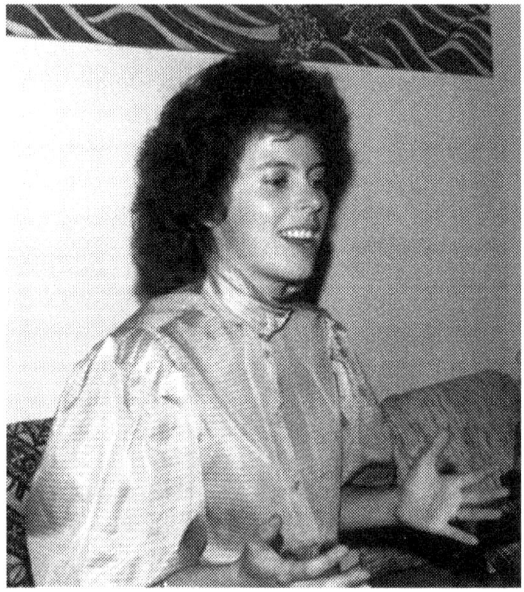

I arrived at the Department of Pharmacology at The University of Michigan in June 1977 with the experience of 3.5 years of doctoral work in biochemistry at West Virginia University and 2.5 years of postdoctoral work in preclinical pharmacology at The National Institutes of Mental Health. I was 27 years old. I had never taken a pharmacology course. Most of the graduate students at the time were older than me. I was the first female tenure-track full time academic in the Department of Pharmacology at the University of Michigan. I was young, naïve and thankfully energetic.

I grew with the Department. I learned pharmacology and loved it. I learned to teach and loved it. I learned to care about, respect and work with my male colleagues. Getting started was difficult because my research did not really integrate with any particular faculty member's research at the time. Nevertheless, from the first one or two years of my hiring, I had continuous funding from NSF, NIMH and NIDA for 24 years.

I owed great debts in my development to many of my colleagues. I was hired by Bert LaDu, who I have always greatly admired and respected. Marshal Shlafer and Ron Holz began their academic careers with me in 1977 and their camaraderie and intellectual support were essential. Wendell Weber and Ben Lucchesi, both masters of the art, taught me to teach. Eventually I learned that less was more in the classroom. I like to think that their efforts finally paid off. My first teaching assignments were antihistamines and gastrointestinal drugs, topics I still regard with fondness and interest, though I no longer teach them. Bill Pratt taught me how to write a grant. The intense push given to me by Ray Ruddon, my second chair, helped me not only to develop scientifically and attain tenure, but to learn how much I enjoyed working with graduate students. It was Ray that appointed me to the Graduate Programs Committee, which I eventually chaired for many years. I had large shoes to fill in that position, those of Ray Counsell, to whom I also owe a great debt for his superb job of teaching me about the graduate program.

And so the years passed, and I went from being the 'new kid' to one of the senior citizens. Along the way, other new faculty joined the department and I continued to learn from them. In particular, Steve Fisher and Rick Neubig taught me a great deal about signal transduction, receptors and science in general.

A true inspiration in my development in neuropharmacology was Ed Domino. His adoration of science in general, and the discipline of neuropharmacology in particular, is infectious. Ed has helped me be a better teacher of neuropharmacology, and I would like to infect the students with the same wonderment

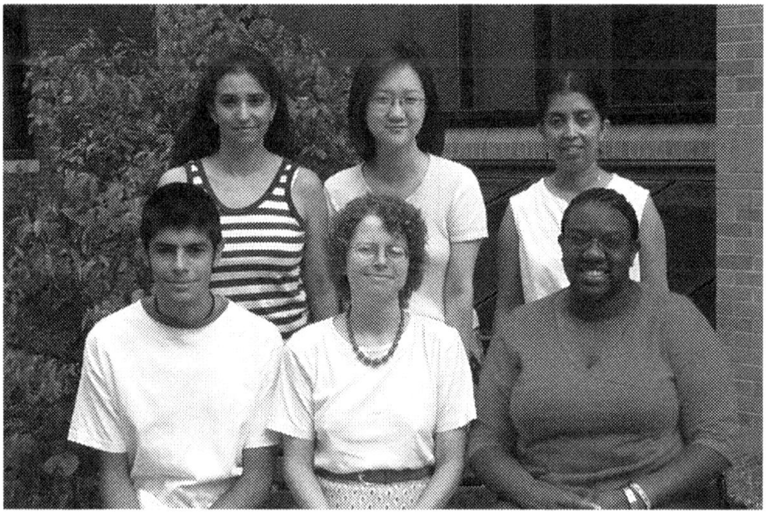

Dr. Gnegy and lab staff, ca. 1999.

of the topic that he continues to give me.

My research had always been focused on the calcium-binding protein, calmodulin, and changes elicited in the protein and its location as a consequence of psychotropic drugs. In pursuing that line of research, I began to work with the drug amphetamine, which I first used as only a tool. It has now become a passion, fueled by extensive collaboration with Terry Robinson, a professor of psychobiology. My fascination with that drug is now boundless. Switching my research from a study of calmodulin to a focus on amphetamine and the workings of the catecholamine transporter has been a wonderful but difficult transition. Most of the difficulty came in convincing the NIH that one can function meaningfully in a new field. This nearly drove me to leave science, but the confidence of my new chair, Paul Hollenberg kept me going. He has worked miracles in keeping the entire Department together.

Amphetamine, as a subject, was worth the initial difficulties. Acutely, amphetamine is the key tool to teach one about the workings and regulation of the catecholamine transporter, a subject that is not as clear-cut as has been believed for the past 30 years. The consequences of repeated amphetamine are equally fascinating, involving the development of plasticity states or learning that may underlie craving. I must thank Jim Woods for introducing me to the University of Michigan Substance Abuse Research Center, through which I have learned much about the fascinating world of drug addiction. And recently, my lab has found that amphetamine can stimulate neurite growth, which could have beneficial consequences for neurologic diseases such as stroke and Parkinson's Disease.

In looking back at my 26 years at the University of Michigan, I would like to think that I have made significant contributions to the Department in the areas of teaching, research and mentoring. My work with graduate students has been especially fulfilling and I am always so proud of their successes. I have personally trained many young men and women in my laboratory. While I am naturally driven to help develop careers for young women, and give them suitable "role modeling," I am, of course, equally proud of my successful male students. My successes are reflected in the accomplishments of my students who will go out in the world and make their own discoveries.

Memoirs: 1977-1982

David W. Hein, Ph.D.

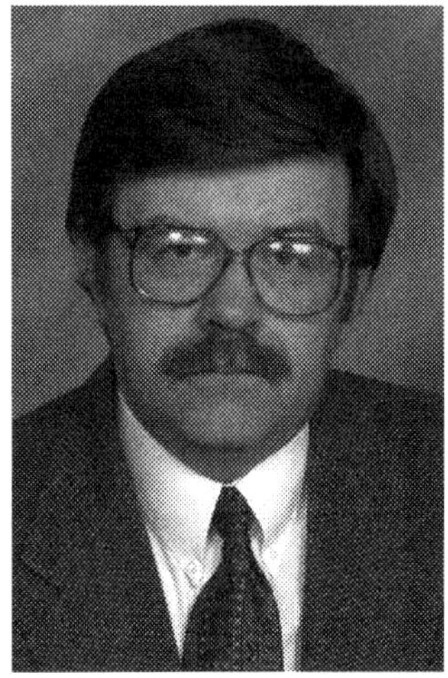

I was accepted into the Ph.D. program at Michigan for the fall semester of 1977. After interviewing with various faculty members during the summer, I decided that Dr. Wendell Weber's research in pharmacogenetics was of greatest interest to me and would be where I would start my laboratory rotations. Other graduate students in the lab at the time included Rob Tannen, Charlene McQueen (a Ph.D. candidate in the human genetics program), and Irene Glowinski. A visiting scientist from Japan, Dr. Masaharu Hirata, also began in Dr. Weber's lab in the fall of 1977; Dr. Weber assigned me to work under Dr. Hirata. Masa, as we called him, was an extremely hard-working, skilled protein chemist. I feel very fortunate to have learned protein chemistry under his patient and very skilled mentorship. Three publications emanated from that work during the 1977-78 academic year. Masa assimilated well into American culture, and I had the distinct pleasure of teaching him about football. It was fun to accompany him to the U of M football games.

I also enjoyed my second laboratory rotation with Dr. Ray Counsell, investigating the relative affinities of various novel drugs to bind to estrogen receptors. At that time, the graduate committees felt that students should do a third rotation in a different area to add breadth. Very reluctantly, I decided to work in Dr. James Woods' lab doing drug discrimination work. I thought I would hate it and would just put in my time. Much to my surprise, however, I really enjoyed the work and had a super rotation there that I extended well past the end of the semester. A number of publications resulted from that laboratory rotation as well.

I then returned to Dr. Weber's lab where I completed my dissertation in 1982. Dr. Weber was a model mentor and I am glad to have been able to learn under his direction. The other members of my dissertation committee (Drs. Bert La Du, George Brewer, and Herb Cornish) were also extremely helpful. One of the projects of my dissertation was to screen for genetic variation of acetylation capacity in inbred hamsters. We found two strains that were slow acetylators; one of these was discontinued by the distributor. Dr. Weber was kind enough to let me take the hamsters with me when I moved to my first position as assistant professor at Morehouse School of Medicine in Atlanta. I took this position without having done a postdoc, but Dr. Weber was very supportive and visited me there that first year and for a few years thereafter.

I have remained active in research investigations on the pharmacogenetics of N-acetylation. I am pleased to have organized a symposium on this topic in honor of Dr. Weber, at the ASBMB and ASPET annual meeting in June, 2000.

My Path to Michigan and My Early Days Here

Marshal Shlafer, Ph.D.

In 1976 I was in my second postdoc year (actually I was a research assistant professor) and it was time to get a real job. I was in Pharmacology at Miami, Florida, working in the lab of the Chair, Roger Palmer. Roger was a Markle Scholar, knowledgeable and skilled and immersed daily in research, teaching, and clinical medicine. He was as hard-playing and flamboyant as he was brilliant. Everyone in the department seemed to have that work hard/ play hard trait.

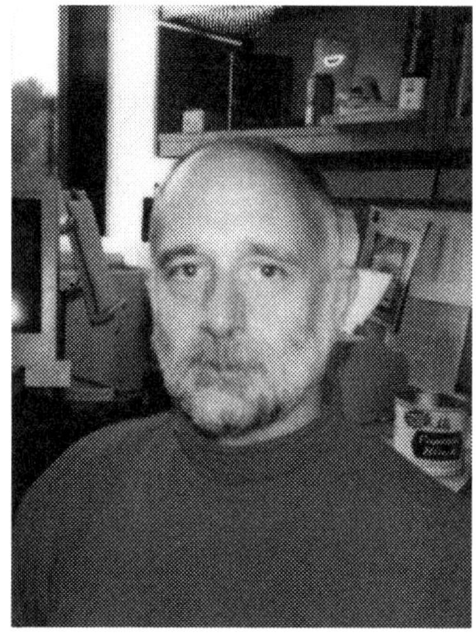

As my mentor, Roger tried to hone many of my career skills sometimes in very unorthodox ways. One facet was preparation to teach medical students, for which my first real assignment was looming. The boss figured I should learn straight from him, so I sat in the back of a packed room listening, watching, and taking notes. Midway through the hour, Roger's two secretaries dashed across the stage on their spiked high heels, obviously clothed only in lab coats that they opened wide, facing him, as they streaked by the lectern. Roger blushed a bit but was otherwise absolutely unflustered, even though his lecture guests were a total surprise to him. He continued with his lecture without dropping a beat. Afterwards, as we walked back to the lab, Roger acted as if nothing unusual had happened. He said "Champ, all you gotta do is what I do..." but, he cautioned me to "probably hold off on the streakers until I was really comfortable in front of large audiences."

Palmer also critiqued my writing style on manuscripts, sometimes mercilessly. Then, one day, I brought him a copy of the latest issue of NEJM. In it, Michael Crichton had written an elegant article entitled "Medical Obfuscation." Among the many examples of poor medical writing was a lengthy quote from one of Roger's review articles, on nitroprusside, which had also been published in the Journal. That was the end of my writing lessons from Roger.

I applied for four faculty jobs, got three interviews. One was at Ohio State. They had a reputation and tradition like Michigan — in football, that is. I liked the people I met, and the opportunities for growth for the department and for me personally. I was intrigued by one faculty member who kept a charcoal grill in his lab and used it to cook lunch for his folks. OSU was to become my first real job offer, but I cooled to it when I was asked, rather explicitly, to promise I'd do a good job at teaching. I hadn't really thought much about a predilection for or skill in teaching (research was tops in my mind), but I certainly knew I wouldn't try to do any aspect of my job poorly; I didn't like being asked to promise to do well. I replied to the chair in basically those words, and that was the end of becoming a Buckeye.

My next interview was with Bill Waddell in Louisville. Bill was a consummate and soft-spoken gentleman, like a true Southerner, who put me at ease immediately. His was a small but growing department in what I still considered "down south," and having gotten my Ph.D. down in Dixie (Augusta, Georgia) that appealed to me. Bill articulated a big but doable vision for the department's future, in research and education, and he was clear on what roles he wanted me to play in it. It sounded great, and frankly my insecurities led me to think I'd do much better in a small and growing school than in some highly visible and established Big 10 place. At the next FASEB meeting Bill took me around to the vendors to assemble a huge shopping list of equipment I'd need for my lab. I came close to going to Louisville. Very close.

But before Bill and I hooked up at FASEB, I'd visited Michigan. In fact, when I left Louisville after my interview I flew straight to Detroit, where Hank Swain greeted me in his green VW microbus. (Was this the Midwest or Woodstock, I wondered.) As we drove past the Blue Front I began seeing many people who looked like what I'd been accustomed to seeing in my college days back in the 60s. Hank picked up one sort of freakish-looking guy who was thumbing a ride. Déjà vu, and it seemed good.

Hank dropped me off at Campus Inn to relax for a bit before escorting me to the sadly long-gone Oyster Bar and Spaghetti Factory. I could quickly sense Hank's genuine sincerity and enthusiasm for the department, the med school, and people in general. Then the discussion got to teaching. Rather than being admonished about teaching, or asked to make a needless promise, Hank simply asked whether I was interested and committed, and why. I answered as sincerely as he had asked. I also recall Hank saying something like, "If you can make a lecture on laxatives interesting and dynamic [and have the students learn], you're doing it right." Yes, too many times I'd sat through exceedingly dull, monotone, and tedious turn-off lectures (in pharmacology and other disciplines) on subjects that, later on my own, I found exciting. Without knowing it, making lectures stimulating for my students (we're not talking about a class of laxatives here, folks), sharing my enthusiasm with them, and venturing a bit off the path to bring in important asides, would prove to be a component in whatever success I'd enjoy as a teacher. Hank, and Ed Domino, come to mind as our departmental exemplars of that approach.

Although Hank was the main human motive force in my decision to join Michigan (he and Vicki certainly won over my wife Jeannie too. They went so far as to find us a rental house right across the street from theirs, one where our two dogs would be as welcomed as we), Hank wasn't the only one. The Michigan tradition in pharmacology was a big factor, and I knew it. When I was a grad student, knowing something about the history of pharmacology was essential. It was still a time when even most graduate students appreciated (if not held in awe) the founding fathers and those who came later to make seminal discoveries. (Hell, in the preliminary exams for my Ph.D. degree, the history of pharmacology was a must-know topic, just like the druggie stuff, or biochemistry, or anatomy for that matter. No doubt, having Ray Ahlquist, the "inventor" of the adrenergic receptors, as my grad school chair, teacher, and curmudgeon, was a big factor in my reverence for things historic).

I had started to perceive myself as a pharmacologist someday, and even conjured an impression of what being a pharmacologist, in the fullest sense, ought to be. I knew who John Jacob Abel was, what he did, and where. Michigan was the home, the seed, for pharmacology in America. Although I was intimidated by the thought of probably forever being a small fish in a place steeped with such tradition, and home to so much talent (and many sharks, I'd later learn), just being a faculty member here was a big thing for me.

I sensed the hospitality and sincerity of the relatively new "New York gang" that I met: Bert La Du, Wendell Weber, and Vince Zannoni. There were others, including Ben Lucchesi, Ed Domino, Ray Counsell, and of course Hank, who just seemed friendly and sincere. There was a group of bright and gregarious grad students, among them but not limited to Tim Geary, Irene Glowinski, Wally Vogel, Fulton Crews, Lindsay Hough, and Germaine

Gwynn. And I wasn't put off by some of our more cynical or pot-stirring faculty; or by one future colleague who responded to my suggestion of going out for a beer and learning more about each others' interests and families by saying "Oh, no! We need to talk science!" I was starting to sense that Michigan was monolithically "science," and it worried me. I was young, still relatively newly married, and wanted a "other" facet of life for us besides my science. When push came to shove, time to choose where to go, it was the Michigan tradition — the "aura" — and the challenges of it, that sealed my decision. Besides, I had to settle down sometime.

When Jeannie and I came back to Ann Arbor for a second visit, we quickly realized things were very different from what we'd been experiencing for the past two years. Compared with the Miami folks, who were productive scientists by day and so collectively free-wheeling at night, Michigan seemed the poster child of the conservative (certainly not in a political sense) Midwest. No streakers in any lecture halls here; no St. Patrick's parties where all the food and drink was green (we're not talking cheap corned beef and beer, either), and the department picked up the tab; no departmental retreats in Bimini. So what. We'd make it here too. At least I promised myself and Jeannie to give it my best shot.

When I settled in on the 7th floor my neighbors were Ben, Bert, Wendell, Vince, Peggy Gnegy, and Ray Counsell. At least for me, from the outset there was virtually no protected time for research. I was thrown into the teaching fray from the start, sharing with Ray Counsell the responsibility for running "Pharm 404" and 405— what was much like 659 and 660 now: a two-term and rather complete survey course for pharmacy students (that was before the B.S. in pharmacy program was replaced with the PharmD-only pathway). There was also some guest-lecturing, mainly in Ben's nursing course and not long later a bit in the M2 year.

I diversified my lecture repertoire, but it was something I did far more out of curiosity than by intent or perceived future need. But it didn't take long until I saw how it could help. I recall getting to work early one snowy morning — it may have been shortly after the '78 blizzard — and running into a worried Wendell Weber, who ran the M2 course. His lecturer, a pulmonologist who was scheduled to do the asthma presentation that day, just called to say he was snowed in at O'Hare and couldn't make it back. The lecture was only a couple of hours from the time Wendell bumped into me. What was he to do? No problem. I got my notes together (having given the lecture once or twice to other classes) and gave it a go. I've been giving that M2 lecture (and now, many more) ever since.

There was no let-up in teaching, and soon I didn't want any. There was a modest but growing amount of teaching for me in the M2 year, much more in Ben's nursing course. Perhaps because Ben kept giving me more assignments (because he traveled more), and certainly because my wife was a nurse (she instilled some sort of "bonding thing" between the nursing students and me), I ultimately asked to take over that course in the early '80s, just a few years after I started teaching in it, and was granted the wish. Finally I could schedule things my way, not worried about lecturers having other commitments; rely on only a few others (now mainly Jon Maybaum and Donna Shewach) to do the areas I knew little about; and give two graduate students what is, essentially, the only opportunity for them to give a "formal lecture" to a large class. I could assign myself what I wanted to teach, how and when I wanted, and self-impose impetus to learn more by having to teach and integrate content more.

I picked up on Ben's prior admonitions to the nursing students to buck stereotype that "nurses only follow doctors' orders; never question the doctor." I drove into their heads not just facts but also understanding and thinking (and assessment) skills to prepare them for what I still view as their essential roles as a critical professional link in the checks and balances system of safe, effective drug therapy. Sounds fancy and pie in the sky, but I believed it more and more, especially as my wife would come home from her night shift (I did night-duty kid care) and relate (no names mentioned, of course) the many times a skilled, knowledgeable, and thinking nurse "saved the doctor's ass" — and the patient's too. And now, of course, we see such statistics as those published by the Institute of Medicine, highlighting the magnitude of the iatrogenic medication error problem — something I've been emphasizing to students long before the IOM released their latest data, and trying to keep them from being a part of the problem.

Not long after I took over Pharm 210 the nursing school took over many basic science courses that had been given by medical school departments, preferring to have their own faculty do them. They tried to do that with pharmacology, too, but after word leaked my former students caused such a ruckus, and course evaluations were so strong, that the nursing school quickly backed off and we kept the course. That was probably 15 years ago. I've run it since, gotten a 25% increase in lecture time approved by their curriculum committee at a time when other courses were just holding their own or getting cut back, and students' winter term schedules were already "heavy."

I honestly believe all the Pharm 210 students get their money's worth. And, it's fun and educational and challenging and on-target for them professionally. I don't know why, but when I was putting my text book for the course together, the publisher held many focus groups nation-wide. Pharmacology was almost universally cited by faculty as "the course I hate to teach most" and, by students, as "the course I hate to take the most." Funny. Neither I or my students seem to feel that way.

I still juggled teaching with research, the latter being an area in which I was only modestly successful (by Michigan standards) based on independent publications, having 8 or so years of my own RO-1, getting on a cardiovascular study section at NIH, and getting a joint appointment in Thoracic Surgery. Christina Myers, John Forder, then Chris Mack, got their Ph.D.s in my lab. They were wonderful students, as was Larry Bush, for whom Ben and I served as co-mentors; Sue Warren (now an M.D.) and Paula Kane (at Upjohn) received their M.S. degrees in my lab.

While the research was exciting and challenging, the medical and service teaching became more so, and my assignments grew and diversified. A few years later I received the Kaiser Permanente Award from the medical school and the Elizabeth Crosby Award from Galens, and got my nursing pharmacology book (a 1,400 page tome) published. It soon won an American Medical Book Writers award and was a top seller nationwide for about half a dozen years.

Actually there was group recognition of my teaching in the early '80s, years before I got the Kaiser and Crosby Awards. Each year, at least back then, the sophomore nursing class was feted with a Striping Ceremony (I wondered if they had a stripping ceremony down in Miami) to mark the successful completion of all the sophomore requirements, and official start of their clinical phase. The class voted one of "their" faculty — the implicit assumption being one of their nursing faculty — to give the keynote address in front of parents and other relatives, significant others (an unknown term then), all the Nursing School deans, and most of the nursing faculty. They had picked me: medical school faculty — an outsider. It was a big deal for all, and the ceremony was held in a decorated auditorium, complete with 3-piece music ensemble, on a Sunday, everyone dressed in their Sunday best.

The thrust of my presentation, besides the obligatory congratulation, was to reiterate my belief that continuing to learn all sorts of things — and wanting to learn — was essential to providing optimal nursing care (of any sort) to their future patients. I wanted the parents, especially, to hear that. I told the students that in two years they'd be getting some letters to put after their names (B.S.N. and soon after, R. N.) but that those were merely letters — they or any other letters they might get only meant that they had met minimum qualifications for a degree. They had to go beyond the minimum and want to do so.

As it was, this ceremony occurred in the

midst of a rather lengthy, messy, and highly publicized (even on national TV) strike by U-hospital nurses. No one coming to the ceremony could miss the long picket lines in the area. The strike was over salary, really nothing more, and since the essence of my talk was about the preeminent role of self-education as the way to care for patients (not money!), I paused, pointed towards the hospital, and remarked "those other nurses over there are showing how much they care about their patients by walking out on them; they're using their union and their union leaders, not their education or their clinical skills, to care for themselves first, and what they seem to care about most now is money."

I was sincere in my message, and intentionally blunt, but I happened to overlook one minor point: a goodly number of parents who were paying for their kids' educations belonged to such organizations as the UAW and the AFL-CIO, and many of the moms and nursing faculty too were Michigan Nursing Association union members. It wasn't a good way to end the talk, but I said what I believed and was glad I did. Parenthetically, my wife was rather pleased. From day one in her regular employment as a nurse here, she refused the requirement to join the union and reluctantly paid what amounted to a fine for that minority of people who were anti-union. An aside: I was the last non-nursing faculty member (and might have been the first) to be the keynote speaker at this affair, and the whole idea of a striping ceremony came to an end not long after.

The birth of my book took an interesting path too, with all sorts of lessons about life. Hank Swain and others often received publishers' requests to review sample chapters for prospective nursing pharmacology texts. Since I directed the course here they passed them on to me. Invariably, the chapters were either laden with touchy-feely nursing things with hardly any sound or accurate basic pharmacology content (these were the manuscripts prepared by nursing faculty); or they were high-level science, riddled with chemical structures (nurses don't need to know that), with virtually nothing to give the prospective nursing student any insight about what to do with all the information (these were written by either pharmacists or pharmacologists). There was nothing that blended and interrelated both pharmacology and nursing in what I felt was the needed way.

My critiques were scathing, but I think on target; and they often exceeded the length of the chapters I was reviewing. For reasons that escape me now (OK, it was arrogance) I wrote a "here's how it ought to be done" sample chapter for the publisher that ultimately would do my book. I wasn't expecting any response other than a check and maybe a thank you, don't call us, we'll call you. Instead, I got a trip to the publisher's office outside San Francisco, and a firm offer to sign a book contract.

I was at Michigan and research was important to me and the institution. I said, "yes, but..." Before I signed any agreement I had to get my NIH competing renewal funded. I got it, and so then said they'd have to provide me with a computer and word processing software of my choice, and probably some secretarial support, hoping that upping the ante would put them off and get me off the hook for some major work for years. They said they'd have to go up the corporate ladder for a decision and it might take two weeks. They called back saying "no problem" the same day. Soon thereafter I had a new IBM PC, a daisy-wheel printer, and a big monitor on my desk. I asked Ray Ruddon, our Chair at the time, if I could go ahead with the project. I wasn't looking for glory; I wasn't looking for more work; I wasn't asking to cut back in the lab or with teaching; and despite eventually having to send three kids through college someday, I really wasn't interested in making money.

By choice I was the only person from here to work on the first edition. There was a co-author in Massachusetts who did little to help; nearly nothing. She had her own best-selling anatomy and physiology book to revise, and so she basically lent her name, her old PhD degree and her very new B.S.N. (it was a marketing aid to lend credibility in the nursing world, to sell more books), and (don't hit me), her gender, as forms of help. There were about a dozen contributors of this or that from around the country, but really only one, save a male psychiatric nurse, had much pharmacology knowledge to back up varying degrees of clinical skills and expertise. Except for the psych nurse, there was almost no help with writing chapters (I assigned more than 30 of the 50 or so total to me as sole author anyway) or revising them to my satisfaction. I didn't want the various chapters to look or read like a patchwork of different styles and orientations, so I basically did a front-to-back rewrite of the whole damned thing. And I won't even go into the advanced charges against royalties for indexing, art work, and the like, which started me wondering whether, when all was said and done, I'd be owing the publisher money.

Soon after the book hit the market, teachers found it complete, authoritative, and on-target, as did many students from around the US who wrote or called too. It quickly made inroads in the large market and hit the number one slot. It got to a second edition (to which Jon Maybaum contributed the revised cancer chapters, and Lori Mangels those on antibiotics), and continued doing well, but the publisher and I came to a philosophic impasse when talk of the third edition (which started as soon as the second came off the press) got serious. The publisher wanted me to include all the "trendy stuff" in nursing (separate expansive sections on age, gender, ethnicity, and nursing research, of which there wasn't too much if rigor counted; with each month that passed, what was in vogue kept changing like a moving target). That would be fine — we managed that in the first two editions — were it not for the demand that I cut back radically the sound pharmacology content. I refused, for it was the basic science content that the students needed and I wanted to provide. They wanted me to write it at a lower level "because students can't and don't like to read anymore." (These students will call themselves educated professionals??) They wanted it thinner and lighter so students would find it easier to carry to class (mine never needed their books in class!). They wanted structures for most of the drugs: it looks more erudite and authoritative. Same went with including a detailed bibliographic citation list in every chapter (as opposed to my short lists of selected readings, annotated so someone could actually see why looking at the original source might be worthwhile). They wanted dosage calculations and metric "conversions." They wanted a female co-author (I dumped the original one) because I was a male in a female-dominated profession (talk about sexism! Could I say something like that?), and even urged me to put my wife down as co-author — even though she didn't want to work on the book, didn't know all that much pharmacology herself, and — "even if she doesn't contribute at all" (and it's intellectual fraud at ones institution to list authors who didn't really contribute anything).

No! I'm trying to educate. I'm not going to aim low because that's all kids want. No structures, because with precious few exceptions they won't know, or need to know, what to make of them. No metrology or dosage calculations: that's math, or medical-surgical nursing stuff, but it ain't pharmacology. No pandering to the special interest group-of-the-month. Some time later I read Charles J. Sykes' book, Dumbing Down our Kids: Why American Children Feel Good About Themselves but Can't Read, Write, or Add. Suddenly it all made sense.

As the teaching grew I had to grow tough skin to respond to sneers that I didn't publish in JBC; I was a Neanderthal for being interested in systemic pharmacology and what regulated contractility or other functional aspects of the intact heart; I was "stupid and suicidal" for not "going molecular." That, plus what I perceived as political back-stabbing BS in the NIH peer review process (I saw it first hand when I was on study section and suffered from it when my own grants were reviewed), and finally "disappearing" for five years in medical school dean-hell, basically put an end to my interest in research, at least for the immediate future.

Vignettes: "I Remember When..."

Staff and Students of the 1970s and Beyond

As the wife of a medical school dean...
Joan Gronvall Bailey, 1970-1983

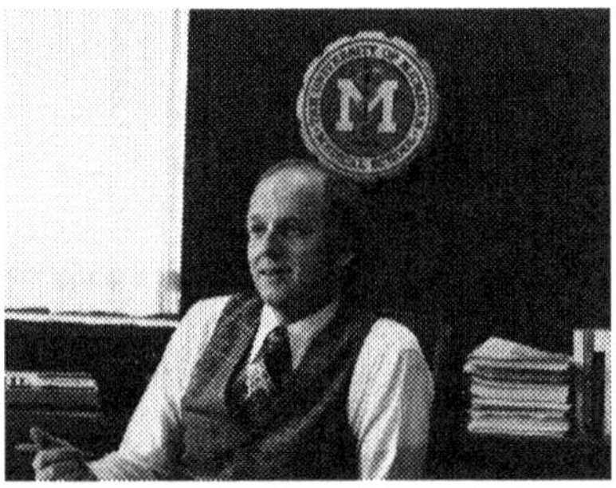

As the wife of a medical school dean, I found myself putting a lot of time and effort into the recruitment of Department chairs. John and I thought it important to host dinners at our home for recruits; these dinners added a flavor of warmth and welcome, a personal touch, to each visit. They also gave a visiting candidate a better feel for people and home environment.

We always invited other faculty members besides someone from the search committee and from the dean's office. We tried to balance guests from the basic and the medical sciences, and, depending on the candidate's interests, we would invite someone from outside the medical school. For instance, if we knew a candidate was interested in music, we would invite a faculty member from the music school to join us for the evening. We had some lively discussions!

Mike Radtke, Ph.D., 1972-1977

I remember when the new chairman, Bert La Du, arrived from the New York area (NYU), bringing two scientists with him (Vince and Wendell) to breathe new life into the Department of Pharmacology. I was surprised that Vince did not own a car and that Wendell collected orchids.

I lived on a 100-year-old farm on East Joy Road, which was just gravel. I tended a huge garden there that provided weeding therapy most spring and summer nights. It was very idyllic in 1974, with fresh vegetables on the table, a short commute, adequate parking in a lot below Medical Science Building I, and an interesting new line of research. I remember some graduate students, Irene, Rita and Barbara, dressing up in costumes at Halloween.

I remember the day that I live-trapped several wild white-footed deer mice in my cold basement and farm out-buildings and brought them into the lab to phenotype them according to their N-acetyl transferase activity. These mice caused quite a challenge, since they could jump about two feet straight up into the air and out of the orange juice containers we kept them in!

Barbara Waszczak, Ph.D., 1973-1978

I don't have time to write a chapter on why I came, stayed, etc., although I'm daily

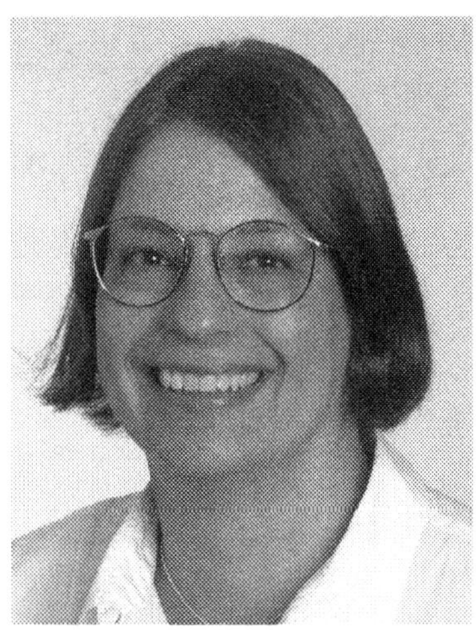

glad that I did! I remain very proud to be a graduate of the Pharmacology Department at Michigan — the best in the world! I enjoy any and all news of the Department, especially newsletters with pictures. I would also be pleased to come back for a grand reunion of all present and past members of the Department. I attended the centennial celebration about a decade ago, and I think its time to have another such event!

Charlene A. McQueen, Ph.D., 1974-1978

I first met Wendell W. Weber, Bert La Du and Vincent Zannoni when I was a graduate student at New York University. Our paths crossed again in 1974 at the University of Michigan where I was then enrolled as a Ph.D. student in the Department of Human Genetics. The area of pharmacogenetics intrigued me. When it came time to choose my dissertation topic, I approached Dr. Weber and he invited me to join his group. There was only one hurdle. I was not a student in the departmental program. I found myself negotiating the maze of becoming what would now be considered an interdisciplinary student. At that time what I was doing didn't have a name, a program or guidelines. All of us persevered and the result was that I had Dr. George Brewer and Dr. Weber as co-advisors. While I may not have always recognized it at the time, it was a superb environment. Since I am now involved in training graduate students, I have a much better appreciation of my educational experience in Ann Arbor.

James A. Grubman, M.S., 1974-1976

My two years at Michigan were stressful but ultimately very educational. The coursework in neuroanatomy, pathology, and medical pharmacology laid the groundwork for later success in fields of psychology coordinated with medicine, i.e., medical psychology and neuropsychology. I have had an extra knowledge base most psychologists do not have, and I have been able to integrate my pharmacology training with everyday clinical practice concerning the psychotropic medications used with patients. With the growing momentum to train psychologists to prescribe medications, my pharmacology background may be very helpful.

My contacts with other Michigan pharmacology students has been very limited since I earned my degree. My experience during my graduate training was difficult due to being a non-traditional student, and it took me many years to place that period of my life in the proper perspective. I still greatly appreciate the support and guidance of Dr. Jim Woods, in whose lab I primarily worked.

Jesus A. Garcia-Sevilla, M.D., Ph.D., 1979-1981

Editor's note: Jesus received an M.D. from the University of Valencia in 1970 and a Ph.D. from the Autonomous University of Barcelona in 1973. He was then an instructor and assistant professor at the latter University. After further postdoctoral research at the University of Gothenburg in the Department of Pharmacology in 1976-78 and at Synthelabo Research in Paris in 1978-79, he came to our Department in 1979-1981. He was the first International University of Michigan Pharmacology Fellow Awardee supported by the funds of the Michigan Japanese Fellows Society. During his stay in Ann Arbor Jesus worked with Dr. C.B. Smith. They studied platelet alpha 2 adrenoceptor in patients with major depression, and the regulation of adrenergic alpha 2 receptors by antidepressant drugs. Jesus returned to Leioa, Spain as an associate professor of pharmacology at the University of Basque Country from 1981-1983, and then as professor and chairman of that department from 1983-91. He received the Dr. Antonio Esteve Foundation Award in Pharmacology in 1989 and again in 1995. He was also president of the Spanish Pharmacological Society from 1993-1995. His current research interests include neuropsychopharmacology, opioid, imidazoline and alpha 2 receptors in affective disorders and drug addiction. These research interests were expanded at the Unite de Recherché Clinique at the Universite de Geneve in Switzerland and a subsequent return to his home laboratory in Spain.

1970

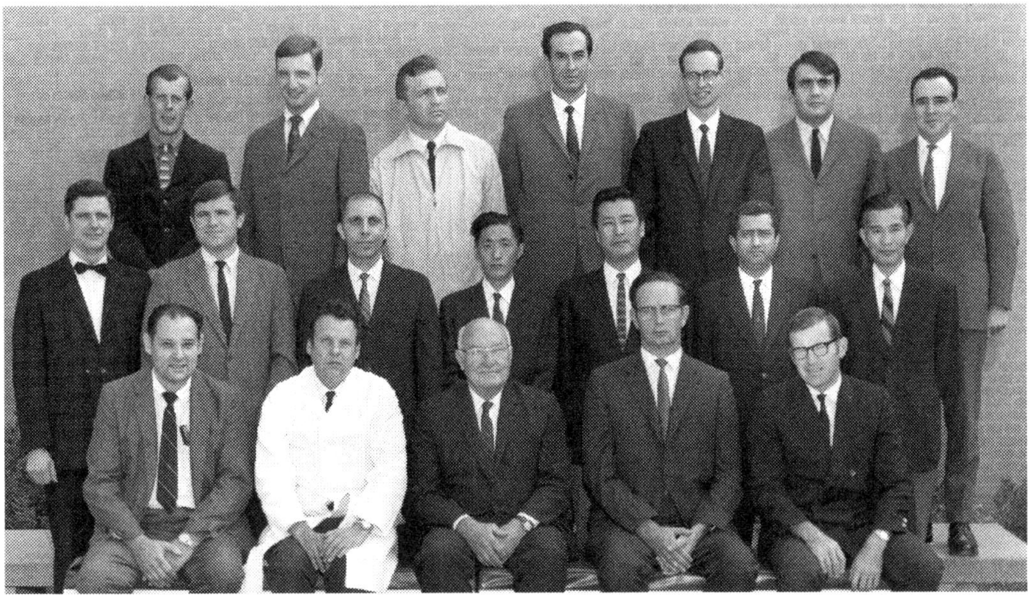

Front row: E. Domino, E. Carr, M. Seevers, H.Swain, R. Ruddon
Second row: C. Hug, J. Johnson, B. Lucchesi, E. Hasegawa, I. Matsuoka, K. Ahmad, F. Ikomi
Third row: I. MacLeod, L. Whitsitt, F. Medzihradsky, M. Medina, C. Smith, J. Woods, J. Villarreal

1971

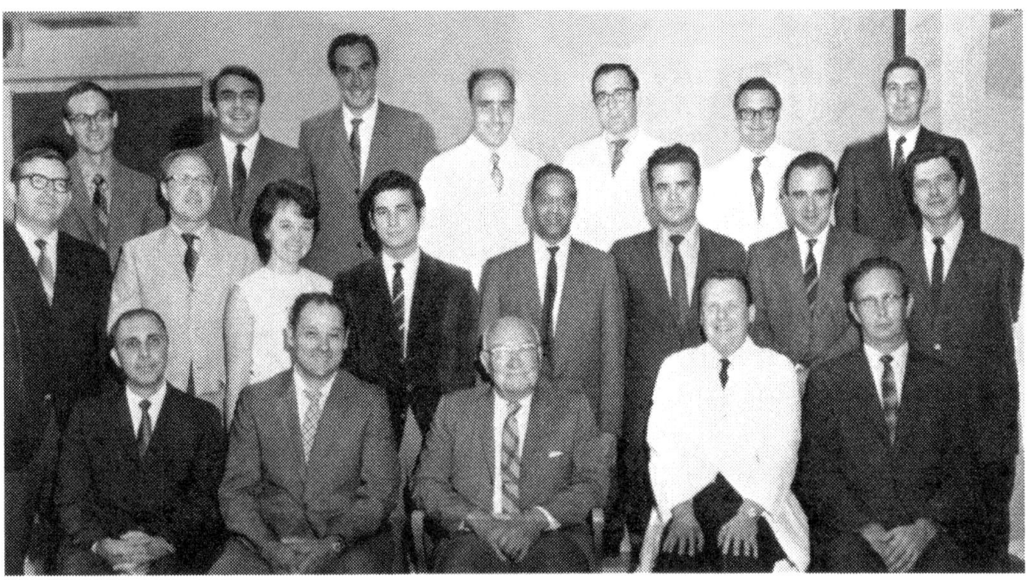

Front row: B. Lucchesi, E. Domino, M. Seevers, E. Carr, H. Swain
Second row: R. Ruddon, T. Tephly, K. Olson, J. Luciani, S. Damle, M. Guzman, J. Villarreal, C. Hug
Third row: C. Smith, J. Woods, M. Medina, A. Bartolini, M. Newman, G. Royer, W. Murray

1972

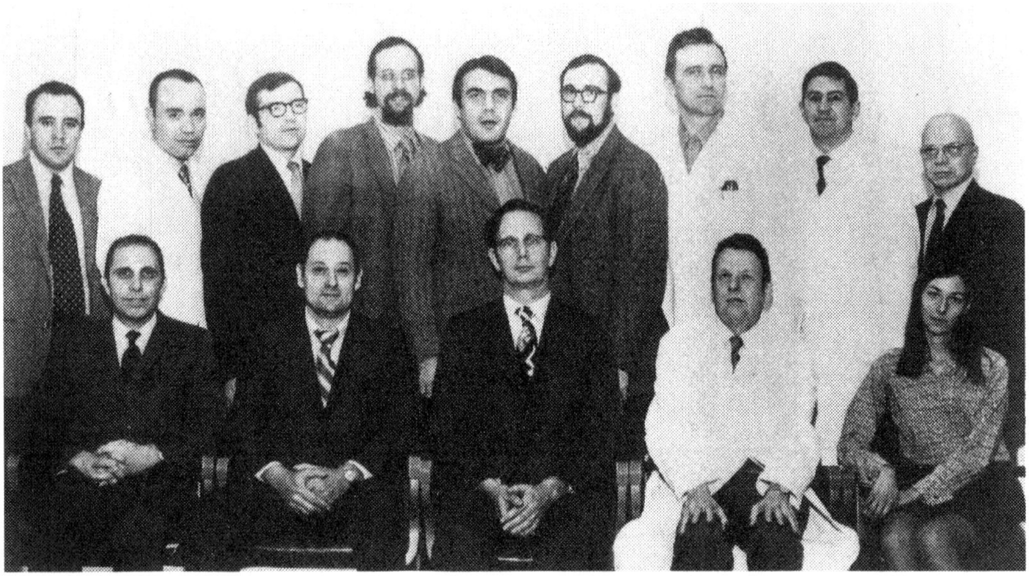

Front row: B. Lucchesi, E.Domino, H. Swain, E. Carr, M. Stitzer
Second row: J. Villarreal, G. Curtis, R. Ruddon, C. Smith, J. Woods, M. Newman, F. Medzihradsky, W. Murray, K. Cochran

1973

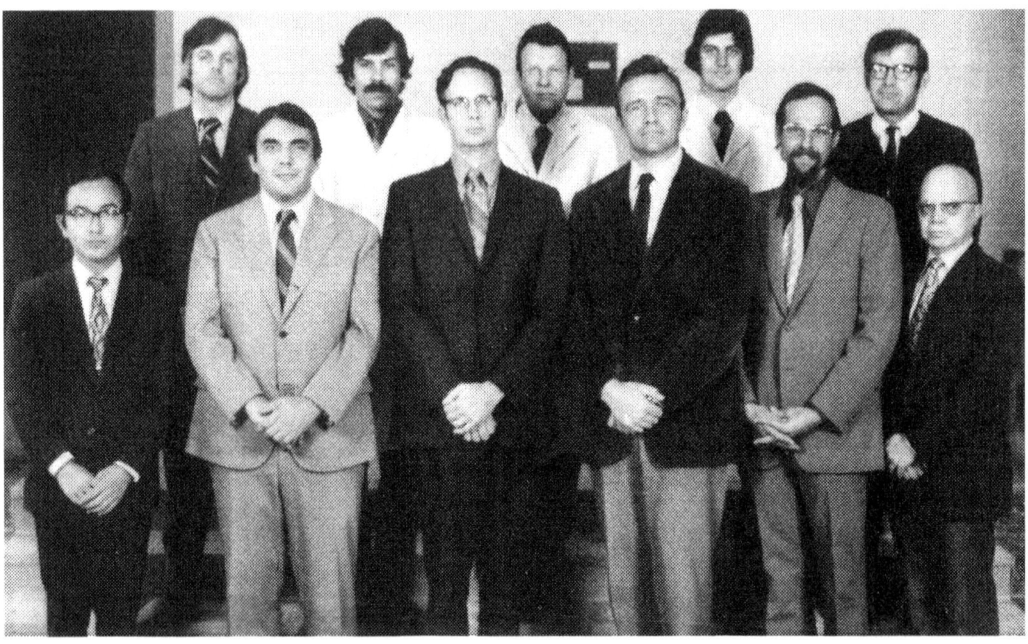

Front row: H. Fukushima, J. Woods, H. Swain, F. Medzihradsky, C. Smith, K. Cochran
Second row: D. Heitz, D. Downs, E. Carr, I. Marshall, R. Ruddon

1974

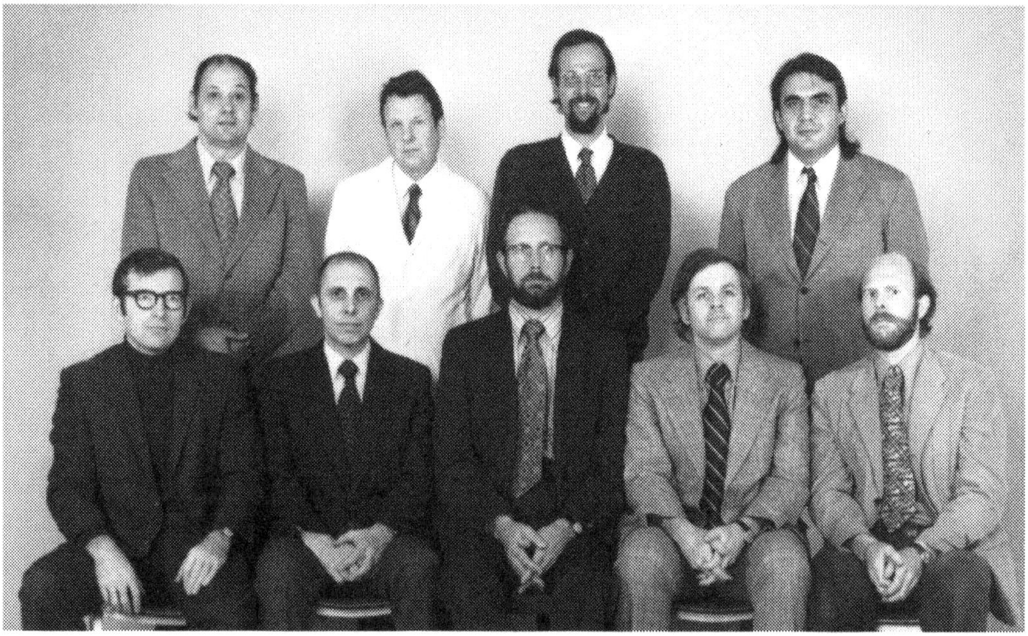

Front row: R. Ruddon, B. Lucchesi, H. Swain, D. Heitz, W. Pratt
Second row: E. Domino, E. Carr, C. Smith, J. Woods

1979

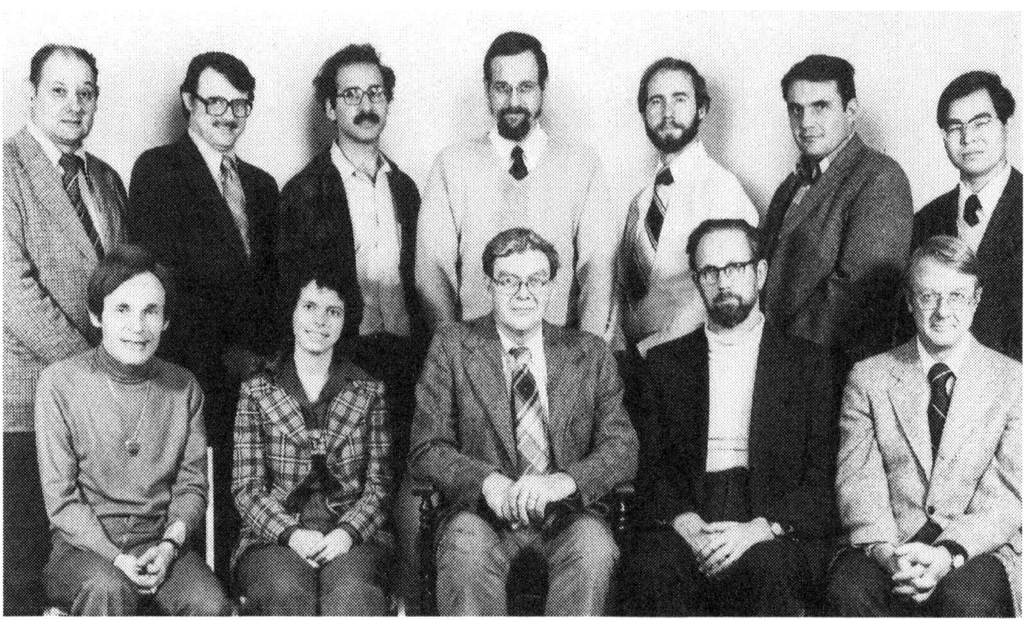

Front row: V. Zannoni, M. Gnegy, B. La Du, H. Swain, W. Weber
Second row: E. Domino, R. Counsell, R. Holz, C. Smith, H. Eckerson, J. Woods, T. Ueda

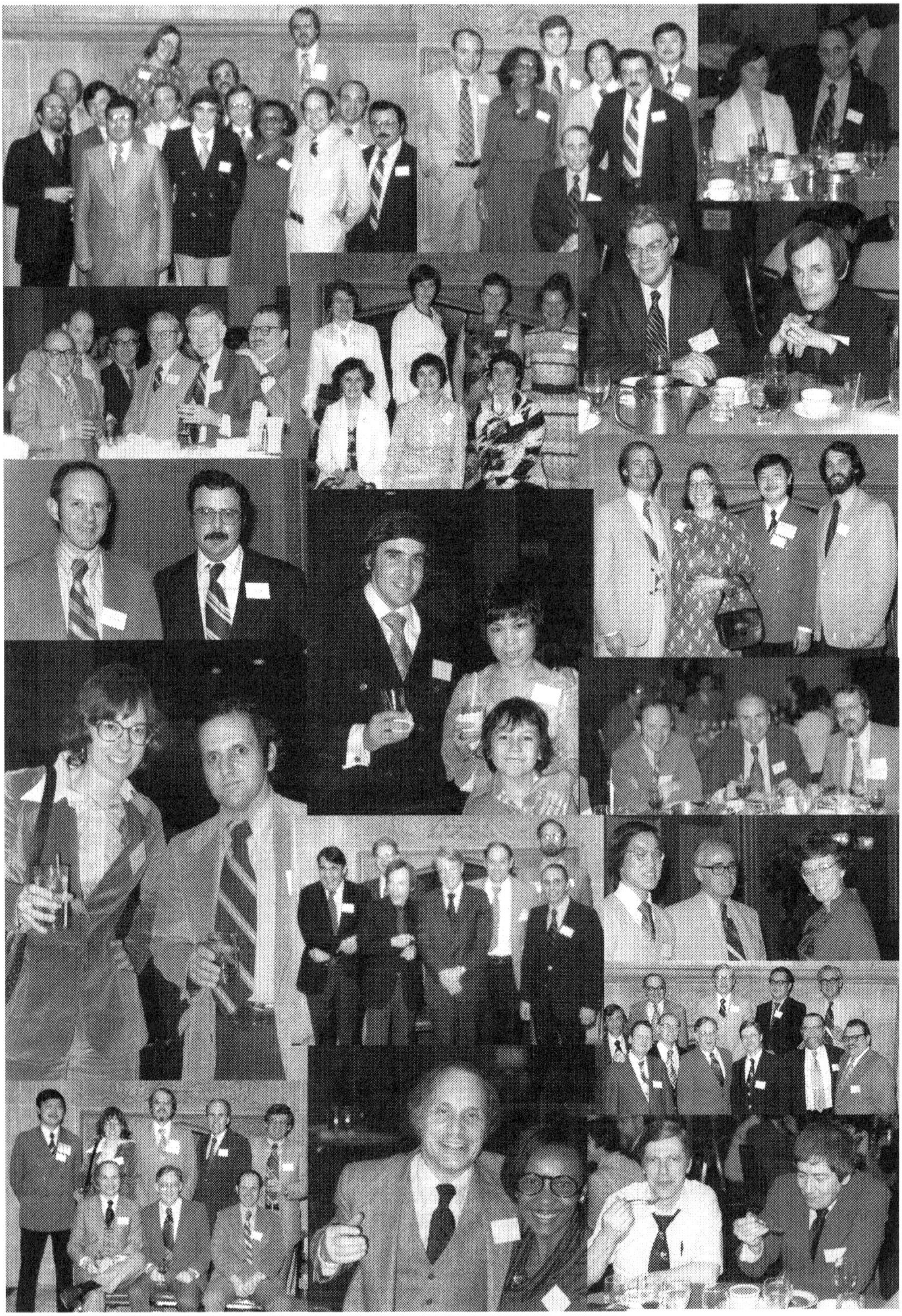

19

A Brief Memoir from Dr. Domino's Lab

Zbyszek Kaminski, Ph.D.

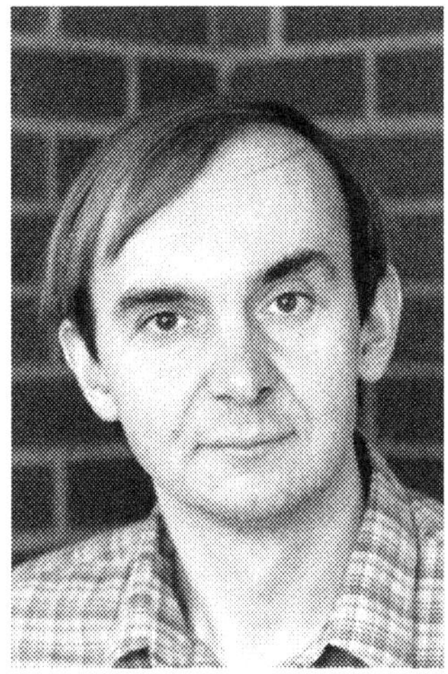

Just after I had completed my Ph.D. work in Poland, I was obligated to find a place abroad to perform my postdoctoral studies—it was essential in order for me to continue my scientific career. Hence, I wrote numerous letters to various laboratories located throughout the USA, and actually received a few positive responses very quickly. Without much delay, I selected one of the offers, and in autumn of 1983, I arrived in Ann Arbor. It became rather quickly evident that I would not be able to stand the conditions, and especially my boss in this laboratory, for long. Fortunately for me, the memories of that time at my first laboratory are now largely suppressed in my mind, so I will refrain from mentioning any more details about it.

Nevertheless, because of the situation I was forced to choose between two possibilities — either to return to Poland immediately or to find a new post at the University of Michigan. With the help of my Polish friends from Ann Arbor, I found Dr. Domino's lab. Actually, by that time, I had already visited his laboratory a few times, as one of my friends who worked there asked me to build for him a precise and reliable electronic thermostat, which he urgently needed for his work on brain tissue slices. Because I was not only a biochemist, but also a skilled electronics amateur, I designed and built the requested instrumentation very rapidly, to the satisfaction of both my friend and Dr. Domino.

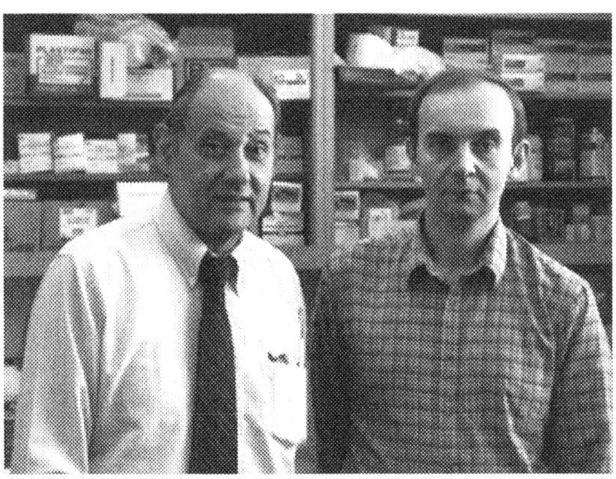

Working together...

Just a few days later, I visited Dr. Domino's lab again and asked him if it was possible to get a position in his laboratory. Dr. Domino had no objections, and after a short time period I began to work in his lab. This part of my story seems to be of especial importance, since I have never before or since met such a person. Dr. Domino has such an exceptional personal culture and great tolerance for other people. He not only gave me a great deal of freedom with my work there, but also did not indulged in any formalities, so I was able to order anything (glassware, reagents, etc.) that was nec-

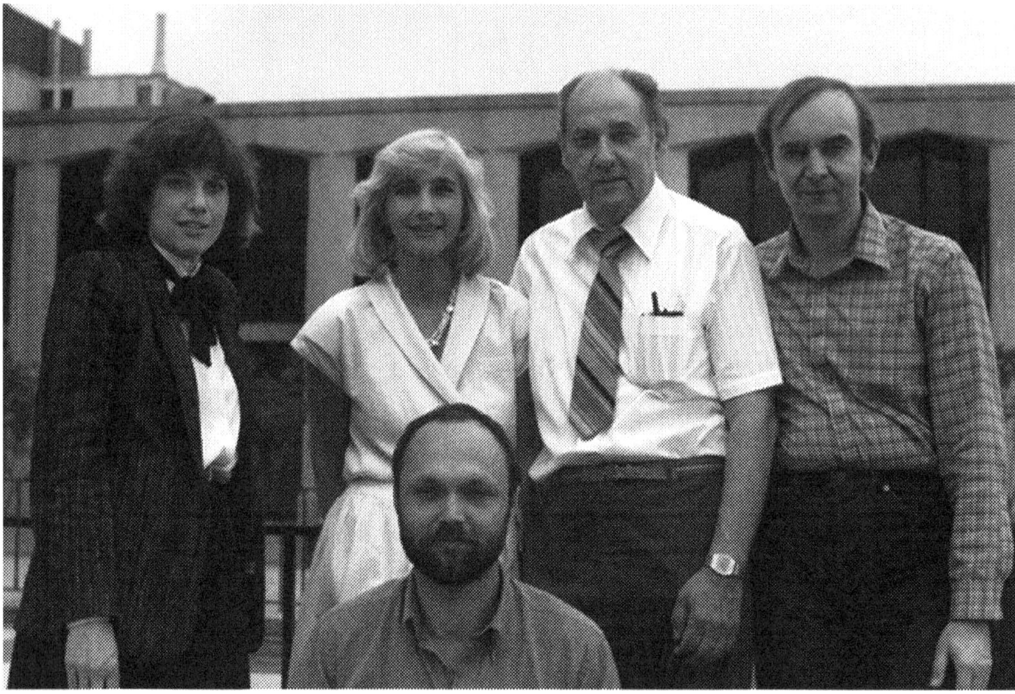

Ed Domino with his postdoctoral fellows: Rebecca Head, Helena Król, Zbyszek Kaminski and Roman Pohorecki, ca. 1983

essary to conduct my project. Moreover, he was not overly concerned with the work pace, so I was not pushed to work any faster than was necessary. Nor was I required to show him the partial results of my current work. He also allowed me to use a very advanced HP computer, located in the lab, which actually had been purchased for quite different purposes. With the use of this particular computer I was able to write a program for kinetic and pharmacokinetic constants calculation, and the results of my research were later published in a specialized scientific computer journal. Because I was also allowed to continue my biochemical research related to the Ph.D. work I had pursued in Poland, within six months I had compiled enough data to write a publication, which appeared in a renowned scientific periodical.

Dr. Domino's help has actually gone much further, as he taught me how to correctly use English and demonstrated the way scientific publications should be written. Those lessons proved very valuable; when I returned to Poland I was able to write my own scientific papers in English. Within one year after I started to work in Dr. Domino's lab, I had to return to Poland. However, I must say that the time I spent in Dr. Domino's lab I still consider to be the best of my scientific career.

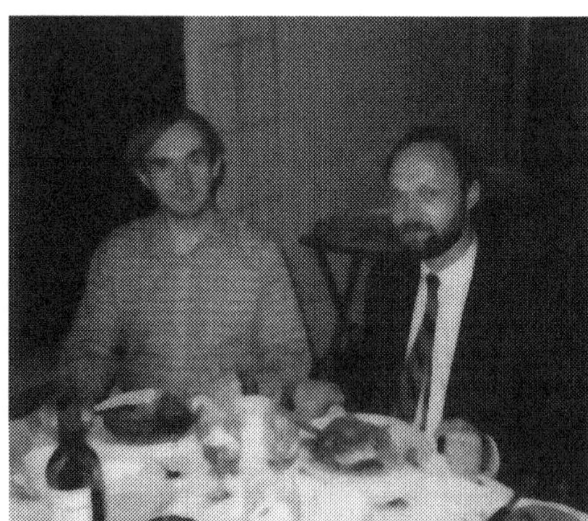

Zbyszek Kaminski and Roman Pohorecki

Thoughts on UM Pharmacology

Jan Kitzen, Ph.D.

Why I Came to Michigan

In 1985, the pharmaceutical industry was beginning to lose interest in developing drugs for the treatment of hypertension. Since this was my area of specialization, and I had never done any postdoctoral work, I thought that it was time to learn some new areas of cardiovascular pharmacology, if I were to be able to adapt to the new climate of change.

I had heard of Dr. Lucchesi many years ago as a graduate student at the University of Iowa, and I seemed to be noticing papers from his laboratory on a fairly regular basis in the mid-1980s. At this time, the area of myocardial ischemia and reperfusion injury was gaining popularity in experimental cardiology. I decided to call Dr. Lucchesi one day to ask him if it would be possible for me to come to work in his laboratory. I was delighted to hear him say "I may have something for you," and over the course of the next few months, we worked something out. I was able to join his laboratory in the fall of 1986.

Most Memorable Moment

One day Dr. Lucchesi had a phone call from Dr. Mel Marcus at the University of Iowa. Dr. Marcus had heard that "an old guy" had come to work for Ben. Ben remarked, "Oh yes, Jan Kitzen, previously from Hoechst-Roussel Labs, just joined my lab this fall." What Dr. Marcus was actually inquiring about was the fact that Dr. Martin Winbury, had joined the lab as a consultant-expert. Dr. Winbury was well known for his pioneering work on nitroglycerin and the coronary circulation, and had recently retired from Warner Lambert; he was in his upper 70s at the time. We thought it was amusing that Ben considered me, at age 36, to be the "old guy". Martin and I developed a

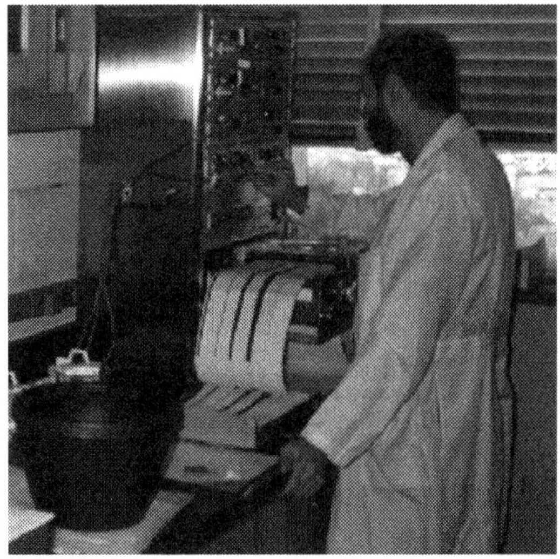

nice relationship during my time at Michigan.

Where is Pharmacology Headed?

There is no question that with the advances made in genome research (pharmacogenomics), a whole new approach to drug development is now upon us. This promises to be an exciting new arena for new drugs. However, the down side is that, even with the incredible potential to develop new types of therapies never before possible, the need to test these new products in conventional types of models for safety and efficacy is still necessary.

Unfortunately, there is now a shortage of people who are trained in whole animal pharmacology, and thus, it may be difficult to conduct the appropriate types of studies needed for regulatory approval of new products. There is still a need for people who are trained in the classical methods used in pharmacology, methods such as those that are well known in pharmacology at the University of Michigan.

Reflections of a Research Associate

Sue Wade, B.A.

I graduated from Western Michigan University in April 1976 with a double major in biology and math (statistics) and a minor in chemistry. While waiting for my husband Phil to finish up his degree, I took some graduate courses at Western, was a teaching assistant in the math department and also worked part-time as a lab assistant at Upjohn. When Phil graduated in December, we left Michigan to fulfill his military obligation. During our more than nine-year association with first the Army and then the Coast Guard, we moved from Kentucky to Georgia to Arizona to Alabama and finally to Cape Cod, MA. Needless to say, my aspirations of a career in science fell by the wayside.

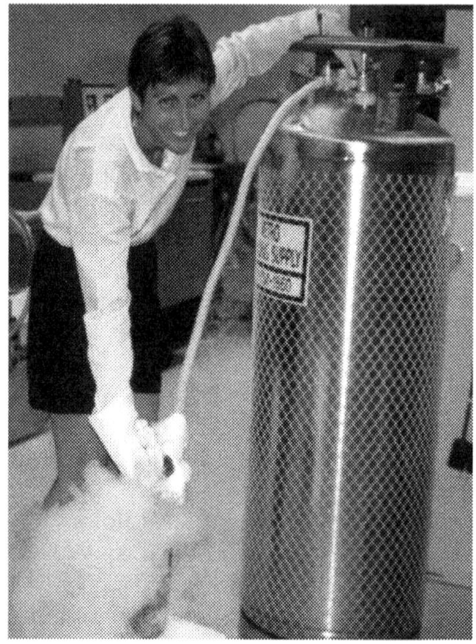

Despite our vow never to return to Michigan, a civilian job opportunity for Phil brought us back to the Detroit/Ann Arbor area, where, for the first time in more than 10 years, many science-related job opportunities existed for me. My first objective was to get my foot in the door and try to pick up again in a very fast-moving field that I had been out of for so many years. Since my most recent work experience on Cape Cod was as a teller, loan clerk, and branch manager for the local credit union, I took a position as a teller here in Ann Arbor while still looking for a job more related to science.

That opportunity came in June 1987, when I was hired as a part-time lab assistant in Rick Neubig's lab. I worked 20 hours per week washing glassware, making buffers, and processing the human blood platelets we received from the Red Cross. My research and lab responsibilities gradually expanded as my hours increased, and I was promoted to Research Assistant.

When I first joined the Neubig lab, we occupied two small labs on the sixth floor of Med Sci I. We later added a third room and eventually moved to a single large lab on the seventh floor. Our final move was to our current space in MSRB III.

I have seen many students, staff and faculty come and go during my 16-plus years in the lab. Although science is very frustrating a lot of the time, I am still learning new things, and every once in a while something really does work like it is supposed to. At one time I did consider going back to school; I even took the GRE. I decided, however, that the experience I had gained on the job was more valuable than an advanced degree ever would be. I guess the reason I have stayed here for so long is that I enjoy the flexibility, the diversity, the challenges and the experiences I am exposed to. For the most part, the positive experiences over the years have far out-numbered the negative ones, and I hope to continue to be a part of the department's history over the next several years.

The Years 1989-1990, Present and Future

Mitsuhiro Yoshioka, M.D., Ph.D.

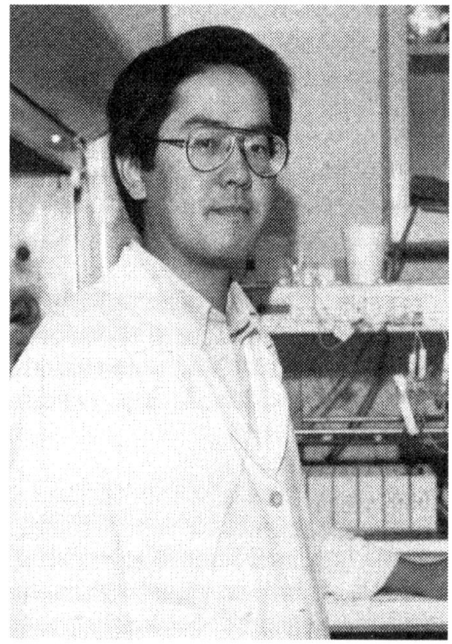

In the summer of 1989, I had joined a glorious family of the Department of Pharmacology at the University of Michigan as a Maurice H. Seevers International Fellow. I had been studying, as a cardiovascular pharmacologist in Japan, the role of the serotonergic systems in the regulation of blood pressure in the central nervous system. My supervisor, Professor Hideya Saito, who chaired the First Department of Pharmacology at Hokkaido University School of Medicine from 1975 to 1997, recommended me as a candidate for a Maurice H. Seevers International Fellow. Professor Emeritus Tsuneyoshi Tanabe who was a former Seevers International Fellow during 1959-1957 also recommended me; he passed away in the winter of 1996.

Though their good offices, I received the fellowship and I took part in Dr. Smith's laboratory. When I arrived in Ann Arbor (this was the first time I came to the US) there was a funny event. I needed some US cash to have McDonalds' hamburgers but I had only travelers checks. I wanted to exchange my travelers checks for cash, and entered a bank. I think it was First of America Bank at the front of Medical Science Building I. I asked a young beautiful clerk, "Please cash my $50 travelers check". She replied with smile," How would you like it?" Unfortunately I could not understand her meaning at that time, but I had to say something as soon as possible. I hesitated to reply; at last I answered " I like it very much." The result is easy to figure out with no explanation. I should say "five $10 bills, please." This was a reason why I was attending the English Language Institute to learn English.

In the laboratory of Dr. Charles B. Smith, I had been further evaluating serotonergic mechanisms in the central nervous system. He and his colleagues had shown previously that drugs and treatments used to manage melancholia and a variety of other psychiatric disorders decrease the density of alpha 2-adrenoceptors located in specific areas of the rat brain and produce a functional sub-sensitivity of those alpha 2-adrenoceptors that regulate the release of norepinephrine from both neurons in the rat brain and from peripheral noradrenergic neurons in the rat heart. During the year that I worked with Dr. Smith, we demonstrated that alpha 2-adrenoceptors located on serotonergic neurons in the hippocampus and the dorsal raphe nucleus of the rat brain also regulate the release of 5-hydroxytryptamine (serotonin). From the peripheral to the central nervous system the change in direction indicates awareness of the most critical areas of contemporary pharmacological research. In this context, I spent a most valuable time in his laboratory.

At that time, Dr. Raymond W. Ruddon was a Maurice H. Seevers Professor and Chairman, but he was to move to Nebraska Medical Center. When Dr. Hosoya and his wife stopped in Ann Arbor for a few hours in the autumn of 1989, Dr. Ruddon, Dr. Woods and Dr. Swain gathered at Mrs. Seevers' home and had a wonderful time to chat with Dr. Hosoya. I could fortunately share the time with the VIPs.

During my working in the US, everyday I carried my lunch "onigiri" which is made by steamed rice and a most common Japanese lunch. Usually I ate onigiri with "miso-soup". This is also a very traditional Japanese soup. I recall that at every lunch time the atmosphere of his laboratory changed to a Japanese style. I did not know whether my colleagues liked it or not.

Since coming back to Japan, I have kept in touch with Dr. Smith for the next era. In 1992 Dr. Smith received a Japan Society for the Promotion of Science (JSPS) Fellowship for Research in Japan. The JSPS Fellowship for Research in Japan was established in 1959 to promote international cooperation and mutual understanding in scientific research; it is operated as a Japanese government subsidy. The program presupposes the existence of contacts between scientists in Japan and in other countries, a condition considered favorable to the promotion of future scientific cooperation and exchange.

During his staying in our laboratory, he conducted a new project using the technique of in vivo microdialysis in which a dialysis probe was inserted stereotaxically into the hippocampus of the awake, unrestrained rat. This study was the first demonstration that an antidepressant drug causes a subsensitivity of alpha 2-adrenoceptors on serotonergic neurons in the rat brain in vivo similar to that observed previously for alpha 2-adrenoceptors on noradrenergic neurons in a variety of in vitro preparations. Other experiments that were conducted during his stay were related to the characterization of opioid receptors that regulate the release of 5-HT from rat hippocampal neurons during in vivo microdialysis. These studies involved the use of agonists and antagonists that are highly specific for mu and kappa and delta opioid receptors and indicate that the mu-opioid receptor is the opioid receptor that predominantly regulates neuronal release of serotonin in that area of the rat brain.

In the spring of 1997, Dr. Smith organized a symposium entitled, "Interactions of Neuronal Systems at Presynaptic Receptors" at Pharmacology '97 in honor of my supervisor Professor Hideya Saito. This symposium was held under the auspices of the Neuropharmacology Division of the American Society for Pharmacology and Experimental Therapeutics. Dr. Peggie J. Hollingsworth edited the proceedings of the Symposium. Her talents always surprised us and helped us for everything. These events were unforgettable for not only Professor Saito but also our Department.

The collaboration that already existed between our group at the Department of Pharmacology, Hokkaido University School of Medicine and the group of the University of Michigan Medical School has been strengthened greatly. I look forward to years of productive collaboration and exchange of scientists and scientific information between our two groups.

Vignettes: "I Remember When..."

Staff and Students of the 1980s and Beyond

Susan L. Pocotte, Ph.D., 1980-1985

As I reflect on how fortunate I am to have received my doctorate from such a prestigious department, I can not help but smile at how I entered the program. Due to my own naivete, UM was not my first choice. I "ended up" at the UM Department of Pharmacology because it was the only program to offer me a full NIH training grant stipend. My tenure at UM was the most stimulating, rewarding and at times difficult period of my life. The high expectations of the faculty were appropriate and prepared me well for the subsequent successful positions in science and academia I have held. I am convinced that holding a degree from the UM Department of Pharmacology opened doors for me that would have remained closed had I graduated from my first choice university!

My most cherished memory is that of my experience with my mentor Dr. Ronald W. Holz. I am forever grateful for his support during my graduate experience at UM. His enthusiasm, passion for scientific discovery, fairness, and generosity with praise was a perfect environment for a student to safely create and grow into a young scientist. I hope that I have been able to demonstrate some of these same qualities to my students in the classroom and laboratory. To this day, as I try to motivate my students, I find myself repeating one of Dr. Holz's common phrases, "Now let me ask you this..."

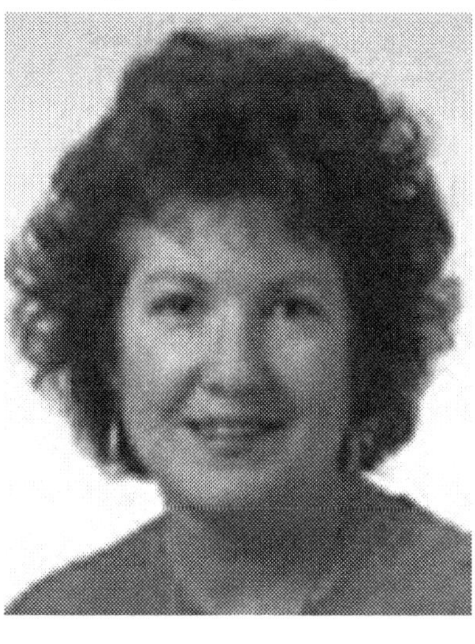

Recently, I was asked the age-old question, "If you had to do it all over again, would you?" Absolutely. A doctorate in pharmacology affords one a diverse choice of careers. In addition, it is easier to understand and work among the multiple fields of the biomedical sciences. Thus far, I have exploited this opportunity. My short journey has been fun and varied— multiple areas of biomedical research, adjunct faculty, continuing education seminars, Complementary medicine clinical service, etc. As of this writing, I recently blazed a new trail. I am the first Ph.D. without an R.N. degree to be hired as faculty by the School of Nursing at the Medical College of Ohio. In fact, a non-R.N. faculty in a school of nursing is rare anywhere. I have the pleasure of using my collective experience to serve as a bridge between holistic nursing and the medical approach to health care in both the classroom and clinical research.

Ante Simonic, M.D., Ph.D., 1982-1983

As a Fulbright Scholar, I was in the Department working with Edward F. Domino from 1982-1983. I had an excellent time with Dr. Domino and his coworkers. We were working with PCP and related drugs in rats and monkeys, measuring EEG and gross behavior effects. Also, we investigated the effects of various cholinergic agonists, classic convulsants, and anticonvulsants. We developed a hypocholinergic animal model of Alzheimer's

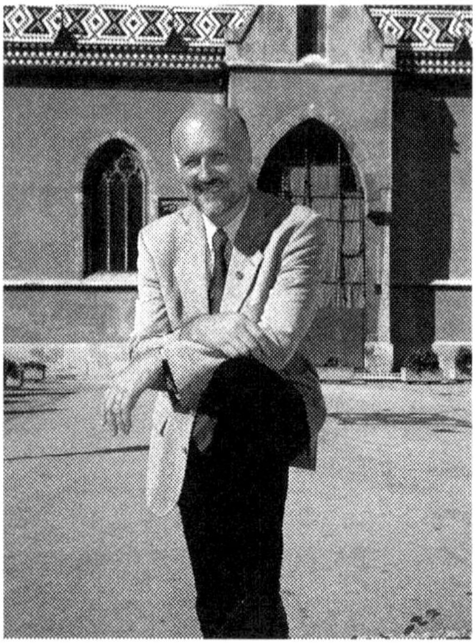

Disease, by producing bilateral electrolytic lesions of the nucleus basalis in rats.

My wife, son, and daughter joined me for my stay in Ann Arbor. We all had an excellent time, and enjoyed the year very much. I thank everyone in the Department for their help, especially my teacher and friend Edward F. Domino.

Editor's note: Ante Simonic was born on September 19, 1949 in Rijeka, Croatia. In 1973 he received his M.D. from the University of Rijeka. In 1977 he received his M.S. and in 1980 his Ph.D. all at the same institution. Dr. Simonic spent a year here at University of Michigan.

His primary research theme here at Michigan was cholinergic neurotransmission in the CNS, Alzheimer's Disease. In 1987, he became Professor and Chairman of the Department of Pharmacology at the Medical School of Rijeka. From 1991-1994, he was Dean of the Medical School of Rijeka.

Dr. Simonic was member of the Croatian Physiological Society, Croatian Pharmacological Society, International Union of Pharmacological Societies, European Union of Pharmacological Societies, Collegium Internationale Neuro-Psychopharmacologicum, European College of Neuropsychopharmacology, and the Calcium Club.

Dr. Simonic was the recipient of the Prize in Scientific Activity from the Croatian Physiological Society in both 1981 and 1984. In 1987, he received the Medical School of Rijeka Award. From 1991-1993, he was president of the Croatian Pharmacological Society.

Dr. Simonic's areas of interest are spinal cord trauma, ischemia and hypoxia of the brain, Alzheimer's disease, convulsive disorders, calcium channel blockers, nootropics, and cholinergic drug. He is now Deputy Prime Minister of Croatia.

Cynthia L. Cooper, Ph.D., 1987-1990

I worked with Dr. Ron Holz from 1987-1990 for a second postdoctoral fellowship. Ron was a very supportive mentor for me and allowed me to pursue my own ideas. This was my first time to experience that type of independence, and although I was not a very productive scientist by publication standards, I learned much more about my strengths and weaknesses as a scientist. In addition, I was supported by all the faculty of UM Pharmacology who displayed a high level of collegiality and professionalism.

Every Friday seminar (I think they were on Fridays) was like going to a national science meeting and hearing top-notch experts or first-year graduate students communicate their ideas in a very professional manner. The seminars were well-attended, which allowed for lively informal discussions on the most current research topics. I learned what PCR was for the first time during a student seminar. I actually thought she had invented the technology for part of the presentation.

I will always value my time at UM because the research experience gave me the confidence I needed to apply for and pursue an academic position where I have become a PI in a small research lab at the predominately undergraduate Truman State University in Missouri. Although my teaching load is large and research is not the largest part of my job, I am able to involve many undergraduate students in meaningful research projects that get them started on their own careers that range from attending medical and graduate school to teaching science (K-12) to working for biotechnology companies. Thank you Ron and thank you UM Pharmacology.

Paul T. Hoff, M.D., 1987-1993

It's been 12 years since I last roamed the halls of Med Sci I. The Department has changed a lot since then, but I'm happy to hear that many of the same faces remain. Upon finishing my master's degree with Dr. Lucchesi, I attended Medical School at U of M and finished in 1993. I am now at St. Joseph Hospital in Ann Arbor practicing general otolaryngology, and hold a clinical appointment in the Department of Otolaryngology at the University of Michigan.

My four years in the Department of Pharmacology were very productive and formative years. I will always consider Dr. Lucchesi to be one of my greatest role models. His work ethic and high expectations, as well as his generosity in allowing his research assistants to participate in all levels of scientific discovery, will always be remembered.

Peter Wick, Ph.D., 1987-1995

Having been in the midst of such a large community of dedicated scientists is something I've come to appreciate more and more with every passing year. I'd like to thank Ron Holz, Mary Bittner, Bill Pratt and so many others for their guidance and inspiration. Looking back on all my time in the Department of Pharmacology I would have to say the most important thing I came away with was the ability to learn from experimental failures and move on. After two years as a postdoc at Northeastern University studying dopamine D4 receptors, I set out on a career in biomedical software. Not having any prior training in that field, it was having that outlook that made all the difference. Along the way I've worked on systems for secure collection and analysis of clinical trial data to high-throughput genomic screening software and my own software aimed at helping patients adhere to complex medical regimens at home.

My experiences at Michigan also inspired me to begin life-long work at raising money for medical research. In 1997 I co-founded a group called Team Friends of Frada (www.friendsoffrada.org) that has gathered close to $100,000 for the Jimmy Fund/Dana-Farber Cancer Institute and the National MS Society in our first 7 years. Keep up the good work, everybody.

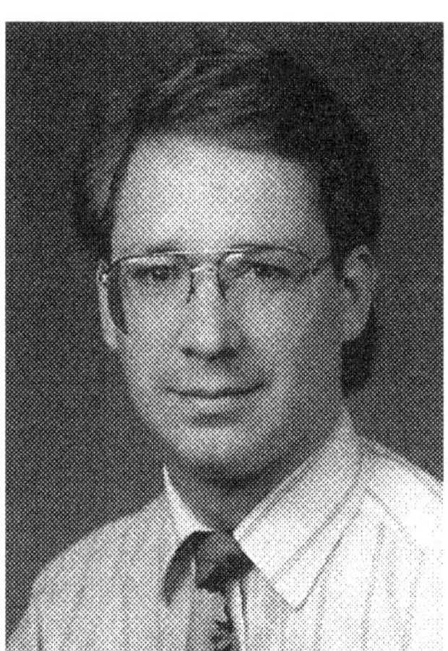

Donalyn Scheuner, Ph.D., 1989-1992

I received my Ph.D. from the Department of Pharmacology at the University of Michigan in 1992 and I conducted my research under the mentorship of Dr. Ronald Holz. My educational experience was an excellent one as I benefited greatly from the keen intellect and motivation of Dr. Holz. My educational experience was also impacted significantly by the members of the Department who participated in my oral defense, contributed to my thesis committee, provided course instruction, and

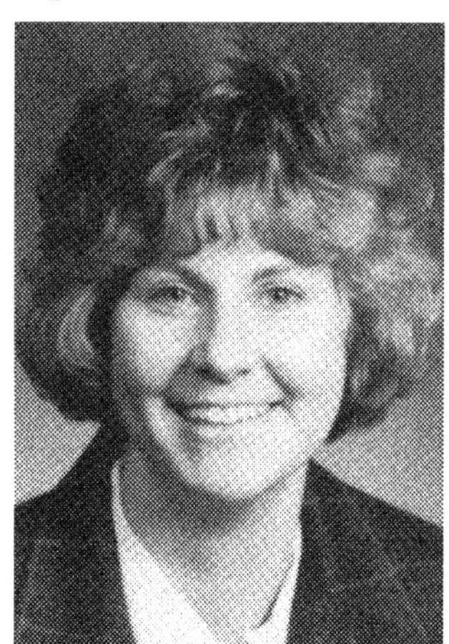

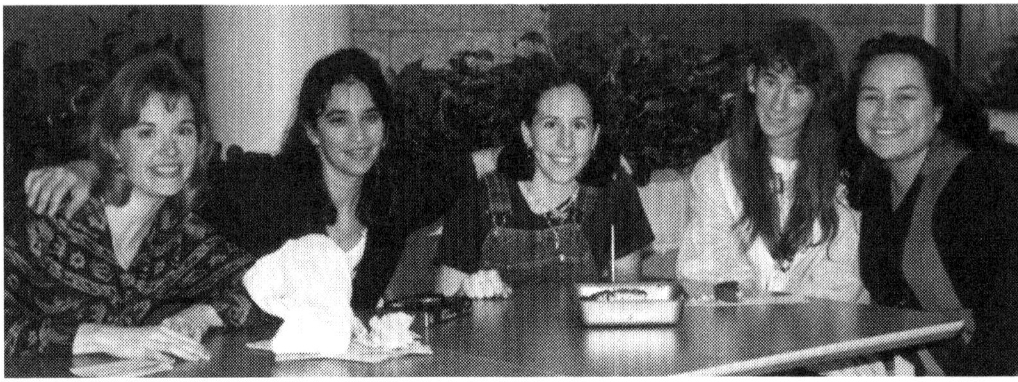

Jill, Lana , Sara, Marry , and Keike celebrating Marry's birthday, ca. 1995.

also organized a rigorous student seminar program. My intellectual development was shaped by many caring, dedicated, and talented scientists that served as excellent role models. In particular, I am thankful to have benefited from the instruction and guidance of Peggy Gnegy, Steve Fisher, Rick Neubig, Ted Ueda, Bill Pratt, Ben Lucchesi, Ed Domino, and the chairmen Ray Ruddon and Ray Counsell. In reflecting upon my graduate experiences, I have thought many times that I am privileged to have been trained by Ron Holz and to have been a member of a department where the science was rigorous and innovative and where there was a strong program for the training of young scientists.

As I am nearing the end of my postdoctoral training, it is my ambition to obtain a position where I am able to fully realize my potential as a scientist incorporating all that I have observed and learned from my mentors, role models, and fellow peers.

Marry Vaughan, 1989-present

I started working here in the Department on Oct. 1, 1989, when I stopped in to visit my sister, Theresa Vaughan, who was working in Oksana Lockridge's lab. Oksana asked me if I want to be dishwasher for her and Dr. La Du. After a while, other labs asked me to wash their dishes, and now I am the dishwasher for almost every lab in the Department, as well as a couple other labs in other departments.

Although I don't have any degrees or honors, awards, or papers, and I really don't know much about science, I do keep all those dishes clean, so everyone can do their experiments. Not an easy job, everyone finds out when I go on vacation. Once when the distilled water was out, I carried a full carboy of water, all the way from Kresge II to MSRB III, without a cart, so there would be water for experiments. Maybe not the smartest thing I've done, but some people are still impressed, years later.

Over the years, I must have put thousands of pipet tips in those empty boxes, and have done all the things that nobody else wants to do, like scrub mold out of the cold rooms and autoclave all those stinky bags of waste and liquid waste, from the tissue culture rooms. I've defrosted freezers, collected the mail and brought the packages to the labs (the hard way, without a cart), made the coffee, labeled tubes from like 1 to a million, with tubes 1a, 1b...and made lots of copies on the copy machine. Sometimes, I've copied entire books, one page at a time.

Also, in Dr. Lockridge's lab and Dr. La Du's lab, I learned how to make gels, the big ones, with the big glass plates, from the old days. I quickly became a gel-making expert, cranking out perfect, bubble-free gels, one after another. I also poured lots of plates, did filter lifts, made lots of buffer and medium, and even did DNA sequencing once. Now, in addition to being a dishwasher/lab assistant, I'm also the pharmacology photographer and sort of a travel agent for part of the second floor.

Aside from trying to find a parking space, I've really enjoyed working in the pharmacology department for all these years, and I hope I can stay for many more.

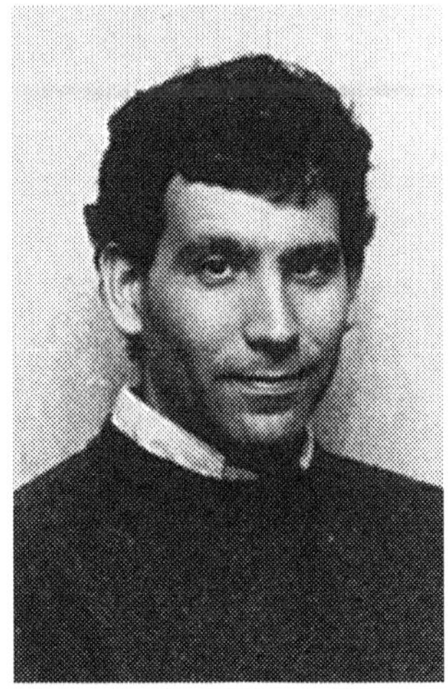

Jonathan Maybaum, Ph.D., 1983-present

As an undergraduate student at M.I.T., I was on course to become an organic chemist. However, by my senior year I was looking for a more biologically applied outlet for my interests in chemical structures and properties. Taking the advice of a postdoc in the lab where I was doing a research project, I applied to the program in Pharmaceutical Chemistry at UCSF. In the summer of 1976 I boarded a "hippie bus" called the Green Tortoise for my move from Cambridge to San Francisco.

When I got there, I probably surprised them by choosing the Pharmaceutics subprogram, rather than Medicinal Chemistry. Actually, the lab that I went into (directed by Dr. Wolfgang Sadée) was not easily identifiable as being focused on either Pharmaceutics or Medicinal Chemistry— it really was more of a Pharmacology training experience (although I did not realize it at the time). Dr. Sadée's lab was the most divergent that I have ever seen in that it was involved in two very different areas: antineoplastic antimetabolites and opiate receptors. I worked in the antimetabolite area and was able to finish my Ph.D. thesis work in just under four years. It was a wonderfully collegial and interesting group. One of the postdocs in the lab during this time was Kary Mullis, who later won the Nobel Prize for inventing PCR. In a Scientific American article, Kary later noted that he was actually thinking about some technical issues in my project (nucleoside triphosphate thermal stability) when his mind wandered in the direction that led him to PCR.

During my last year in the Sadée lab we hosted Dr. H. George Mandel for a sabbatical visit. Dr. Mandel was the Chair of Pharmacology at George Washington University at that time and he recruited me to come to his lab for post-doctoral training. I was given great autonomy during my time at GW, and I developed a project that was aimed at understanding how incorporation of 6-thioguanine into DNA could eventually cause cells to die. This was where I first started to focus on downstream determinants of cell death. My work resulted in the discovery of a lesion that I named "Unilateral Chromatid Damage."

Late in 1982 I applied for several faculty positions, including one in Pharmacology at the University of Michigan. Upon returning from that interview, I got a fortune cookie that said: "Fortune lies in a north westerly direction. Take advantage of it." And so I did.

I arrived at UM in June, 1983, and started up my lab in the Upjohn Center for Clinical Pharmacology as a member of the Cancer Pharmacology Program, directed by Dr. Bill Ensminger. Not long after that, Dr. Ted Lawrence was recruited into the Department of Radiation Oncology, in nearby space. Bill and Ted became (and are still) two of my closest collaborators, and we successfully organized a Program Project grant that was centered on radiosensitization. This brought my research direction back to the direction of thymidylate synthase inhibitors (which I had studied in graduate school), as they comprise an important class of clinical radiosensitizers.

At The McNeil Symposium, 1983

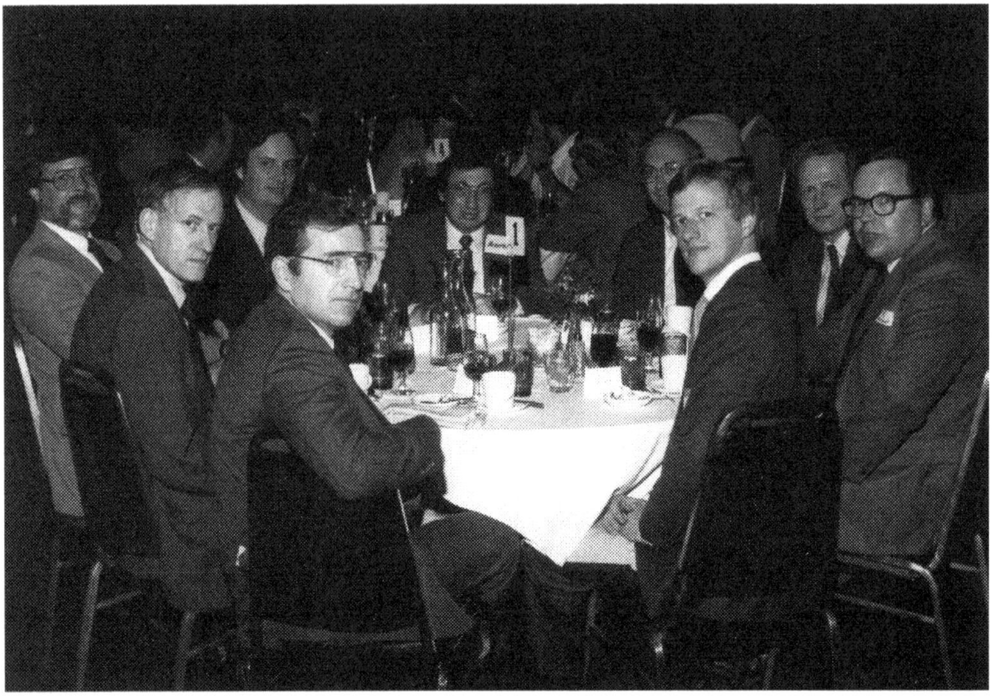

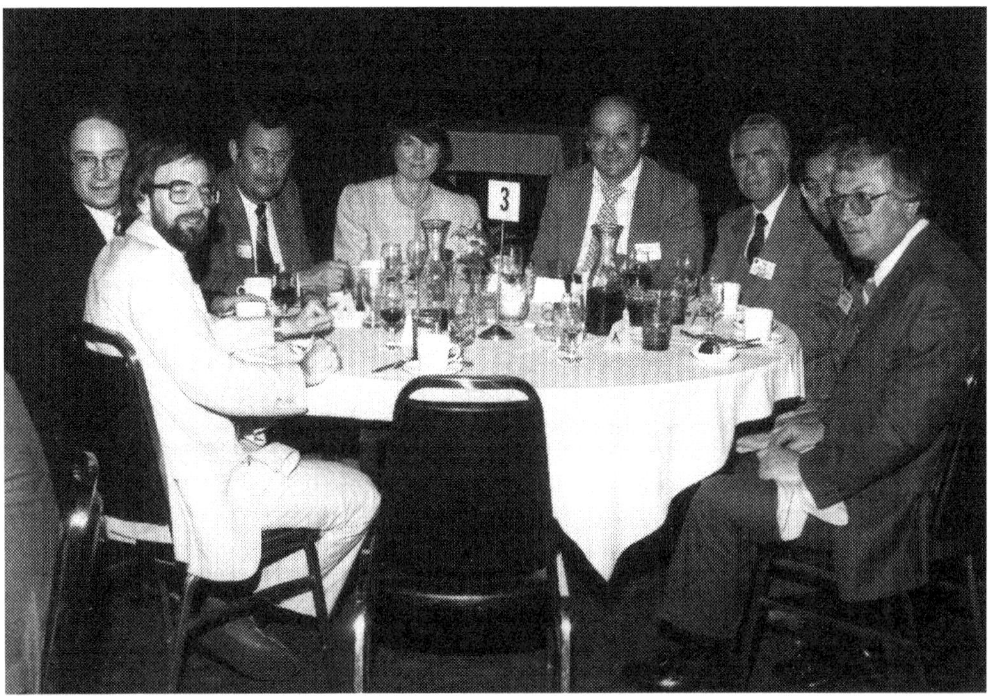

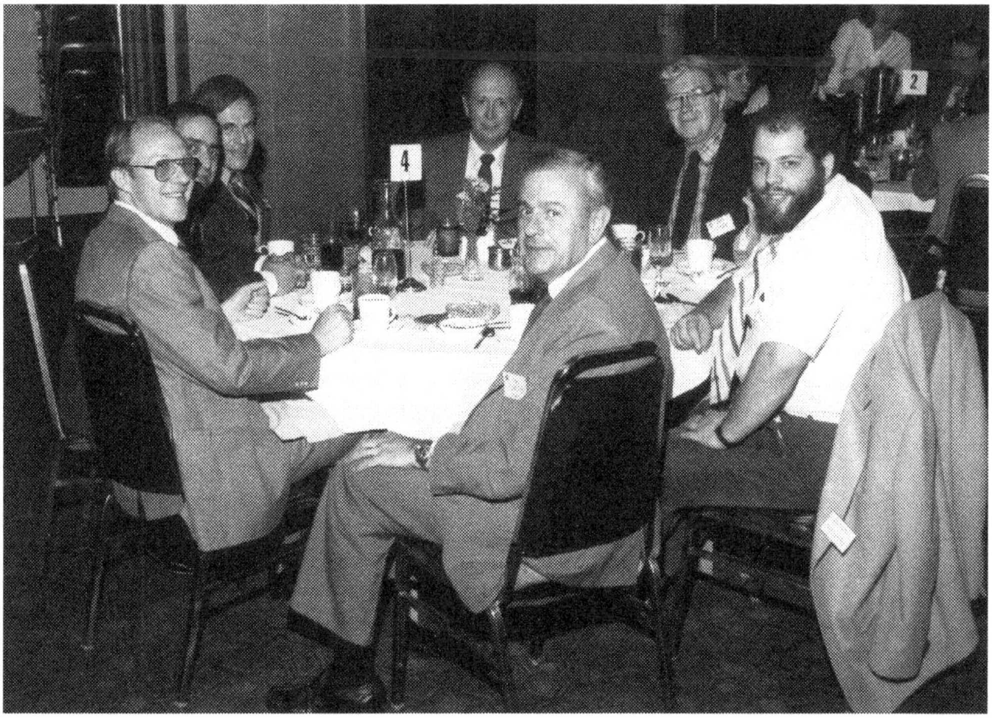

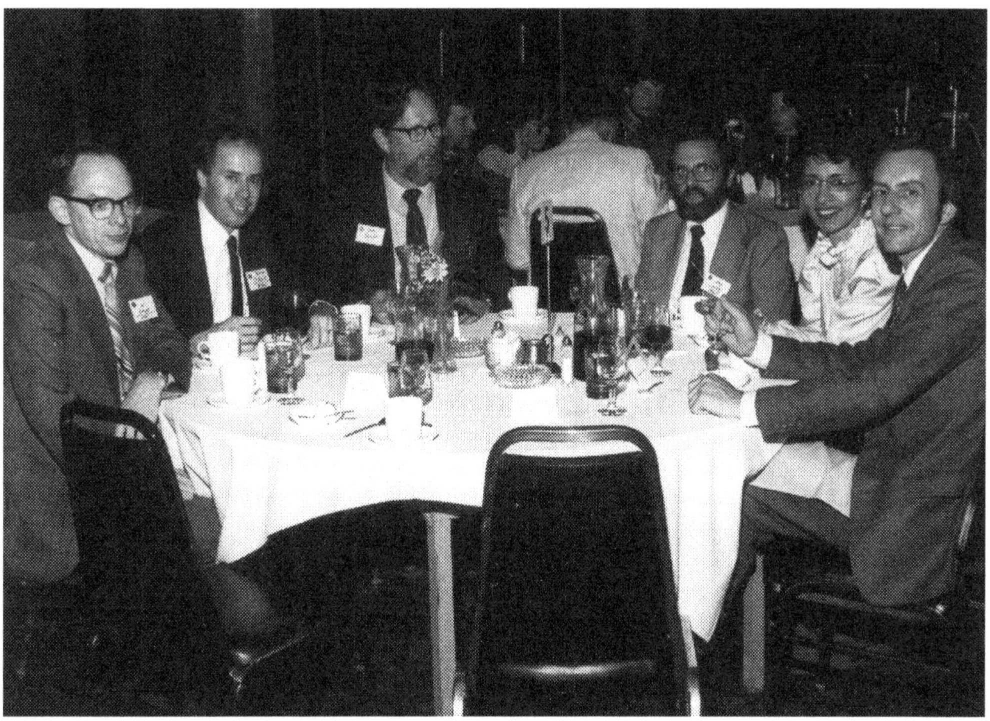

1981

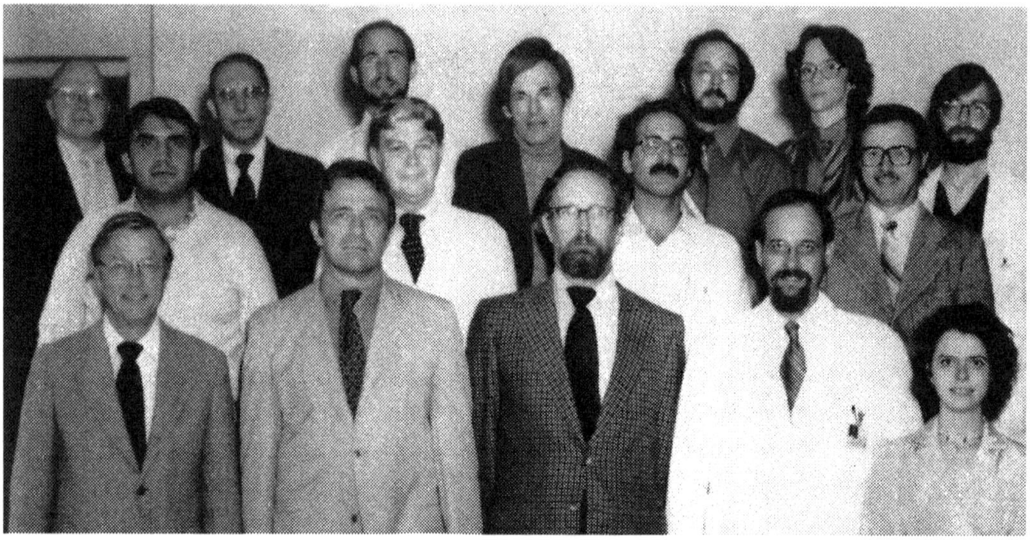

Front row: W. Webber, F. Medzihradsky, H. Swain, C. Smith, M. Gnegy
Second row: J. Woods, B. La Du, R. Holz, R. Counsell
Third row: K. Cochran, B. Lucchesi, H. Eckerson, V. Zannoni, M. Shlafer, A. Young, J. Katz

1983

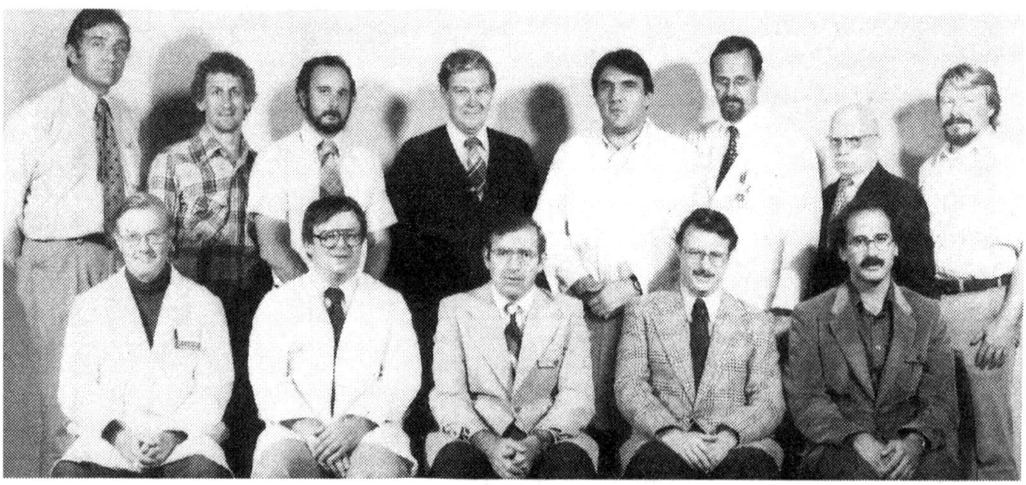

Front row: W. Weber, W. Ensminger, R.Ruddon, R. Counsell, R. Holz
Second row: F. Medzihradsky, T. Landefeld, M. Shlafer, B. La Du, J. Woods, C. Smith, K. Cochran, R. Simpson

1984

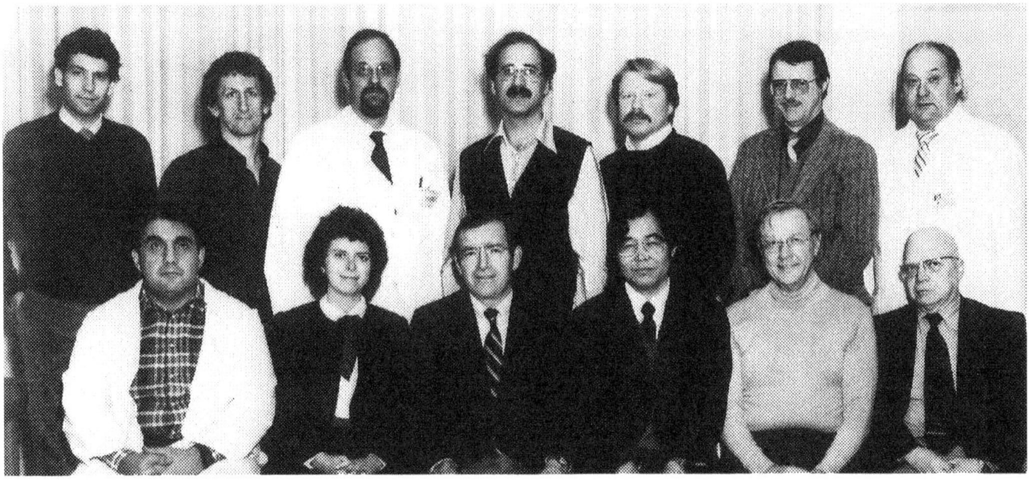

Front row: J. Wood, M. Gnegy, R. Ruddon, T. Ueda, W. Weber, K. Cochran
Second row: J. Maybaum, T. Landefeld, C. Smith, R. Holz, R. Simpson, R. Counsell, E. Domino

1986

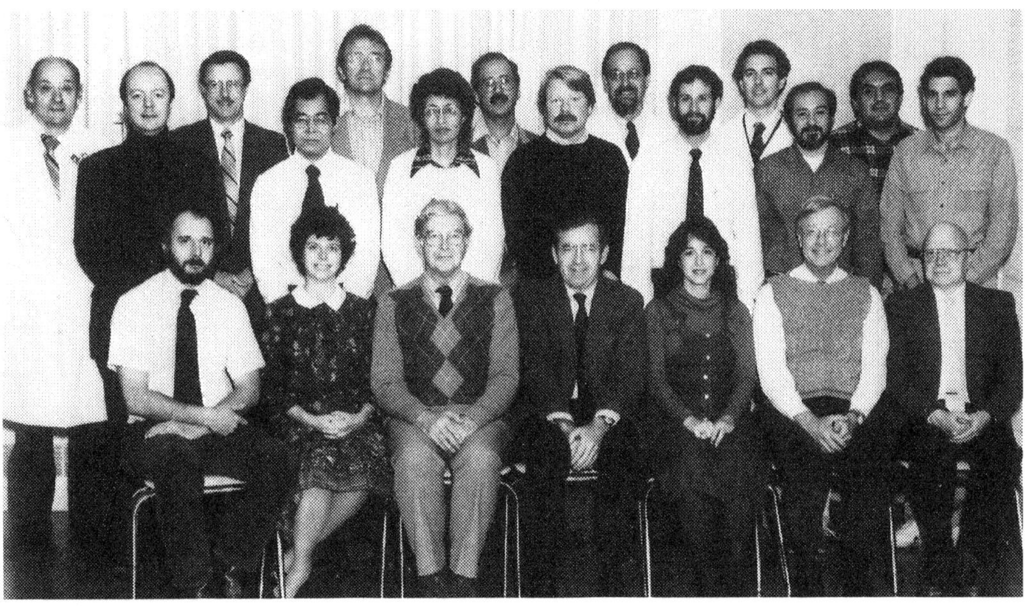

Front row: M. Shlafer, M. Gnegy, B. La Du, R. Ruddon, D. Gmerek, W. Weber, K. Cochran
Second row: E. Domino, S. Fisher, R. Counsell, T. Ueda, F. Medzihradsky, P. Hollingsworth, R. Holz, R. Simpson, C. Smith, R. Neubig, J. Lynch, W. Mancini, J. Woods, J. Maybaum

1987

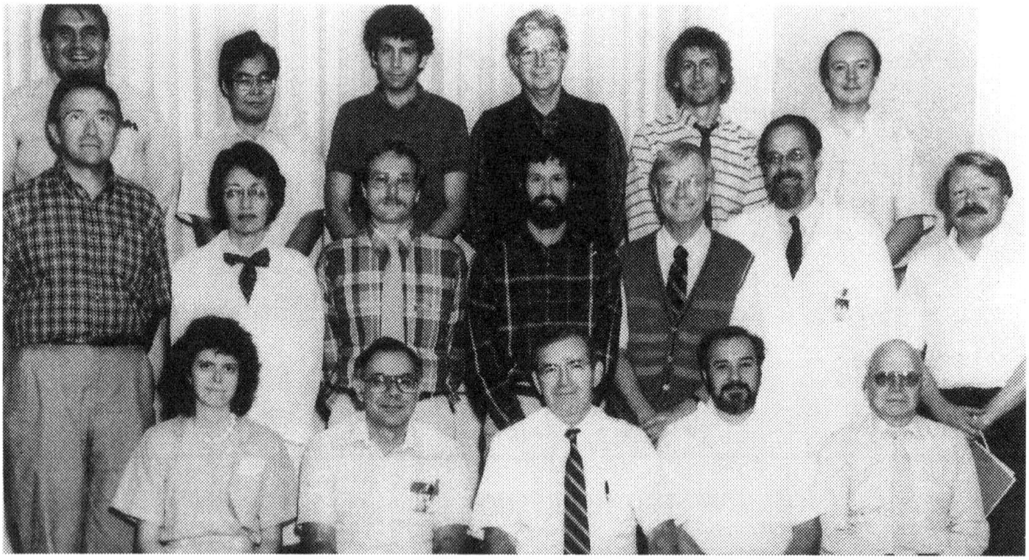

Front row: M. Gnegy, F. Perini, R. Ruddon, W. Mancini, K. Cochran
Second row: F. Medzihradsky, P. Hollingsworth, M. Longino, R. Neubig, W. Weber, C. Smith, R. Simpson
Third row: J. Woods, T. Ueda, J. Maybaum, B. La Du, T. Landefeld, S. Fisher

1989

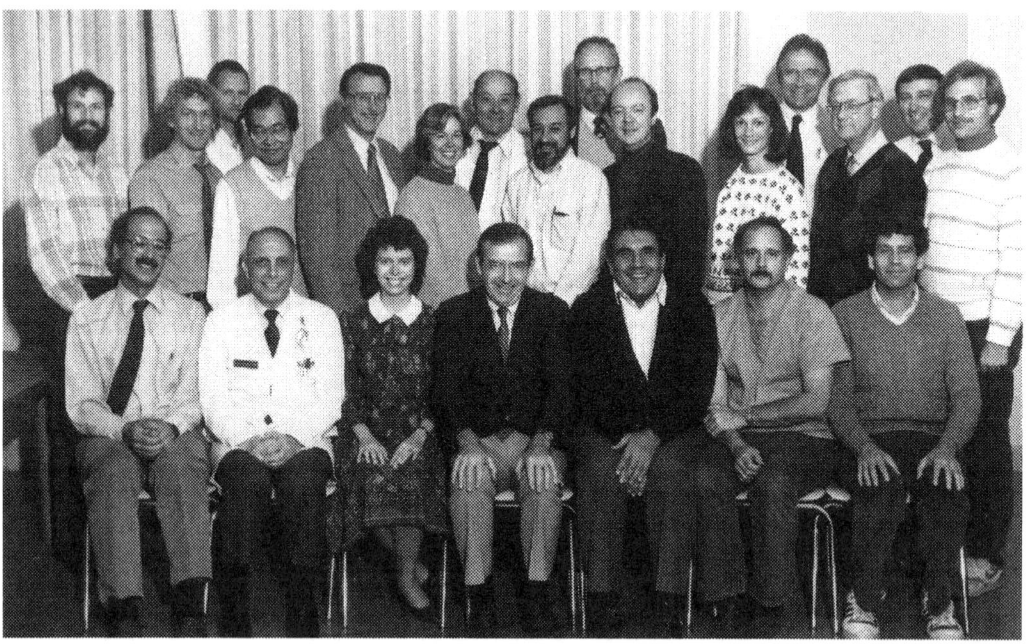

Front row: R. Holz, B. Lucchesi, M. Gnegy, R. Ruddon, J. Woods, M. Shlafer, J. Maybaum
Second row: R. Neubig, T. Landefeld, C. France, T. Ueda, R. Counsell, G. Winger, E. Domino, W. Mancini, H. Swain, S. Fisher, D. Shewach, F. Medzihradsky, W. Weber, W. Piper, M. Longino

20

Memoirs: 1995-2001

Jillian Helen Broadbear, Ph.D.

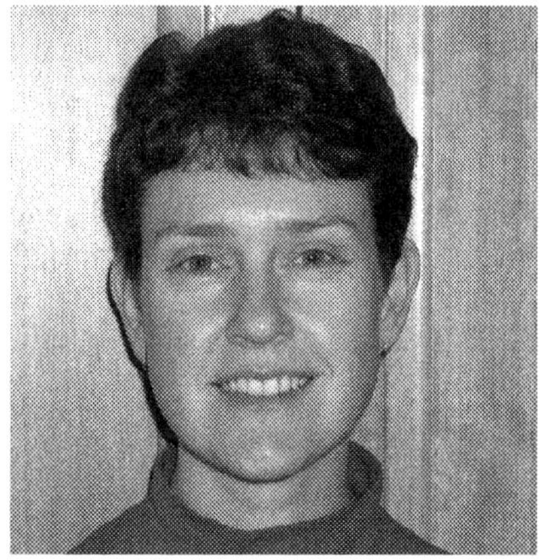

Born and educated in Melbourne, Australia (B.Sc. Monash University, 1987), I first visited Ann Arbor and the U of M while on vacation in the fall of 1990. At that time I was a research assistant in the Department of Clinical Pharmacology (Hypertension) at the Austin Hospital, a campus of the University of Melbourne. I was very impressed by Ann Arbor and with campus life, and interviewed informally at Parke-Davis (now Pfizer). I also left a copy of my resume in the UM Pharmacology office. Two days before I was due to return to Australia, I was contacted by Dr. Charles France, a senior post-doctoral researcher and laboratory manager working with Dr. James Woods in the Behavioral Pharmacology Unit. I met with Charles France, as well as with Dr. Gail Winger, senior research scientist, and we discussed possible job opportunities.

I left for Australia the following day, uncertain of when or whether I would be returning to Ann Arbor. However, through the persistence of my future husband, John Cookson (who would receive a Ph.D. from the University of Michigan Department of Nuclear Engineering, Materials, in 1996) and Gail Winger's advocacy, I received a job offer by phone from Jim Woods in March 1992. In April, I started work as a research assistant in a newly created position that involved the screening of codeinones and morphinones synthesized by Dr. John Lewis (U of Bristol, UK). My job was to measure them to determine their opioid activity and selectivity in mouse models of analgesia. I worked on this project for a little over two years, and had the opportunity to attend my first meeting (CPDD, Toronto, 1994) and to author my first paper, under the guidance of Dr. S. Stevens Negus, who had taken the place of Charles France prior to my arrival.

By this time, both Steve Negus and John Lewis had encouraged me to consider applying for graduate school. I took their advice, and in the fall of 1994, I became a student in the biopsychology program, with Jim Woods (who has a joint appointment in the psychology department) as my advisor. The biopsych program is very flexible, and I was able to take classes in pharmacology, biochemistry and neuroanatomy in addition to psychology. In the year after I attained candidacy, 1996, my first child Kathryn, was born and I commenced work on the project that would become my thesis work.

I moved from mice and opioids to Rhesus monkeys and cocaine self-administration, in Gail Winger's laboratory. The project was an idea that had been expressed in Gail's grant and was a perfect thesis project! The title of my thesis was "Cocaine self-administration and hypothalamic-pituitary-adrenal (HPA) axis activity in rhesus monkeys," and I defended in December 1998. The supposition for this work was based on rat data published outside our lab, whose hypothesis was that the release of stress hormones plays a causative role in stimulant-related behavior. We explored this hypothesis by doing a number of pharmacological manipulations of the HPA axis in rhesus monkeys that had a history of cocaine self-injection (delivered via an indwelling intravenous catheter following lever presses generated by the monkey). Cocaine dose dependently stimulates the HPA axis, and although it was possible to selectively suppress the HPA axis at each level of hormone release, none of these manipulations affected cocaine-maintained drug self-administration behavior. Jim Woods and Gail Winger offered me a postdoctoral research position that enabled me to continue this work. In 1999, my second daughter, Sophie, was born, and we published four papers from my dissertation. An important question that remained unanswered was whether it was the CNS effects of CRH itself that influenced drug-maintained behavior. CRH is the primary hormone released in the HPA axis response to stress. The tools for investigating this question were only then becoming available.

My postdoc years were focused on the investigation of several CRH receptor antagonists, and although the role of the central release of CRH in cocaine-maintained behavior has not yet been elicidated (due to unsuitability of the compounds that we tested), several interesting studies were completed. For instance, during our investigation of antalarmin, a CRH antagonist, we found to our surprise that antalarmin itself had reinforcing properties! We also examined the HPA effects of self-administered drugs from different classes — an opioid, stimulant, benzodiazepine, barbiturate, NMDA-antagonist, and ethanol — and found that although each of these drugs has reinforcing properties, they varied widely in their effects on the HPA axis. This implies that there is no unifying role for the HPA axis that underlies the reinforcing properties of drugs of abuse.

In March of 2001, I contacted Professor Iain Clarke at Prince Henry's Medical Institute of Research (PHMIR) in Melbourne, whom I had met at the ISPNE conference in Melbourne the previous year. My family and I were planning to return to Australia at the end of 2002 and I needed to find out what sort of opportunities might be available. I attached my CV and, to my amazement, was offered a position on return email! Iain Clarke and I met in Melbourne in April and Iain agreed to hold the position for me until January 2002.

Having arrived in the Pharmacology Department more than a decade before, with the expectation of a research assistantship and a stay of no more than two years, I left instead armed with an advanced degree and a new appreciation for the excitement and rewards that come with a life in pharmacological research! I am exceedingly grateful for the many opportunities that Jim Woods and Gail Winger put in my path, and will treasure my Ann Arbor years.

I am currently employed as a senior research officer at Monash University (Physiology), examining the interaction between the HPA axis and antidepressant treatment. Although geographically I'm back where I started, my association with the Pharmacology Department at the University of Michigan radically transformed my outlook, expectations and abilities.

Vignettes: "I Remember When..."

Staff and Students of the 1990s and Beyond

Shawn C. Black, Ph.D., 1990-1994

In the Department of Pharmacology at the University of Michigan, my primary experience was as a postdoctoral fellow in the lab of Dr. Ben Lucchesi. As Ben has been a faculty member at Michigan since my Ph.D. mentor, Dr. John H. McNeill (dean of Faculty of Pharmaceutical Sciences at the University of British Columbia) was a graduate student at Michigan, for me working with Ben was an opportunity to learn not only of current and future directions of pharmacology, but to also learn of the history and evolution of the Department. These discussions were corroborated, and refuted, by Dr. Zannoni, a regular visitor to Ben's always-full and free coffee pot.

Through my understanding of some of the history of the evolution of the Department, I gained a greater appreciation for its contributions to pharmacological research. The number of Department alumni attending the 100th anniversary celebration and associated Wolverine football game also contributed to the realization of the depth and breadth of the influence of Michigan on pharmacology in the United States, Canada, and elsewhere. From a personal perspective, my interest in pharmacology was stimulated by two alumni of the Department, Drs. John McNeill and Jack Diamond, who lectured to me while I attended UBC. Also from a Canadian perspective, while at Michigan I had the opportunity to listen to Dr. Mark Nickerson speak and it was interesting to learn that he left Michigan to play a major role in the building of the Department of Pharmacology at the University of Manitoba, and that he also later became chairman at McGill University.

While the research experience of Ben's lab inculcated a view and approach to pharmacological research that remains with me in my current research, memories of Michigan also include Drs. Ray Counsell and Marshal Shlafer who provided me with a very rewarding lecturing opportunity while I was at Michigan. Having studied as a postdoctoral fellow, lectured to nursing students, and lived in Ann Arbor, I now understand why John McNeil, as a dean at UBC, wore Michigan attire when I visited his home as a graduate student one Saturday afternoon long before I understood the meaning of "Go Blue." Lastly, my Michigan experience includes the birth of our daughter at U of M Hospital. This is our life-long link to Michigan Pharmacology.

Lourdes Estrada, Ph.D., 1991-1997

As of my experience in the Department, I must treasure the enduring friendships with students as well as faculty that I made through the years at the Department. Dr. Weber and Dr. Pratt were instrumental in my dissertation work and are still very supportive of the development of my career. I will always be thankful to them.

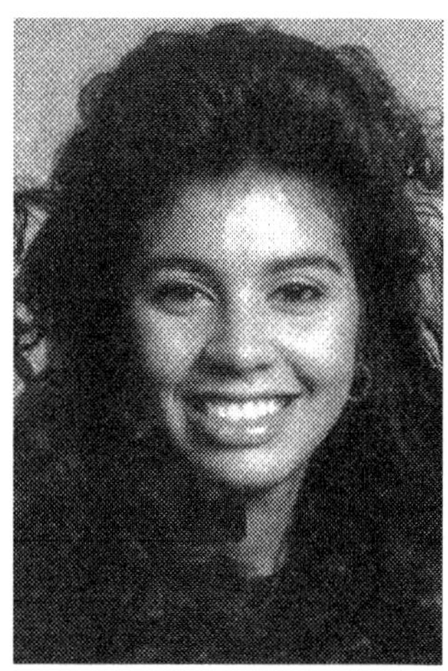

Kevin Wang, Ph.D., 1997-present

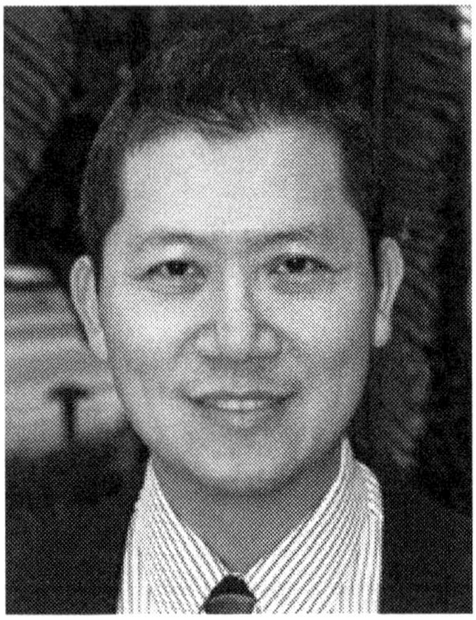

In February 1991, after two years of postdoctoral training, I was excited to finally start my career as a senior scientist at Parke-Davis in Ann Arbor (which eventually merged with Pfizer in 2000). In the next five to six years, I became increasingly drawn to the collaborative work and scientific exchange with faculty members at the neighboring University of Michigan Pharmacology Department. My frequent interactions with Drs. Margaret Gnegy and Stephen Fisher, and the chairman Dr. Paul Hollenberg, along with my love for the educational aspect of research, had prompted me to seek an adjunct appointment within the Pharmacology Department.

In January 1997, I was officially appointed an adjunct assistant professor of pharmacology. In those days, beside my own research activity at Pfizer, I kept myself engaged in UM Pharmacology events such as mentoring graduate students (Kim McGinnis, Ph.D., graduated in 1999; and YangHae Park, M.S., is a current Ph.D. candidate) and postdoctoral fellows (Dr. Iradj Hajimohammadreza, from 1993-95; Dr. Rand Posmantur, from 1996-98; Dr. Neeta Mukerjee in 1999-2000; Dr. Yuanhui Huang, from 1999-present); co-organizing the annual UM-Pfizer Pharmacology Poster Day; and coordinating and teaching Pharm 503, Industrial Pharmacology, which overviewed the pathway from drug target identification to clinical application. Through these channels, I wanted to pass on my industrial research experience to the next generation of UM pharmacologists!

In July 2002 I joined the Department of Psychiatry at the University of Florida, College of Medicine as an associate professor of psychiatry and neuroscience at the McKnight Brain Institute in Gainesville, FL.

Jyoti Malhotra, Ph.D., 1998-present

I earned my Ph.D. in India and came to the United States to do my postdoctoral training. My postdoctoral career started in the laboratory of Michael Hortsch in the Department of Anatomy and Cell Biology, now renamed Cell and Developmental Biology. I worked on neural cell adhesion molecules and their link to the cytoskeleton. The experience in Dr. Hortsch's lab was very rewarding intellectually, and was also productive, which pushed my career a step further.

I moved into the Department of Pharmacology in the lab of Lori Isom, as a senior postdoc, and continued my work on the cell adhesion field. I now worked on a very novel idea of characterizing sodium channel subunits as cell adhesion molecules, and their role in localization of sodium channels in both brain and heart. The postdoc experience was very productive and I was promoted to research faculty in the Department of Pharmacology. It has been a great experience working in the Department of Pharmacology, especially in Lori Isom's lab; Dr. Isom has been very supportive. It has been pleasure to have Paul Hollenberg as the chair. He has supported me all along, promoting me to faculty level and writing very strong letters for my independent grant applications. The UM Pharmacology Department is ranked very high in the country, and with such strong old and new faculty in the Department, it will stay at the top.

1990

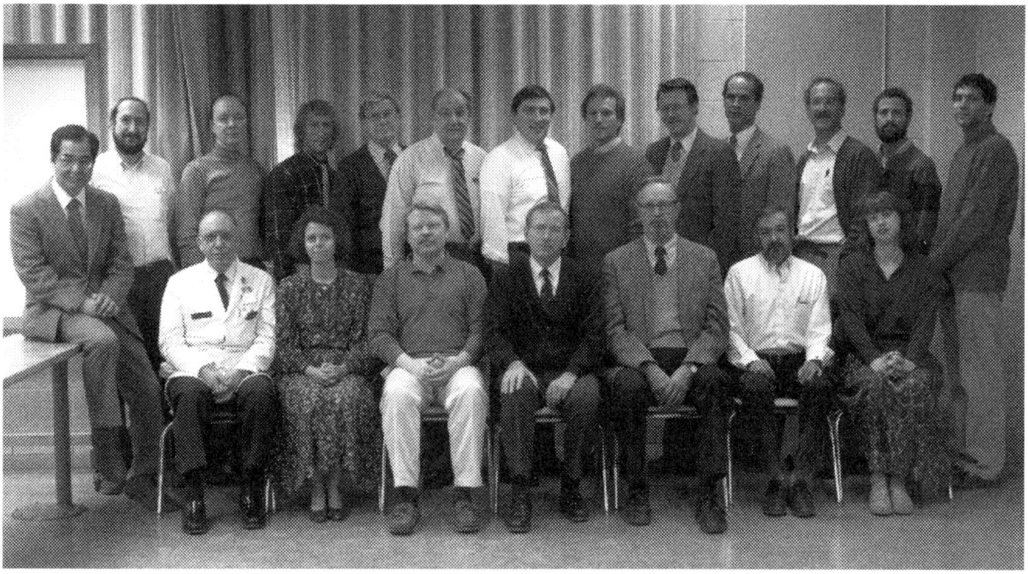

Front row: B. Lucchesi, M. Gnegy, R. Simpson, R. Ruddon, H. Swain, W. Mancini, M. Bittner
Second row: T. Ueda, D. Brenner, S. Fisher, T. Landefeld, B. La Du, E. Domino,W. Piper, M. Longino, R. Counsell, R. Newton, R. Holz, R. Neubig, J. Maybaum

1991

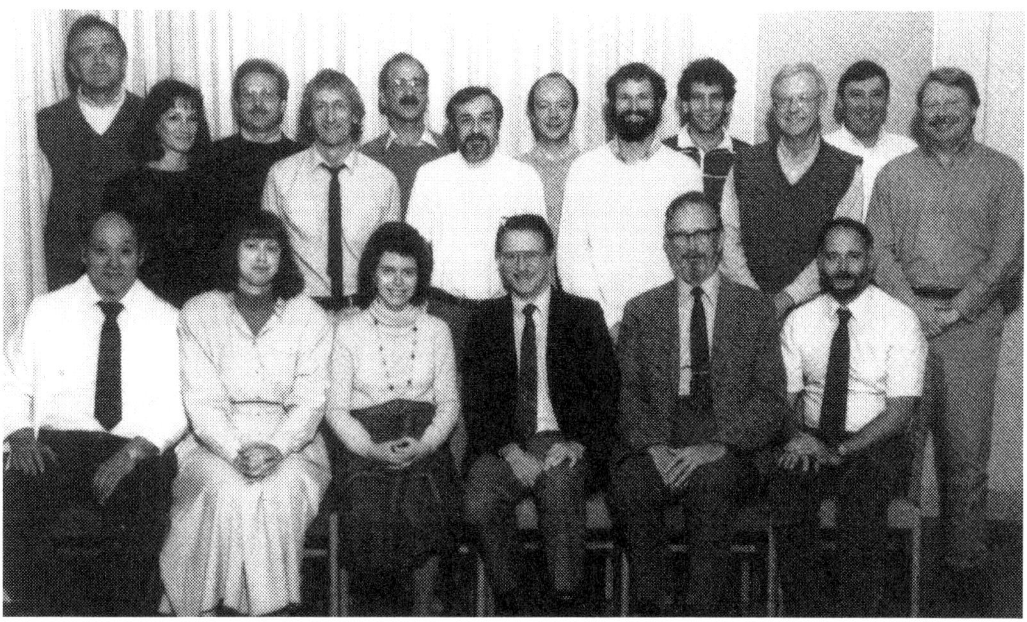

Front row: E. Domino, M. Bittner, M. Gnegy, R. Counsell, H. Swain, M, Shlafer
Second row: D. Shewach, T. Landefeld, W. Mancini, R. Neubig, W. Weber, R. Simpson
Third row: F. Medzihradsky, M. Longino, R. Holz, S. Fisher, J. Maybaum, W. Piper

1992

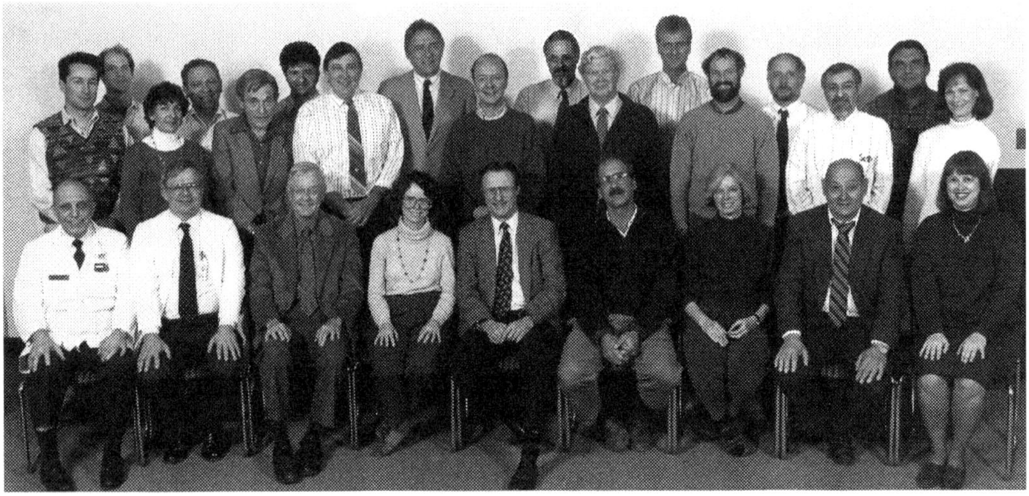

Front row: B. Lucchesi, W. Ensminger, W. Weber, M. Gnegy, R. Counsell, R. Holz, G. Winger, E. Domino, M. Bittner
Second row: S. Black, M Sommerman, V. Zannoni, W. Piper, S. Fisher, B. La Du, R. Neubig, W, Mancini,, D. Shewach
Third row: S. Negus, G. Levy, E. Butelman, F. Medzihradsky, C. Smith, G. Zernig, M. Shlafer, J. Woods

1994

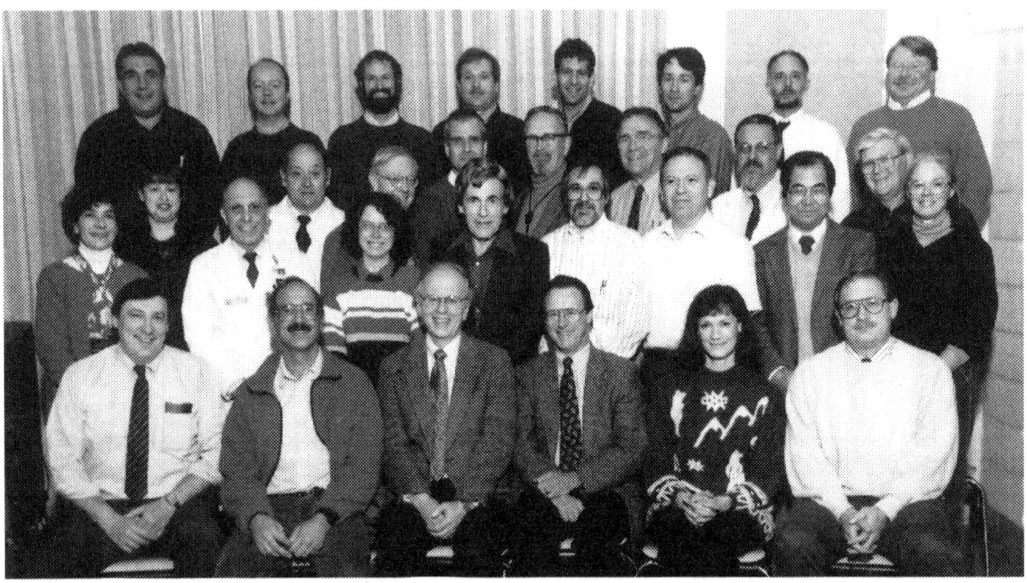

Front row: W. Piper, R. Holz, P. Hollenberg, R. Counsell, D. Shewach, C. Harris
Second row: M. Sommerman, B. Lucchesi, M. Gnegy, V. Zannoni,W. Mancini, G. Levy, T. Ueda, G. Winger
Third row: M. Bittner, E. Domino, W. Weber, G. Zernig, H. Swain, F. Medzihradsky, C. Smith, B. La Du
Fourth row: J. Woods, S. Fisher, R. Neubig, M. Longino, J. Maybaum, S. Black, M. Shlafer, R. Simpson

1997

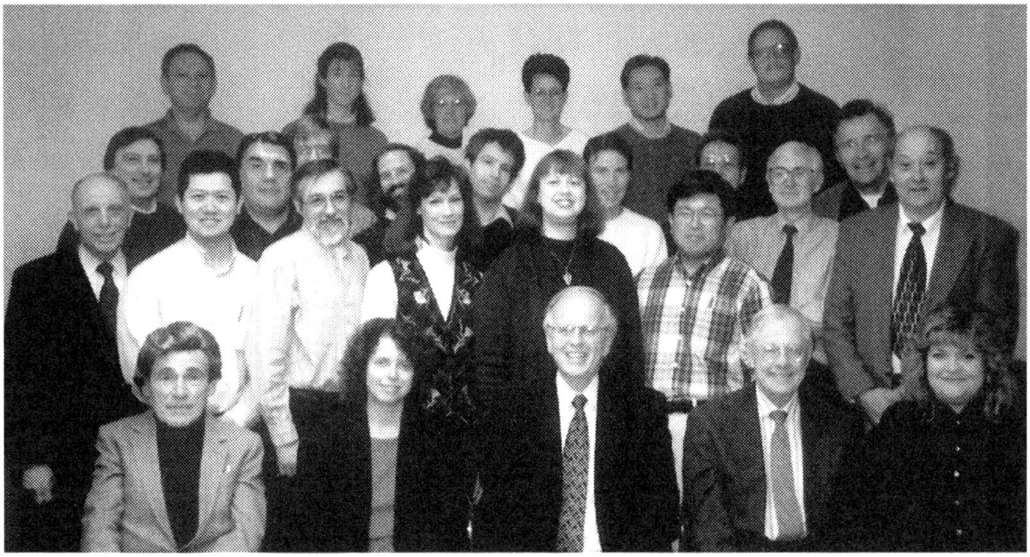

Front row: V. Zannoni, M. Gnegy, P. Hollenberg, W. Weber, L. Isom
Second row: B. Lucchesi, K. Wang, W. Mancini , D. Shewach, M. Bittner, S. Kishioka, E. Domino
Third row: W. Piper, J. Woods, K. Bently, R. Neubig, J. Maybaum, Eric Pakarinen, Mark Longino, J. Traynor, F. Medzihradsky
Fourth row: G. Levy, A. Remmers, G. Winger, L. Roberts-Kirchhoff, Y. Osawa, C. Harris

1999

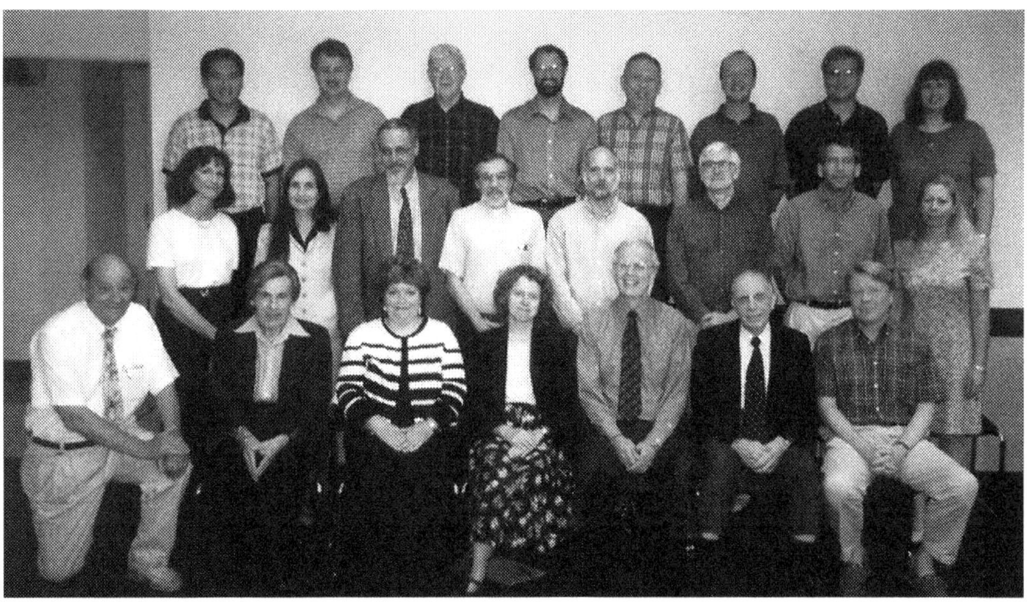

Front row: E. Domino, V. Zannoni, L. Isom, M. Gnegy, P. Hollenberg, B. Lucchesi, R. Simpson
Second row: D. Shewach, H. Baghdoyan, C. Smith, W. Mancini, M. Shlafer, J. Traynor, J. Maybaum, U. Kent
Third row: Y. Osawa, J. Stitzel, B. La Du, R. Neubig, G. Levy, S. Fisher, M. Longino, M. Bittner

2000

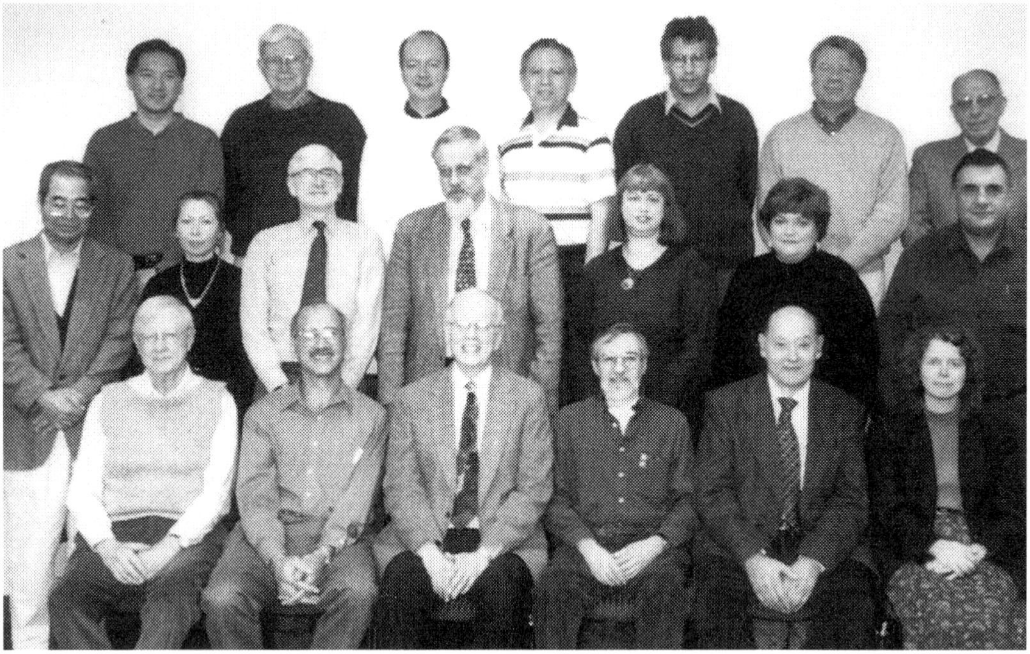

Front row: W. Weber, R. Holz, P. Hollenberg, W. Mancini, E. Domino, M. Gnegy
Second row: T. Ueda, U. Kent, J. Traynor, C. Smith, M. Bittner, L. Isom, J. Woods
Third row: Y. Osawa, B. La Du, S. Fisher, G. Levy, J. Maybaum, R. Simpson, B. Lucchesi

2002

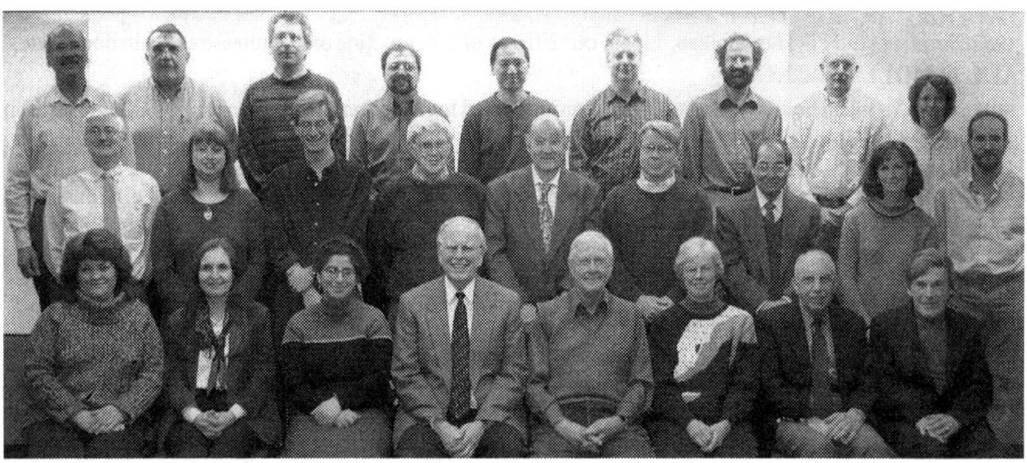

Front row: L. Isom, H. Baghdoyan, J. Malhotra, P. Hollenberg, W. Weber, G. Winger, B. Lucchesi, V. Zannoni
Second row: J. Traynor, M. Bittner, K. Bently, B. La Du, E. Domino, R. Simpson, T. Ueda, D. Shewach, J. Iniguez-Lluhi
Third row: R. Holz, J. Woods, J. Maybaum, D. Dragonov, Y. Osawa, J. Stitzel, R. Neubig, M Shlafer, M. Gnegy

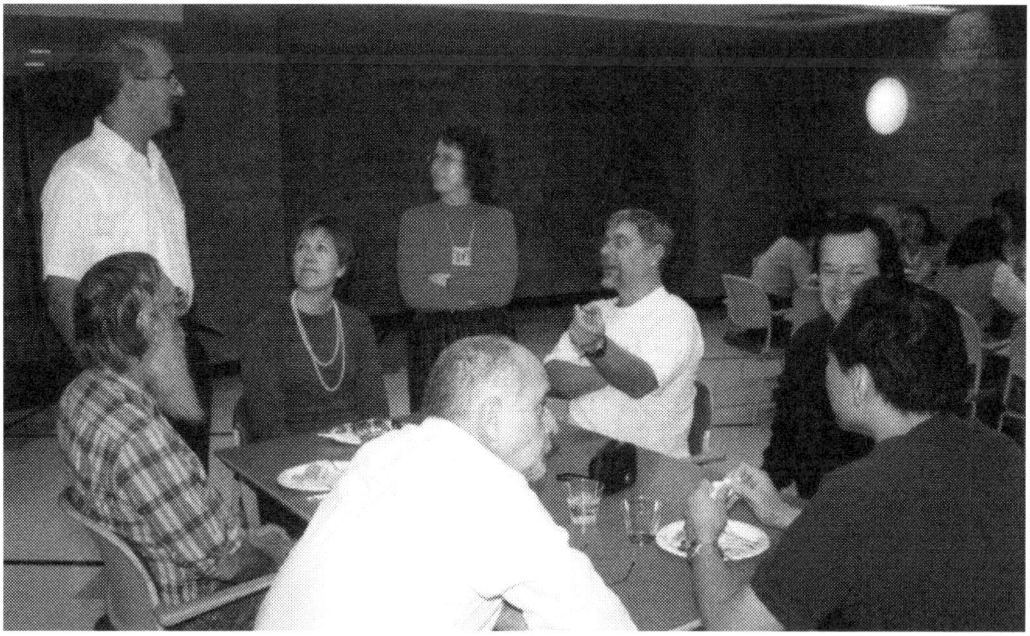

Tom Larmee responding to Ron Holz's comments; some are listening but the others are engaged in small talk.

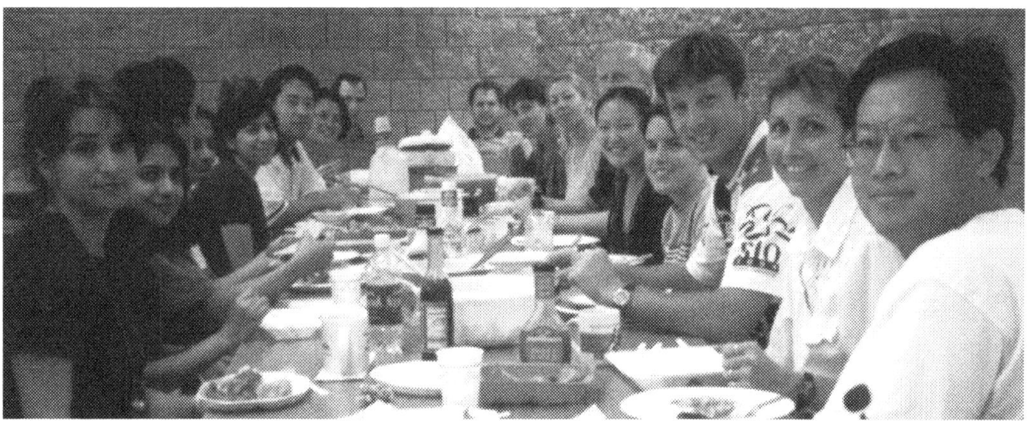

A Departmental party

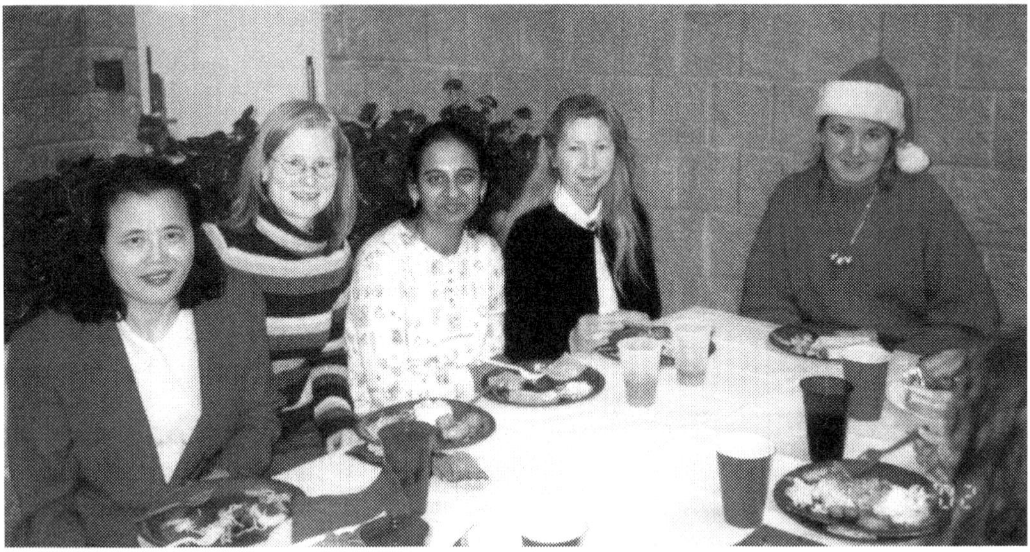

A Departmental Christmas party

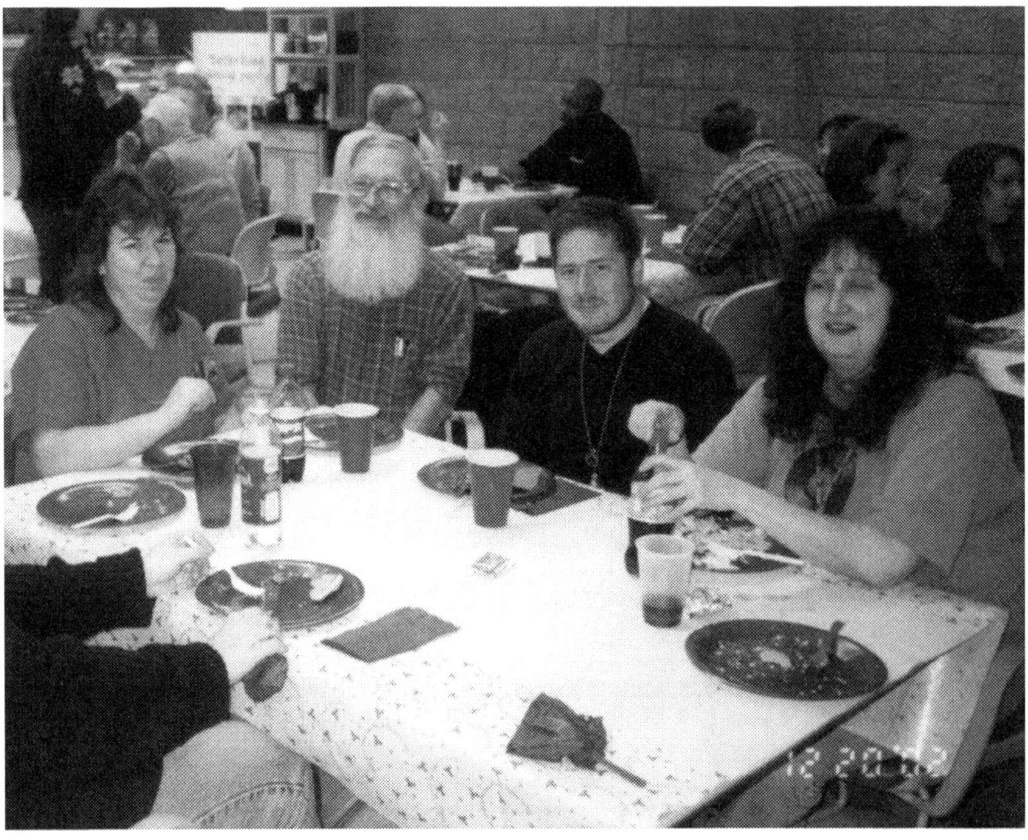

A Departmental Christmas party

21

Connections Between Industry and Academia

Harvey R. Kaplan, Ph.D.

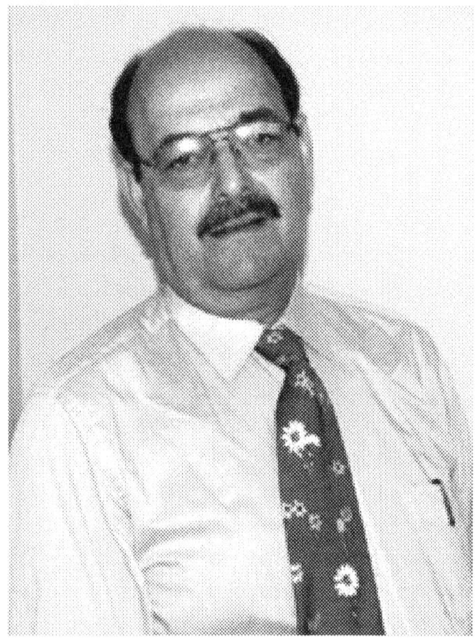

Introduction

I value my association with the University of Michigan, the Department of Pharmacology, and Warner-Lambert/ Parke-Davis (now Pfizer); each has played an important role in shaping the different phases of my career in pharmacology. Now, semi-retired, I continue to value these connections and remain active as a member of the local scientific community.

The pharmaceutical industry has had a long and interesting history with the Department of Pharmacology. I will provide some background only on my career and interactions with the Department, its faculty and graduates. I will also reflect on how the field of pharmacology has evolved over the past 25 years and where I believe it will be going in the future.

In 1962, my first visit to the University of Michigan Department of Pharmacology and the Parke-Davis Company was as an undergraduate pharmacy student in Philadelphia, at Philadelphia College of Pharmacy and Science (now the University of the Sciences in Philadelphia, USP). These two Michigan institutions would eventually have an important role in shaping my future.

While I always considered both academia and the pharmaceutical industry as viable career options, I decided upon a career in industry, expecting to reside in the Northeast, the "epicenter" of the pharmaceutical industry ("big pharma"). My interest in "big pharma" evolved; I was exposed to the industry throughout my undergraduate, graduate and postdoctoral training. As an undergraduate, I interacted with adjunct instructors and professors from industry. In graduate school, the faculty and fellow graduate students had strong and positive associations with the pharmaceutical industry, and as a postdoctoral student at the University of Pittsburgh there were also strong industry affiliations. Each academic-industrial connection provided valuable insights to the many challenges and opportunities in the industry.

Also, as a graduate student I worked on several industry-related and funded projects that further stimulated my interest in drug discovery. As a NIH postdoctoral fellow, I gained experience and expanded my knowledge and interests in cardiovascular pharmacology. When I joined the pharmaceutical industry in the '60s, it was the era of second and third generation beta blockers, renewed interests in the renin-angiotensin system, central and peripheral control of the cardiovascular system, stereo-selective drugs, the arachidonic acid cascade/prostaglandins, etc. It was a great time to be a cardiovascular "drug hunter" and I felt I had the training to do so! It was during this period that I first met Drs. Ben Lucchesi, Martin Winbury, and many other prominent cardiovascular pharmacologists in academia and industry.

After my postdoc, in 1967, I joined the pharmacology department at the Warner-Lambert Research Institute, which was headed by Martin Winbury who is now in his retirement years as a Lecturer in Dr. Lucchesi's laboratory. I retained a strong interest in academia and a desire to build strong industrial-academic relationships, a carryover from my years as a student.

After I had spent 10 years at the Warner Lambert Research Institute, which was the research arm of the Warner-Lambert Company, the company merged with Parke-Davis in 1978. The newly merged company consolidated its R & D operations in Ann Arbor. Unlike today's mergers, this one took several years to complete due to special circumstances. It required all the cultural adjustments associated with a merger, including the relocation to the Midwest and a major lifestyle change for my family and me. Moving to Ann Arbor in the late 1970s did, however, provide the opportunity to build strong ties with a prestigious academic institution. The University of Michigan was geographically convenient and academically strong in the cardiovascular sciences.

When I relocated to Ann Arbor I headed up cardiovascular pharmacology in the new company. I had already established several professional relationships with University of Michigan scientists, e.g., Ben Lucchesi (pharmacology), David Bohr (physiology), Stevo Julius (hypertension), and Bert Pitt (cardiology), to name a few. I had also interacted with several U of M Pharmacology graduates, not located in Ann Arbor any longer, who had joined the pharmaceutical industry, including Mike Antonaccio (at that time at Ciba-Geigy), Mitch Steinberg (with Lilly), Don DuCharme (at Upjohn, now Pharmacia, to be acquired by Pfizer), Tom Baum (with Schering), and numerous others. Other U of M graduates in academia were also part of my network of scientific colleagues with excellent relationships to the pharmaceutical industry, e.g., Mike Brody (at Iowa) and Ben Zimmerman (at Minnesota). Even my first boss in industry, at the Warner-Lambert Research Institute, Martin Winbury, moved to Ann Arbor, and, although he retired from Parke-Davis shortly thereafter, he continued to serve as a mentor to students in pharmacology at the University of Michigan.

In brief, throughout my career I have had the opportunity to interact with several U of M graduates and faculty who have had distinguished careers in pharmacology in both academia and industry; I continue to value these relationships.

I became an adjunct professor in 1982. This proved to be an unexpectedly long and complicated process! At that time (in the '70s and early '80s), industrial-academic relationships at the University of Michigan and elsewhere were much less productive than they are today. There appeared to be a bias by many academics in positions of influence against those of us having or seeking careers in the pharmaceutical industry, and to some extent those trained in schools of pharmacy and not in medical schools. This bias also existed in the Pharmacology Society.

However, attitudes were changing, and greatly improved during my career. I was strongly encouraged by the leadership of both institutions to pursue my interests in pharmacology at the University of Michigan. At that time, Ray Ruddon was chairman of pharmacology at U of M, and Jerry Weisbach was the new president of Parke-Davis research. For reasons that were unclear to me, relatively few scientists from Parke-Davis pursued opportunities to strengthen ties with the University and the Department.

In 2000, Parke-Davis was acquired by Pfizer, and I elected to retire from my full time career in industry. I still remain active in the scientific community, retaining my passion for pharmacology and maintaining ties to both of these institutions.

Challenges for an Industrial Pharmacologist

I became a member of the American Society of Pharmacology and Experimental Therapeutics (ASPET) in 1972. It was a time when membership in ASPET was an important credential and milestone for pharmacologists who had completed their formal training. Membership denoted peer recognition as an independent researcher. Today, membership criteria for ASPET have become more inclusive and less of a hurdle, especially for those in industry. This occurred in part because of the realization that interest in ASPET had waned (especially in industry) because of the emergence of new organizations that better met the emerging specialized needs of the more recent graduates. However, over the past few years there has been a revitalization of ASPET and a desire to meet the diverse needs of scientists in both industry and academia.

Early in my career there were then unspoken and unwritten "rules" that resulted in a less-than-equal stature for the industrial pharmacologist (as compared to the academic). Happily and fortunately, the attitude that careers in industry are somewhat tainted or otherwise inferior is not at issue today.

Parke-Davis and University of Michigan Interactions

When I joined the Department as an adjunct faculty, relationships between these two institutions were very spotty and really not "institutionalized" to any great extent until the '90s. There were, of course, exceptions.

Certain key events led to a transformation in the Michigan/Parke-Davis relationships. Ronnie Cresswell and Pedro Cuatrecasas provided strong scientific-leadership leadership for Parke-Davis in the '90s and were strong advocates for interactions between the two institutions. Also, Parke-Davis was about to be transformed as a company because of the pending commercial success of Lipitor. This Parke-Davis asset was the primary reason for Pfizer's aggressive pursuit of the company. This led to the acquisition of Parke-Davis by Pfizer. The commercial success of this drug transformed the company. In some ways the impact of a single drug (Lipitor) was analogous to the impact of the antibiotic Chloromycetin (chloramphenicol) on the success of Parke-Davis in the 50s, when the old Parke-Davis organization achieved its number one ranking in the pharmaceutical industry. Today, Pfizer is the number one company in the world, having recently acquired Pharmacia, which had earlier acquired Upjohn (Kalamazoo, Michigan).

More recently, Gil Omenn, then executive vice president for Medical Affairs at the U of M, made it a priority to strengthen the relationship between University of Michigan and Pfizer. This relationship exemplified both the highest standards of corporate responsibility and the importance for the University of Michigan to maintain its continued excellence in higher education and research.

Several new initiatives are evolving at the U of M that will further strengthen the relationships between scientists and companies such as in U of M's Life Sciences Institute, the Michigan Economic Development Corporation and Life Sciences Corridor Initiatives. Just recently, Alan Saltiel, a former Parke-Davis colleague was appointed director of the Life Science Insititute at the U of M. There is a high value placed on the quality, diversity, and number of interactions across the various colleges at the University of Michigan — in the physical and biological sciences, in the pharmaceutical sciences, in medicine, and in the College of Engineering. The opportunity to collaborate closely with the scientific community at the University of Michigan is a major and mutual asset to both institutions. The state-funded Life Sciences Corridor program is fostering strong collaborations not only between the industry and academia, but also among other Michigan colleges, universities and institutes in the "corridor".

Pfizer recently acquired large parcels of land from the University of Michigan and ERIM (Environmental Research Institute of Michigan) that will enable the company to greatly expand its R & D operations in Ann Arbor. There is a revitalization of the life sciences industries at both the local and state level that are benefiting all in the scientific community. The commitment to the Life Sciences is further exemplified by the new President of the U of M, Dr. Mary Sue Coleman herself a Ph.D. in biochemistry. Interactions between Pfizer and the Department of Pharmacology continue today, and the Pharmacology Department is poised to continue its excellent relationships with Pfizer.

During the past two decades in which I have been affiliated with the Department, the scope of interactions has included: scientist to scientist relationships (too numerous to mention), seminars/retreats, journal clubs and discussion groups, adjunct appointments, research agreements, technology transfer, clinical trials, post-doctoral programs, internships, teaching, space and facility sharing, recruitment activities and spousal placement, collaborations and consultantships, joint scientific publications, poster days, career days, and many others. I catalogued many of these interactions in 1993 for an informal presentation to the University of Michigan Biomedical Research Council (BMRC), and then updated this document several times to serve as background and a source for reviewing current initiatives and identifying both opportunities and barriers for enhancing the value of these activities. An annual update would be a useful document.

I had the opportunity to develop and then co-coordinate Pharmacology 503, a course in Drug Discovery and Development. It provided a forum for students to learn about careers in the pharmaceutical industry. The course featured guest lecturers from the research-based pharmaceutical and biotechnology industries and described technologies and procedures for the discovery and development of new pharmaceuticals. In addition, it featured case studies, a tour of the Parke-Davis facility and a career opportunities workshop to enlighten students about the different career paths within the pharmaceutical/ biotech industries. The course will be given again this year (2003).

Where the Field of Pharmacology is Going From an Industry Perspective

When I began my career, it was a time when "me-too" drugs were prevalent. These second-generation drugs had the potential to become commercially successful (e.g., beta-blockers, angiotensin converting enzyme inhibitors, etc.). In the '60s and '70s and well into the 80s, innovation alone created the demand for new drugs— safety and efficacy were key, and incremental advances in same class drugs having some unique features were often adequate enough to ensure commercial success. Health care costs and the cost of new drugs were not anywhere near the issue they are today.

It was not until the '90s that "value" truly entered into the equation, linking innovation and cost inasmuch that innovation, per se, was not necessarily the key attribute to ensure commercial success, but rather it was value (innovation/cost). Today the worldwide economic slowdown and increased pressures from states, insurers, and escalating health expenditures are all putting tremendous pressure on the pharmaceutical industry. Pharmacoeconomic factors are becoming increasingly more important at a time when the cost of research is soaring. A recent study from Tufts researchers indicated that it cost $231 million to develop a new drug in 1987. If the cost had risen at the rate of inflation, it would have reached $318 million in 2000, but the costs have exploded to more than $800 million today!

The rate of change in the science and cost of enabling technology has had a major impact on the development of new chemical/medical entities, and underscores the importance of patents to protect the intellectual property of the innovator. The increased competition and global communication have greatly lessened the time for the innovator to own the market. Patent expirations, generic drugs, direct to consumer marketing, and the regulatory environment are among the current issues impacting the future. The pharmaceutical industry is facing a public relations crisis and needs to do a better job in communicating with the public.

As we look to the future we clearly see the emergence of gene-based therapies targeted for selected patient populations. Pharmacology will be focusing on disease prevention, modification, and cures based on the knowledge derived from expressed genes (and their proteins) and an analysis of individuals' genetic profiles— we have entered the era of functional genomics/proteomics that will lead to customized therapy and drugs. The skill sets and armamentarium of technologies have also changed dramatically; consider the thousands of new drug targets. Miniaturization of technologies have resulted in ultra high throughput screening (and other enabling technologies) and "industrialization" of the drug screening and development process. Further, innovation remains the key to the value added by new medicines.

Biotechnology firms are also consolidating to ensure critical mass, a stronger pipeline of products, and efficiency of scale. The cost savings of new drug development have not as yet been realized, and costs continue to dominate health delivery discussions. Today the industry has consolidated and "big pharma" has formed strategic alliances with small biotech companies that are often founded/staffed by academics. More and more scientists (in both academia and the pharmaceutical industry) have to deal with the business of science to advance their careers.

Since the horrific events of September 11, 2001, pharmacology will likely assume new and expanded roles in the area of "biodefense." In Michigan, there are several life-science corridor grant proposals competing for funding from the state. World health issues, such as the AIDS epidemic and malaria, are having an impact on the demand and supply of affordable drugs in poor countries.

Time and money are always at issue, in both industry and academia, and competition is fierce in industry. The cost of discovery, development and commercialization of new drugs has clearly outstripped the rate of inflation two to three-fold. Intellectual property rights have always been key to innovation and are being challenged by nations unable to deliver health care or new drugs; consider the AIDS epidemic. Patent expirations underscore the need for innovative pharmaceuticals.

Successful companies have to integrate critical but costly new enabling technologies and manage multiple alliances with biotechnology companies. Genomics and validation of targets (functional genomics) will be key for future successful drugs. The industry will continuously be compelled to do things better, faster, and cheaper. This focus on speed will drive organization and reorganization and further consolidation in the industry will likely occur in 2003. Surrogate endpoints will be necessary to measure potential benefits of new drugs in chronic diseases to speed up the drug discovery and development process and contain costs. There will be an ever-increasing need to acquire, analyze, and otherwise manage the avalanche of information from the new science and methods. There is a need to deal with the issue of patient access to innovative pharmaceuticals at a time when so many people remain undiagnosed, untreated and/or undertreated. There are great challenges and opportunities ahead.

The Local Scientific Community

Because of the location of the University of Michigan and Pfizer (and other scientific companies like Esperion Therapeutics and academic centers of excellence) there is a special opportunity for all that work in this scientific community to benefit.

Editor's note: On December 22, 2003 it was announced that Pfizer will acquire Esperion Therapeutics for 1.3 billion dollars. It's founder, President and CEO, Roger Newton is an adjunct member of the Department of Pharmacology (see Research Interests section).

Reflections on Academia and Industry: How Pharmacology Found Me

Martin M. Winbury, Ph.D.

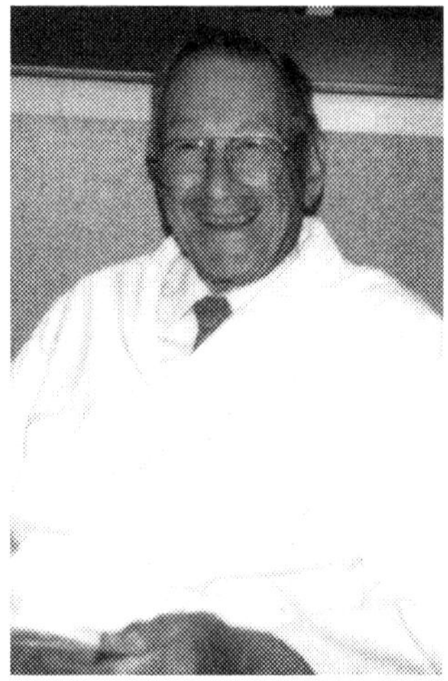

This is a story of the odyssey of a biologist who started graduate school in plant physiology, then zoology and biochemistry, and finally found pharmacology in an industrial setting. Were it not for the industrial position at Merck Institute for Therapeutic Research in Rahway, NJ, I would have been in some other area of biological research. It was my good fortune to obtain my first position in industry at the Merck Institute, which was organized in the German and Austrian fashion as a true research institute not with the objective of developing products for commercial purposes. At that time Merck and Company was under the control of the Merck family and primarily was a producer of fine chemicals including many amino acids. They were preparing solutions of amino acids to be marketed for intravenous alimentation. The Institute was under the direction of Dr. Hans Molitor, a pharmacologist from the University of Vienna. Included in the personnel of the Institute was Dr. Klaus Unna, also from Vienna; an American, Dr. Phoebe Crittenden; and a consultant, Dr. Ernst Pick, who was Dr. Molitor's mentor and in his mid-80s at the time. These people introduced me to pharmacology at an early stage of my career. I am thankful to them for the opportunity afforded me. Fortunately, Molitor ran the Institute in a democratic fashion and encouraged us to continue graduate studies at the local universities. Although we had 48-hour work weeks, we were allowed flex time so that it was possible to take classes during the day.

My first position was in biochemistry working on the nutritional efficacy of dehydrated rations using rats. Being curious about what was going on in other sections of the Institute, I observed animal studies in the laboratories of Dr. Unna and Dr. Crittenden, and came to realize that pharmacology was much more interesting than biochemistry. Dr. Molitor permitted me to switch to pharmacology working with Dr. Crittenden, and suggested studies on amino acids marketed by Merck. My introduction to pharmacology came from the contact with and advice and encouragement from Drs. Crittenden, Unna, and Pick. One could not have found better mentors, since all had had classical training and experience in many fields of pharmacology. It was a unique opportunity for a novice who knew little about the field but had a basic curiosity. The work that was completed resulted in a publication in JPET on the basic amino acids.

A move to GD Searle and Company in Skokie, IL, put me under Dr. Walter Hambourger, who had been trained in pharmacology by Dr. Torald Sollmann at Western Reserve Medical School. Hambourger introduced me to the history of pharmacology, knowledge he had acquired under Dr. Sollmann. The Chicago area universities' pharmacology departments had an active seminar program and encouraged the pharmaceutical companies to participate in their programs. In particular, we had close contact with the pharmacology department at the University of Illinois College of Medicine, and were invited to participate in a statistics course which was in its infancy then. This group was headed by Dr. Carl Pfeiffer; a number of people on his staff or in graduate studies there ultimately moved to the University of Michigan. Included were Ed Domino, Henry Swain, Ted Brody, and Harry Hardman. Also at Illinois at that time was Dr. Klaus Unna, who had been at the Merck Institute. I also was in contact with Dr. E.M.K. Geiling at the University of Chicago and with various staff members at Northwestern University and Chicago Medical School. The Chicago chapter of the Society for Biology and Experimental Medicine was also very active, and the group at Searle frequently attended the meetings and established contacts with our academic colleagues that developed into cooperative enterprises.

I returned to New Jersey, first at Schering Corporation, then at Warner Lambert. When Warner Lambert acquired Parke-Davis, I spent the final years of my career in Ann Arbor. After I retired, Dr. Lucchesi offered me an opportunity to maintain contact with young people as a lecturer in his group. While here I have seen the development of many pharmacologists and the expansion of the Department. My memories of the Department range from the time of Seevers, Nickerson, Chenoweth, Swain, Brody, on up through more recent years. The Department has had many famous pharmacologists as faculty members, as well as graduate students who are now leaders in the field. It is a pleasure and an honor to be associated with this Department, and to see the development of young people as graduate students.

Technology Transfer Policy at the University

Mark Maynard, B.A., Program Coordinator

The mission of UM Tech Transfer is to effectively transfer University technologies to the market so as to generate benefits for the University, the community and the general public. A group of Tech Team members offer a full set of services to ensure effective technology transfer. Professionals at the university and the central office work closely with researchers and faculty to provide advice about potential tech transfer issues during research activities and to assist in the invention disclosure process. Providing guidance in planning an effective patent copyright or trademark strategy, the Tech Team competently handles all implementation details during the implementation process. The UM tech team take to proactive assistance in analyzing potential opportunities to form a start-up with UM technology and encourage this interaction during the early disclosure process. Their skilled New Business Development Staff also provide hands-on business assistance, project planning and links to funding and people resources.

The Tech Team assists in technical and market assessments while actively marketing UM technologies to industry partners. This creates secrecy, evaluation, material transfer, option and license agreements with these industry partners to effectively get their technology into commercial use. With two full-time tech transfer staff attorneys, in partnering with the Office of the General Counsel, the Tech Team provides legal guidance and assistance for all of the UM Tech Transfer activities. Having the business support and administrative staff, UM Tech Transfer is able to provide information and guidance to conduct business and expedite decisions by utilizing both internal and external partners. UM Tech

Transfer also advises interested parties on UM policies and procedures including conflict of interest issues.

Results from the UM Tech Transfer research is deployed, which in turn improves our quality of life. Tech transfer activities lead to valuable educational experiences for the students, which augment classroom teachings. Commercialization efforts of the Tech Team often lead to expanded University research opportunities. This technology commercialization is able to create many job opportunities for students upon graduating from the university. These job opportunities lead to positive economic development for the community, the state and the general public.

In fiscal year 2003 UM Tech Transfer took in six invention disclosures from the Department of Pharmacology. During that year, six percent of all disclosures taken in from the University of Michigan Medical School as a whole were from researchers and faculty in Pharmacology.

University-wide, UM Tech Transfer took in 257 invention disclosures durring fiscal year 2003, representing an eight percent increase over the previous year. During that same period of time, the office signed 76 agreements with industry partners licensing UM technologies for commercialization, and launched nine new startup companies. This activity in licensing reflects a 23 percent increase in activity over the previous year, an example of Departmental UM Tech Transfer.

On October 1, 2003, Dr. Raymond E. Counsell received the first Technology Transfer Career Achievement Award in recognition of his accomplishments and dedication.

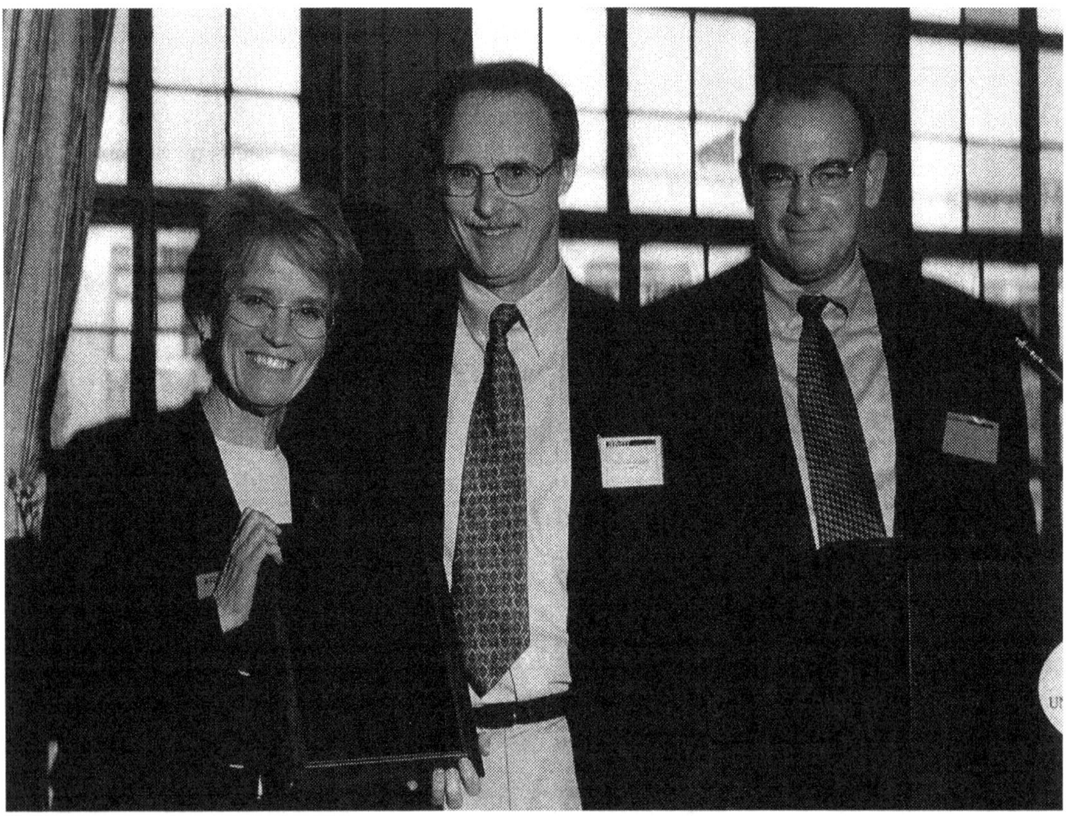

Mary Sue Coleman, UM President, Ray Counsell, and Marvin G. Parnes, Associate Vice President for Research, October 1, 2003

22

Highlights of The Department

As one of the world's major research facilities, the University of Michigan is one of only two public institutions consistently ranked among the top ten universities in the United States. The University of Michigan Ann Arbor campus consists of seventeen schools and colleges serving approximately 39,031 students of which about 14,500 are graduate students. Its main campus is in Ann Arbor, but it also has small campuses in Dearborn and Flint. In the sciences, the University offers a wide variety of graduate courses and is ranked very high in the United States for sponsored research funding. Scientists from all over the world are attracted to the University by the availability of virtually any research technology, one of the largest library systems in the United States, and one of the largest concentrations of computers in a campus or corporation.

Directly adjacent to the University's main campus is the University of Michigan medical campus. The medical campus contains the University Hospital and the Schools of Medicine, Nursing, and Public Health; and is home to more than fifteen graduate programs in the biomedical sciences.

The University of Michigan's Department of Pharmacology has a distinguished tradition of research, graduate training, and education of health science professionals including: medical, dental, pharmacy, and nursing areas of interest. The Department of Pharmacology is located in the Medical Science Research Building III (MSRB III) within the medical campus as part of the medical school. The Department of Pharmacology occupies floors A, 1, and 2 of the MSRB III; other laboratories are located in the adjacent buildings that house the Upjohn Center for Clinical Pharmacology, the Mental Health Research Institute, and other units.

Ann Arbor Today

Located in an area of southeastern Michigan, known for its lakes and scenic parks, rests Ann Arbor with the last census population of 114,024, of whom about 38,000 are students. The University plays a major role in attracting people from all over the world to live in the city. This diversity of perspective contributes to the city's reputation as a major educational and cultural center. Ann Arbor consists of a small downtown containing hundreds of restaurants spanning all ethnic cuisines; 83 parks, nature preserves and recreational areas; beautiful tree-lined streets and an extensive system of bike paths. Along with Cambridge, MA, Madison, WI, and Berkeley, CA, Ann Arbor is one of the major university cities in the United States. With four musical series, a renowned School of Music, the largest art fair in the country, professional and student theater, opera, and dance productions, it is no surprise that the University of Michigan and Ann Arbor have been named the premier cultural environments among all American campuses.

The Department Today

Today, the Department of Pharmacology has 50 full-time faculty, some of whom maintain joint appointments in other departments or programs within the Medical School or in other schools. The Department faculty teaches several basic courses administered to more than 600 students annually. We are primarily a research department and the great majority of faculty time is devoted to research.

The Department has modern facilities and equipment for performing all of the routine procedures of molecular biology, biochemistry, and both cellular and organ system physiology. The Taubman Medical Library and core facilities for electron microscopy, confocal imaging studies, nucleic acid synthesis, and peptide sequencing and synthesis are immediately adjacent to the Department offices. Core facilities for the production of transgenic and gene "knockout" animals are also readily available. Included here is a brief description of only some of the research currently being conducted in the laboratories of the faculty of the Department of Pharmacology.

Addiction Research

For almost 50 years, the Department has contained a primate center for the study of opioids and other substances with abuse liability. This Center has made major contributions to the study of the abuse liability of investigational compounds with analgesic properties. Compounds from a wide variety of sources (e. g., the World Health Organization, the National Institute on Drug Abuse, and academic chemists) are assessed through this program. The findings have led to the introduction of new analgesics with reduced human abuse liability and to the identification of the abuse liability of potential new therapeutics. Through both teaching and research, the investigators in this unit also contribute significantly to a university-wide Center on Substance Abuse. A large number of students, both graduate and postdoctoral have received addiction research training in the department. The Departmental Center is under the direction of Dr. Woods, who is interested in the behavioral effects of opioids and phencyclidine-related agents. A variety of behavioral techniques are used to study these drugs in rhesus monkeys, rodents, and birds. Drs. John Traynor and Gail Winger are key members of the Center whose expertise in molecular to behavioral methods are at the cutting edge of substance abuse research. The phenomena of tolerance and dependence are investigated at the biochemical level with receptor binding assays as well as at the behavioral level. Together with faculty from other departments and programs, the investigators in addiction research provide a multi-disciplinary approach to a difficult pharmacological, medical, and social problem.

Cancer Research

The Cancer Pharmacology Program at the University of Michigan comprises a broad spectrum of investigators from the Department of Pharmacology, the College of Pharmacy, and clinical departments in the Medical School. It focuses on developing experimental approaches to the clinical treatment of cancer through research that bridges the fields of molecular carcinogenesis, biochemical pharmacology, radiation biology and clinical pharmacology. The mechanistic concepts developed in cultured cells are examined in animal models and then taken to clinical trials. Dr. Ensminger focuses on the delivery and disposition of anticancer drugs. Because of the anatomy of hepatic blood flow and the relatively high intrinsic tolerance of normal liver cells to several anticancer drugs, tumors in the liver can be treated by pumping drugs directly into that organ through a cannula implanted in the hepatic artery. Dr. Ensminger is an expert in this form of regional drug delivery and combines this approach with gene therapy and activation of drugs by ultrasound to develop new combined modality therapies for treatment of cancers restricted to specific regions that, like the liver, can be exposed selectively to drugs. Two major interests of investigators in the Cancer Pharmacology Program are the study of cell killing by nucleoside analogs and the enhancement of cell killing by X-irradiation. The nucleoside analogs require activation within the cancer cell by phosphorylation to nucleotides that then interfere with DNA synthesis to cause cell death. Dr. Shewach develops methods of enhancing drug activation, both by biochemical manipulation of existing enzymes in the activation pathway and by using gene transfer techniques to express enzymes not normally present in humans but which are superior activators of the nucleoside analogs. Such gene transfer techniques can be used in cultured cells to overcome drug resistance, an approach that is being used by several investigators in the program. In a second line of investigation, Dr. Shewach is studying the way in which the nucleoside analog gemcitabine sensitizes cells to the lethal effects of X-irradiation. Dr. Maybaum is interested in the mechanisms by which nucleoside analogs and some other anticancer drugs initiate the process of apoptosis, or programmed cell death. Although the biochemical pathways of drug damage are often very well defined, the damage itself triggers the expression of genes that initiate and carry out the death process and these events are being probed with the tools of molecular biology. Dr. Lee's lab is interested in how receptor tyrosine kinases protect hematopoietic cells from apoptosis or programmed cell death. To address this, her lab constructs growth factor receptor mutants that are defective in mitogenesis and then genetically complements their biological defects with specific downstream signaling molecules. A significant thrust is in determining how phosphatidylinositol 3-kinase and protein kinase B/Akt contribute to the growth factor survival program. Studies on carcinogenesis are being carried out by Drs. Hollenberg and Brenner. Dr. Hollenberg is developing specific inactivators of different forms of P450 that activate carcinogens, the ultimate goal being to protect subpopulations exposed to specific carcinogens from developing cancer. Dr. Brenner conducts both laboratory and clinical studies aimed at lowering the incidence of carcinogenesis in susceptible populations by the long-term administration of chemopreventive agents. Certain carcinogens (e. g., dioxin), anticancer drugs (e. g., steroids) and differentiation promoting agents (e. g., vitamin D 3) act through nuclear receptors that regulate gene expression. Dr. Simpson's laboratory studies the mechanism by which 1,25-dihydroxy-vitamin D 3 promotes cell differentiation in vitro, with the ultimate goal of using differentiation promoters as a means of cancer treatment.

The Cancer Pharmacology Program is part of the University of Michigan Cancer Center, which is one of 25 national centers for research on and treatment of cancer. The Cancer Center includes the new cancer hospital adjacent to the basic science laboratories, the NIH-funded Cancer Biology Training Program, which funds several pharmacology graduate students, and over a hundred different laboratories that reflect a broad range of expertise and interest. Most Pharmacology Department faculty members who are in the Cancer Pharmacology Program have laboratories located in the Upjohn Center for Clinical Pharmacology, which is located in the center of the Medical Campus.

Cardiovascular Research

Cardiovascular disease is the major cause of death in the United States. The development of a basic understanding of the pathophysiology of cardiovascular disease and the development of new drugs and their preclinical testing has been a long-term focus of the Department of Pharmacology. Dr. Lucchesi's laboratory is a major training site for students, postdoctoral fellows and clinician scientists. This large and highly regarded laboratory receives a large amount of its support from pharmaceutical manufacturers, and its trainees are especially attractive candidates for research and development positions in the drug industry. One major area of interest in the Lucchesi laboratory is to identify, characterize, and evaluate drugs that prevent ventricular fibrillation, the most lethal of all cardiac rhythm disturbances. A person suffering from a heart attack suffers myocardial damage, both during the ischemic phase when blood flow to regions of the heart is diminished or absent, and during the reperfusion phase when blood flow is increased again as a result of drug treatment and/or angioplasty. Dr. Lucchesi's laboratory has developed models for analyzing the pathophysiological basis for myocardial injury and the pharmacological protection of the ischemic heart. Major patho-physiological studies focus on the role of the immune system in causing myocardial damage, for example, through leukocyte-derived oxygen free radicals and through complement mediated membrane damage. In that a heart attack usually results from coronary artery thrombosis resulting from platelet aggregation and platelet interaction with the vascular endothelium, a third focus of the laboratory is on the pharmacological control of the coronary circulation through drugs that prevent thrombosis. Dr. Osawa is interested in the effects of active radical forms of oxygen on cells and tissues. Free radicals, such as nitric oxide and superoxide, and other chemically reactive compounds play important roles in a variety of pathological and physiological processes, including myocardial ischemia and reperfusion injury. Dr. Osawa's laboratory focuses on the effects of free radicals on biological systems at the molecular level, with the focus on developing rational treatments of conditions due to inappropriate free radical formation. The medulla of the adrenal gland secretes adrenalin and other substances that increase blood pressure and control other responses of the cardiovascular system. Dr. Holz studies the fundamental process by which these vasoactive compounds are secreted from adrenal cells. One of the types of receptors that controls blood pressure is the 2 class of adrenergic receptors, and Dr. Neubig investigates the coupling of 2 receptors to the G-protein effectors that mediate responses. Dr. Simpson was the first to demonstrate direct effects of vitamin D 3 in regulating cardiovascular function. At the cellular level, he studies the effect of vitamin D 3 in promoting the differentiation of cardiac myocytes in culture. These studies utilize molecular biological probes to monitor hormone-induced changes in myocyte gene expression. Dr. Shayman's laboratory investigates the role of phospholipid and lipid metabolism in renal disease and lipid storage diseases. Through the efforts of these faculty members, their students and collaborators, the department is making important contributions to both the fundamental understanding of problems associated with cardiovascular disease and the development of new therapies.

Drug Metabolism/Gene Expression

The study of drug metabolism is a major area of emphasis in the department. Dr. Hollenberg's laboratory studies the microsomal P450-dependent mixed-function oxidases, which are responsible for metabolic activation and/or detoxication of many drugs, toxins and xenobiotics. Using several forms of purified P450 in a reconstituted system consisting of NADPH-P450 reductase, phospholipid and cytochrome P450, the Hollenberg laboratory studies the mechanisms of oxygen activation and substrate oxygenation and the way in which other components of the endoplasmic reticulum affect the catalytic activity of P450. Mechanism-based inactivators are being used to investigate the structures of the active sites of P450. Dr. Osawa is studying the mechanisms by which free radicals, such as nitric oxide and superoxide, interact with cellular targets and the regulation of oxidative enzymes, such as nitric oxide synthase and prostaglandin synthase, that are responsible for generation of these reactive intermediates. Dr. Brenner is interested in drug kinetics and disposition. Using a rabbit model, which he has developed to study pharmacokinetics in normal and in hepatic or renal disease states, he evaluates the resulting changes in drug metabolism and toxicity. Two laboratories utilize the techniques of molecular biology to study how hormones and differentiation factors regulate gene expression. Operating through nuclear receptors the calciotropic hormone 1,25-dihydroxy-vitamin D 3 regulates the growth and maturation of a variety of cell types. Dr. Simpson's laboratory has shown that 1,25-dihydroxy-vitamin D 3 controls the transcription of genes for protein kinase C and c-myc proto-oncogene. His research is directed at identifying the cellular processes in which these gene products participate and how these genes alter cell function. Dr. Iñiguez is studying the N-terminal regulatory domain of the receptor and the proteins with which the domain interacts to determine transcription activation. A second project explores the control of synergy by a protein motif found in steroid receptors and in other regulators, such as the proto-oncogenes cMyb and ETS-1. Deletion of this motif results in transcriptional synergy, and the molecular mechanism of the control is being examined. Dr. Pratt's laboratory studies the way in which the steroid binding activity and cytoplasmic-nuclear trafficking of the glucocorticoid receptor are controlled by the ubiquitous protein chaperone hsp90. The study of how drugs, hormones and xenobiotics regulate gene expression is not limited to the laboratories described here. These are general questions pursued in several of the laboratories in the groups focusing on signal transduction, cancer pharmacology and cardiovascular pharmacology, and many graduate students carry out their thesis work in this general area.

Signal Transduction/Neuropharmacology

The Department's largest area of research is in neuropharmacology. Several of the laboratories in this area are working on the fundamental mechanisms by which neurotransmitter binding to receptors is transduced into the molecular events that determine the cell response. At the receptor level, Dr. Isom utilizes the techniques of molecular biology to study the functional domains of voltage-sensitive sodium ion channels and their auxiliary beta-subunits. Of particular current interest is the interaction of beta-subunits with extracellular matrix. Dr. Esteban's laboratory studies the cellular and molecular mechanisms by which synaptic connections in the brain are remodeled in response to neuronal activity. This process, known as synaptic plasticity, is widely accepted as the cellular basis for learning and memory. Dr. Esteban's lab combines molecular biology together with electrophysiology and imaging to understand how individual molecules contribute to synaptic function and plasticity. Dr. Neubig's laboratory studies receptor-mediated signal transduction via the G protein transducers. Using fluorescently labeled G protein subunits, receptors, and RGS proteins, he studies protein-protein interactions in this signaling system. He also uses peptides derived from the a2A adrenergic receptor to determine specific sites of receptor-G protein interaction, with the goal of developing potential inhibitors or activators of G protein signaling. Dr. Sunahara's laboratory also studies G protein-coupled receptor pathways. He utilizes biochemical and structural biological approaches to study the mechanisms that regulate the cAMP signaling cascade, from hormone binding to the degradation of second messengers. Dr. Iñiguez is studying the N-terminal regulatory domain of the receptor and the proteins with which the domain interacts to determine transcription activation. A second project explores the control of synergy by a protein motif found in steroid receptors and in other regulators, such as the proto-oncogenes cMyb and ETS-1. Deletion of this motif results in transcriptional synergy, and the molecular mechanism of the control is being examined. Dr. Bentley's laboratory is concerned with cellular signal transduction integration involving PDE genes regulating cGMP in response to NGF. Receptor-mediated inositol lipid breakdown by phospholipase C occurs throughout the nervous system and leads to the production of the second messengers inositol triphosphate and diacylglycerol with subsequent linkage to calcium signaling and protein phosphorylation. Dr. Fisher's laboratory studies the way in which muscarinic cholinergic receptors couple to phosphoinositide hydrolysis. Dr. Lee is studying the mechanism by which receptor tyrosine kinases activate the phosphatidylinositol 3-kinase pathway and the role of Src family kinases in this process. Much of the role of calcium in transducing signals is determined by the calcium-binding protein calmodulin. Dr. Gnegy's laboratory is interested in the adaptive changes in calmodulin and protein kinases in brain regions following repeated amphetamine administration and the role of these kinases in regulating dopamine transporter function. Drs. Holz and Ueda carry out fundamental studies on the process of neurotransmitter secretion from vesicles. Dr. Holz's laboratory uses biochemical, molecular genetic and biophysical techniques to study the effects of specific proteins on regulated exocytosis in adrenal chromaffin cells and other model systems. Dr. Ueda's laboratory studies the neurotransmitter vesicles of the synapse with special focus on how glutamate uptake into and release from brain synaptic vesicles is regulated and the role of protein phosphorylation in synaptic vesicle function. Four laboratories in the neuropharmacology area are studying the effects of drug administration on brain function and behavior. Dr. Baghdoyan studies the role of muscarinic acetylcholine receptors in generation of the rapid eye movement phase of sleep. Dr. Domino's laboratory is concerned with the role of nicotinic cholinergic mechanisms in brain function involving animals and human volunteers. Translation of research findings in animal to clinical pharmacology in human volunteers is a major focus of Dr. Domino's interest and research. Dr. Smith has been evaluating the way disease states, such as affective and anxiety disorders, as well as administration of a variety of psychoactive drugs are related to abnormalities of synaptic transmission. Dr. Woods' laboratory focuses on the relationship between drug binding to receptors and the behavioral effects of the drugs using a variety of unconditioned and conditioned behaviors in birds, rodents and primates. Taken together, the laboratories in the signal transduction/neuropharmacology area provide graduate students with a broad range of research choices from the most specific molecular approaches to the most integrated systems measuring the effects of drugs on animal behavior.

Editor's note: Additional (especially joint) appointee faculty have not been added to the above description of research interests and activities. However, in the following pages, each faculty member was requested to provide a detailed description of his or her research interests. In addition, photographs of the personnel involved (when available) are enclosed. Due to time constraints and other personal factors, some faculty research interests and personnel photos are unavoidably missing.

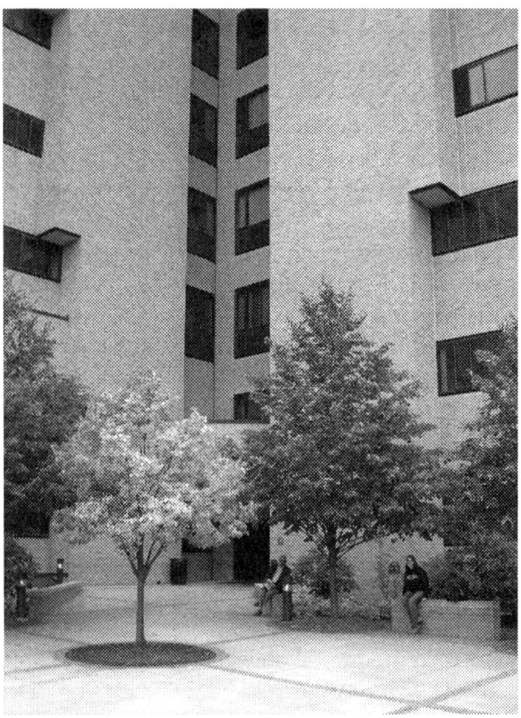

The north/west entrance to MSRB III where many take a brief time out

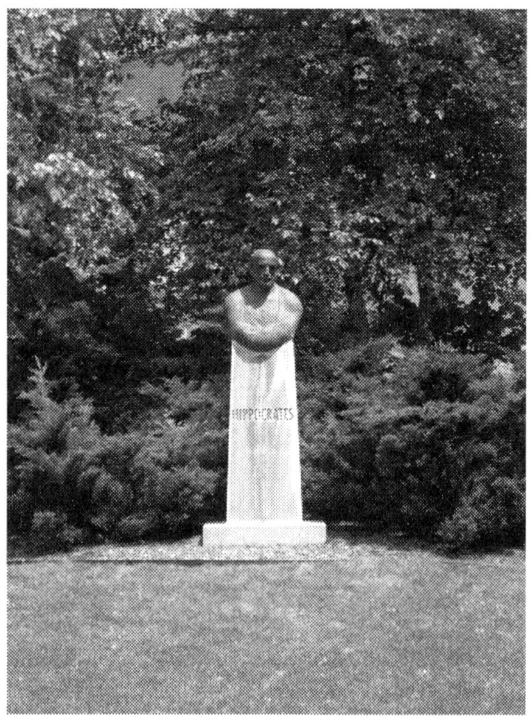

Hippocrates courtyard between the Taubman Medical Library and MSRB III

Dr. Helen A. Baghdoyan's Research Interests

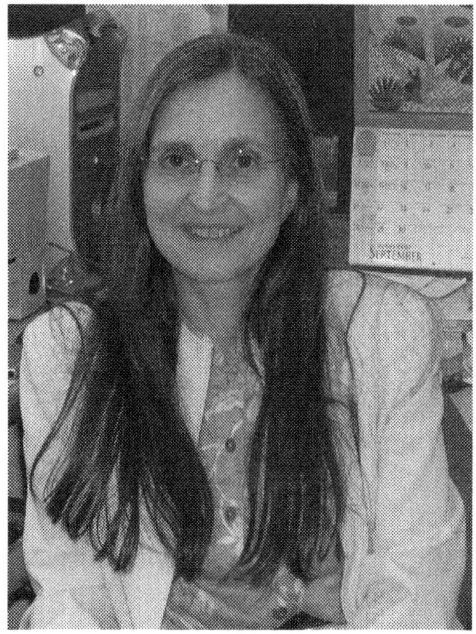

Helen A. Baghdoyan, Ph.D. is Professor of Anesthesiology and Professor of Pharmacology. Following completion of her Ph.D. in Neuropsychopharmacology in 1980, Dr. Baghdoyan joined the Laboratory of Neurophysiology at the Harvard Medical School as a postdoctoral fellow, sponsored by a National Research Service Award. She was promoted to Assistant Professor, and in 1987 she was recruited to The Pennsylvania State University College of Medicine as Assistant Professor of Anesthesia and Pharmacology. In 1993 she was awarded tenure and promoted to Associate Professor, and in 1998, Dr. Baghdoyan became the first woman in the Department of Anesthesia at Penn State to become a full Professor. In 1999, Dr. Baghdoyan was recruited to the University of Michigan by the Departments of Anesthesiology and Pharmacology.

Dr. Helen Baghdoyan's research is concerned with characterizing the neuronal mechanisms regulating sleep and anesthesia. Her studies span from the behavioral to the molecular level. Her work is funded by the National Institute of Mental Health and the National Heart, Lung, and Blood Institute. The neurotransmitters acetylcholine (ACh) and gamma-aminobutyric acid (GABA) play key roles in generating the rapid eye movement phase of sleep, as well as waking consciousness. The peptide neurotransmitter hypocretin (orexin) is also thought to be important for the generation of normal wakefulness. Dr. Baghdoyan's research program seeks to determine how anesthetic drugs, endogenous neurotransmitters, and neurotransmitter receptors alter 1) the release of ACh and GABA, and 2) G protein mediated signal transduction pathways activated by ACh and hypocretin.

Dr. Baghdoyan recently served as a member of the Advisory Committee for Appointments, Promotion, and Tenure in the Medical School. She teaches School of Medicine and School of Pharmacy students, and co-directs a course entitled "Sleep: Neurobiology, Medicine, and Society," offered to graduate students through the Program in Neuroscience and to advanced undergraduate students through the Department of Psychology.

Dr. Baghdoyan was honored by the Sleep Research Society at its meeting in Chicago, Illinois, in June 2003. She gave a major historical review of the role of acetylcholine in the brain mechanisms of rapid eye movement (REM) or dream sleep.

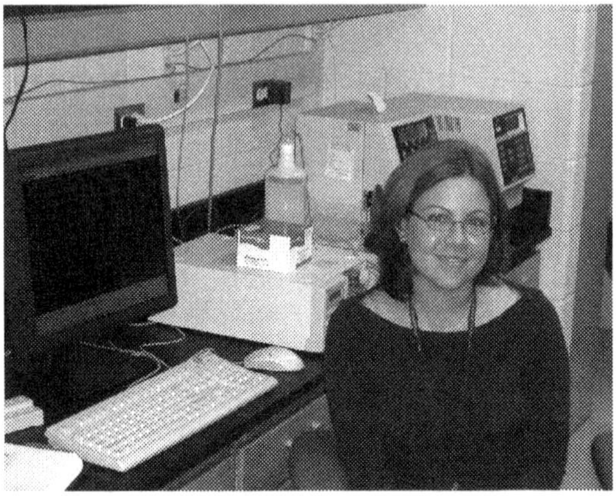

Haideliza Soto-Calderon

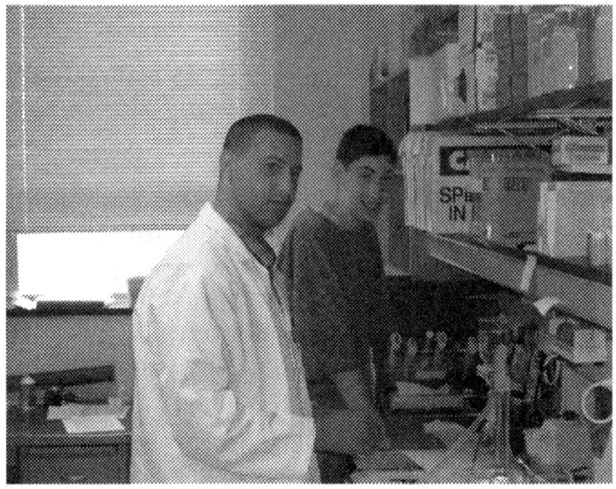

Dr. Nadir Osman and Eric Skulsky

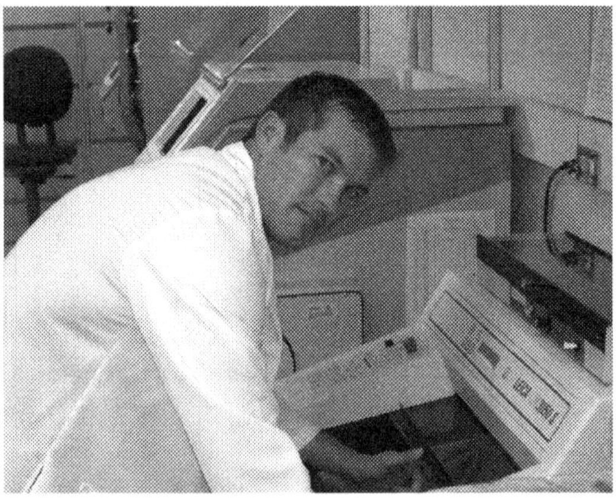

Adam Hill

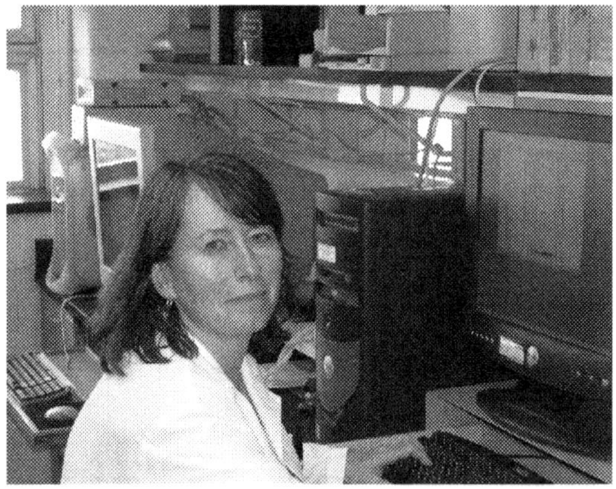

Mary Norat

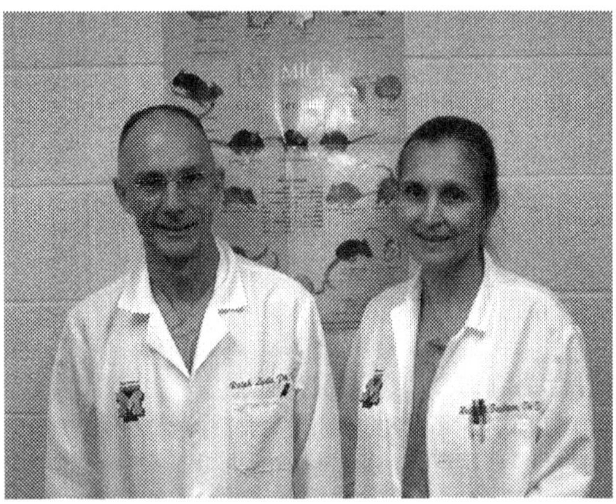

Dr. Ralph Lydic and Dr. Helen Baghdoyan

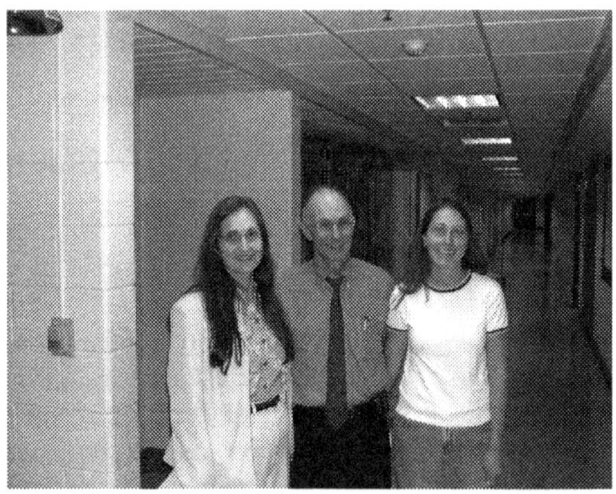

Dr. Helen Baghdoyan, Dr. Ralph Lydic and Christal Coleman

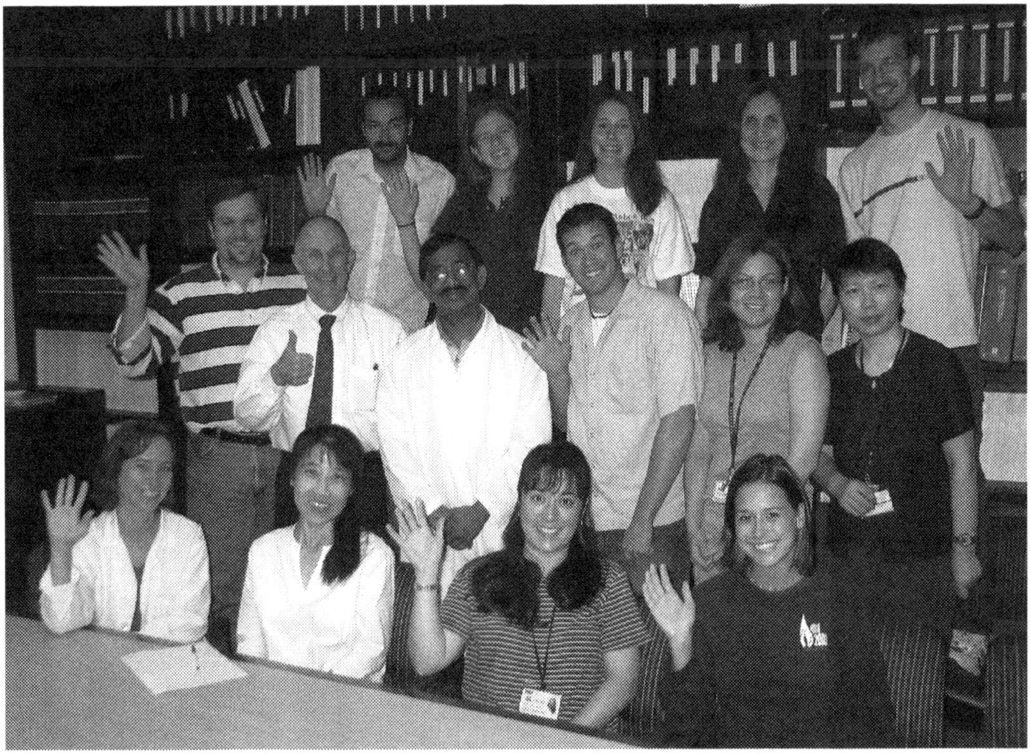

Front row: Dr. Christina Puscau, Dr. Fang Liu, Dr. Jacqueline Vazquez, Lindsey Morgan
Middle row: Dr. Chris Douglas, Dr. Ralph Lydic, Dr. Subhash Datta, Adam Hill, Haideliza Soto-Calderon, Sha Jiang
Back row: Jonathan Morrow, Karen Wiesenauer, Christal Coleman, Dr. Helen Baghdoyan, Rene Bernard

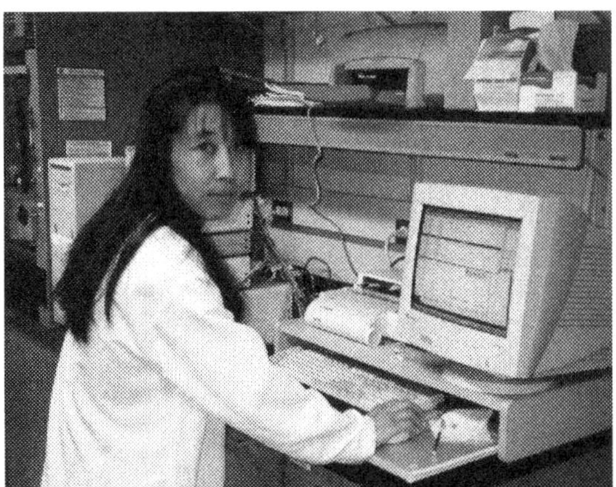

Dr. Fang Liu

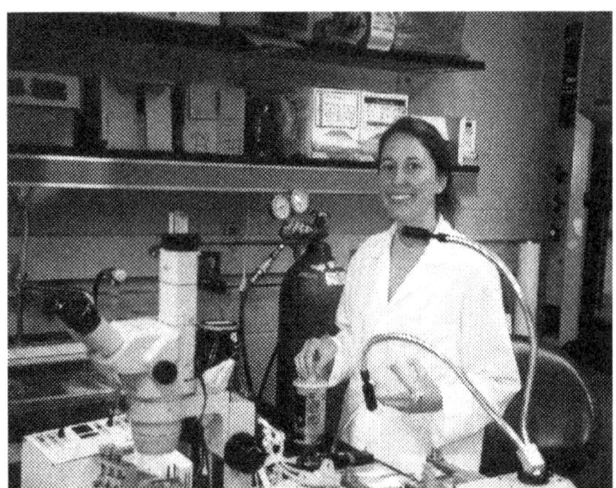

Christal Coleman

Dr. J. Kelley Bentley's Research Interests

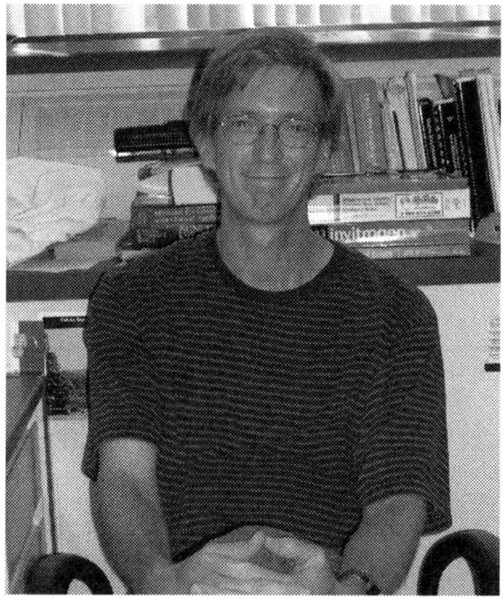

The biochemistry of cyclic nucleotide crosstalk has been the focus of my research. As a student of Dr. David L. Garbers at Vanderbilt University, I studied the mechanism of action of sperm cell chemotactic and chemokinetic factors and the role of phosphorylation in the regulation of sperm cell guanylyl cyclase by the egg peptides speract and resact.

My postdoctoral training was with Drs. Jim Hurley and Joe Beavo at the University of Washington. In Dr. Hurley's laboratory, I cloned and expressed inhibitory subunits of the retinal cyclic GMP (cGMP) phosphodiesterase interacting with transducin, and developed antibodies to these proteins. On entering Dr. Beavo's laboratory, I cloned, sequenced, and expressed a calmodulin-stimulated phosphodiesterase (PDE 1B), I also compared the localization of mRNA and different kinetic parameters for the three different known PDE 1 genes, PDE 1A, 1B, and 1C.

My long term goals are to resolve the genetic and protein structural basis for cyclic nucleotide metabolic regulation in neuronal and cardiovascular function, to examine PDE structural interaction with other cellular proteins, to develop proteomic approaches for the study of signal transduction interactions, and to develop the therapeutic potential of this gene family in neurodegenerative and cardiovascular disease. For example, cyclic AMP, cGMP, or PDE inhibitors keep neurons functioning normally in diabetic neuropathy.

Recently I have studied how nerve growth factor (NGF) may regulate cyclic nucleotide metabolism as a "switch" to facilitate neuronal gene transcription. Data in the NGF responsive PC12 cell (with cGMP-stimulated PDE 2) and other data for the cAMP specific PDE 4 suggest that protein serine/threonine and tyrosine kinase/phosphatase systems are involved in the regulation of cyclic nucleotide metabolism. PDE inhibitors, cAMP, or cGMP cause differentiation of PC12 cells in a manner similar to NGF. NGF greatly augments receptor mediated cAMP production. One PC12 protein involved is the cGMP- stimulated cNMP phosphodiesterase, PDE 2. NGF differentiation of PC12 cells into a sympathetic neuronal phenotype is reversibly accompanied by a reduction in PDE2 activity.

Phosphorylation hypothetically causes PDE 2 to interact with specific regulatory proteins and recent data suggests similar mechanisms may regulate PDE2 in cortical steroid-producing cells as well. I am identifying the phosphoprotein substrates for phosphorylation that regulate cNMP metabolism through protein interaction. I will extend this work into genetic knockouts and the introduction of dominant negative transgenes into specific cells and mice to understand how different phosphodiesterase regulatory proteins regulate neuronal and cardiovascular function.

Dr. Dean E. Brenner's Research Interests

Dr. Brenner is interested in understanding the pharmacodynamics of cancer chemoprevention and cancer treatment drugs. Two projects are currently active. Chemoprevention is a new area of research that focuses on the clinical pharmacology of cancer chemoprevention agents. It is the development of drugs for the purposes of preventing cancer in people who have known epidemiologic or biochemical risk factors for cancer.

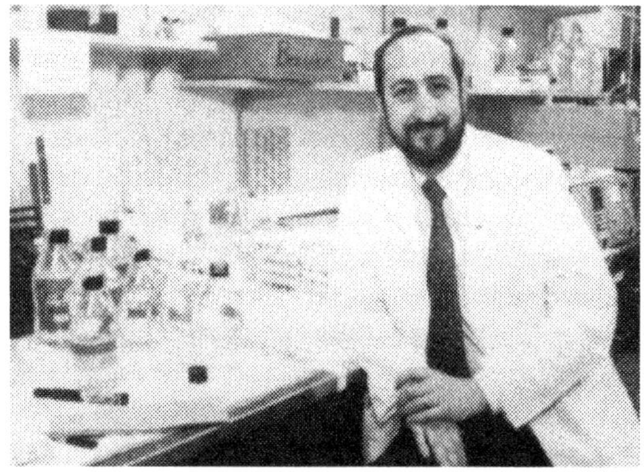

Key enzymes of metabolizing and important cellular biochemical enzymes have been identified that activate pre-carcinogens or promote cells that have been initiated by cancer causing agents. Chemopreventive drug development uses drugs and nutritional extracts that inhibit enzymes that convert pre-carcinogens to carcinogens, enhance a cell's ability to detoxify carcinogens, or inhibit proliferation of cells that are pre-malignant. He is exploring drug modulation of cyclooxygenase in colon epithelium. He uses probes of cyclooxygenase gene expression and protein levels to detect drug effect in colon epithelium. He is also using lectin markers of pre-malignant change of colon cells to detect reversal of cellular malignant expression. He tests, in humans and in animals, a wide range of drugs and nutritional constituents that have the potential of reversing cells that lead to cancerous change.

The second project involves anti-cancer drugs which are metabolized and excreted by the liver. Dr. Brenner is studying individual genetics that determine cellular concentrations of key anti-cancer drug metabolizing enzymes, the reductases. He hypothesizes that individual cellular concentrations of reductases (polymorphisms) may predict an individual's ability to metabolize anti-cancer drugs and thus, respond or experience severe toxicity from an anti-cancer drug. He is using cDNA probes of key cellular reductases to assess cellular reductase expression, gene expression, and cellular reductase concentrations in humans and rabbits. His group expects to correlate gene expression of metabolizing enzymes to in vivo metabolism and toxicity in humans.

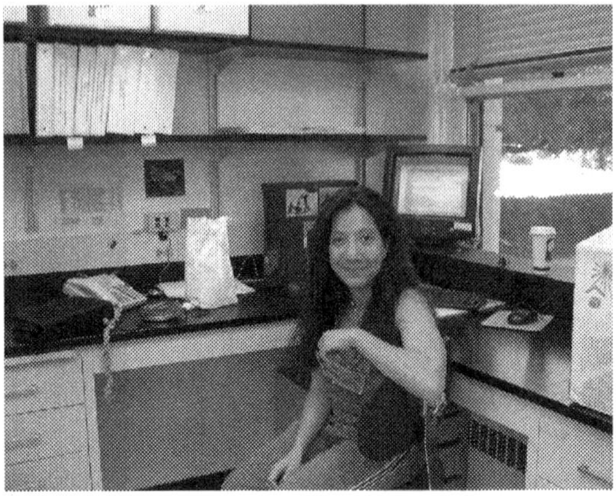

Courtney Streeter

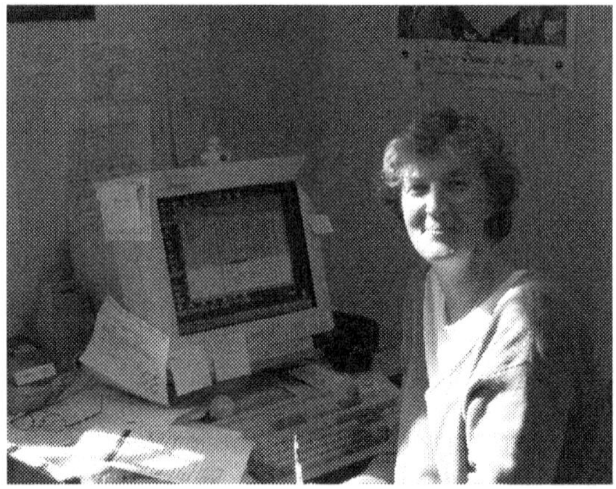

Laurie Fortlage

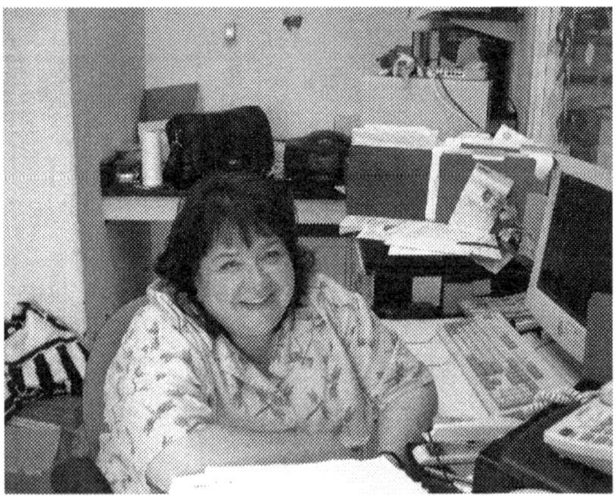

Mary Jo Beck

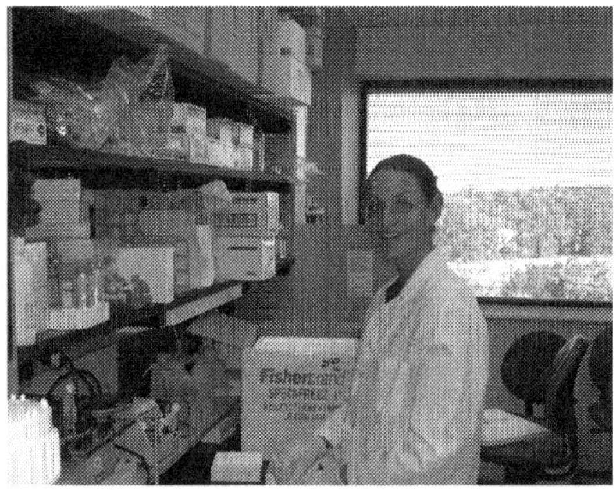

Mary Jo Hofmeister

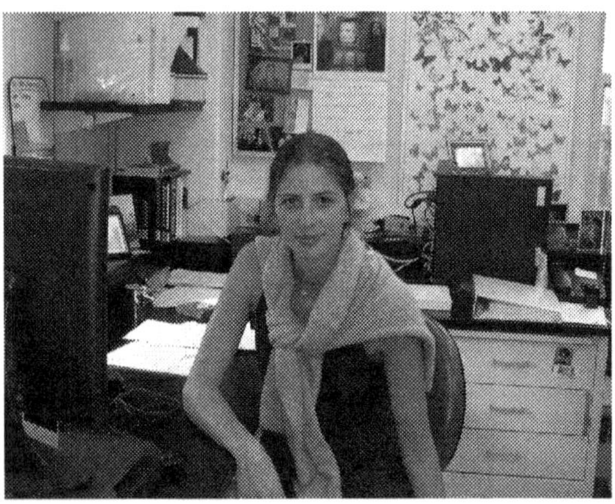

Sandra Murray

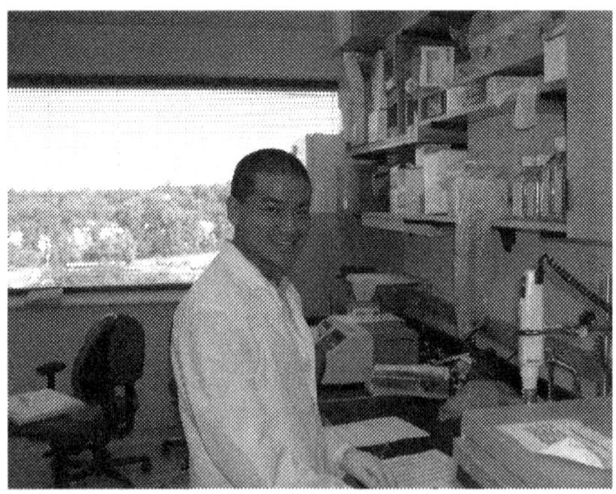

Timothy Liao

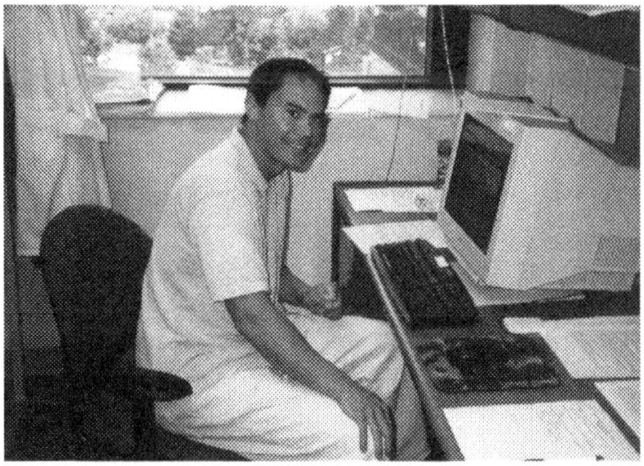

Christopher Lao

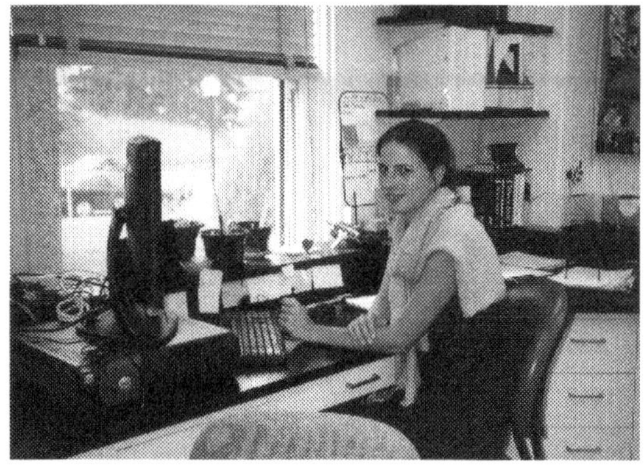

Sandra Murray

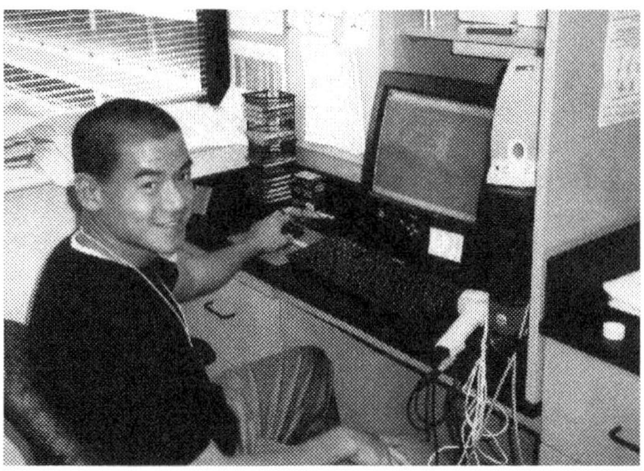

Timothy Liao

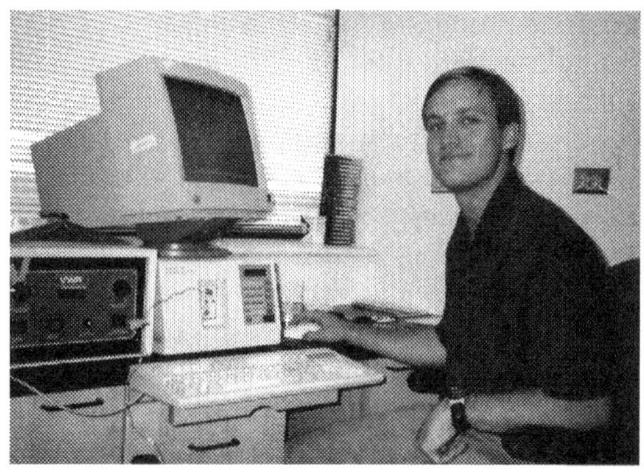

Jeff Braziunas

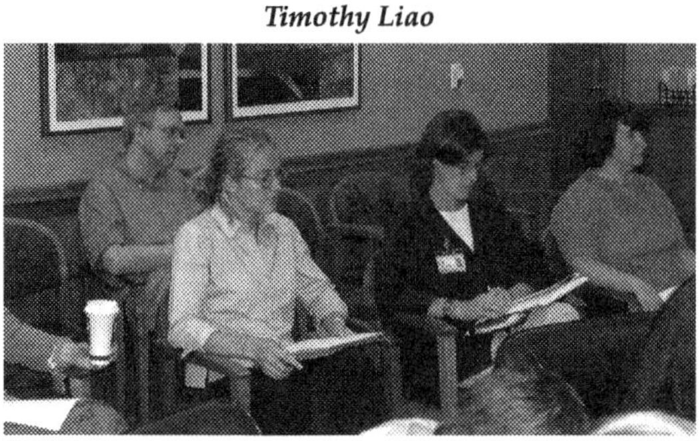

Daniel Normolle, Amy Blume, Joanne Bailey, Suzanna Zick

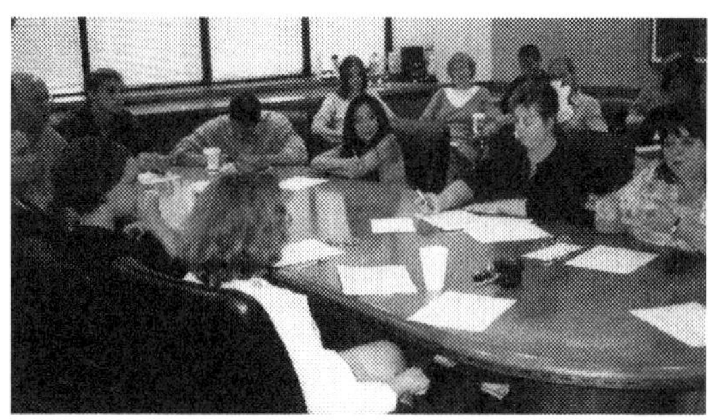

A Brenner Lab meeting

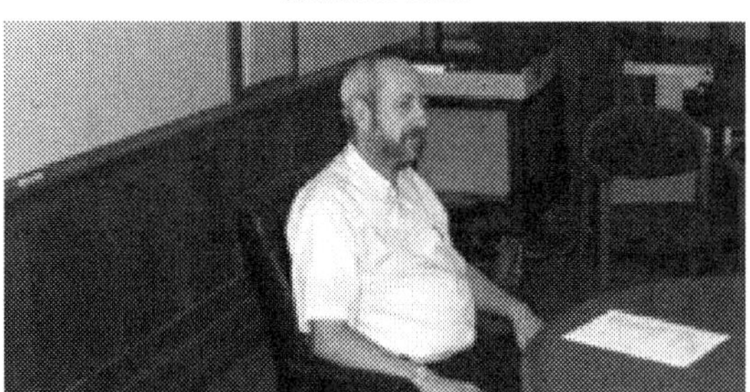

Dr. Brenner

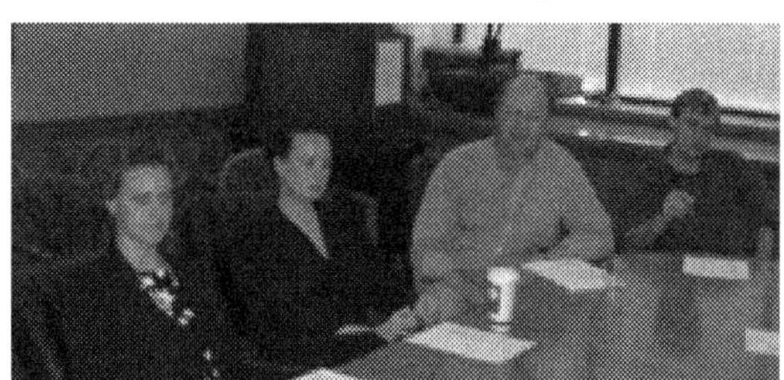

Martha Boggs, Tracy Eaton, Mack Ruffin, Jeff Braziunas

Dr. Christine Canman's Research Interests

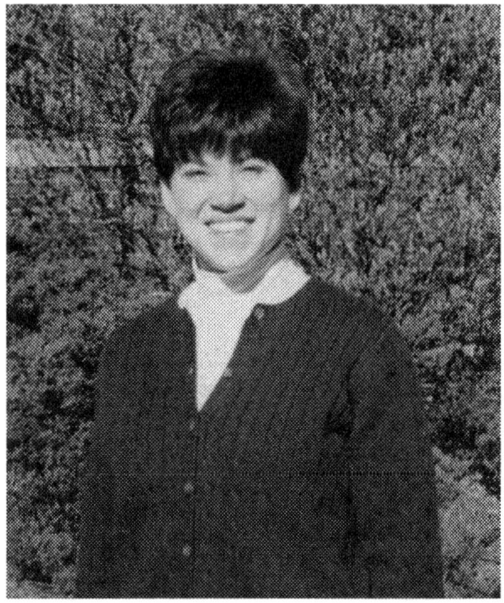

Never did I imagine that after receiving my Ph.D. in Pharmacology back in 1992 that in twelve years I would once again be walking through the labs in the Upjohn Center where I had spent the majority of my early adulthood doing graduate research. Except now I am walking the same corridors as an Assistant Professor of Pharmacology rather than graduate student of Pharmacology.

My interests in Pharmacology first surfaced while taking a microbial pathogens course as an undergraduate student at the University of Illinois, Champaign-Urbana. I enjoyed learning the mechanisms by which antibiotics killed or slowed the growth of bacteria. After receiving my Bachelor's degree in microbiology from Illinois in 1987, I continued my pursuit of understanding how drugs work by becoming a graduate student of Pharmacology here at Michigan. I decided to do my thesis project, the "Role of DNA fragmentation in fluoropyrimidine-induced cytotoxicity", with Jonathan Maybaum. Instead of focusing on how antibiotics kill bacteria, I now devoted my days to understanding how chemotherapeutic agents work. Using pulsed-field gel electrophoresis, I characterized various patterns of DNA fragmentation thought to be caused by misincorporation of uracil into DNA as a consequence of thymidylate synthase inhibition and dUTP accumulation in human colorectal tumor cells. I also found that high levels of dUTPase activity within a tumor cell correlated with low dUTP pool accumulation, DNA damage, and insensitivity to cell death following thymidylate synthase inhibition. My interests in cell cycle regulation, radiation biology, and DNA repair matured during this period of my career.

With these growing interests in DNA repair and cell cycle control (the cyclins were discovered while I was a graduate student), I ultimately found the perfect postdoctoral position. In 1993, I joined the laboratory of Michael B. Kastan M.D., Ph.D. at Johns Hopkins University in Baltimore, Maryland. Dr. Kastan was the first to recognize that the p53 tumor suppressor gene product was regulated by DNA damage and that enhanced transcriptional activity by p53 promoted cells to arrest in the G1 phase of the cell cycle prior to the initiation of DNA synthesis. My first project involved investigating the molecular factors that influence whether a cell undergoes p53-dependent G1 arrest or apoptosis in response to ionizing radiation (IR). These studies involved developing a model system in which the presence or absence of growth factors could determine which p53-dependent response was observed. I also participated in studies demonstrating that the p53 tumor suppressor gene product is phosphorylated on Serine 15 in response to IR. This led to my personal pursuit of showing that the ATM kinase directly phosphorylates p53 on serine 15 and that ATM increases its specific activity in irradiated cells. This was the first demonstration that ATM, the gene mutated in the devastating cancer-prone disease Ataxia-telangiectasia, possesses intrinsic kinase activity.

I continued my interests in DNA damage cell cycle checkpoint pathways as an Assistant Member at St. Jude Children's Research Hospital in 1998. A major focus of my lab was studying how ATM activates the Chk2 kinase in cells exposed to DNA damage. We found that ATM directly phosphorylates Chk2 at T68 when cells are exposed to IR and that this event was necessary for efficient activation of Chk2 enzyme activity. We also explored how T68 phosphorylation by ATM affects Chk2 kinase activity by demonstrating that the Forkhead-associated (FHA) domain of Chk2 is necessary for efficient autophosphorylationn and that the FHA domain of Chk2 binds to the phosphorylated T68 of another Chk2 molecule thereby facilitating trans-autophosphorylation between multiple Chk2 molecules. Then an unexpected opportunity emerged at Pfizer Global Research and Development in Ann Arbor where I could experience first hand how cancer drugs were developed from the ground up.

In 2002, I surprised many by moving to Ann Arbor to work at Pfizer. I served as co-chair on several projects including one whose goal was to discover selective IGF1R (insulin-like growth factor 1 receptor) kinase inhibitors. Inappropriate expression of this kinase is believed to promote tumor genesis and resistance to chemotherapeutic agents by increasing the threshold of cancer cells to apoptotic cell death. We never identified a chemical series that was selective for IGF1R over the insulin receptor (the insulin receptor possesses an extremely high degree of similarity to IGF1R in the ATP-binding site of the catalytic domain) and that had not already been described in patents written by the competition. I learned that it is not easy to discover a new drug though I did get to participate in efforts to develop a new and improved ErbB kinase inhibitor. This compound will eventually get its chance in the clinic and holds great promise in targeted therapy of tumors overexpressing this growth-factor-like kinase. Unfortunately, the merger with Pharmacia resulted in the end of cancer drug discovery in Ann Arbor and I found myself without a job. In the summer of 2003, I began interviewing for a faculty position in the Department of Pharmacology at Michigan.

Maintaining genetic fidelity is crucial for cell viability and limiting the propagation of mutations that lead to cancer. I plan on continuing my research in academia by studying how mammalian cells utilize highly conserved pathways to sense DNA damage, recruit repair and signaling proteins to DNA lesions, and generate signals to downstream effectors that regulate apoptosis and progression through the cell cycle. I will also expand my studies to include investigating how cells sense and relay checkpoint signals in response to incomplete or stalled DNA replication forks, the primary mechanism of action of most common anti-cancer agents. By characterizing these pathways in more detail, we may be able to identify new targets for discovery efforts since modulating these pathways to our advantage could sensitize tumor cells to current DNA-directed cancer therapy strategies. My two-year sabbatical in industry has certainly broadened my perspective how basic science leads to new drug discovery in cancer and I also had a chance to really learn what Pharmacology is all about and how it is applied thus increasing my enthusiasm for teaching the subject.

Dr. Thomas E. Carey's Research Interests

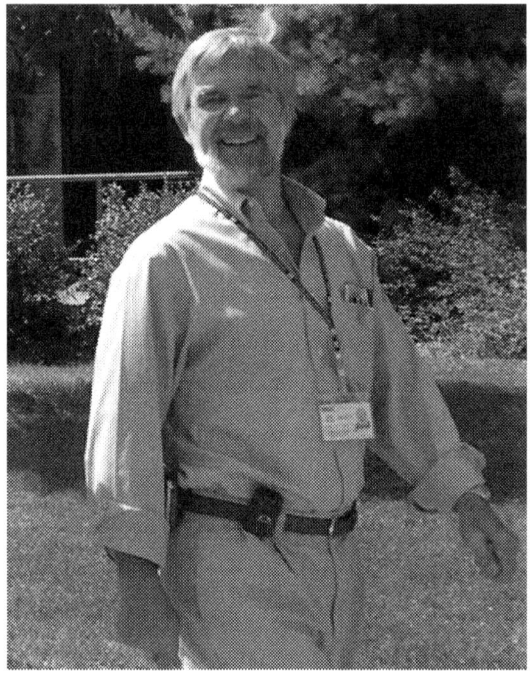

Dr. Carey directs the research activities of two research laboratories, one in the Cancer Center and the other in the Kresge Hearing Research Institute. The cancer lab investigates genetic mechanisms of tumor progression in patients with head and neck cancer as well as genetic changes associated with resistance to cancer therapy. The hearing research lab studies the basis for and mechanisms of autoimmune hearing loss.

In the hearing research lab we recently discovered, characterized and cloned the gene for an inner ear antigen that is the target of antibody induced hearing loss in a guinea pig model system. The antigen was found to be a homologue of the human CTL2 protein, a member of the choline transporter-like family of ten transmembrane domain proteins. We are currently investigating the function of this protein and attempting to determine the mechanism by which antibodies that bind to this protein cause damage to the organ of Corti. CTL2 is an abundant protein in the inner ear and it is also expressed in the human inner ear. Patients suspected to have autoimmune hearing loss have antibodies that stain the inner ear with the same distribution as CTL2. We are using this knowledge to develop an improved test for diagnosis of autoimmune hearing loss and to monitor patients at risk of further autoimmune damage.

In the head and neck cancer research lab we previously discovered a pattern of consistent loss of the long arm of chromosome 18 in tumors from patients with the most aggressive disease. The most frequently lost region contains a G-protein coupled receptor gene that encodes the galanin receptor 1 (GALR1). We postulated that reduction in GALR1 gene dosage might affect the growth behavior of squamous cell carcinomas. Further investigation demonstrated that there are two other galanin receptors, GALR2 and GALR3. All three of these receptors are expressed in normal keratinocytes as is the ligand, galanin, a 30 amino acid neuropeptide. Galanin and GALR2 had already been implicated in aggressive growth of small cell lung cancers. Thus, reduced expression of which signals through the Gi pathway, might down-regulate cell proliferation, and that GALR2 which signals through G12 might stimulate proliferation. Current experiments support these hypotheses.

Using tumor tissues we identified a pattern of gene expression that predicts preservation of the larynx in patients treated with chemotherapy and radiation. In the laboratory we used our well characterized cell lines to confirm that tumors with mutant p53 are more sensitive to platinum-based chemotherapy than are those tumors with wild type p53. Subsequently we found that the cell survival pathways affect drug resistance. We are currently investigating new agents developed by our colleague, Shaomeng Wang, that specifically attack the Bcl-2 family of cell survival proteins as a means of overcoming drug resistance. We have shown that such agents can trigger very high levels of apoptosis in the most drug resistant cell lines. We are testing the mechanisms responsible for our findings and developing testing protocols to predict response to therapy. We are also developing combination treatment protocols in vitro and in vivo to overcome resistance to standard chemotherapy, reduce morbidity, and increase survival. One of the new agents is a BH3 mimetic for Bcl-xL. It shows excellent promise in both in vitro and in vivo models and may enter the clinic soon.

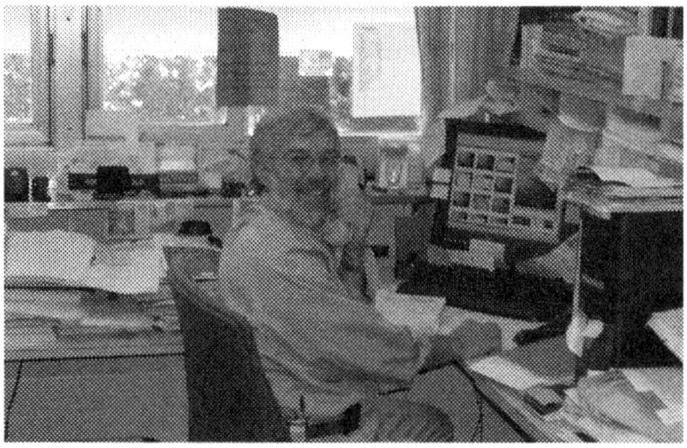

Tom Carey

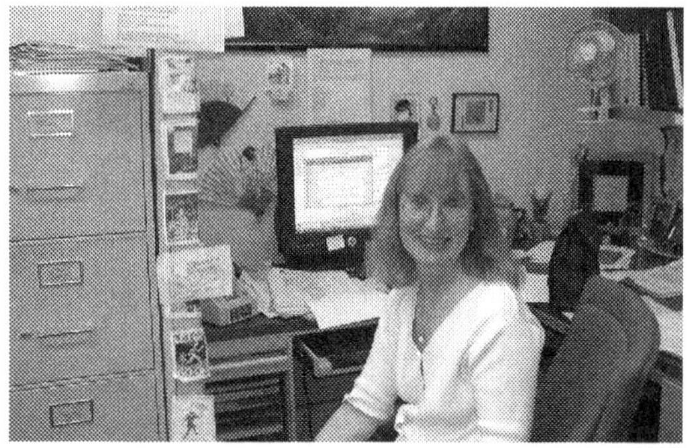

Margie Conlon

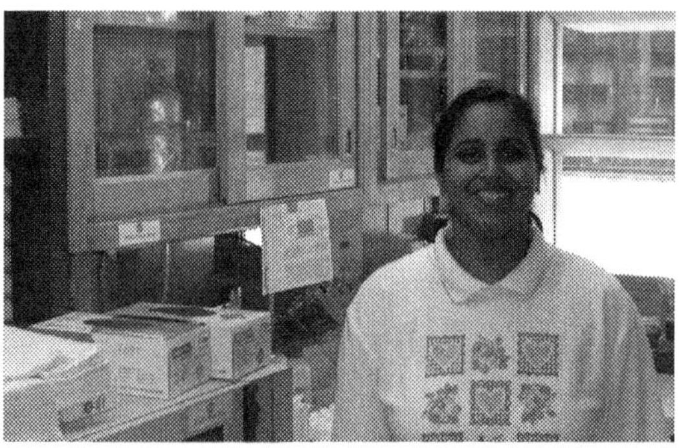

Sushma Yarlagadda

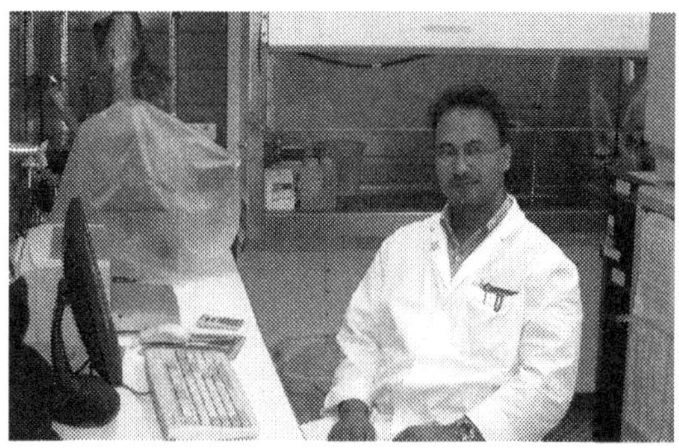

Mozaffarul Islam

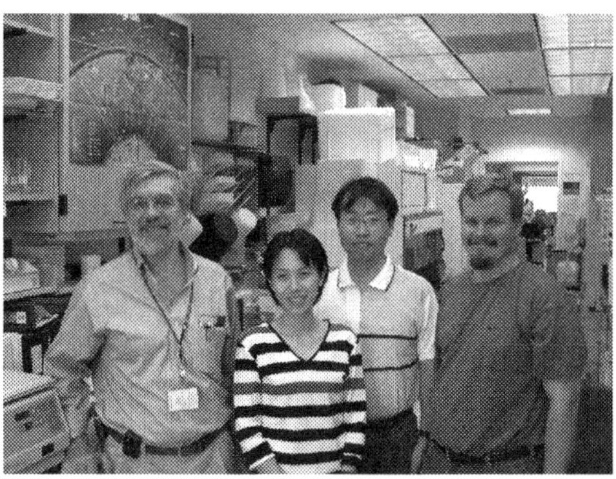

Tom Carey, Yuki Misawa, Kiyoshi Misawa, Andy Cole

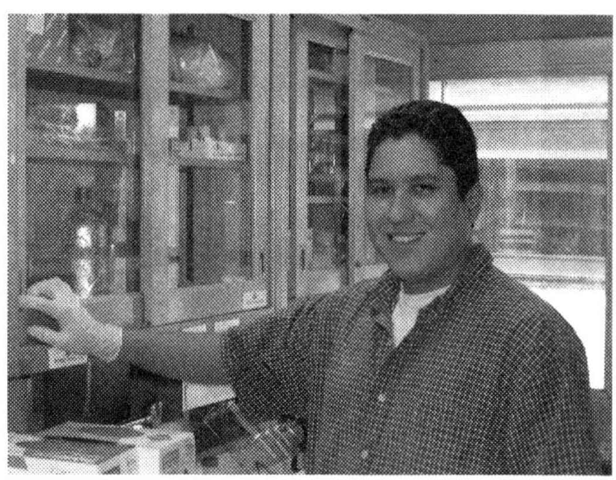

Jairo Matthews

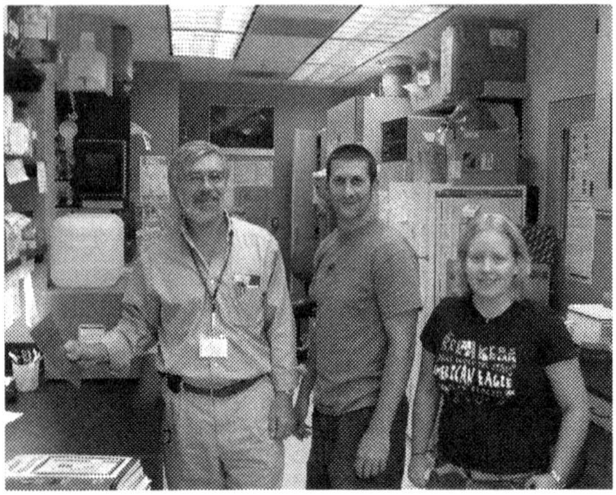

Tom Carey, Josh Bauer, Stephanie McLean

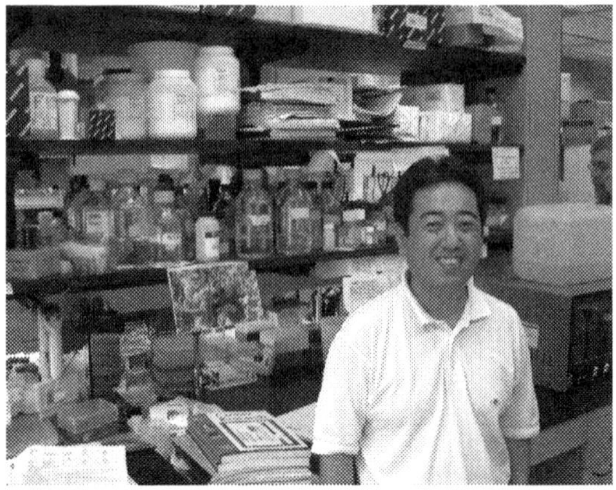

Takeharu Kanazawa

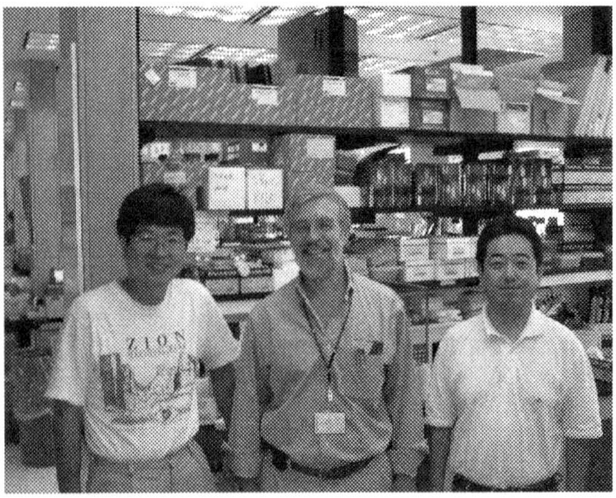

Satoru Takebayashi, Tom Carey, Takeharu Kanazawa

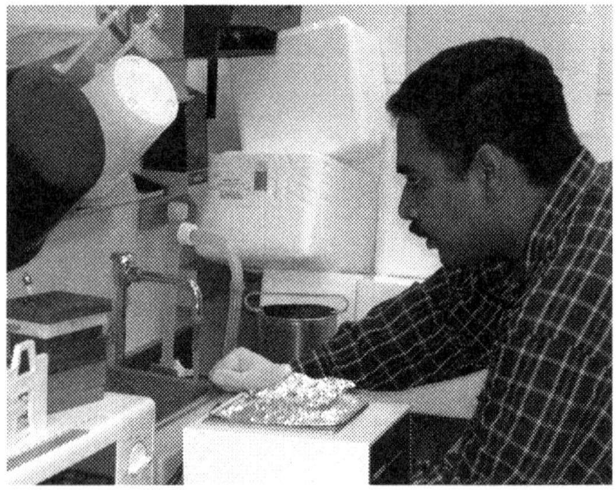

Pavan Kommareddi

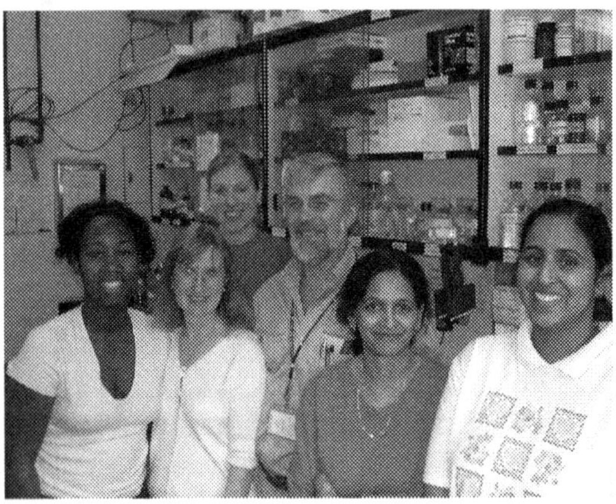

Charla Harvey, Margie Conlon, Andrea Braunz, Tom Carey, Thanku Nair, Sushma Yarlagadda

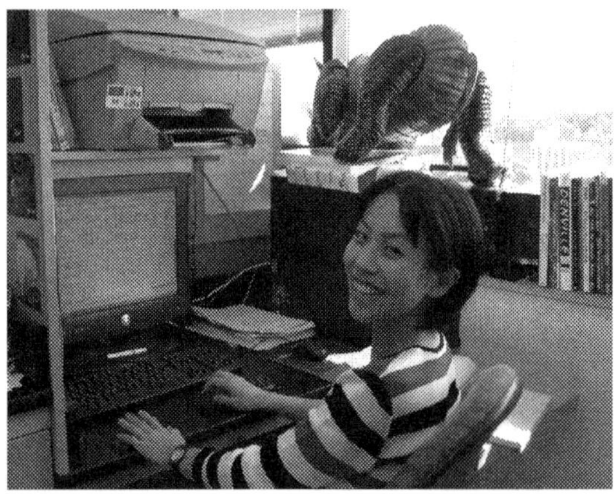

Yuki Misawa

Dr. Raymond E. Counsell's Research Interests

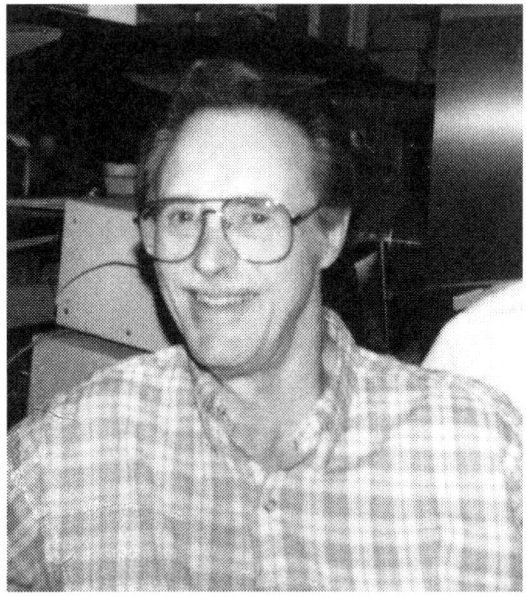

Dr. Counsell's laboratory is closed. He continues to be interested in targeting therapeutic or diagnostic agents to specific tissues or sites of action which is of fundamental concern to pharmacology. His diverse research interests have encompassed synthesis and evaluation of chemical regulators of biological processes, including steroid hormone biogenesis, and development and characterization of radiologic imaging agents for the early diagnosis of disease.

In recent years his interests expanded to include not only radiodiagnostic but also agents and site-selective drug-delivery vehicles. His publication record includes more than 160 articles in peer reviewed journal, 20 book chapters, and numerous abstracts. He is listed as the inventor or co-inventor on more than 50 issued patents. He has been a visiting research professor in Italy, Sweden, Belgium, and Japan. In addition, he has served as a drug and chemical industry consultant and as a member of the editorial boards of the Journal of Pharmaceutical Sciences, Annual Reports in Medicinal Chemistry, the Journal of Medicinal Chemistry, and the Quarterly Journal of Nuclear Medicine. He has received numerous honors, including an American Cancer Society Eleanor Roosevelt International Fellowship, a Fogarty Senior International Fellowship, and the Czerniak Prize of Nuclear Medicine and Radiopharmacology, as well as the T.O. Soine Memorial Award and the Alumni Outstanding Achievement Award from the University of Minnesota. Ray has served on NIH Study Sections, NIH and DOE committees, and numerous University of Michigan advisory and review committees, and is a member of many national and international professional societies.

The legacy of Dr. Counsell's 37 years of teaching and research at the University of Michigan was sustained by the former graduate and undergraduate students, postdoctoral fellows, and research associates and assistants who have built upon the lessons learned in Ray's laboratory to become leaders and innovators in the drug industry, academia, and consulting as small business entrepreneurs.

A major focus involves the evaluation of various strategies for achieving such site-specific delivery of drug molecules. Various hypotheses are tested by first designing and synthesizing an appropriate molecule, which is then radiolabeled for tissue distribution and metabolic fate studies in experimental animals. Studies included analysis of methods for achieving selective accumulation of agents in such tissues as tumors, adrenal cortex, liver, myocardium and atherosclerotic lesions. Targeting via receptor-mediated endocytosis is a specific area of interest. In cases where selective localization is achieved, follow-up experiments are performed to ascertain the nature of the physiologic or biochemical process or processes involved. Although agents arising from such studies can play important roles as pharmacological tools, they have potential clinical value as noninvasive imaging agents in Nuclear Medicine and Radiology. For example, several radioiodinated analogs of cholesterol and adrenergic drugs that are now widely used for the noninvasive diagnosis of various adrenal diseases evolved from such studies.

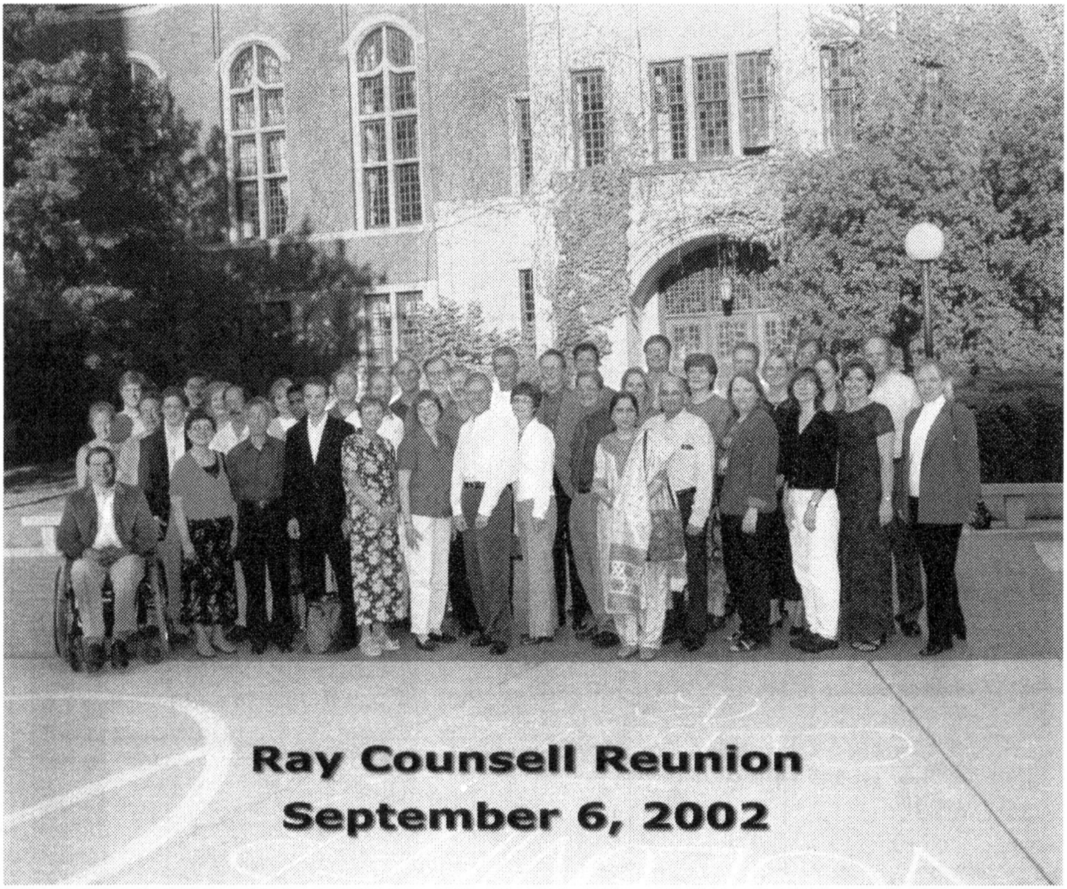

Front row: Mark DeGalan, Susan Hare, Matt Lu, Anatoly Pinchuk, Liz Counsell, Jane Aldrich, Bernardo Beyer, Suzanne Venton, Mike Mimnaugh, Usha Ranade, Vasant Ranade, Susan Schwendner, Laura DeForge, Sue Brueggemeier, Nancy Auestad

Back row: Carol Counsell, Steve Counsell, Will Klausmeier, Mark Rampy, Len Mattano, Susan Mattano, Che Cheng Huang, Chris Longino, Ramesh Gopalswampy, Marc Longino, Bob Seevers, Roger Newton, Larry Hare, Landis Keyes, Duane Venton, Ray Counsell, Doug Bakan, Edie Quenby Brown, Ron Counsell, Nancy Korn, Jamey Weichert, Cathy Counsell Martin, Mike Darby, Laura Russell, Bob Bruegemeier

Dr. Edward F. Domino's Research Interests

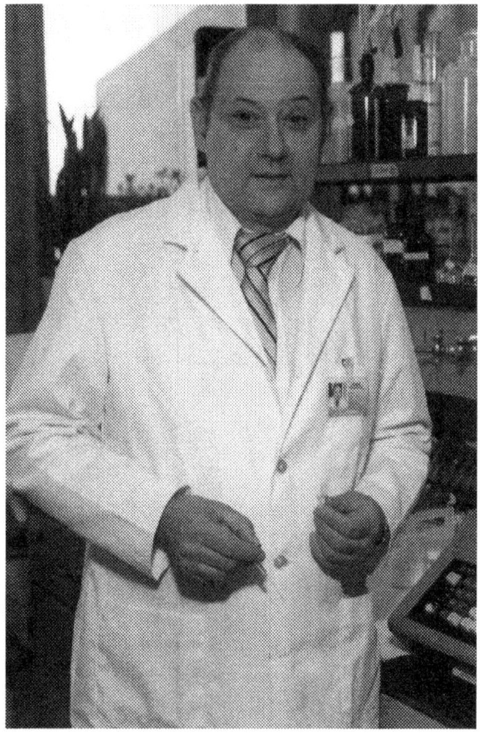

Dr. Domino's interests are broad in both basic and clinical pharmacology. Over the years specific research problems include:

1. Drugs affecting levels of consciousness (anesthesia, coma, psychotomimetic states, wakefulness, sleeping and dreaming) correlated with EEG and evoked potential topographic brain mapping
2. Neuropsychopharmacology of nicotine and tobacco smoking with PET scanning
3. Drugs of abuse and therapy – methods of assay, pharmacokinetics and clinical implications
4. Parkinson's disease – new methods of treatment
5. Toxic effects of medications as well as environmental pollutants

For any given decade or so research emphasis has varied with available funding from the state and federal governments, industry, private groups, and persons. His laboratory has been funded continuously since 1953. The role of the chemical neurotransmitter, acetylcholine, and its interaction with various drugs, substances of abuse and toxins has been a consistent research theme. Both the muscarnic and nicotinic cholinergic mechanisms in brain function have been explored. Nicotine in particular is an important agent in elaborating the role of nicotinic cholinergic receptors in maintaining arousal with skeletal muscle relaxation.

Current research support involves the role of nicotine in tobacco smoking. Why is it so difficult for smokers to quit when they know the obvious harmful effects of tobacco smoking? Is there more to smoking than nicotine? What are the functions of multiple nicotinic cholinergic receptors? Are there better agonists and antagonists to nicotine? What is the role of the other 4,000 plus chemicals in tobacco smoke?

Current emphasis is on PET studies, but phenotyping/genotyping and its role in tobacco addiction and carcinogenesis are important priorities. Nicotine induced behavioral sensitization is a very intriguing phenomena whose mechanism of action is an exciting area of research. Translational research from in vitro to in vivo animal to human studies is an essential activity of our laboratory. Basic research findings, whenever possible, are extended to studies involving human volunteers. Students, postdoctoral fellows, and technicians are key members of a research team which involves collaboration with other faculty members in pharmacy, psychiatry, radiology, and nuclear medicine.

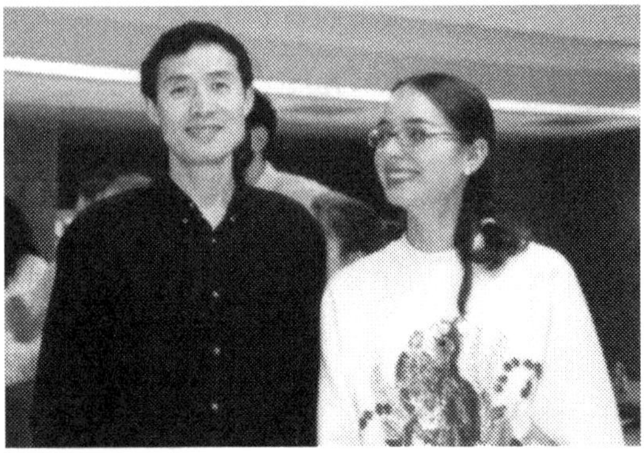

Lisong Ni and Kari Fedewa

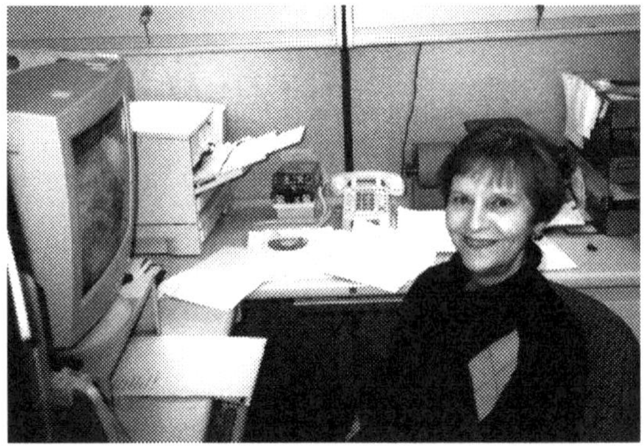

Ellen Howard at work

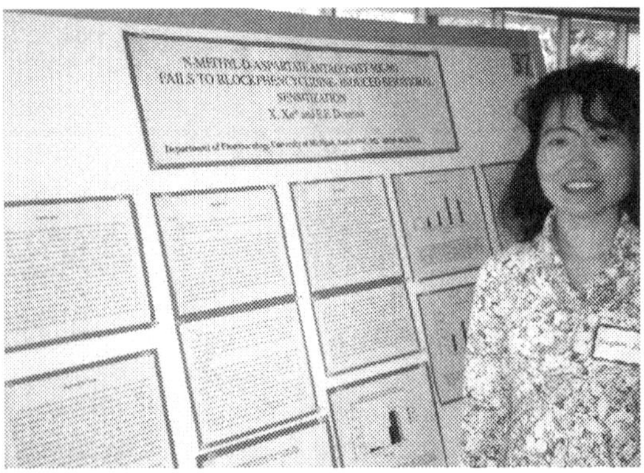

Xiao Juan Xu at her poster.

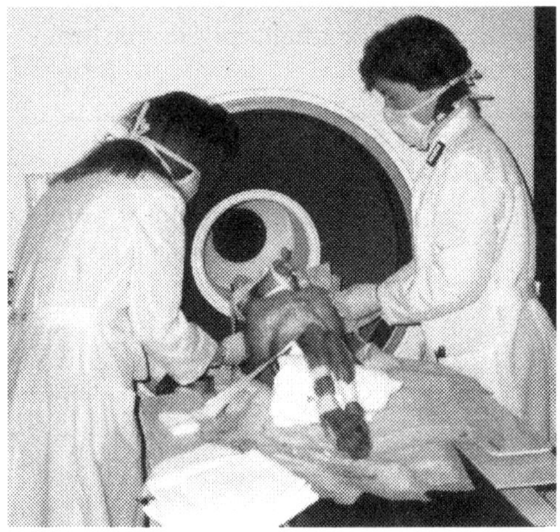

An anesthesized Scarlet being placed in the animal PET scanner

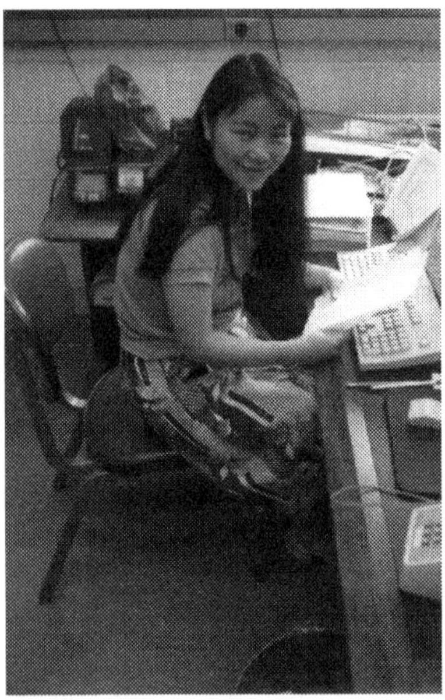

Yingfan Zhang doing computer analysis of EEG

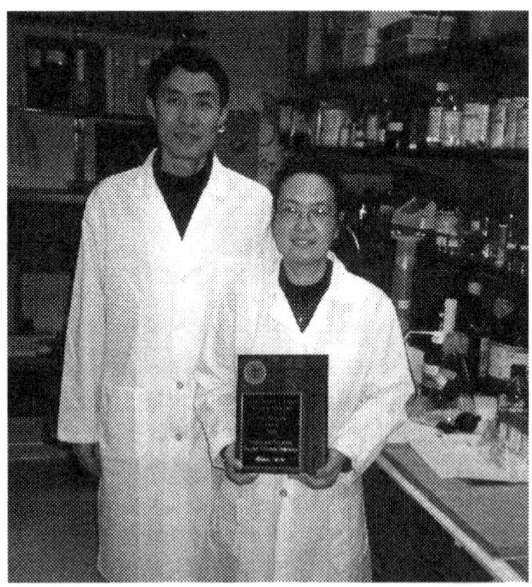

Lisong Ni and Huilei Zhang with an award from Eastern Michigan University

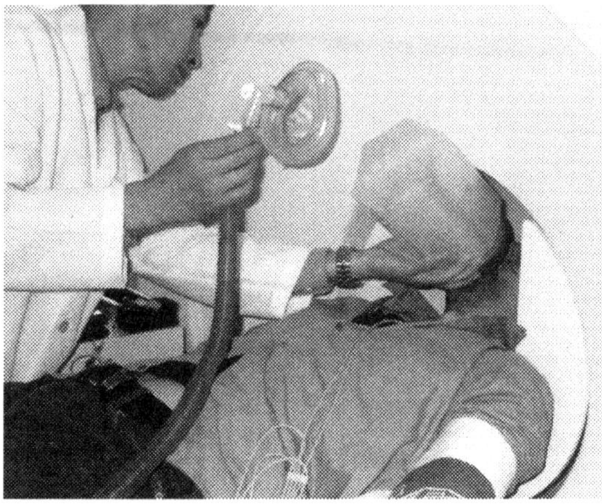

A unique (but approved) way to smoke a cigarette in the PET facility of University Hospital

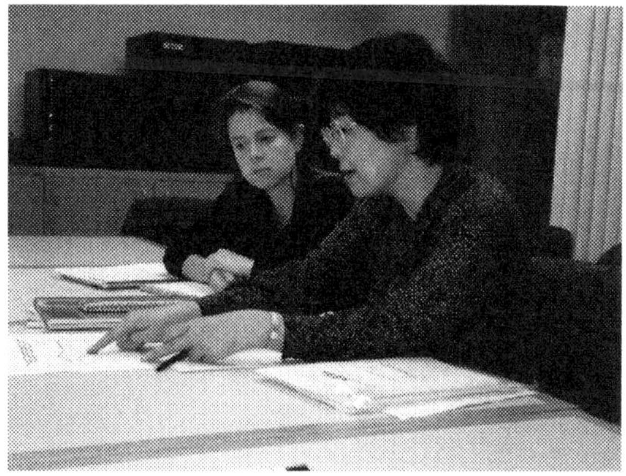

Marina Emborg with Dr. Kono

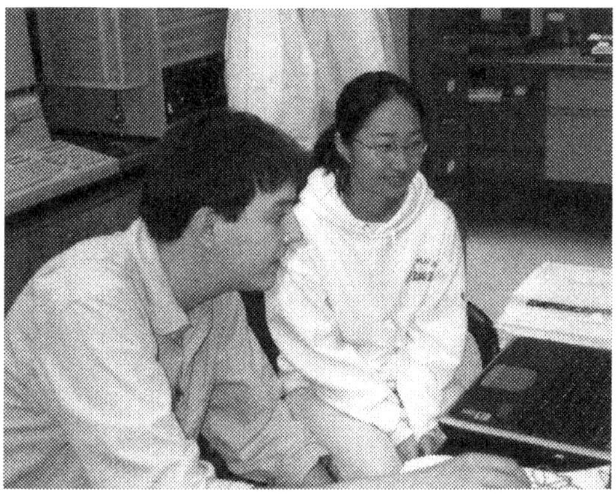

Christopher Buchanan and Jane Ni getting this book composed

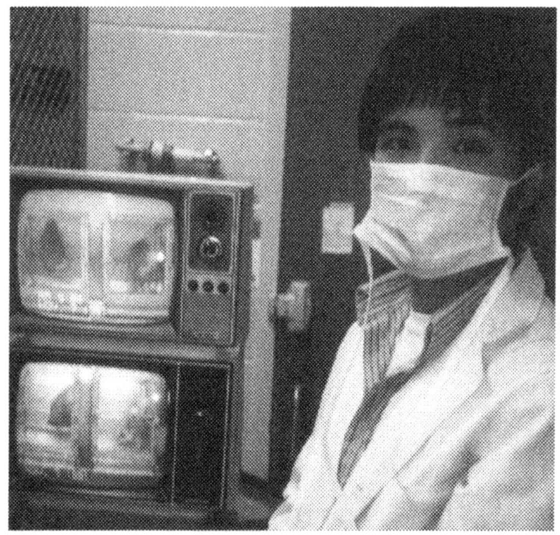

Jonathan Sheng with Flash, Margie, Lilbet and Tibet on TV monitors

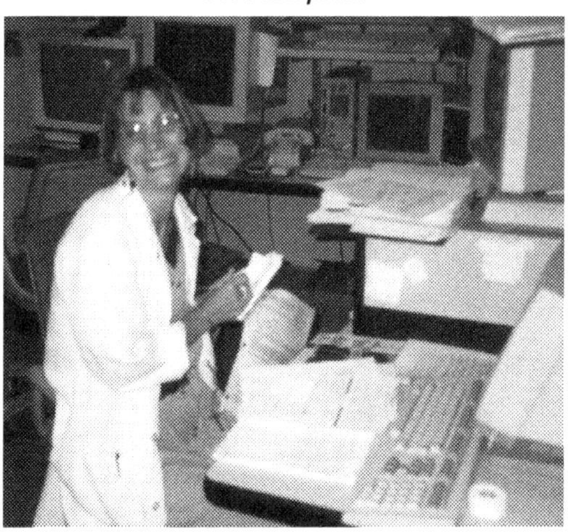

Jill Rothley, who hates the smell of burning tobacco

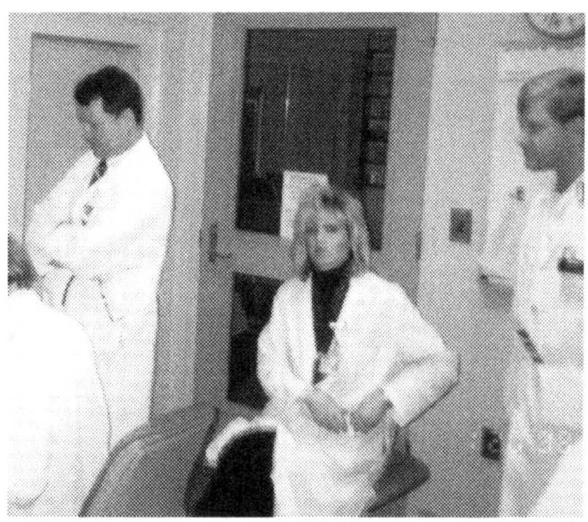

Ed McKenna, Linda Ohl and Jon Kar Zubieta in the PET unit

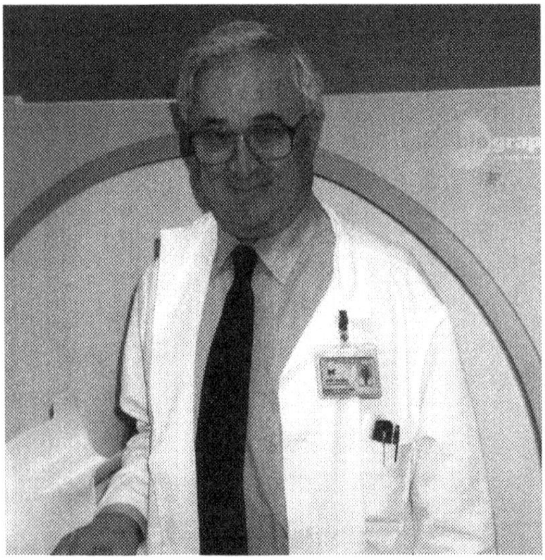

Dr. David E. Kuhl who helped make PET possible

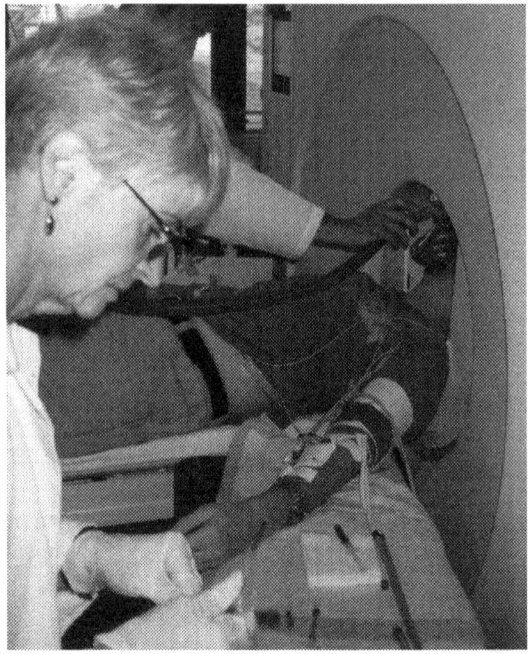

Dr. Sally K. Guthrie drawing blood samples

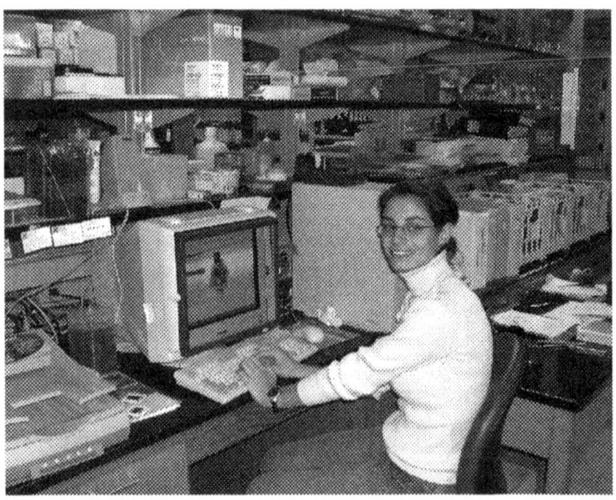

Valerie Burnisky surfing the internet for this book

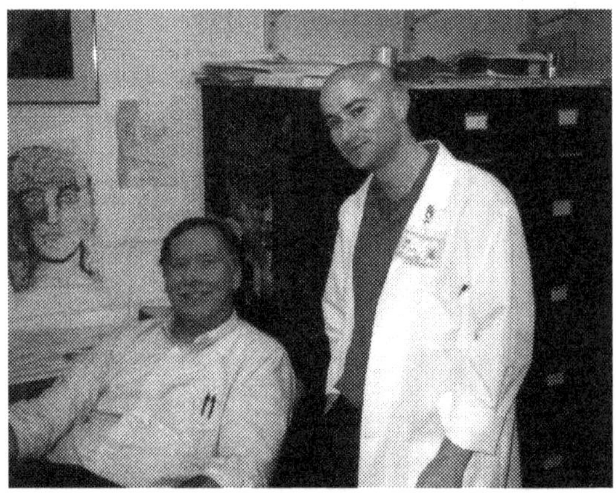

Dr. Robert A. Koeppe with Josh Bueller

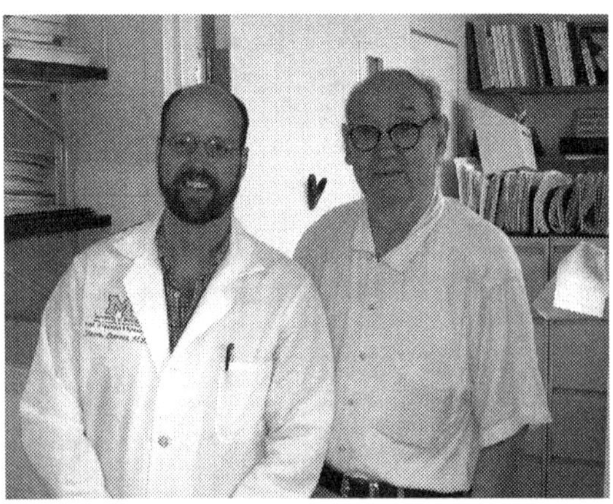

Kicking around research ideas

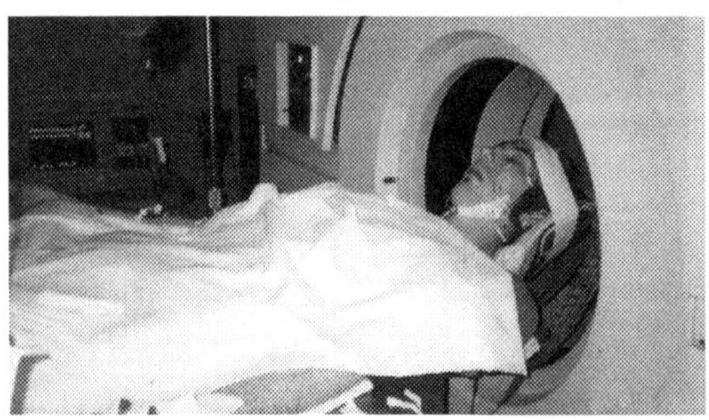

A Japanese volunteer in Domino's joint study in Akita

Dr. William D. Ensminger's Research Interests

Dr. Ensminger's research focuses on more selective drug use in cancer therapy. A major emphasis has been on the mechanisms apparent in increased regional therapeutic effect with primary and metastatic cancer in liver. Studies with the antimetabolite 5-fluoro-2'-deoxyuridine (FUDR) demonstrated that hepatic arterial (HA) infusion of the drug exposed liver tumors to 400-fold higher drug levels than tolerated with standard intravenous infusions.

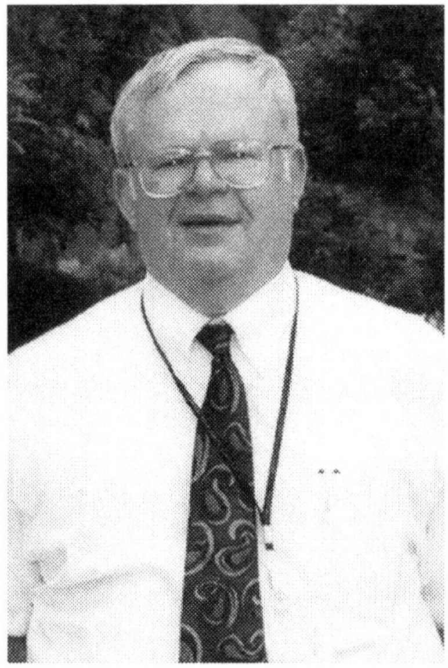

Appropriate methods were developed for administering such infusions to patients on a protracted basis, namely the development of implanted infusion pumps for distribution. The sideport of the infusion pump was, in turn, developed into a mechanism for administering intravenous chemotherapy. Ports were tested in dogs and then in patients and found to be a good method for vascular access, now being utilized in over 100,000 patients per year. Variations in ports have been developed through further dog studies and taken into the clinic.

The use of high dose focal radiotherapy combined with hepatic arterial FUDR is being tested for tolerance and toxicity in patients with liver cancers based upon cell culture studies demonstrating significant radiosensitization with FUDR. Also other studies involve examination of the regional pharmacokinetics of portal venous infusions of amifostine as a radioprotectant for liver cells.

A series of clinical studies with amifostine combined with whole liver radiotherapy have been initiated. In recent years, preclinical studies involving suicide gene therapy for liver cancers have been undertaken. The enzyme cytosine deaminase (CD) converts the antifungal agent flucytosine to the anticancer drug fluorouracil. This is a bacterial and yeast enzyme not found in mammalian cells. An adenoviral vector encoding for the yeast enzyme is being examined in nude rats having human colorectal cancer. The adenoviral vector currently being studied has a CEA promoter, which leads to high activity specifically in CEA-producing colorectal cancer cells.

We found that the use of direct HA vector administration along with starch microspheres to temporarily block the virus solution from being flushed through the microvasculature appears to increase tumor expression selectively by several hundred-fold.

Attempts are underway to produce therapeutic effects in the rat model. Other studies have shown that irradiation can increase viral vector uptake more than 5-fold. It is anticipated that, ultimately, combining HA administrated CD adenoviral vector with focal radiotherapy to liver tumors will be examined in clinical trials. Essentially all of the preclinical cell culture and animal studies conducted in this research program finds outlet in correlative clinical trials.

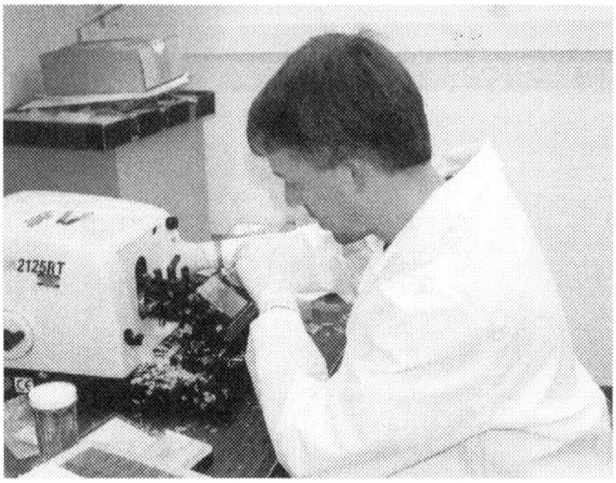

Joshua Parsels

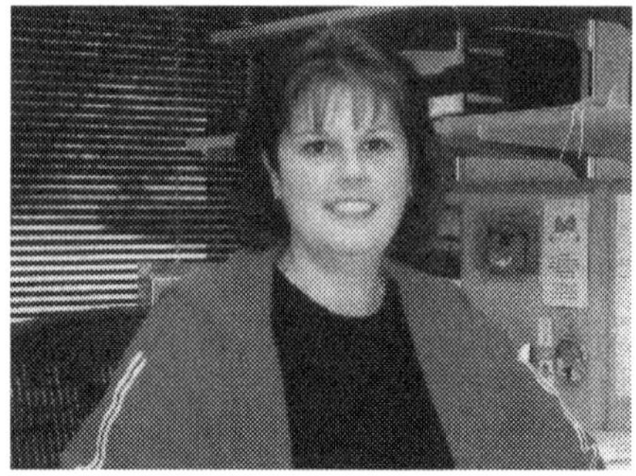

Pam Benci

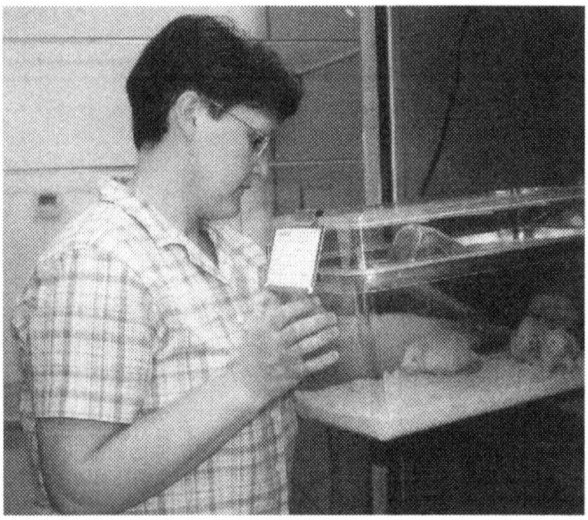

Susan De Remer

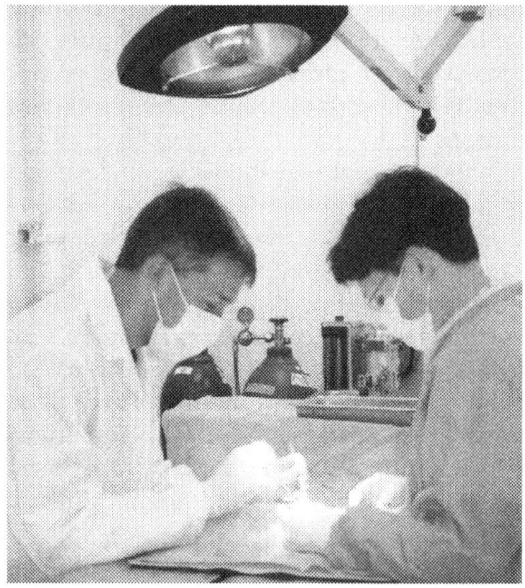

Joshua Parsels and Susan De Remer

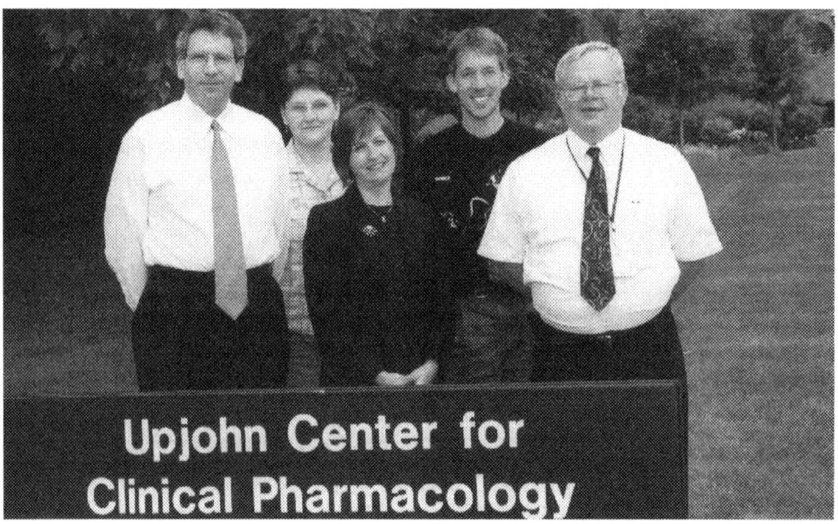

Jon Maybaum, Susan De Remer, Susan Walker, Joshua Parsels, William Ensminger

Dr. José A. Esteban's Research Interests

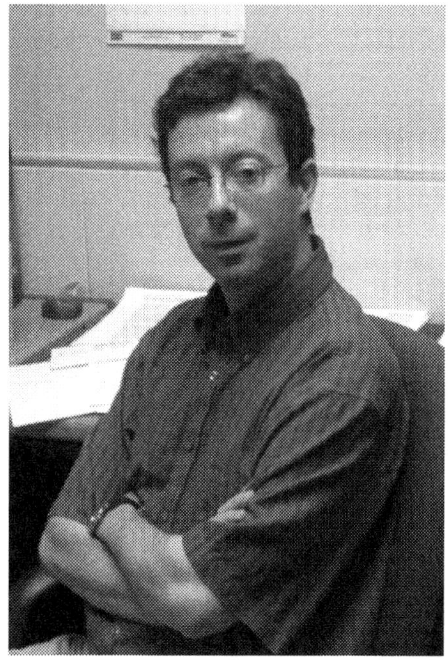

Dr. José Esteban's research involves neurotransmitter receptor trafficking and synaptic plasticity in the brain. Synaptic connections in the brain are continuously remodeled in response to neuronal activity. This process, known as synaptic plasticity, is widely accepted as the cellular basis for learning and memory, and it is also critical for the establishment of functional neuronal circuits during development. Additionally, several neurological and neurodegenerative diseases (such as schizophrenia, epilepsy and Alzheimer's disease) have been correlated with deficits in synaptic plasticity. Research in the laboratory is focused on the cellular and molecular processes responsible for synaptic plasticity, as a way to understand basic mechanisms underlying brain development, learning and memory.

Most excitatory transmission in the brain is mediated by AMPA-type glutamate receptors (AMPA receptors). Therefore, the presence of these receptors at synapses has to be carefully regulated in order to ensure correct neuronal communication. Interestingly, AMPA receptors are not static components of synapses. On the contrary, they are continuously being delivered and removed in and out of synapses in response to neuronal activity. In fact, recent investigations have demonstrated that this dynamic behavior of the AMPA receptors is an important mechanism to modify synaptic strength during plasticity. For instance, brief episodes of intense neuronal activity trigger the addition of new AMPA receptors into the synapse, leading to a long-lasting enhancement of synaptic transmission known as long-term potentiation (LTP). On the contrary, longer or more moderate periods of activity induce the removal of AMPA receptors from synapses, and consequently, lead to long-term depression (LTD). These forms of synaptic plasticity are especially prevalent in the hippocampus, which is one of the brain regions most clearly involved in learning and memory. In fact, LTP and LTD are presumed to be the synaptic mechanisms by which new memories are acquired and stored in the hippocampus.

The research work concentrates on the mechanisms that regulate the trafficking and synaptic targeting of AMPA receptors during synaptic plasticity. The major experimental approach consists of the expression of recombinant receptors and regulatory proteins tagged with GFP in hippocampal slices, using electrophysiology and neuronal imaging as functional assays. This experimental setting preserves the basic connectivity and developmental pattern of the intact hippocampus while allowing pharmacological manipulations and efficient expression of recombinant proteins. His group believes this multidisciplinary experimental approach is essential for the general goal of understanding how individual molecules contribute to neuronal function.

AMPA receptors are hetero-tetrameric molecules composed of different combinations of GluR1 to GluR4 subunits. In hippocampus, most AMPA receptors are composed of GluR1/GluR2 or GluR2/GluR3 combinations, whereas GluR4 is expressed mainly in early postnatal development. Interestingly, the synaptic trafficking of AMPA receptors is determined by their subunit composition. GluR2/3 receptors continuously cycle in and out of synaptic membranes in a process that does not require neuronal activity, whereas GluR1/2 and GluR4 receptors are added in an activity-dependent manner during synaptic plasticity. We are currently investigating the cellular machinery that controls the movement of these two populations of receptors. We have found, for instance, that members of the Rab family of small GTPases are necessary for the synaptic insertion of AMPA receptors both during their activity-independent cycling and also during the regulated delivery that accompanies LTP. In contrast, we have found that some chaperones are specifically required for the recycling of receptors back into synapses during their continuous movement. We are also investigating the mechanisms that control the removal of AMPA receptors from synapses. In this sense, we have found that long-term depression involves the endocytosis of AMPA receptors from the synaptic membrane, and that this process is also mediated by Rab proteins.

These studies are being continued and expanded to characterize other molecular components that control the transport and synaptic targeting of AMPA receptors. Also, we are investigating the signaling transduction cascades that trigger the movement of these receptors in response to neuronal activity. With this combined effort, we are trying to elucidate how the signaling pathways initiated by neuronal activity communicate with the cellular transport machinery to orchestrate the synaptic trafficking of receptors during plasticity.

We hope that this basic research on synaptic plasticity will help us to understand the mechanisms that underlie higher brain functions, like learning and memory, and eventually, develop therapies for the mental disorders that alter them.

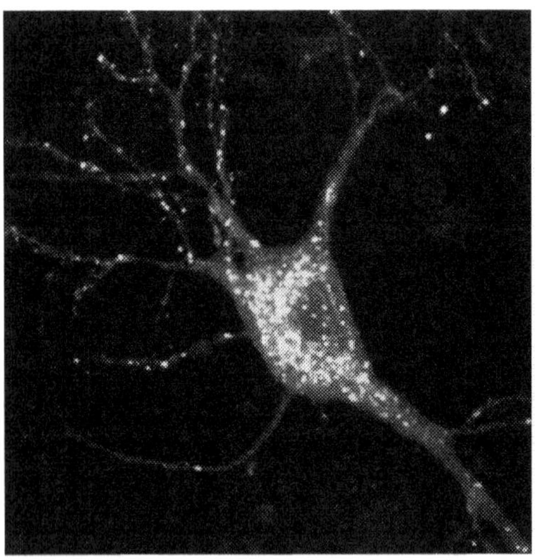

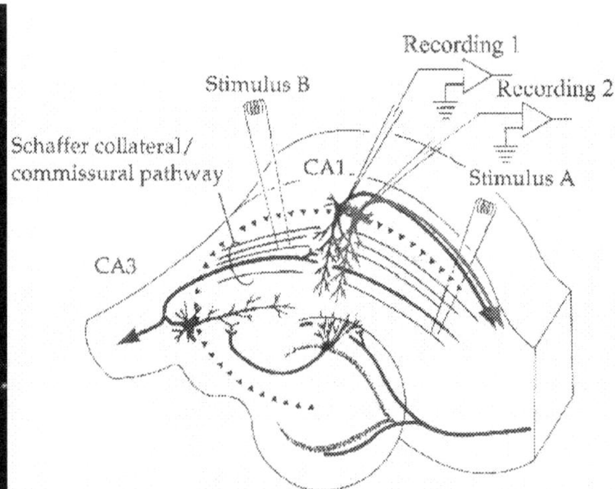

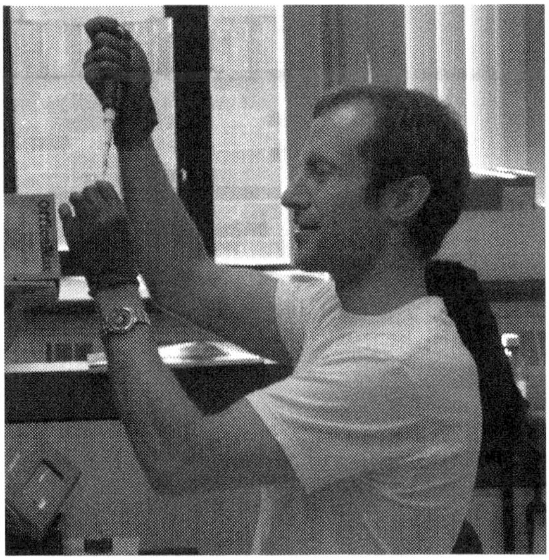

Donald Backos

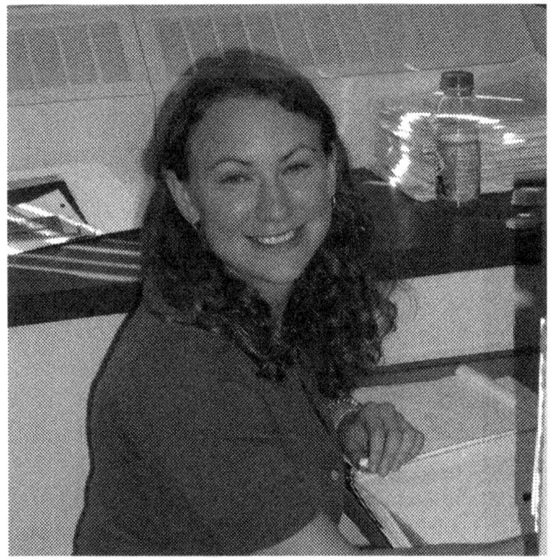

Katie Weiss

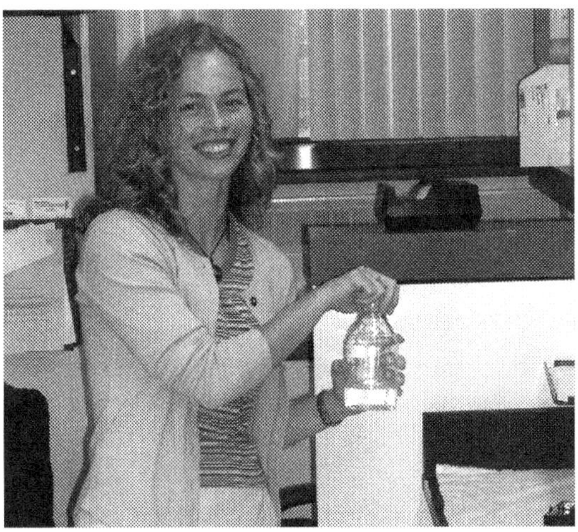

Alana Lysholm

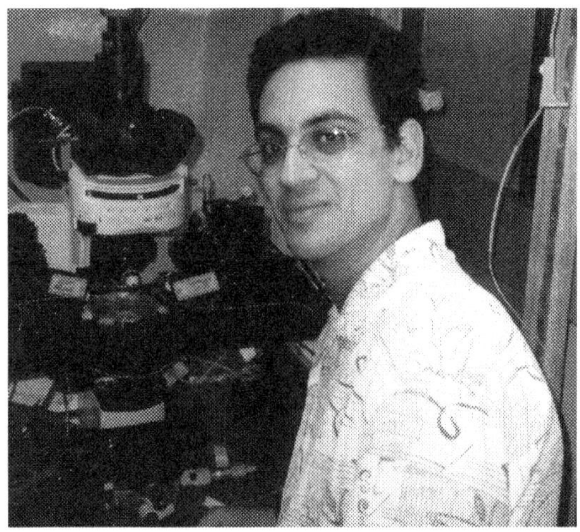

Nashaat Gerges

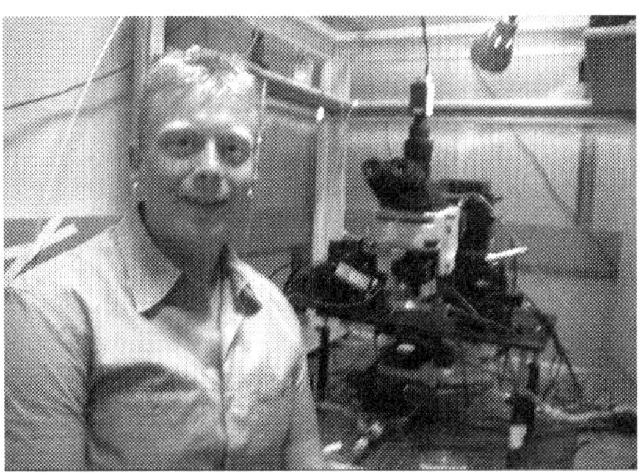

Tyler Brown

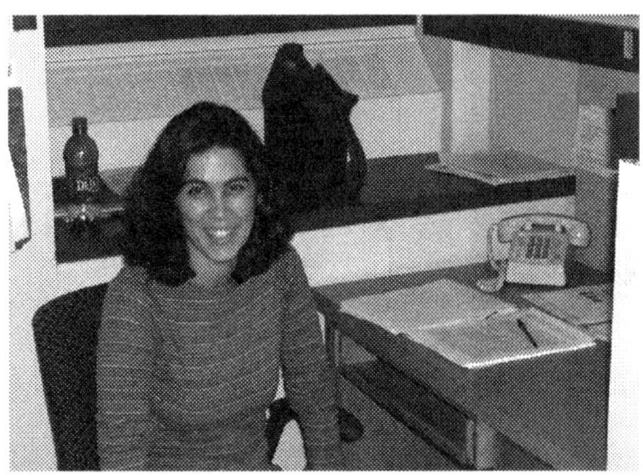

Susana Correia

Dr. Peter S. Fischbach's Research Interests

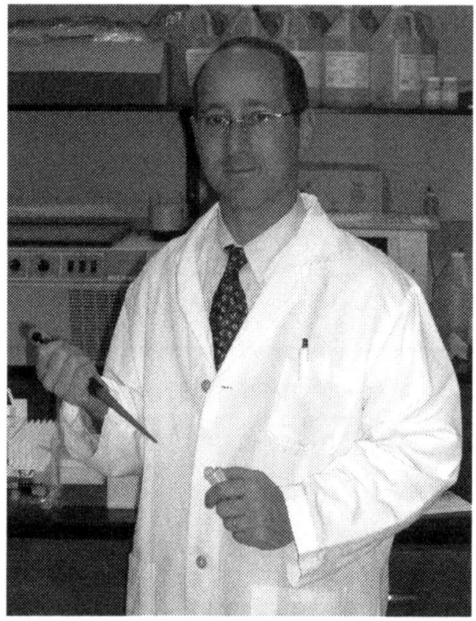

Dr. Fischbach is currently the director of the pediatric electrophysiology laboratory and has been participating in research within the Department of Pharmacology since beginning his pediatric cardiology fellowship in 1996. His laboratory research interests have focused on the mechanisms of arrhythmia formation and maintenance as well as in pharmacological management of arrhythmias. In particular, Dr. Fischbach has been interested in the electrical remodeling that occurs during sustained atrial fibrillation. Atrial fibrillation is the most common tachyarrhythmia in humans causing an increase in the need for hospitalization, increased risk of stroke, and leading to an increase in mortality. Medical therapy has been disappointing using both traditional pharmacological agents as well as interventional therapies such as radiofrequency ablation and implanted pacemakers and cardioverters. Recent experimental results have demonstrated that sustained arrhythmia induces cellular and sub-cellular changes in the atrial muscle referred to as electrical remodeling. These changes include an alteration in the composition of ion channels inhabiting the sarcolemmal membrane. In effect, the medicines that are currently being used to treat atrial fibrillation may be targeting ion channels that are no longer present in the atrial myocardium or have only a minor role in the maintenance of the arrhythmia. In conjunction with Dr. Lori Isom's laboratory, Dr. Fischbach has been examining the alterations in the expression and localization of the voltage gated sodium channel in a canine model of atrial fibrillation as well as from biopsy specimens of humans with and without atrial fibrillation.

Additionally, Dr. Fischbach has been investigation the role the ATP-gated potassium channel (K^+-ATP channel) plays in hypoxia/ischemia related arrhythmias. It is currently known that there are K^+-ATP channels localized to the sarcolemmal and inner mitochondrial membranes. These channels are molecularly distinct and are influenced by different pharmacological agents. Channels residing in the mitochondrial membrane appear to be responsible for chemical and ischemic preconditioning of the heart. The role of the sarcolemmal channels remains a mystery. Using a Langendorff perfused isolated rabbit heart model, the role of the ATP gated potassium channel in the sarcolemmal membrane is currently being investigated.

Clinically, Dr. Fischbach has been examining the use of pacemakers in children. In particularly he is interested in the role of bi-ventricular pacing in children with repaired congenital heart disease. Bi-ventricular pacing has become a powerful new tool for treating heart failure in adults with ischemic and non-ischemic dilated cardiomyopathy. The efficacy of its application and appropriate selection criteria for its use in children has yet to be established however.

Dr. Stephen K. Fisher's Research Interests

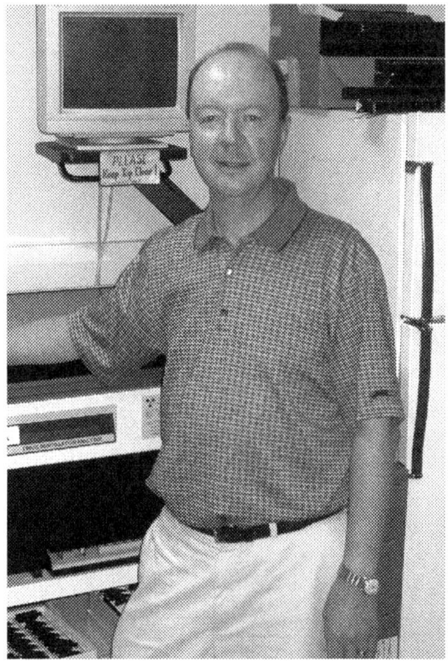

Dr. Fisher's laboratory is concerned with the role of phospholipids in signal transduction at cell-surface receptors. The focus of his laboratory is that of the role played by phosphoinositides (inositol-containing phospholipids) in the cell biology of neural cells. These quantitatively minor phospholipids, which are prevalent within the nervous system, are known to play an important role in signal transduction events at neural membranes since their turnover is linked to the activation of a pharmacologically distinct group of cell-surface receptors. This then leads to activation of phospholipase C and, via the phosphodiesteratic breakdown of phosphatidylinositol 4,5-bisphosphate (PIP_2), the subsequent formation of intracellular second messengers involved in calcium homeostasis and protein phosphorylation. It has also become evident that inositol lipids may play important roles in other aspects of the cell biology of neurons. Elucidation of the roles for phosphoinositides in such functions as the internalization (endocytosis) of cell surface receptors and in maintenance of the actin cytoskeleton have been major research objectives of this laboratory. In the latter context, PIP_2 has been shown to play a key role in the tyrosine phosphorylation of focal adhesion kinase, a protein tyrosine kinase that is enriched in neuronal growth cones and plays a role in their remolding. In addition, regulation of the homeostasis of myo-inositol, a key precursor molecule for phosphoinositide synthesis, has been investigated using human NT2-N neurons.

The availability of inositol may be of major importance to our understanding of the therapeutic efficacy of lithium salts, which, to date, are the most effective form of treatment for manic-depressive psychosis. Most recently we have observed that receptor-stimulated phosphoinositide hydrolysis may facilitate the regulatory changes in brain cell volume following hypoosmotic stress (encountered during hyponatremia, following excessive water intake by athletes and in other clinically relevant conditions). Increases in the volume of brain cells is of major physiological importance because of limitations of the skull. Our results suggest that cell surface receptors, some of which operate via phospholipase C, can increase the release of small organic osmolytes such as inositol, taurine and glutamate from neural cells. Recent data indicate that muscarinic receptor activation significantly enhances the release of osmolytes under conditions of very limited reductions in osmolarity (e.g. 5%), conditions under which the basal release of osmolytes is minimal. Thus receptor activation serves to facilitate osmolyte release and constitutes part of a regulatory volume decrease mechanism that restores the volume of brain cells.

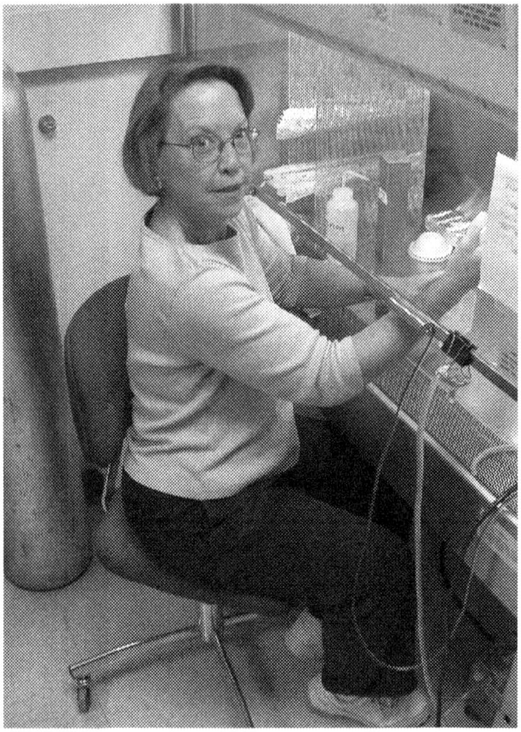

Dr. Heacock subculturing neurotumor cells

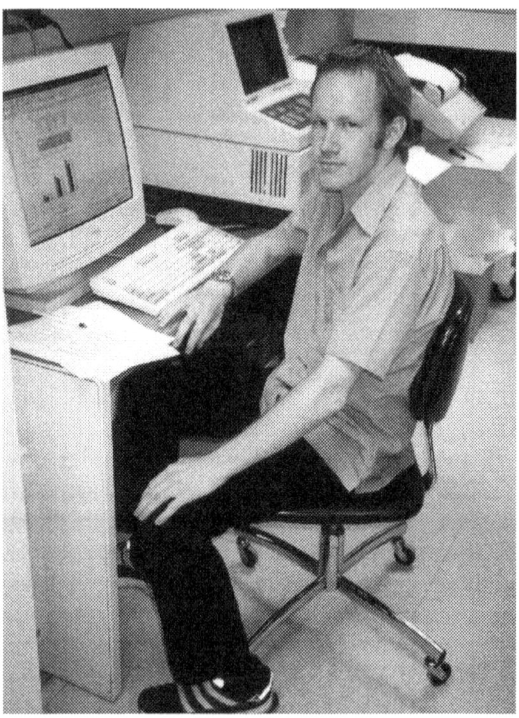

Dan Kerly computing

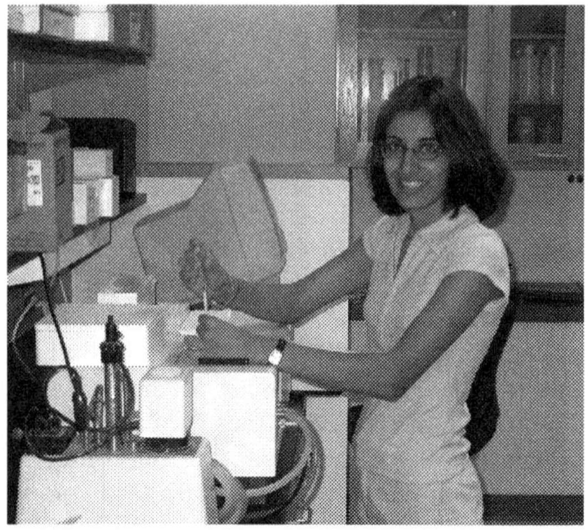

Tooba Cheema monitoring calcium signals in neural cells

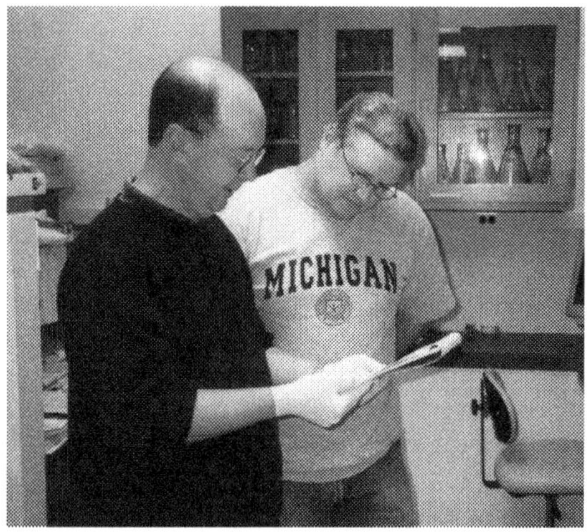

Aaron VanTroostenberghe with Dr. Fisher reviewing data

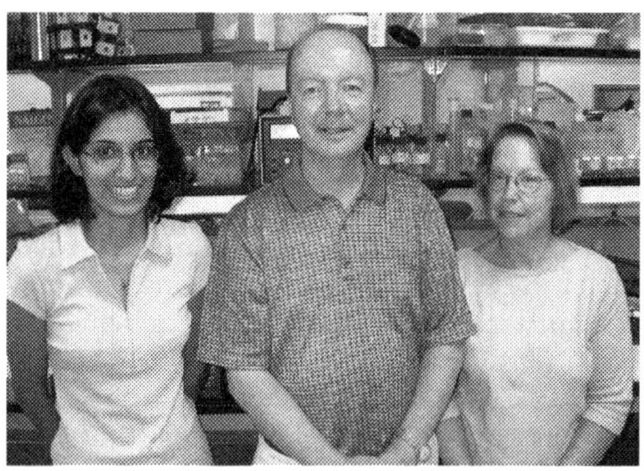

Tooba Cheema (graduate student), Stephen Fisher and Anne Heacock

Dr. Margaret E.Gnegy's Research Interests

Dr. Gnegy's laboratory is interested in three amphetamine-related projects:

1 The mechanism of action of amphetamine at the catecholamine transporter
2 The neurobiological adaptations that occur in the brain following repeated amphetamine
3 The effect of AMPH on cell growth and differentiation.

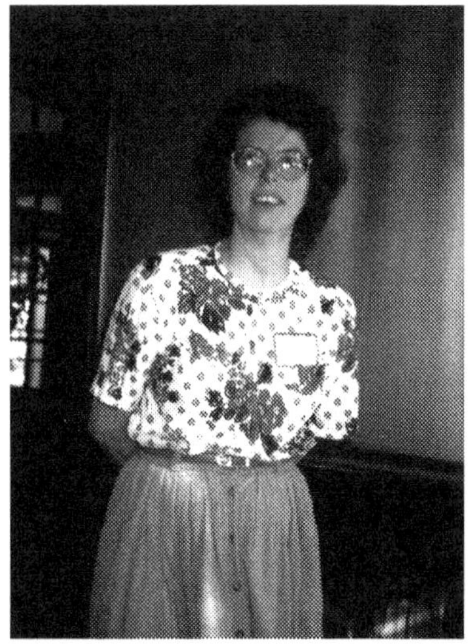

Mechanism of Action of Amphetamine (AMPH) at Plasmalemmal Catecholamine Transporters

Amphetamine (AMPH) and its congener, methamphetamine, are stimulant drugs that elicit hyperactivity, tachycardia, appetite suppression and wakefulness in humans. Repeated use of AMPH can lead to drug addiction and craving, along with anorexia, excessive heart stimulation and stroke. Amphetamines elicit these effects by reversing plasmalemmal dopamine transporters (DAT) or norepinephrine transporters (NET), and eliciting the release of the catecholamines into the synapse. Both DAT and NET are members of a family of Na^+/Cl^- dependent transporters. In order for AMPH, a transporter substrate, to release dopamine it must bind to DAT or NET and be transported into the terminal or cell. Cocaine, a transporter antagonist, increases extracellular dopamine by binding to outward-facing DAT and blocking DA uptake. Many aspects of the mechanism whereby AMPH makes DAT available for binding to DA inside the terminal and reverses the transporter are unknown.

Our data reveal a requirement for protein kinase C (PKC) activation in the mediation of AMPH's effects. Selective PKC inhibitors, such as chelerythrine (above) block AMPH-mediated dopamine release without affecting normal dopamine uptake. This inhibition of AMPH activity has behavioral consequences; a PKC-inhibitor reduced AMPH-mediated locomotor activity. Another novel finding is that intracellular, as opposed to extracellular, Ca^{2+} is required for AMPH-mediated reverse transport. Moreover, direct PKC activation can release dopamine through DAT. This suggests that a PKC-mediated phosphorylation is occurring with AMPH.

Neurobiological Adaptations Following Repeated AMPH

We are investigating the role of a PKC-mediated phosphorylation in AMPH activity by investigating the phosphorylation of DAT by AMPH and PKC activators, and by the use of stable HEK cell lines containing DAT mutants having altered putatative phosphorylation sites.

Repeated treatment with psychomotor stimulants leads to a number of gradually developing neuroadaptations leading to behavioral syndromes of withdrawal and sensitization. Behavioral sensitization to AMPH, expressed as a persistent augmentation of psychomotor stimulant effects to drug challenge, has been detected in humans and laboratory animals. Sensitization to AMPH is induced by an action of the drugs at the cell bodies but an action of the drug in the terminal region is sufficient for its expression. The behavioral sensitization and some neuroadaptations following AMPH administration are characterized by persistence and strengthening with time following discontinuation of drug. One persistent neuroadaptation which develops days following cessation of repeated AMPH is enhanced stimulus-induced DA release.

Following repeated AMPH, dopamine release in striatum and nucleus accumbens is enhanced by stimuli that activate exocytotic release and by stimuli (AMPH) that reverse the plasmalemmal DA transporter, DAT. The fact that this occurs in striatal synaptosomes indicates that a complicated anatomical circuitry is not necessary for the effect. DAT-mediated DA release is normally independent of extracellular Ca^{2+} but following repeated AMPH it becomes dependent upon $Ca^{2+}$and the Ca^{2+} and calmodulin (CaM)-dependent protein kinase II (CaM KII) in addition to PKC. In addition, we have found increased phosphorylation of presynaptic proteins at sites specific for PKC, PKA and CaM KII following repeated AMPH.

We have developed a cell culture model of repeated amphetamine action that demonstrates the enhancement in transporter function following repeated AMPH. Treatment of either rat pheochromocytoma PC 12 cells or human neuroblastoma SH-SY5Y cells with repeated, intermittent amphetamine leads to twice as much AMPH-induced dopamine release as compared to vehicle-treated cells (see above). Cells were given 1 mM of amphetamine for five min a day, five consecutive days followed by 10 drug-free days. Both PC 12 cells and SH-SY5Y cells are nucleated, synthesize and store norepinephrine and dopamine, and readily release dopamine through a transporter. Just as in the rat, the enhanced amphetamine-induced dopamine release was dependent upon extracellular Ca^{2+} and CaM Kinase II. Also, just as in the rat, all AMPH-induced dopamine release is dependent upon PKC activity.

We are investigating the role of different protein kinase activities in the development of the enhanced release as well as the role of a Ca^{2+}/CaM Kinase II-mediated phosphorylation.

Role of AMPH in cell growth and differentiation

In addition to developing an enhancement in dopamine release, repeated treatment of the cells with AMPH followed by 10 drug-free days led to neurite outgrowth. There was a 3-fold increase in the number of cells with neurites, the length of neurites and the amount of the growth-signalling proteins, neurofilament protein and GAP-43 as compared to control cells. The action of AMPH was not synergistic with that of nerve growth factor and was not blocked by antibody to nerve growth factor. The action of AMPH was, however, blocked by PKC inhibitors, suggesting that PKC is important in the development of the neurites in response to amphetamine.

We are presently examining the role of various protein kinases in the development of the AMPH-mediated neurite outgrowth and whether the process resulting in the neurite outgrowth are also those responsible for the development of enhanced AMPH-induced dopamine release.

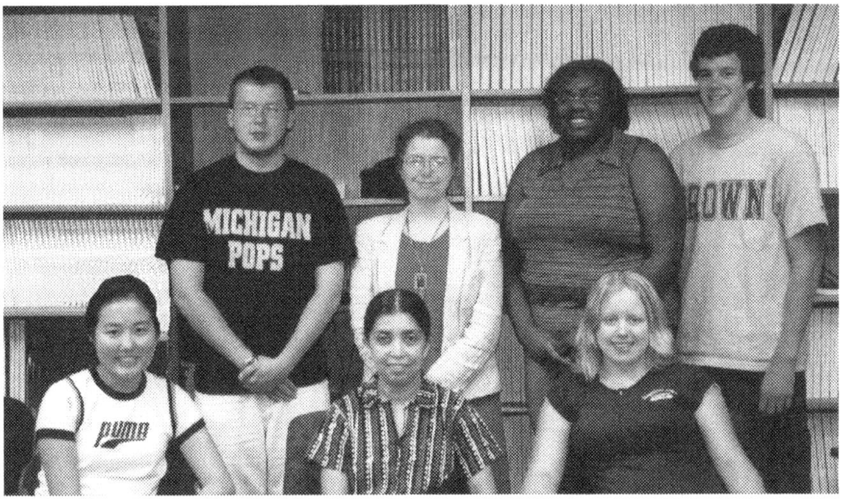

Front row: Christine Chi, Bipasha Guptaroy, Stephanie McLean
Back row: David Lund, Margaret Gnegy, L'Aurelle Johnson, Chris Burke

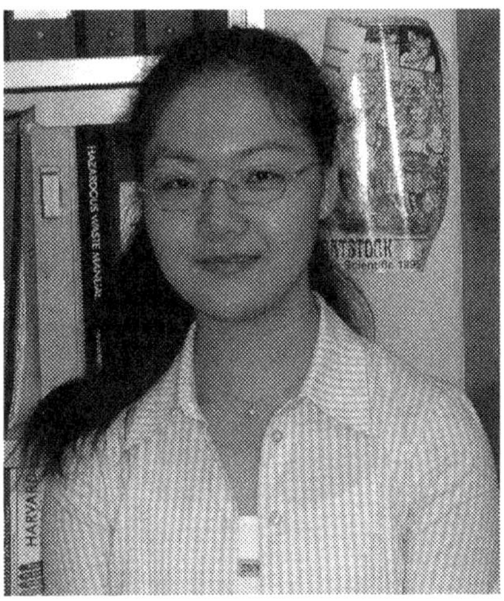

Minjia Zhang

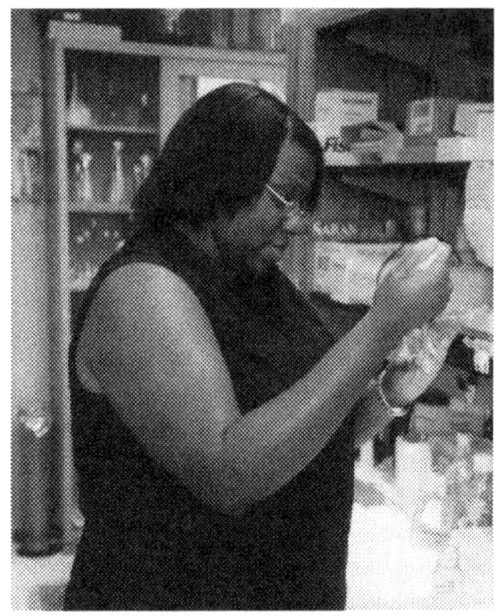

L'Aurelle Johnson

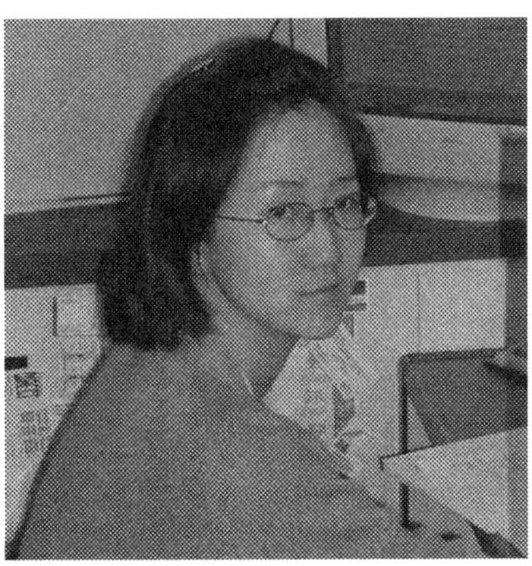

Yanghae Park

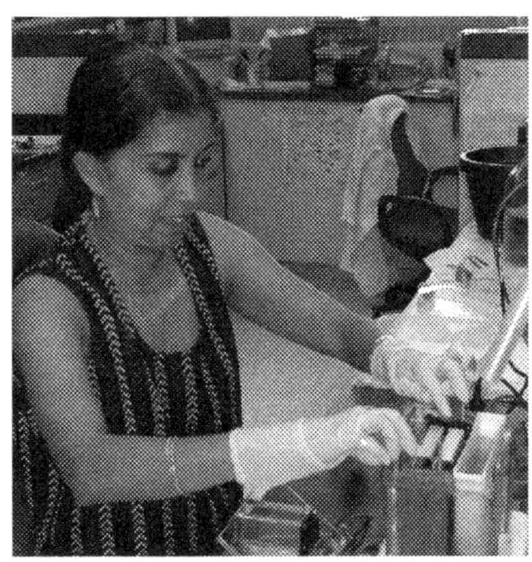

Bipasha Guptaroy

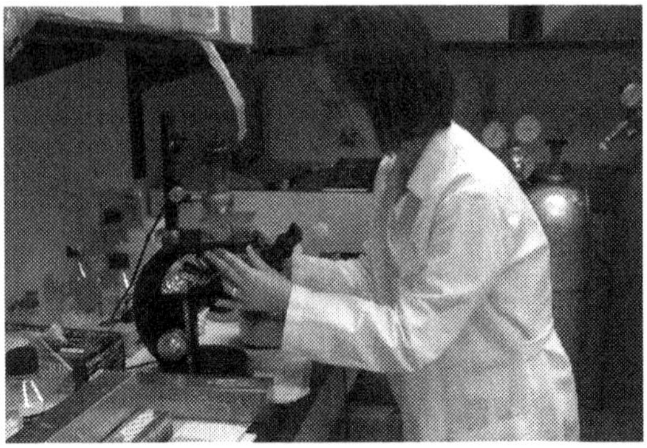

Yanghae Park

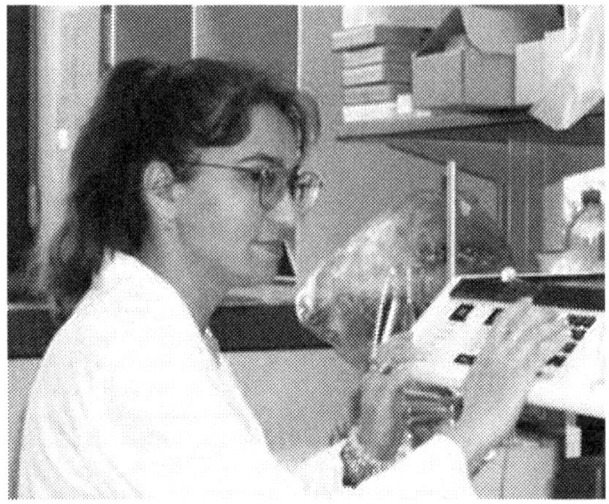

Lana Kantor

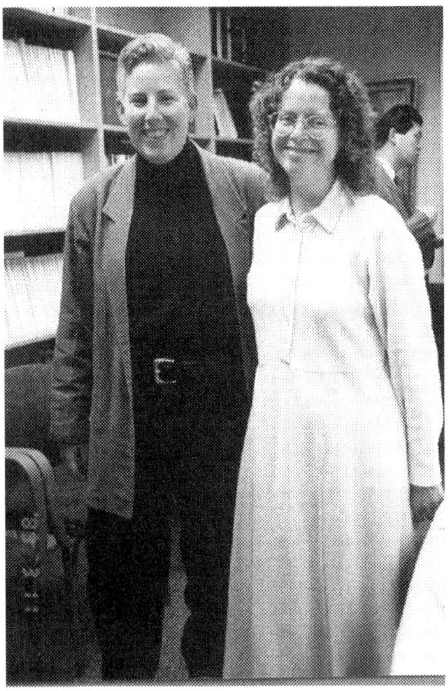

Kim McGinnis and Margaret Gnegy

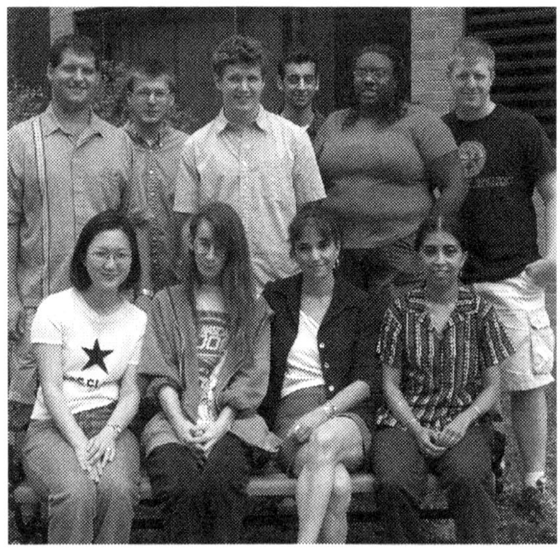

Front row: Yanghae Park, Marry Vaughan, Lana Kantor, Bipasha Guptaroy
Back row: Gabe Knudsen, David Lund, Andy Foster, Wagdi Sidrik, L' Aurelle Johnson, Colin Daining

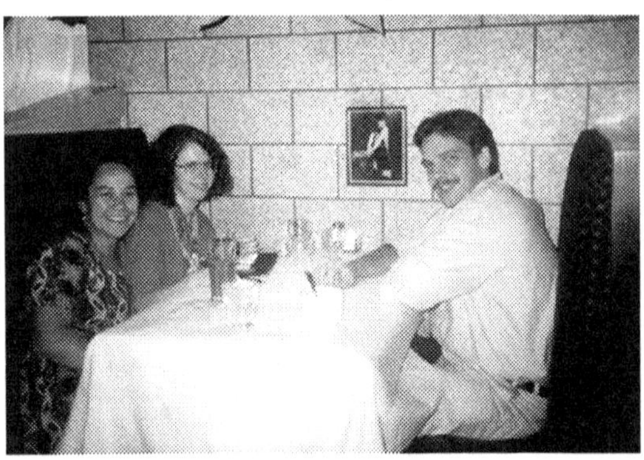

Keiki Hewlett, Margaret Gnegy, Jeffrey Harrison

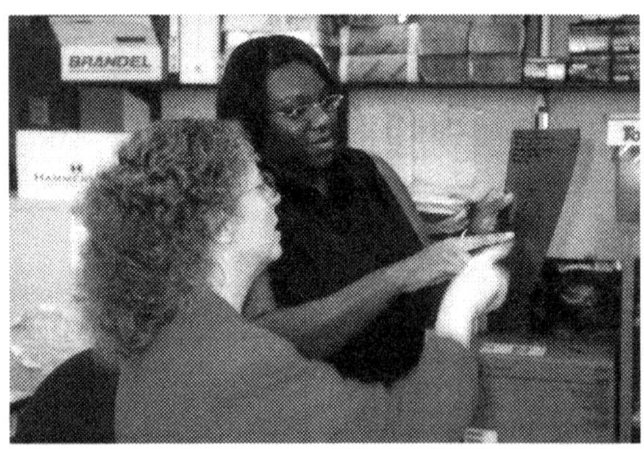

Dr. Gnegy and L'Aurelle Johnson

Dr. Paul F. Hollenberg's Research Interests

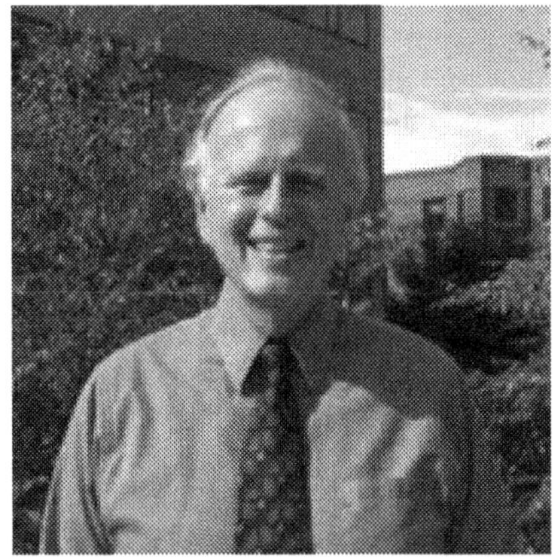

Our laboratory is primarily concerned with investigations of the microsomal cytochrome P450-dependent mixed-function oxidases found in most mammalian tissues. These enzymes catalyze the metabolism of a wide variety of xenobiotics including drugs, anesthetics, pesticides, chemical carcinogens, and organic solvents as well as endogenous compounds of great physiological importance including steroids, fatty acids, retinoids, eicosanoids, and lipid hydroperoxides. They also serve as nitric oxide (NO) synthases. Understanding the catalytic mechanisms, regulation, and roles of the P450s in the metabolism of endogenous and exogenous compounds is of great importance to the fields of pharmacology, endocrinology, toxicology, and oncology.

Epidemiological studies suggest most human cancers are due to exposure to chemicals in the environment that cause cancer. In general, these chemicals are biologically inert and require activation by the drug-metabolizing enzymes in the target tissue to express this carcinogenic potential. Compounds known to cause cancer as a result of metabolic activation by P450 include polycyclic aromatic hydrocarbons, nitrosamines, and aflatoxins. Thus, a primary objective of the laboratory is to gain a better understanding of mechanisms by which cells activate environmental chemicals to reactive forms that cause cancer and ultimately to develop approaches that could be used to protect humans against potentially carcinogenic or toxic chemicals in the environment.

More than 30 different forms of cytochromes P450 have been found in human tissues. Each form exhibits its own unique substrate specificity and even when two different forms metabolize the same substrate, they generally give very different product profiles. For some time, a major interest in our laboratory has been concerned with the relationships between the structures of the active sites of various forms of P450 and their catalytic functions. For these studies we have been using purified P450 2B1 and P450 2B4, the major forms of P450 induced by phenobarbital in rats and rabbits, respectively. We are also studying P450 2E1, a form that is thought to play a major role in the metabolic activation of many low molecular weight carcinogens and other toxic agents.

We have successfully expressed several human P450s and are now studying human P450 3A4, the human liver P450 which appears to play a major role in the metabolism of up to 50% of all drugs currently used in the United States; P450 2B6, another human P450 that plays an important role in the metabolism of a variety of drugs and toxins, and P450 2E1, which is known to play an important role in the metabolic activation and detoxication of many low molecular weight carcinogens and other toxins. We are using mechanism-based inactivators to investigate the structures of active sites of these P450s and to identify the specific amino acid residues in the active sites involved in catalysis or substrate-binding. Mechanism-based inactivators are substrates of an enzyme which, during the course of catalysis, are converted to highly reactive forms which react with moieties in the active site to form covalent adducts, thereby preventing the enzyme from traversing further catalytic cycles.

We are also trying to identify and develop mechanism-based inactivators that are specific for the forms of P450 such as 2E1 that are responsible for the activation of carcinogens, and thus have potential to be used as chemopreventive agents to protect against environmental carcinogens. We are working with a variety of mechanism-based inactivators including mifepristone (RU486), tamoxifen, 17 a-ethinylestradiol, phencyclidine (angel dust), benzyl isothiocyanate, tert-butylisothiocyanate, 7-ethynylcoumarin, and bergamottin. We have identified critical peptide regions and, in some cases, specific amino acid residues in the active sites of P450s 2B1, 2B4, 2B6, 2E1, and 3A4.

Current studies are concerned with: identification of additional active site amino acid(s) and peptide(s) of the enzymes modified during inactivation; determination of the mechanism(s) by which inactivation occurs, and determination of the specificity of each inactivator for protection against different carcinogens in cells expressing various P450s. These studies will provide valuable information for designing inactivators to selectively manipulate the catalytic activity of P450s and may ultimately lead to the development of approaches that may be used to protect people against developing cancer due to carcinogen exposure. Other studies aimed at understanding the relationship between the structure and function of P450 involve site-specific mutagenesis of selected amino acid residues in the P450 active site followed by investigations into changes in the catalytic function of the enzyme. We have performed site-specific mutagenesis studies on P450s 2B1 and 2B2, which differ by only 14 amino acid residues and yet exhibit marked differences in their specificities for some substrates and on P450 2E1. Additional site-specific mutagenesis studies target those amino acid residues that have been identified by the studies using mechanism-based inactivators and will yield valuable information regarding the role(s) of those residues in catalysis and substrate binding.

A second area of interest is concerned with the metabolism of dialkylnitrosamine carcinogens such as N-nitrosodimethylamine (NDMA), N-nitrosodiethylamine (NDEA) and N-nitrosodipropylamine (NDPA). These compounds are of great interest and concern because of widespread human exposure, high carcinogenic potency, and their demonstrated importance in human carcinogenesis. Nitrosamines are readily metabolized by various forms of cytochrome P450 that play a critical role both in their metabolic activation and their detoxication. Our laboratory is currently studying the metabolism of a series of nitrosamines. Areas under investigation include: determination of the metabolic products formed from each nitrosamine; identification of the forms of P450 responsible for the metabolism of each nitrosamine leading to the formation of the various products; elucidation of the role(s) of the various metabolites in cancer induction; and investigations of the effects of modifying agents such as phenobarbital, ethyl alcohol and pyridine on the metabolic activation and detoxication of these nitrosamines.

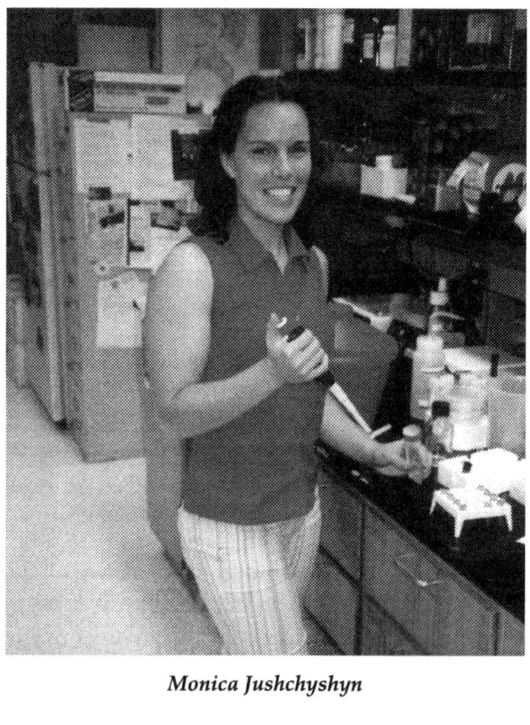

Monica Jushchyshyn

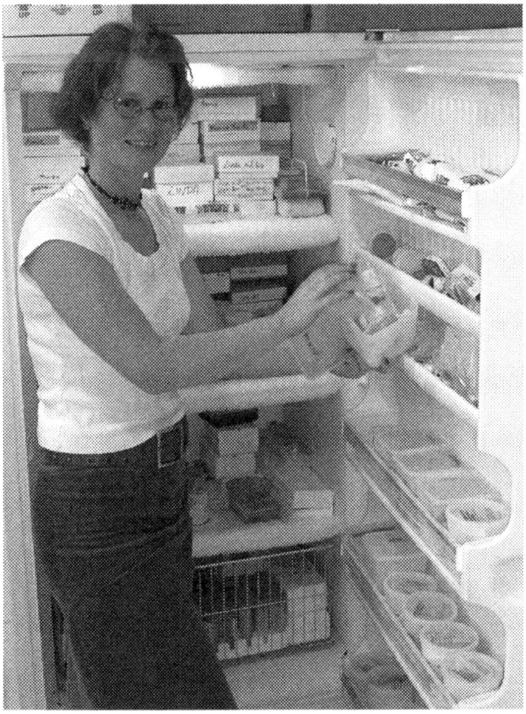

Linda Von Weymarn

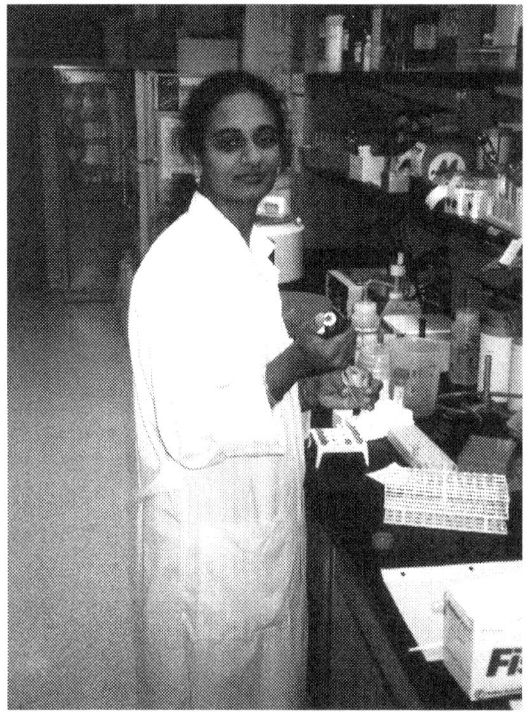

Chitra Sridar

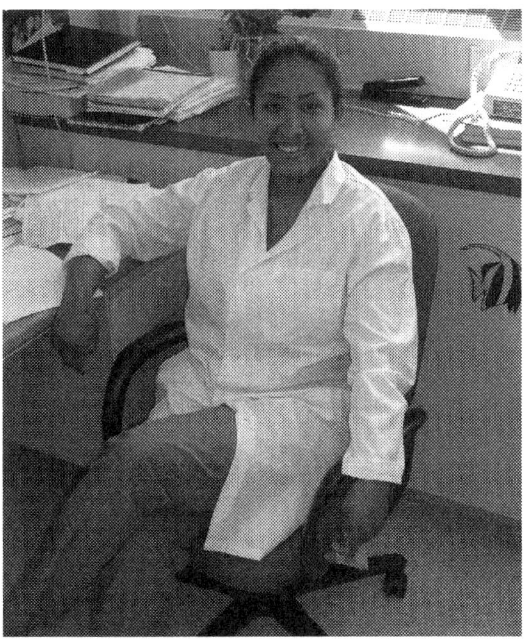

Edith Mensah-Osman

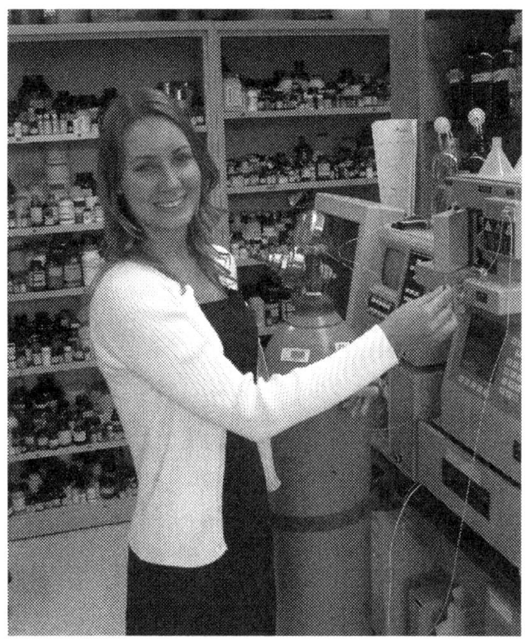

Annie Blobaum

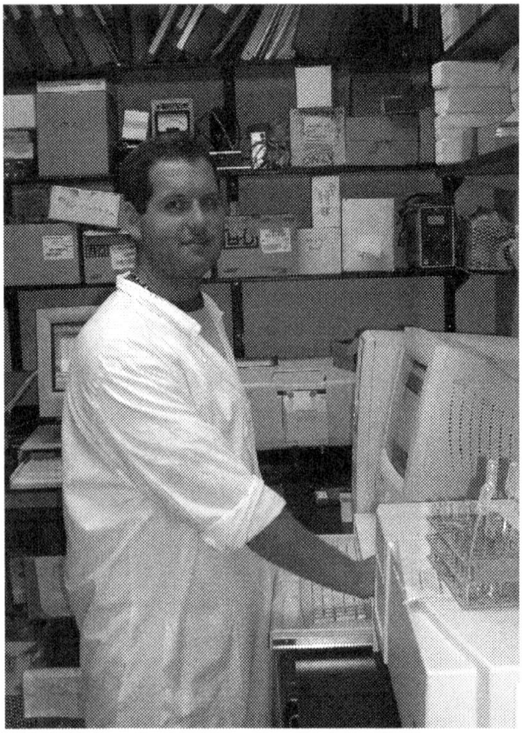

Gabe Knudsen

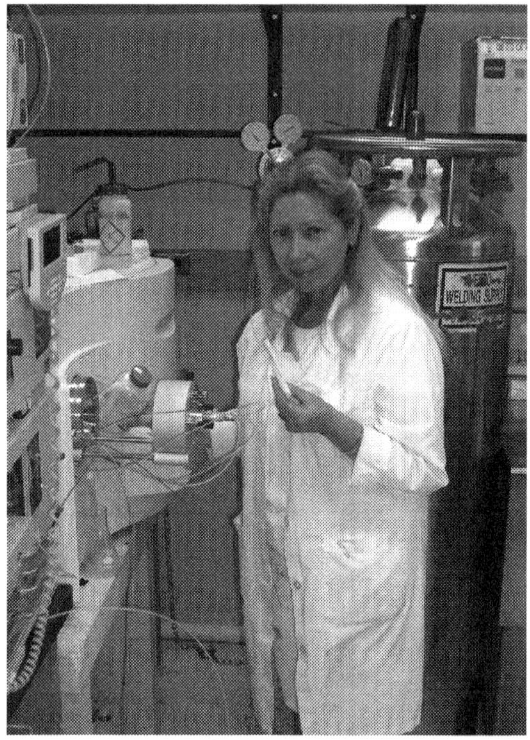

Ute M. Kent

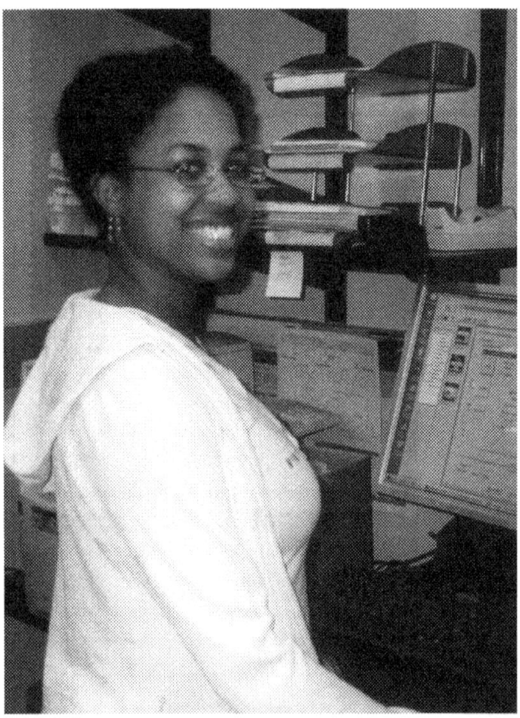

Namandje Bumpus

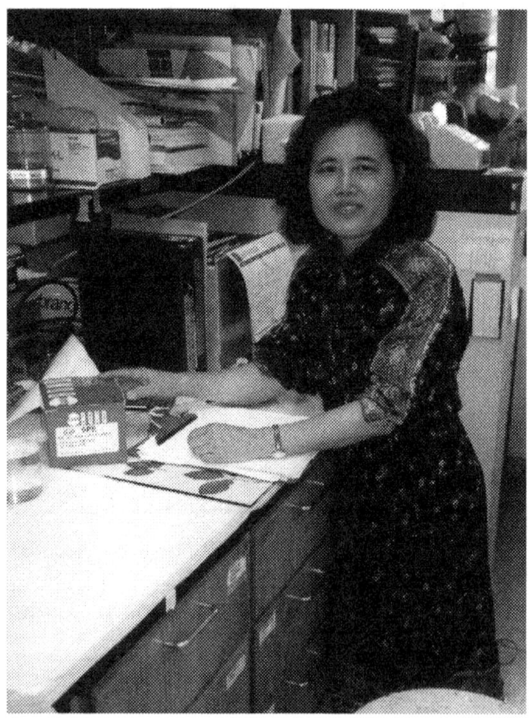

Hsia-Lien Lin

Dr. Ronald W. Holz's Research Interests

Dr. Ronald W. Holz joined the Department of Pharmacology as an Assistant Professor in 1977 and rose through the ranks to full Professor in 1985. He has taught autonomic pharmacology to generations of medical, graduate, pharmacy and nursing students. His research has focused on the biochemical and physiological mechanisms underlying calcium-dependent exocytosis from neuroendocrine cells (adrenal chromaffin cells). Numerous insights into the secretory pathway developed in his laboratory.

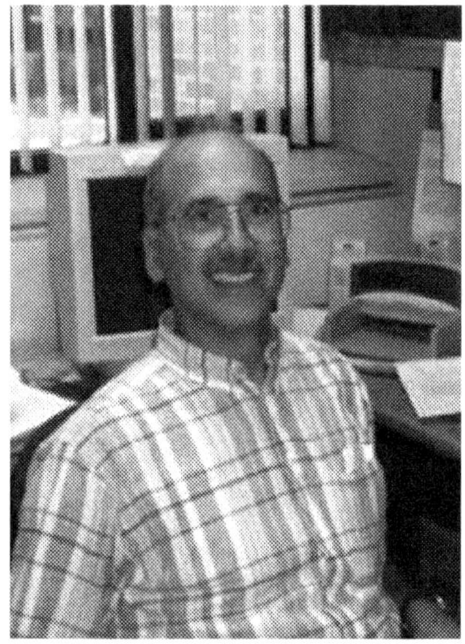

Dr. Holz helped demonstrate the importance of both secretory granule membrane potential and the H^+ chemical gradient in powering catecholamine uptake into chromaffin granules. This H^+ electrochemical gradient, while essential for catecholamine storage, was shown not to be necessary for exocytosis. He helped develop the chromaffin cell culture system into a powerful model for studying exocytosis. He discovered that one could permeabilize the plasma membrane to ions and proteins with low concentrations of digitonin, thus making accessible the cell interior to biochemical manipulation. He demonstrated that one could discern different rate limiting steps in the secretory pathway and separated ATP-dependent priming from the Ca^{2+}-dependent triggering step. His laboratory was the first to recognize the central role of PIP_2 in exocytosis. The polyphosphoinositides were subsequently shown to be essential in many vesicular trafficking pathways. To utilize the enormous potential of molecular biology, a method was devised for transiently expressing exogenous proteins by transfection and detecting their effects on secretion. Secretion from the small fraction of transfected cells in the cultures was detected by measuring the release of co-expressed human growth hormone that had been sorted to secretory granules.

Using this system, the laboratory demonstrated the importance of the low molecular weight GTPase Rab3a on the surface of secretory granules in the secretory pathway. Currently, the role of several Rab3a-binding proteins in secretion including Rabphilin3 and Rim are being investigated.

A new direction of the laboratory is the development and use of a powerful optical technique, total internal reflection fluorescence microscopy (TIRFM), to visualize events in the secretory pathway within 300 nm (the width of a secretory granule) of the plasma membrane. The technique enables in living cells the investigation of biochemical events important for the late steps of exocytosis with high temporal and spatial resolution. Fusion of individual granules with the plasma membrane is being directly visualized and the motion of the granules immediately before fusion is currently being investigated.

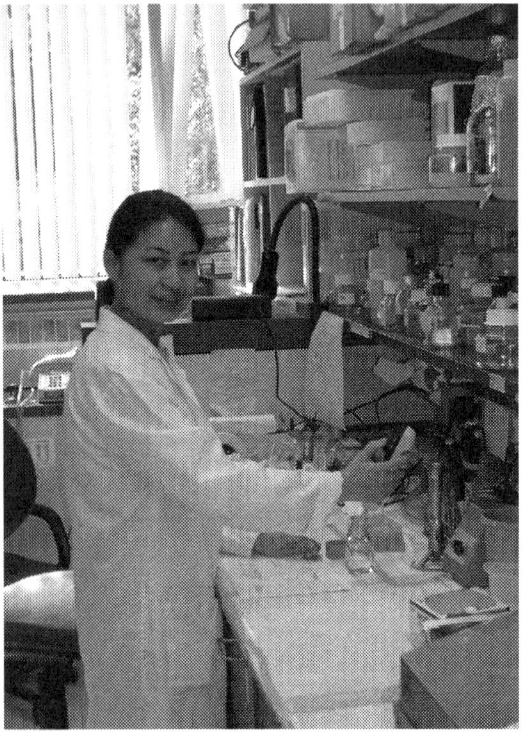

Li Wang

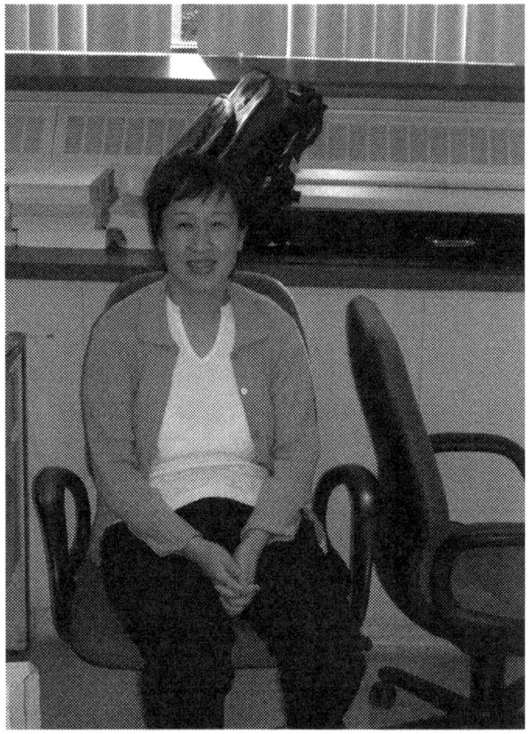

Lei Sun

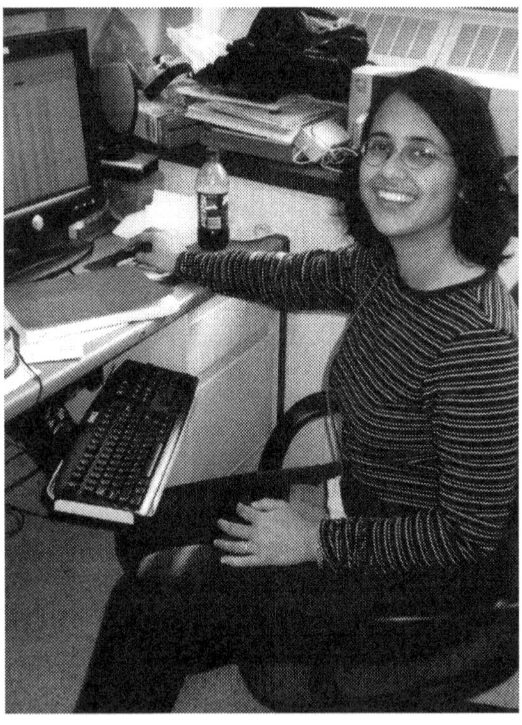

Tania Chakrabarty

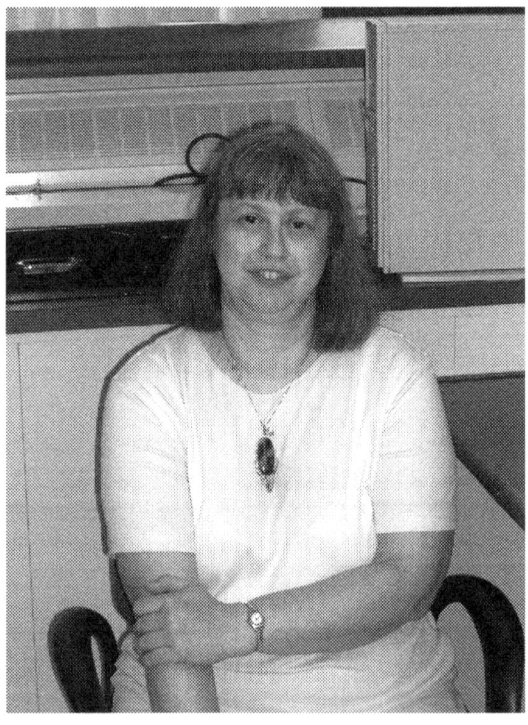

Mary A. Bittner

Dr. Jorge A. Iñiguez-Lluhí's Research Interests

A fundamental property of living cells is their ability to sense cues in their environment, process the information they embody and respond in a physiologically and developmentally appropriate manner. The types of cellular responses mounted during normal and pathologic conditions are ultimately dependent on the accurate expression of a large array of independent genes. The establishment and maintenance of such gene expression programs relies on the complex interplay between specific transcription regulatory factors, the signals they respond to and the regulatory genomic sites where they act.

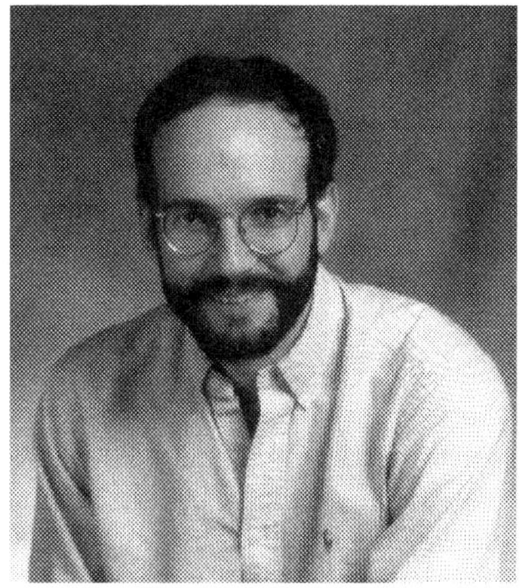

Our interests lie in understanding the molecular basis for the regulatory transactions that transcription factors engage in as they assemble in the vicinity of specific genes and how these operations are integrated to yield the final transcriptional output. We focus on members of the Intracellular Receptor (IR) superfamily as well as other transcription factor classes as paradigms to explore these issues. IRs constitute a large group of transcription regulators includes key mediators of metabolism, reproduction, growth and differentiation and its members mediate the effects of steroid and thyroid hormones and other signaling molecules. Upon agonist binding to a C-terminal ligand-binding domain (LBD), IRs are recruited to specific genomic sites via a central DNA binding domain. Once within the vicinity of a target gene, IRs deploy latent transcriptional regulatory functions and in conjunction with other sequence-specific factors, they nucleate the assembly of multiprotein complexes that activate or repress transcription of nearby promoters. By taking advantage of complementary biochemical, genetic, structural and molecular biological approaches we are exploring (A) the basic mechanisms of transcription, (B) the molecular basis of specific functional interactions among transcription factors, and (C) how these elements of genomic regulatory logic are assembled to give rise to the complex patterns of gene expression in an intact developing tissue.

Determinants and Mechanism of Transcriptional Activation

Many of the functional properties of IRs can be recapitulated in model organisms such as the yeast Saccharomyces cerevisiae. We have exploited the genetic tools available in this organism to define the critical transcriptional activation determinants within the N-terminal regulatory region of the Glucocorticoid Receptor (GR). Through an unbiased genetic screen for mutant receptors with altered transcriptional potential we found that the hydrophobic character of critical residues within a short 16 amino acid region is essential for transcriptional activation. By providing a link between structure and function, these mutants constitute invaluable tools to study both genetically and biochemically the mechanism of action of this domain. Recently, we have exploited these mutants to identify components of the cellular machinery that interpret the activation signal emanating from this region of the receptor. We found that DRIP 150 directly interacts with the N-terminal region of GR and mediates some of its functions. This protein is a specific subunit of a recently described protein complex implicated in transcriptional activation by multiple regulators. We are examining the biochemical and structural properties of this interaction and exploring its functional consequences.

Molecular Basis and Regulation of Transcriptional Synergy

The DNA regulatory regions of a particular gene determine the specific pattern of its expression and invariably contain binding sites for a variety of transcription factors, often in multiple copies. Functional interactions between multiple regulators often yield a more than additive or synergistic output but the mechanisms that enable or control such synergy are not fully understood. I recently identified a novel protein motif responsible for the control of synergy. These short motifs are found in steroid receptors and other regulators such as the proto-oncogenes cMyb and ETS-1. When disrupted, transcriptional synergy is greatly enhanced. This occurs without alterations in DNA binding or in the intrinsic activation potential of the regulators. Deletions of cMyb encompassing the synergy control motif possess enhanced transcriptional activity and are the most common transforming alteration of this proto-oncogene. We are interested in the mechanism of action of these motifs since they represent a higher order element of the genomic regulatory logic. We are using them as probes to identify and understand the molecular basis for the mechanisms that control the outcome of functional interactions among transcription factors.

At a higher level of organization, we are interested in examining how individual transcription factor regulatory interactions contribute to the establishment of gene expression programs in the context of an intact mammalian animal or tissue. Current mouse knock-out or knock-in approaches however, are labor intensive and can be limited since an essential role of the gene of interest during development could preclude analyses in mature organs, and functional redundancy could demand multiple mutations before the emergence of a phenotype.

We are interested in developing alternative genetic approaches to assess the transcriptional and developmental consequences of regulatory proteins at the tissue level. The remarkable regenerating potential of the adult liver and recent advances in both gene targeting and liver stem cell research offer the possibility to use this organ as a genetically accessible experimental system to overcome some of these problems. Furthermore, this tissue is a primary target of glucocorticoids and thus ideally suited to study the consequences of altering individual functional surfaces of the glucocorticoid receptor. In conjunction with novel tools to monitor genome-wide expression, these methods may allow us to examine the contributions of any particular factor to the regulation of gene batteries during normal physiologic function or during regeneration and disease.

The combination of basic studies of fundamental mechanisms of cell regulation with manipulation of whole animal systems is likely to be an essential component of the emerging functional genomics era. By applying innovative approaches, we envision participating in the daunting but increasingly approachable tasks of revealing how the basic elements of genomic regulatory logic are assembled into the higher order structure and hierarchy of genome-wide cis-regulatory networks.

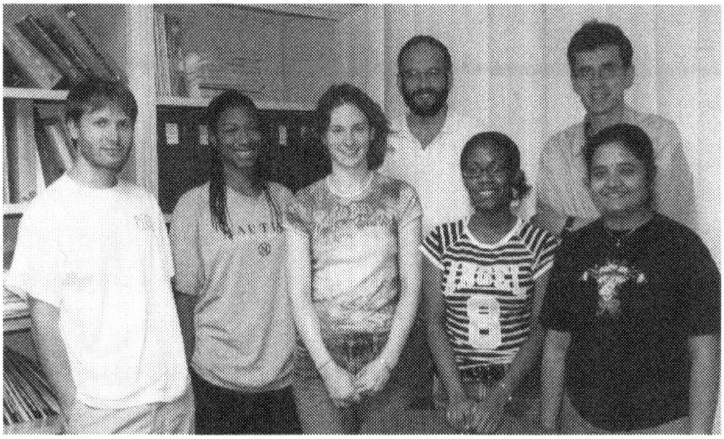

Front row: Sam Holmstrom, Denise Parrott, Katherine Kieckhafer, Brandi Thompson, Lalitha Subramanian Back row: Jorge Iñiguez-Lluhi, Sergey Chupreta

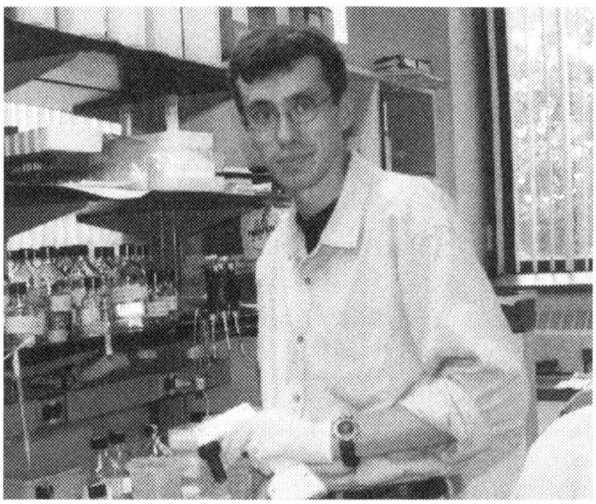

Sergey Chupreta

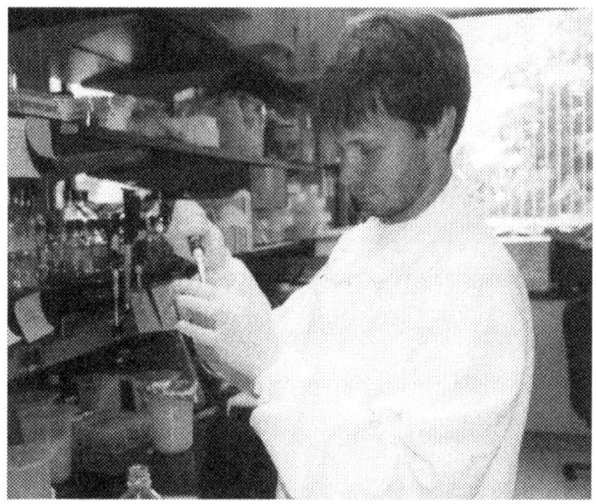

Sam Holmstrom

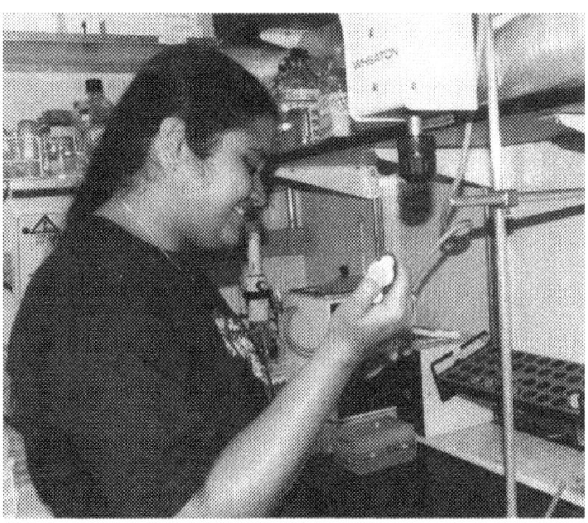

Lalitha Subramanian

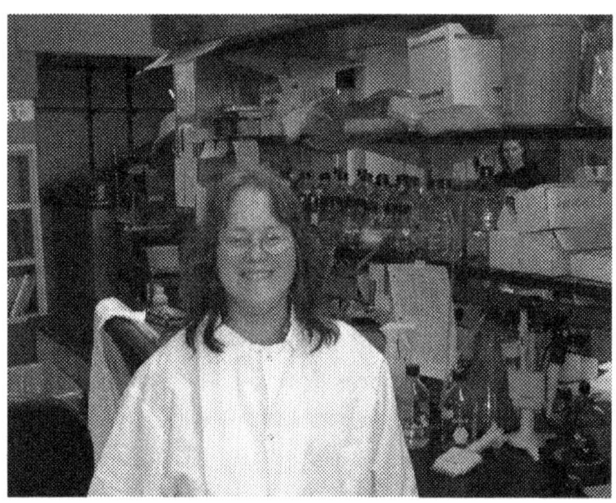

Mary Van Antwerp

Dr. Lori L. Isom's Research Interests

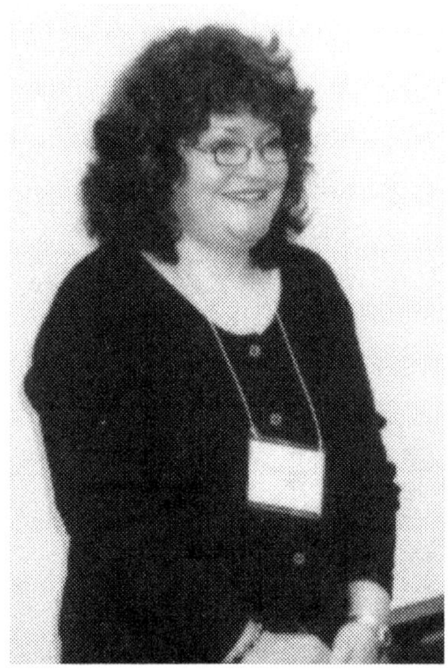

Voltage-gated Na^+ channels are responsible for action potential initiation and conduction in excitable cells. In myelinated neurons, Na^+ channels are clustered at high density in specialized, subcellular domains such as nodes of Ranvier and axon initial segments. What is the mechanism responsible for Na^+ channel localization and clustering? What proteins make up the Na^+ channel signaling complex? We have shown that Na^+ channels are unique among voltage- and ligand-gated ion channels in that they contain auxiliary subunits that not only modulate channel kinetics, but also function as cell adhesion molecules (CAMs) that direct channel insertion into the plasma membrane and channel interaction with other signaling proteins. We propose that, as CAMs, Na^+ channel β subunits act as critical communication links between extra- and intracellular signaling molecules in excitable cells.

Voltage-gated Na^+ channels isolated from mammalian neurons are heterotrimeric protein complexes composed of α and β subunits. The mammalian pore-forming α subunits encode a gene family of at least ten members. The β subunit gene family consists of four members: β1, β2, β3, and β4. β1A, a splice variant of β1 expressed in embryonic brain, has also been described. α subunit cDNAs express functional Na^+ channels in heterologous expression systems such as *Xenopus* oocytes or mammalian fibroblasts. However, for brain α subunits, the currents characteristic of these channels expressed in isolation are quite different from native currents. Co-expression of the β subunits with these channels results in hyperpolarizing shifts in the voltage-dependence of activation and inactivation, changes in channel modal gating behavior resulting in increases in the rates of inactivation and recovery from inactivation, and increases in channel density at the plasma membrane as assessed by ^3H-saxitoxin (STX) binding. Na^+ channel β subunits and the β subunits of voltage-gated Ca^{2+} and K^+ channels are functionally homologous in terms of channel modulation. However, $Ca^{2+}$and K^+ channel β subunits are not structurally homologous to Na^+ channel β subunits and only the Na^+ channel β subunits have been shown to function as CAMs in addition to their roles in channel modulation. Thus, the Na^+ channel β subunits present a unique opportunity to study cell adhesion in terms of electrical signal transduction.

The β1, β1A, β2, β3, and β4 subunits are transmembrane proteins with the type I topology containing an extracellular amino-terminus, a single transmembrane segment, and an intracellular carboxyl terminus. All five β subunit molecules contain a single extracellular immunoglobulin (Ig) domain that is structurally homologous to the V-set of the Ig superfamily and often found in CAMs. This unique property of the Na^+ channel β subunits was first discovered following sequence analysis of β2, revealing that its extracellular domain contained an Ig fold and an extended region with similarity to the CAM contactin. Two distinct regions of the extracellular domain of contactin have greater than 40% amino acid sequence identity with Na^+ channel β2 subunits. Subsequent analysis of the extracellular domains of β1, β1A, and β3 showed a similar homology to the CAM myelin P_0, with β3 showing that highest degree of similarity.

Do β subunits have roles in addition to modulation of channel kinetics? Three key observations provided important early clues: First, β2 expression is required to detect the translocation of newly synthesized Na^+ channels from intracellular stores to the plasma membrane of primary neurons. Second, expression of β2 alone in ooctyes results in dramatic changes in membrane capacitance, and expansion of the surface membrane, through promotion of intracellular vesicle fusion with the microvillus membrane. Third, coexpression of α and β1 in mammalian cells results in a significant increase in the level of cell surface Na^+ channels. These data, coupled with the observation that β2 is homologous to contactin, led our laboratory to ask whether β subunits function as CAMs: Do they interact with extracellular matrix proteins? Do they interact with other CAMs leading to cellular aggregation and cytoskeletal changes? Do they participate in cell migration? If so, what are the implications of these activities on Na^+ channel localization and density in neurons?

β subunits interact with extracellular matrix proteins and influence cell migration. The glial-derived extracellular matrix molecules tenascin-C (TN-C) and tenascin-R (TN-R) play important roles in cellular interactions in developing or injured neurons, such as neuronal migration, neuritogenesis, and neuronal regeneration. β subunits interact with TN-C and TN-R [19, 20]. Incubation of purified Na^+ channels or recombinant β2 with TN-C or TN-R showed saturable and specific binding. Transfected cells expressing β1 or β2 were repelled from TN-R spotted on a nitrocellulose substrate. β subunit-mediated effects in response to TN-R occurred in the absence of α, suggesting that β subunits may function as CAMs independently of the ion channel complex.

β subunits interact homophilically to cause cellular aggregation and ankyrin recruitment. CAMs of the Ig superfamily interact homophilically and heterophilically to transduce signals between adjacent cells or adjacent molecules on the same cell where they participate in, for example, axonal fasciculation, growth cone guidance, and nodal formation. Using the S2 cell model system we tested whether β1 and β2 behave in a similar manner. S2 cells transfected with β1, β2, $Na_v1.2$ + β1, or $Na_v1.2$ + β2 displayed homophilic interactions while cells transfected with $Na_v1.2$ alone did not. Immunocytochemical analysis of the cell aggregates revealed recruitment of ankyrin to sites of cell-cell contact.

The intracellular domains of β1 and β2 are critical for ankyrin recruitment. Mutants lacking the intracellular COOH-terminal domains of β1 and β2, respectively, were transfected into S2 cells. While both cell lines aggregated, ankyrin staining was diffuse and not concentrated to points of cell-cell contact as in cells expressing full-length β subunits. A tyrosine residue in the cytoplasmic domain of β1 is important for ankyrin recruitment. We demonstrated this using β1 mutants replacing β1Y181 with alanine (β1Y181A), phenylalanine (β1Y181F), or glutamate (β1Y181E) or a truncated construct deleting all residues beyond Y181 (β1L182$_{STOP}$). Ankyrin recruitment was observed in β1L182$_{STOP,}$ showing that residues I166-Y181 contain the major ankyrin-recruiting activity of β1. Ankyrin recruitment was abolished in β1Y181E, suggesting that tyrosine phosphorylation of β1 may inhibit β1-ankyrin interactions. Ankyrin$_G$ and β1 associate in transfected cells expressing β1 and ankyrin$_G$ in the absence of α. β1 is recognized by anti-phosphotyrosine antibodies following treatment of these cells with FGF. However, under these conditions, β1 and ankryin$_G$ association is not detectable. Ankyrin$_G$ and β1Y181E do not associate, even in the absence of FGF treatment. β1 subunit-mediated cell adhesion and ankyrin recruitment may contribute to Na^+ channel placement at nodes of Ranvier. Furthermore, phosphorylation of β1Y181 may be a critical regulatory step in this developmental process.

β subunits interact with other signaling molecules in complex with, or perhaps independently of, α. β1 interacts with contactin, a GPI anchored protein expressed by neurons and glia that is thought to play multiple roles in the nervous system and that has significant homology with β2. Contactin is linked to the localization of axonal ion channels through its association with Caspr, a neurexin-family protein that forms part of the axoglial junctions at paranodes, and whose expression precedes Na^+ channel clustering in the optic nerve. Contactin and Na^+ channels can be reciprocally coimmunoprecipitated from brain homogenates. Cells co-transfected with $Na_v1.2$ + β1 + contactin have 3 to 4-fold higher peak Na^+ currents and correspondingly higher saxitoxin binding than cells with $Na_v1.2$ + β1, $Na_v1.2$ + contactin, $Na_v1.2$ + β2 + contactin or $Na_v1.2$ + β1 + β2, suggesting an increased channel surface membrane density. Coimmunoprecipitation from cell lines showed that contactin interacts specifically with β1, and not β2 or α. In the CNS there is a high level of colocalization of Na^+ channels and contactin at nodes of Ranvier. Contactin may thus significantly influence the functional expression and distribution of Na^+ channels in neurons through heterophilic cell adhesive interactions with β1. β1 also interacts with the receptor tyrosine phosphatase β (RPTPβ). RPTPβ, contactin, and Caspr form a complex and localize to the paranodal axolemma in myelinated fibers of the CNS and PNS. An intracellular site on β1, but not β2, binds the intracellular phosphatase domains of RPTPβ. Finally, β1 colocalizes with the L1 family CAM neurofascin-186 at nodes of Ranvier and β1 and β3 associate with neurofascin-186 in a heterologous expression system.

To investigate the functions of Na^+ channel β subunits *in vivo*, we created "knockout" mice. We showed that β2 plays essential roles *in vivo* in maintenance of normal electrical excitability of neurons. β2 is not required for Na^+ channel expression or for life, as the β2 (-/-) mice appear to develop normally, have normal brain, axon, and neuronal morphology as well as normal neurological function, and live typical life spans. However, β2 is required for the normal voltage dependence of inactivation of Na^+ currents and for the maintenance of the normal level of Na^+ channels at the plasma membrane in neuronal cell bodies and in myelinated axons in mice, as shown by our observations of reduced STX binding in cultured neurons

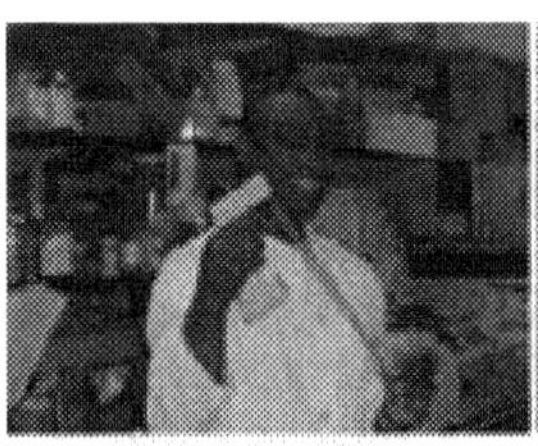
Tigwa Davis

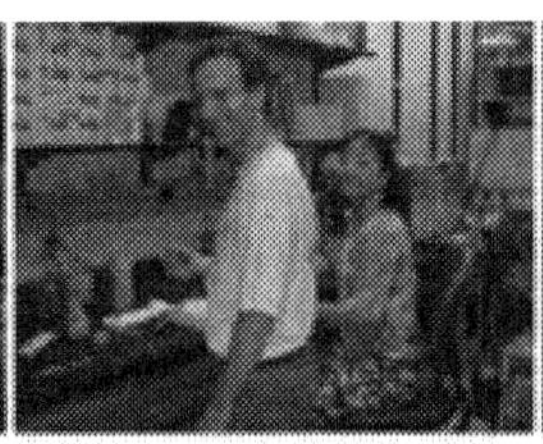
Laurence Meadows and Chunling Chen

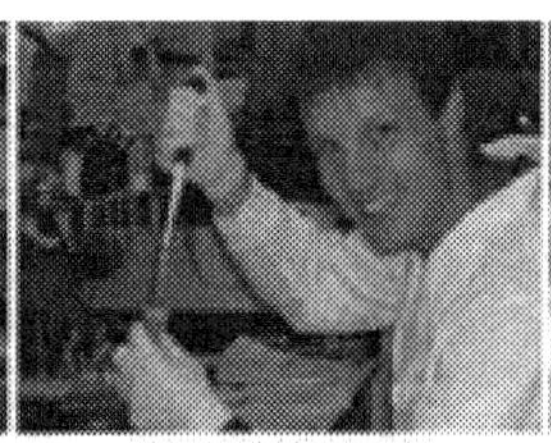
Dyke McEwen

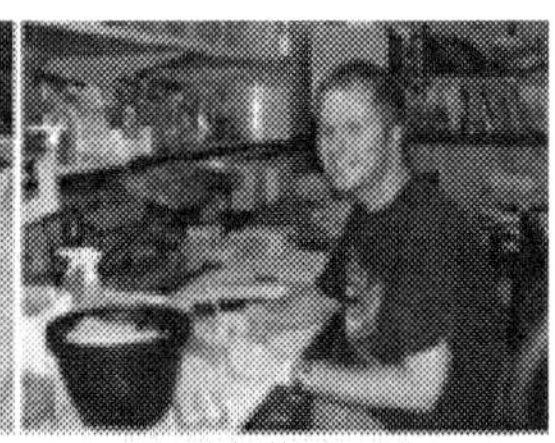
Matt Detrow

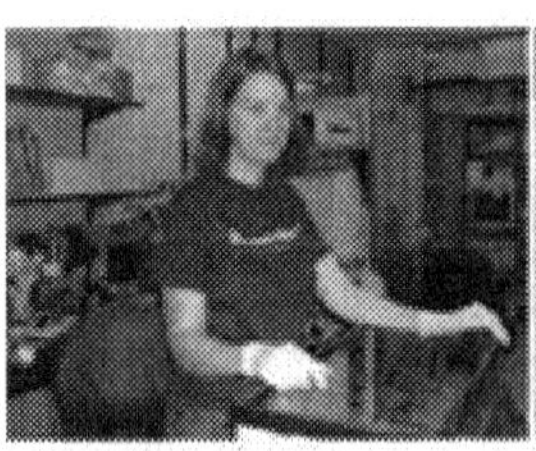
Amanda Hobson

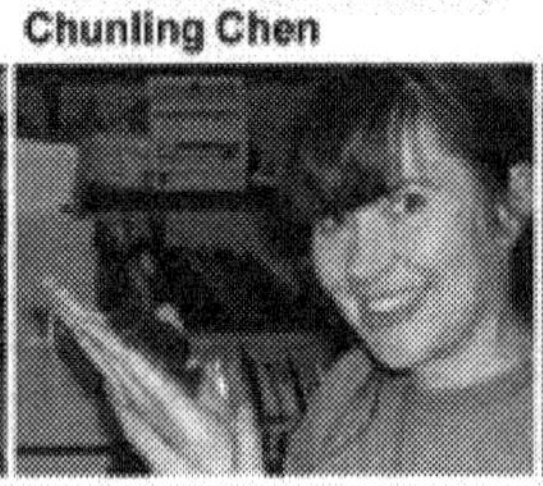
Audrey Speelman and a knockout mouse

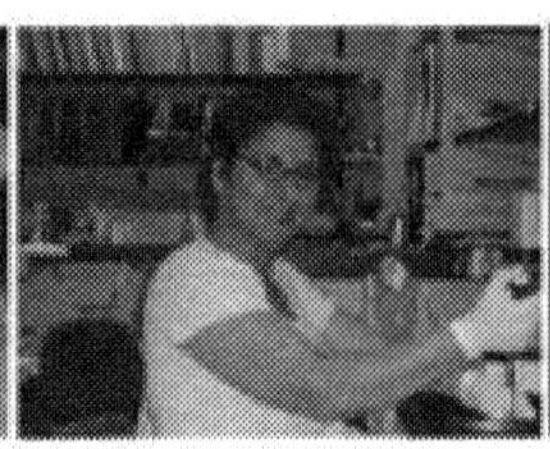
Jyoti Malhotra

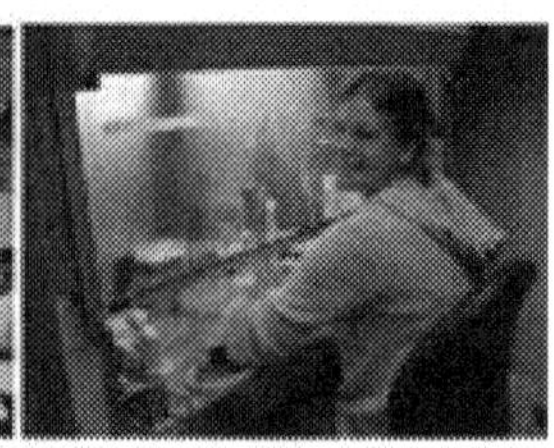
Rebecca Csomos

and reduced Na^+ currents in dissociated hippocampal neurons and optic nerve axons. These defects in electrical excitability at the cellular level lead to hyperexcitability and a reduced threshold for seizures, probably due to reduced excitability of inhibitory interneurons. Thus, normal control of neuronal excitability requires β2 subunits.

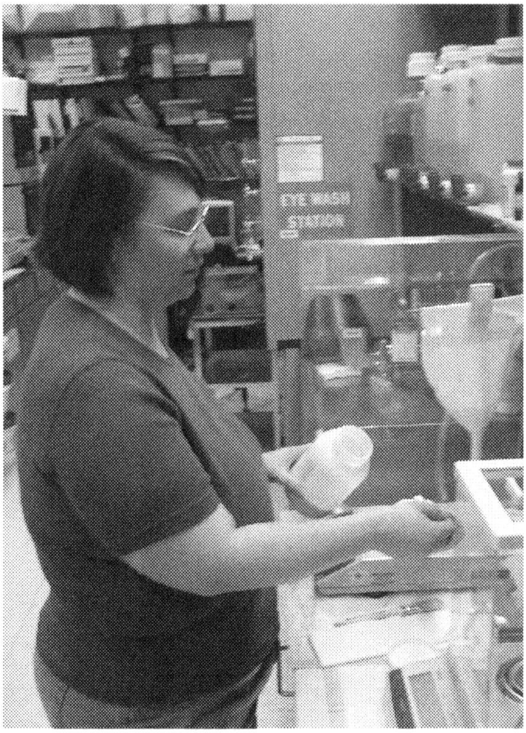

Heather O'Malley

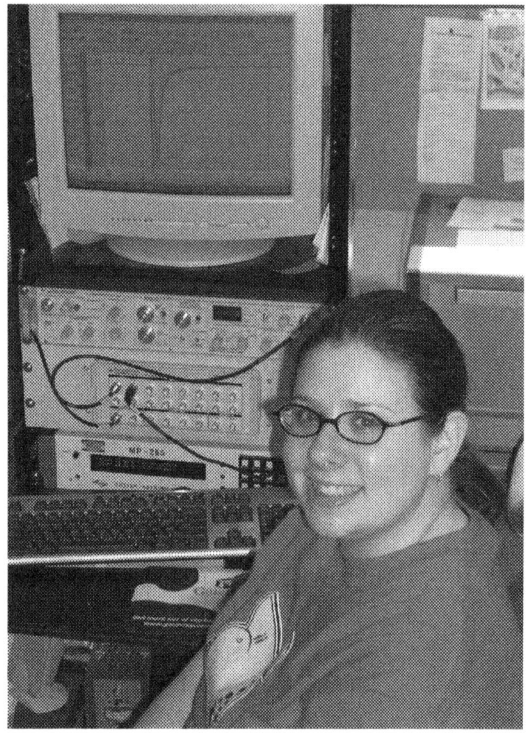

Amanda Evans

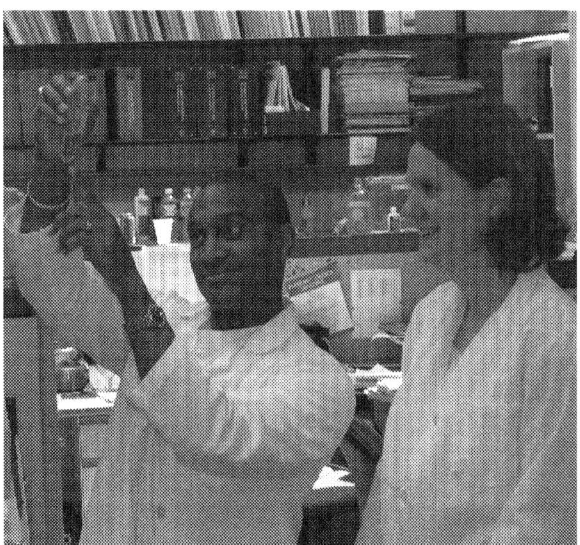

Tigwa Davis and Amanda Hobson

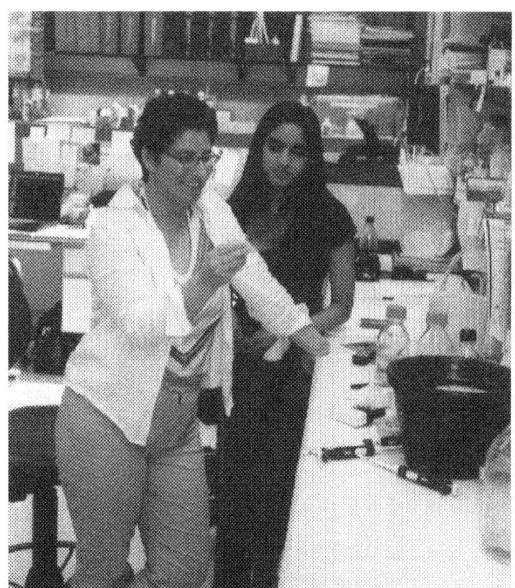

Veena Thyagarajan and Jyoti Dhar Malhotra

Dr. Robert T. Kennedy's Research Interests

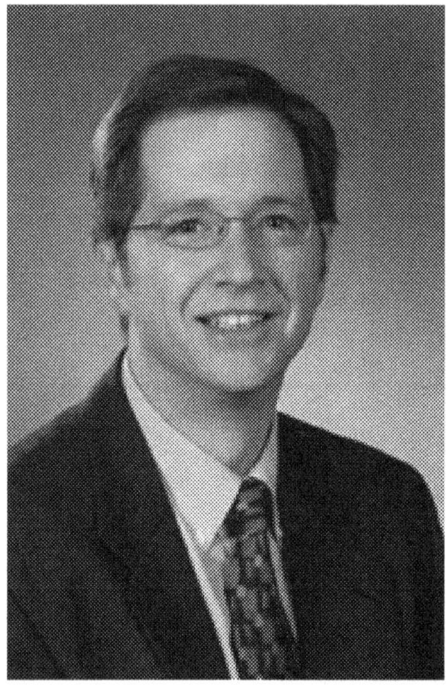

Robert Kennedy joined the University of Michigan faculty as the Hobart H. Willard Professor of Chemistry and a Professor of Pharmacology in August of 2002. His joint appointment was made as part of a University initiative to increase the interaction between the Medical School and College of Literature, Science, and Arts. His research group of 14 graduate students and 6 postdoctoral associates has settled into laboratory space in the Chemistry Building but numerous interactions with the Pharmacology faculty and students are already underway. The laboratories include a class 10,000 clean room, a fast-scanning confocal microscope, 2 mass spectrometers, and numerous "home-built" instruments for in vivo and single cell monitoring of neurotransmitters and hormones. Kennedy group research focuses on analytical chemistry and its application to pharmacology. His group has pioneered the use of capillary electrophoresis (CE), capillary liquid chromatography-mass spectrometry (LC-MS) and microelectrodes for the study of neurotransmitters and hormones at single living cells and in vivo.

An important accomplishment was the development of microelectrodes and a confocal fluorescence method that allowed insulin release to be monitored at single pancreatic beta cells and islets in real time. These methods have been augmented by development of sensors to monitor metabolism in real time. These novel techniques are presently being used to study the mechanisms of secretion and its relationship to diabetes. Of particular interest is the relationship between changes in metabolic rate and secretion that produce oscillatory insulin levels in vivo. Another area of intense investigation is the role of insulin in self-regulating insulin secretion in beta-cells. Using direct measurements and animal models with insulin signaling components knocked-out, it has been demonstrated that insulin can have profound effects on insulin secretion. Defects that arise as a result of the knock-outs mimic those found in Type 2 diabetes. These studies suggest a link between impaired insulin secretion and insulin resistance, two hallmarks of Type 2 diabetes with an ill-defined connection. New directions include development of a simple method to test islets for viability prior to transplants and using a metabolomic approach, i.e. simultaneous measurement of many metabolites, to study beta-cell metabolism.

The Kennedy group also has a significant effort aimed at developing and applying methods for in vivo monitoring neurotransmitters. They have coupled in vivo sampling methods with CE which has allowed multiple transmitters to be monitored on the second time scale. This development has opened the door to numerous studies on the chemical substrates for behavior. This development has also led to collaborative studies related to addiction and sleep in collaboration with numerous faculty on campus. More recently his group has developed a highly sensitive LC-MS method that has allowed neuropeptides to be monitored and discovered in the brain of living rats. Of particular interest has been the observation of bioactivity of previously unknown non-opioid peptides derived from proenkephalin. Future directions include follow-up studies of other novel neuropeptides and development of microfabricated in vivo instruments as a national resource center as part of the UM Center for Neural Communication Technology.

A final area of interest is the development of novel approaches to studying and exploiting bioaffinity interactions. The Kennedy group demonstrated several years ago that it was possible to separate non-covalent complexes in a few seconds by capillary electrophoresis. This led immediately to a new type of immunoassay which has been adopted in clinical as well as basic research applications. Other interactions that have been exploited include receptor-ligand (with help from the Traynor laboratory), GTP-G-protein (thanks to help from the laboratories of Neubig and Sunahara), and aptamer-ligand. Future directions include exploring these methods as drug-screening tools and for identifying intracellular binding interactions.

Professor Kennedy earned a B.S. in Chemistry at the University of Florida in 1984 and a Ph.D. from the University of North Carolina in 1988. After a two-year stint as a NSF postdoctoral fellow, also at North Carolina, he served as a professor of chemistry at the University of Florida for 11 years before moving to Ann Arbor. He has served on the editorial board of several journals including the Journal of Chromatography, The Analyst, and Electrophoresis. He has received several awards including the Presidential Faculty Fellowship, ACS Findeis Award, Benedetti-Pichler Award of the Microchemical Society, NSF National Young Investigator Award, Beckman Young Investigator Award, Lilly Analytical Research Award, and Alfred P. Sloan Fellowship.

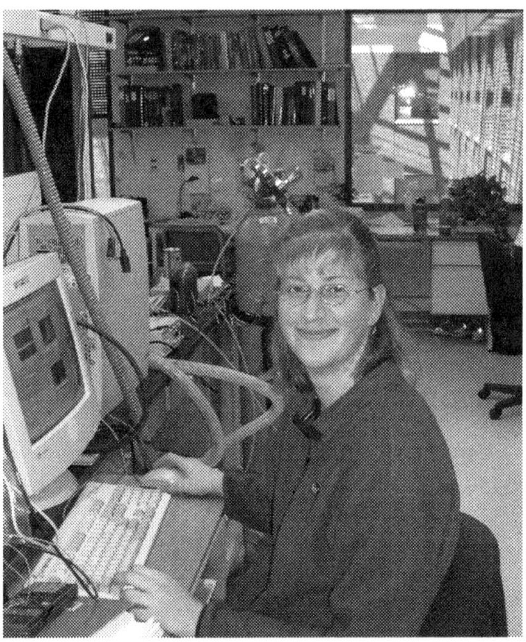

Rebecca Whelan is developing a new capillary electrophoresis-fluorescence anisotropy instrument to monitor receptor-ligand interactions.

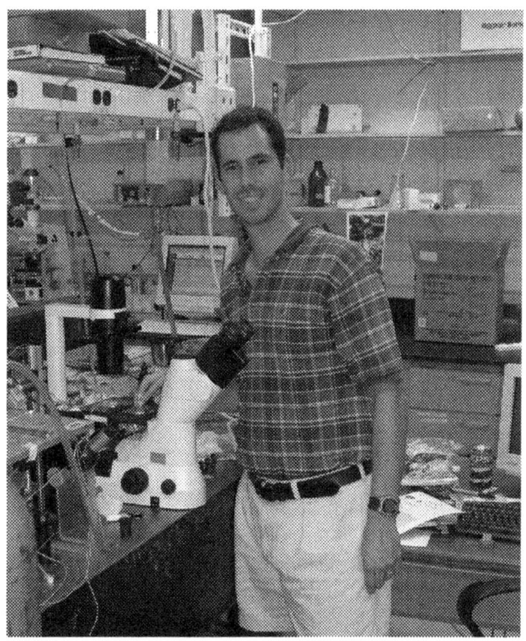

Scott Burns is developing a novel nanoscale pump for sampling from the brain in vivo.

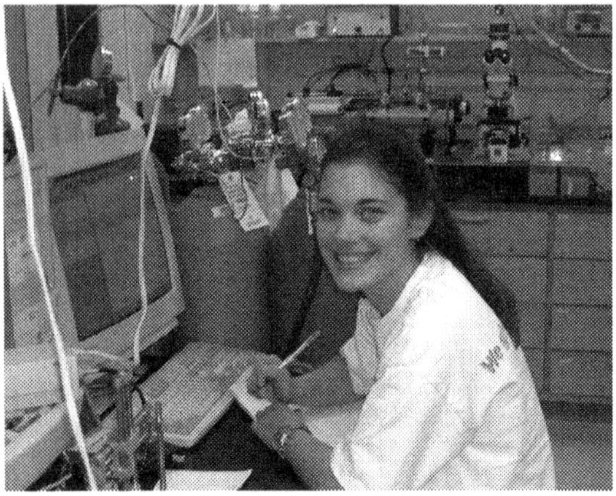

Holly Baseski using a capillary LC-mass spectrometer to monitor opioid peptides in vivo.

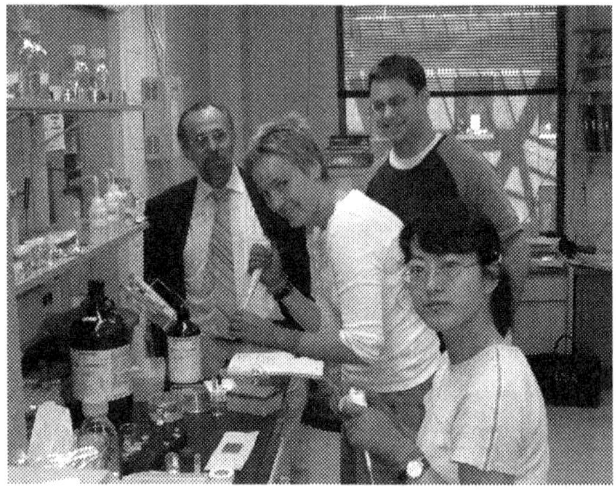

Hui Wei, Jim Edwards, and Kerstin Nolkrantz are developing peptide assays using mass spectrometry.

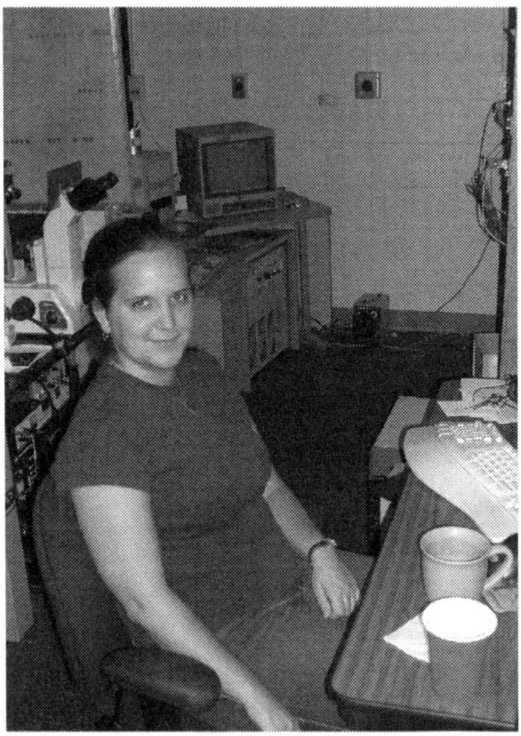

Jennifer Peters is investigating the communication signals involved in generating oscillations of insulin secretion.

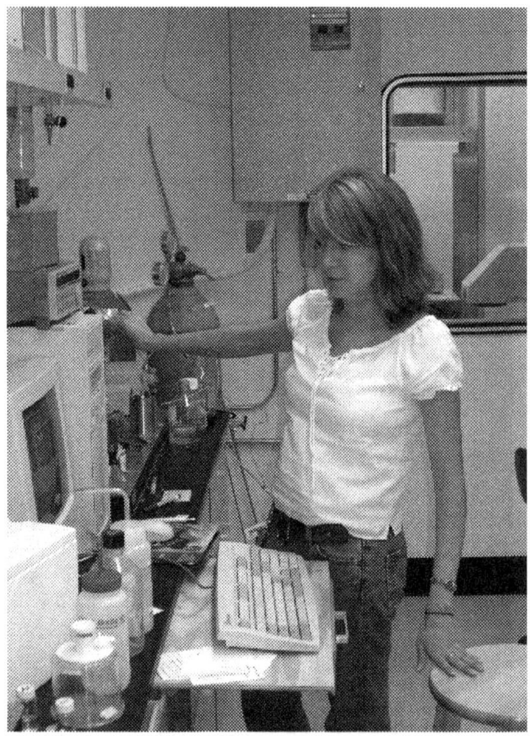

Emily Jameson is developing a novel high-throughput assay for G-proteins and G-protein receptor activation.

Dr. Bert N. La Du's Research Interests

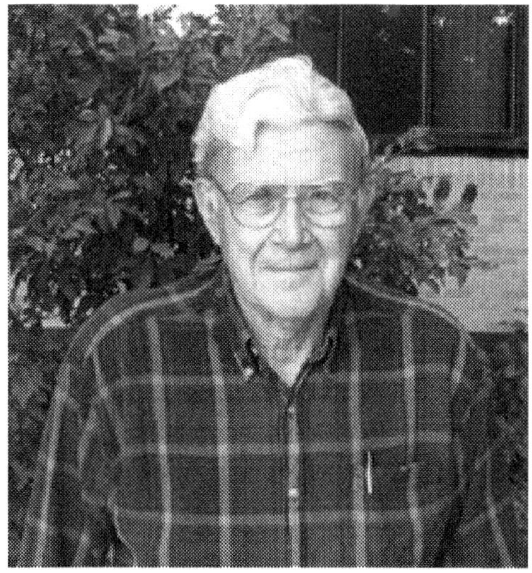

The major research interest in Dr. La Du's laboratory over the past 20 years has been pharmacogenetics. He is particularly concerned about hereditary differences in the human esterases that modify the response to drugs or the sensitivity of individuals to drugs and environmental chemicals that are esters. Plasma butyrylcholinesterase (cholinesterase) is a prototype example since it hydrolyzes succinylcholine, aspirin, heroin and a large number of other esters, and is subject to many genetic modifications. The laboratory, primarily with the excellent work of Dr. Oksana Lockridge and others, cloned and sequenced human BCHE. Over the years the laboratory has developed new methods to identify about 35 variants forms of BCHE that are associated with unusual response to succinylcholine and mivacurium. The laboratory has become a world referral center for the diagnosis and genetic analysis of BCHE variants, and for doing the related individual genotyping and phenotyping testing, and family studies.

In recent years more attention has turned to another human serum enzyme, paraoxonase (PON1). The fact that PON1 is just one member of a family of at least three PONs, (PONs 1, 2 and 3), was discovered in the La Du laboratory. The individual PONs each have different tissue distributions and catalytic properties. The laboratory has expressed and purified all three human PONs and has been able to characterize their similar as well as their distinctive features. The PONs appear to be the main defensive enzymes of mammalian tissues against organophosphates, but neither PONs 2 or 3 have any significant hydrolytic activity against paraoxon, and even that activity for human PON1 is not very potent. It appears more likely that the PON family with its redundancy of enzymatic activities is involved in some important endogenous metabolic reactions, so finding what this may be remains a very important aim for the future. Some recent studies seem to suggest that PON1 is important in protecting LDL from oxidation. All the PON1 in the blood is associated with the HDL fraction, and this may be the main reason why HDL is protective against the development of cardiovascular disease. The La Du laboratory and collaborators are trying to find whether these possibilities can be substantiated.

A recent major interest of our group has been to improve the method of purification of the three member proteins of the paraoxonase (PON) family. Since the three (PONs 1,2 and 3) are very similar in their amino acid composition and physical properties, this has been a difficult problem for many years. Other serum proteins such as apolipoprotein A-1, platelet-activating factor acetylhydrolase and many other proteins stick tightly with PON1 and PON3. The difficulties in purification have led to incorrect assumptions by many investigators about the real catalytic properties of the individual PON enzymes as well as in defining the individual substrate specificity characteristics of the different PONs. Our laboratory is also continuing to study how the quality and quality of the individual paraoxonase isozymes may affect the sensitivity of different individuals to certain drugs, and to environmental chemicals, such as insecticides and other very toxic organophosphates.

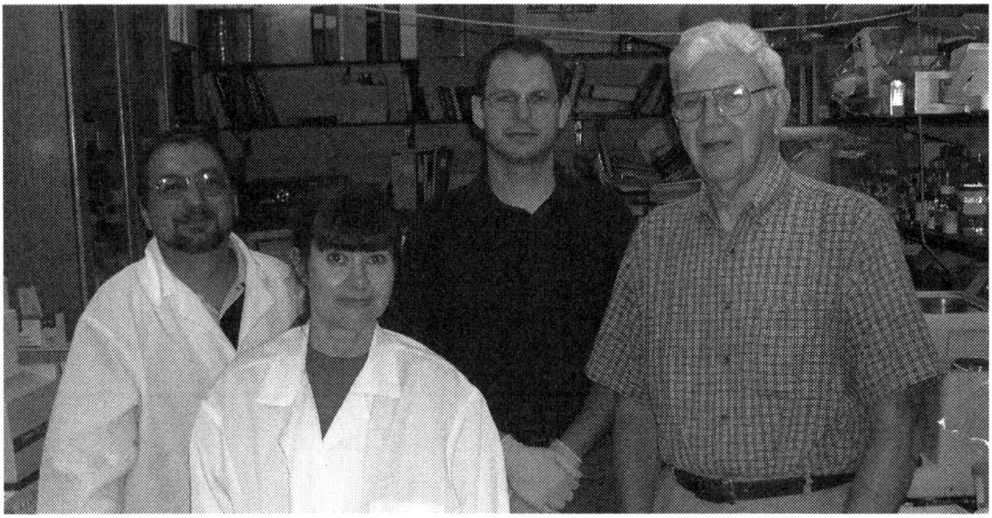

The above photo was taken in the spring of 2003. From the left, are Dr. Dragomir Draganov, who joined the laboratory in the summer of 1998, Audrey Speelman, who started in May of 2002, Dr. John Teiber a post doctoral trainee who had worked in the laboratory in 1995 as a rotating graduate student, and Dr. Bert La Du.

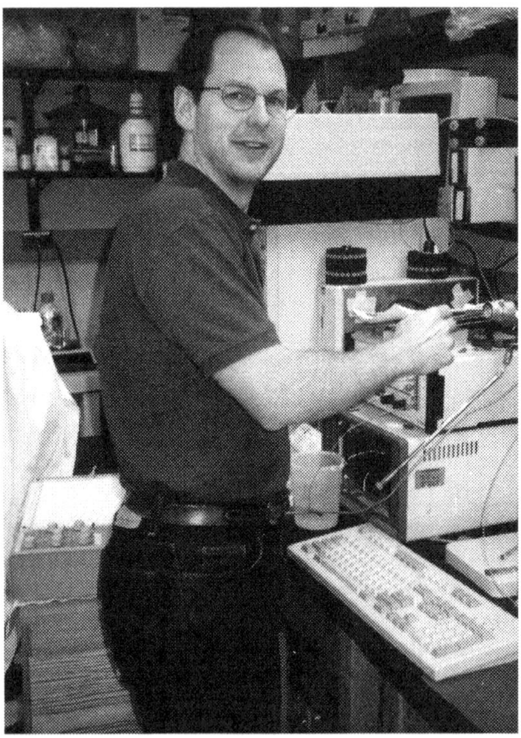

John at work

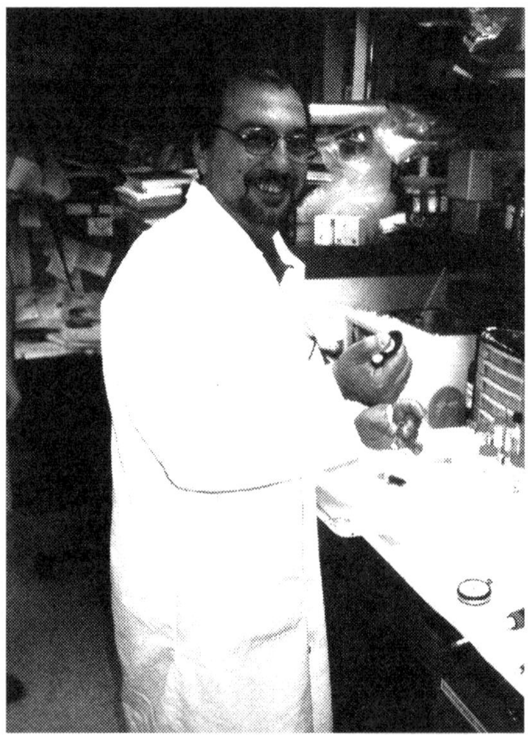

Drago pipetting

Dr. Angel W. Lee's Research Interests

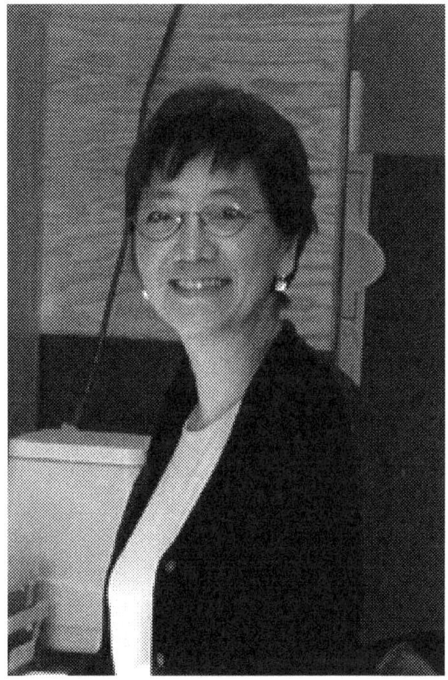

It is important to note that the first draft of the Human Genome Project showed that up to 20% of the 30,000-40,000 genes are involved in signaling. There are more than 520 protein kinases and of these 58 have been identified as receptor tyrosine kinases (RTKs) and 32 as cytosolic protein tyrosine kinases. Protein tyrosine kinases function in a variety of cellular activities, e.g., cell growth, cell cycle progression, differentiation, embryonic development, anti-apoptosis, cell motility and adhesion, gene transcription, angiogenesis, ion channels and the list goes on. We study one of the RTKs. This is the receptor for CSF-1, which stands for Colony Stimulating Factor-1, also known as M-CSF or Macrophage Colony Stimulating Factor. As the name implies, CSF-1 is a key growth factor for cells of the monocyte-macrophage lineage. The CSF-1 receptor is in the same family as the PDGF, kit and flk/flt receptors. We use the CSF-1 receptor as a model for studying the basic mechanisms underlying the control of cell growth (increase in cell size), proliferation (cell division) and survival. Mutations and upregulated expression of RTKs are frequent in human cancers. Moreover the pathways utilized by RTKs are often constitutively active. Hence both RTKs and their downstream effectors are potential targets for anticancer drug therapy.

There are *four* projects in the lab.

Project 1. The role of the juxtamembrane region of the CSF-1R is not known. An YTFI motif had been proposed to bind Src kinases. Using retroviral transduction we establish myeloid cell lines expressing 4 mutant CSF-1R: FTFI. DTFI, YTFS, YTFG. Compared to cells expressing wildtype CSF-1R, the FTFI and DTFI cell lines showed hyperproliferative CSF-1 responses whereas the YTFS and YTFG cell lines showed comparable or reduced growth kinetics. We are currently investigating the possibility that the juxtamembrane region recruits both positive and negative regulators. In addition, the FTFI mutant exhibits delayed downregultion and we are examining how the juxtamembrane region and Scr kinases couple to the endocytic machinery.

Project 2. Gab2 is a docking protein that mediates signaling by hematopoietic growth factor receptors and can contribute to leukemia development. We have previously identified Gab2 as a potential signal amplifier of the CSF-1R-PI 3-kinase (PI3K) pathway. Current work is to use RNAi (RNA interference) to "knock-down" expression of Gab2 and a related molecule Gab3 to determine how these molecules contribute to CSF-1R-dependent mitogenesis.

Project 3. PI3K is a lipid and protein kinase. To determine how PI3K contributes to CSF-1R dependent growth and survival, we have utilized a mitogenically-defective

CSF-1R mutant (ΔKI) that shows reduced PI3K activation. The ΔKI cell line has been separately reconstituted with different molecules (constitutively active PI3K, constitutively active Akt, Bcl-x_l, hexokinase). Our results show that PI3K is essential for CSF-1-dependent growth and survival and that both Akt-dependent and –independent pathways are involved. Moreover, sufficient PI3K activity is needed to maintain adequate metabolism and when this function is compromised, survival may be impaired even when mitochondrial function is essentially intact and caspase activation is suppressed.

Project 4. Using microarrays to analyze our panel of cell lines expressing wildtype and mutant CSF-1R reconstituted with different signaling molecules, we have identified a number of potential downstream effectors. Our goal is to map the signaling pathways that lead to the induction/repression of a subset of these genes, particularly those that may function in the PI3K pathway.

This work is supported by the National Institutes of Health (RO1 CA85368).

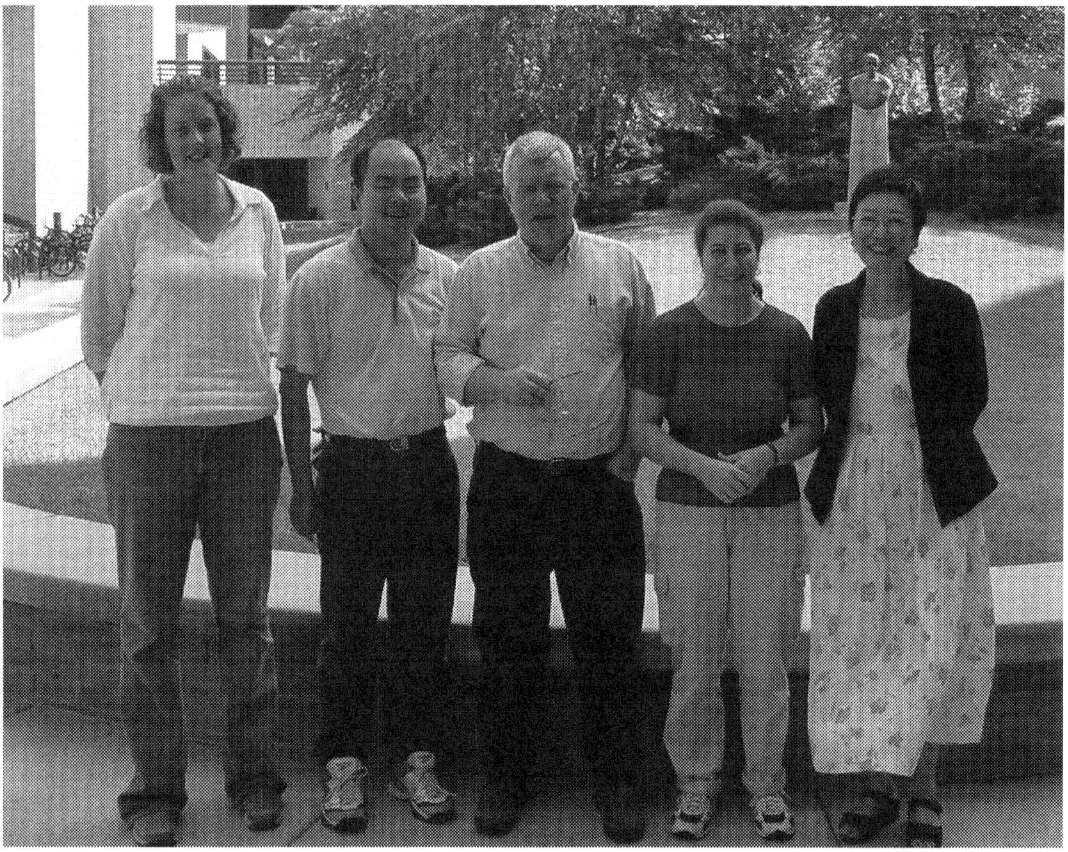

Jessica O'Konek, Yingwei Mao, Mike Hayes, Cindy Rohde, Angel Lee

Dr. Benedict R. Lucchesi's Research Interests

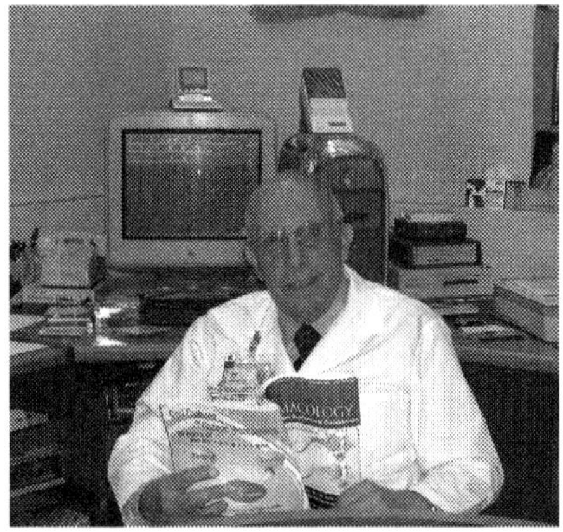

Three major areas of cardiovascular pharmacology are studied in Dr. Lucchesi's laboratory. The investigations are focused on the cellular and electrophysiologic mechanisms related to the sequelae of ischemic heart disease and pharmacologic approaches to its management. Studies are conducted at the cellular and whole organ level with final evaluation in the intact animal. Emphasis is placed on an integrative approach to the study of pharmacologic interventions for the purpose of understanding underlying pathophysiologic mechanisms and drug actions related to ischemic heart disease.

The first research area concerns the cellular and electrophysiologic mechanisms involved in the genesis of reentrant arrhythmias in the ischemic heart and the assessment of pharmacologic interventions for the prevention of ventricular fibrillation or sudden coronary death. The investigations are conducted in open-chest anesthetized, or chronically instrumented ambulatory animals, and with isolated heart preparations. Efforts are underway to correlate specific biochemical and ionic mechanisms with the electrophysiologic disturbances occurring during myocardial ischemia. These studies constitute a unique, integrative approach to understanding the mechanisms of action of antiarrhythmic drugs at various levels of complexity.

A second research area involves the study of pharmacologic interventions that can protect against irreversible ischemic myocardial injury. Physiologic parameters and biochemical alterations associated with myocardial ischemia are assessed both before and during pharmacologic interventions. The cytotoxic influences of mediators of cellular inflammation (oxygen radicals, cytokines, platelet activating factor and neutrophils) are being investigated in in vivo and in vitro models. Current investigations focus on the use of monoclonal antibodies and selected pharmacologic interventions to modulate neutrophil function as well as selected pharmacologic agents known to antagonize one or more mediators of the inflammatory response to injury.

A third area of intense pharmacologic investigation concerns the study of drugs that prevent arterial and venous thrombosis. Critical to this area of investigation is a better knowledge of the physiologic, biochemical and pathologic events causing abnormal interactions among the cellular elements in the blood and the vasculature. In the arterial circulation platelets adhere and aggregate in response to vascular wall injury. Thrombus formation in the venous circulation differs from that in arteries in that fibrin deposition forms the basis for clot formation. The goal is to identify pharmacologic agents for the prevention of obstructive lesions of the arterial and the venous vascular beds. Studies involve the use of platelet specific interventions to prevent formation of occlusive arterial lesions or specific antagonists of the coagulation cascade for prevention of venous thrombosis.

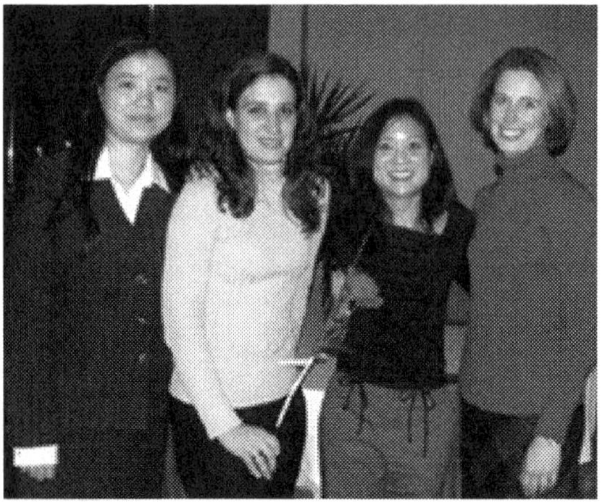

The rose is for Laura.
Ting-Ting Hong, Marta Marchesi, Elaine Tanhehco, Erin Booth

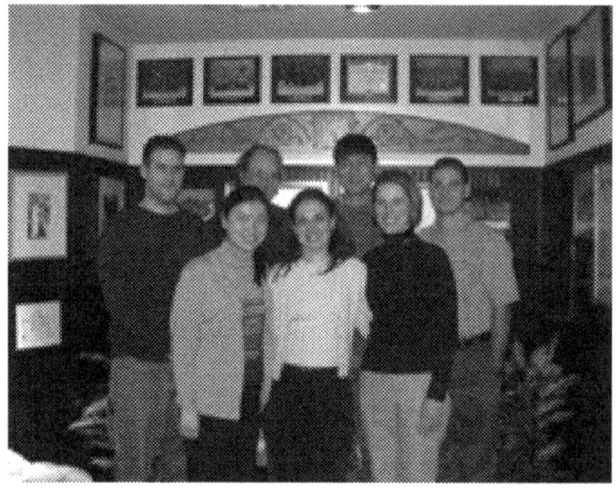

Front: Ting-Ting Hong, Marta Marchesi, Erin Booth
Back: Andrew White, Ed Driscoll, Jinbao Huang, Ryan Wojciechowski

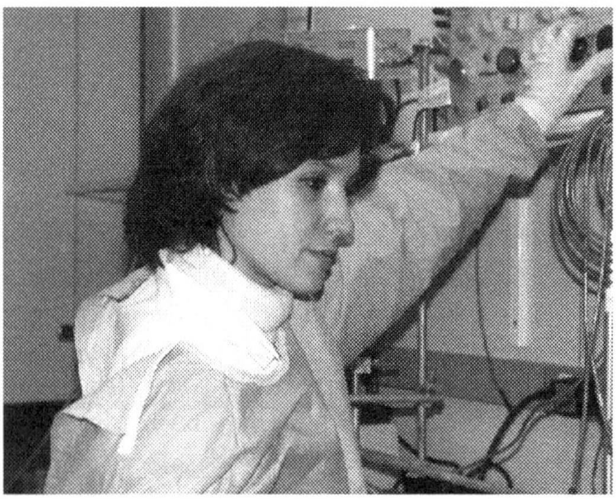

Marta Marchesi

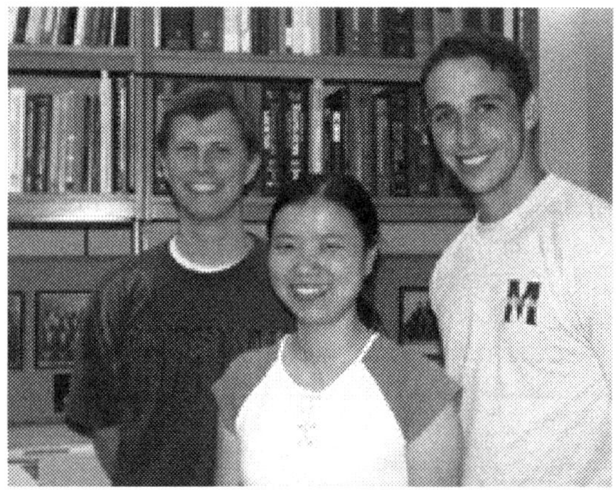

Joseph M. Hendrix, Ting-Ting Hong, Paul DiMusto

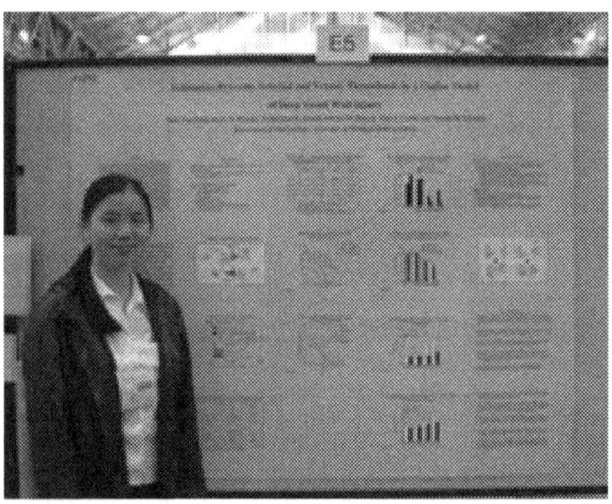

Ting-Ting Hong at her poster

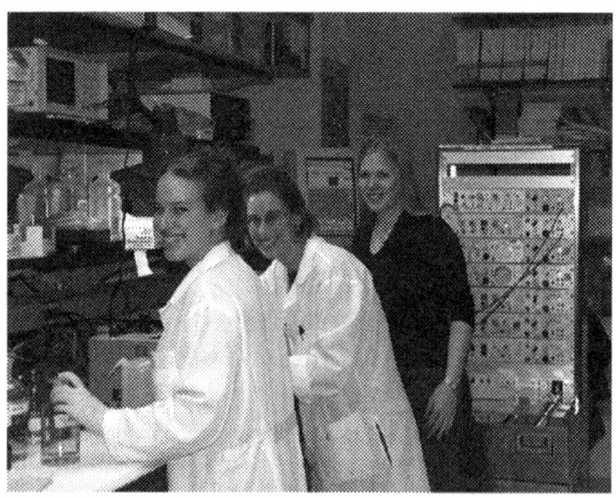

Andrea Knittel, Erin Booth and Jessica Galaska

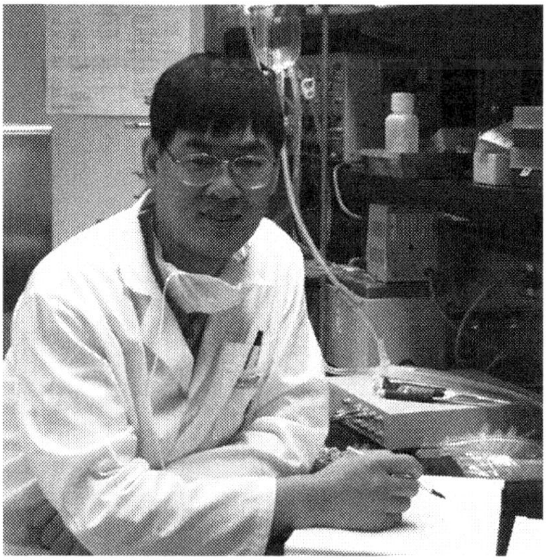

Jinbao Huang

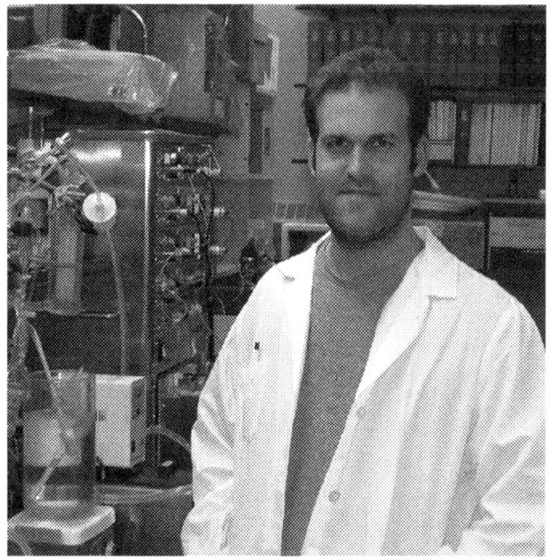

Andrew White

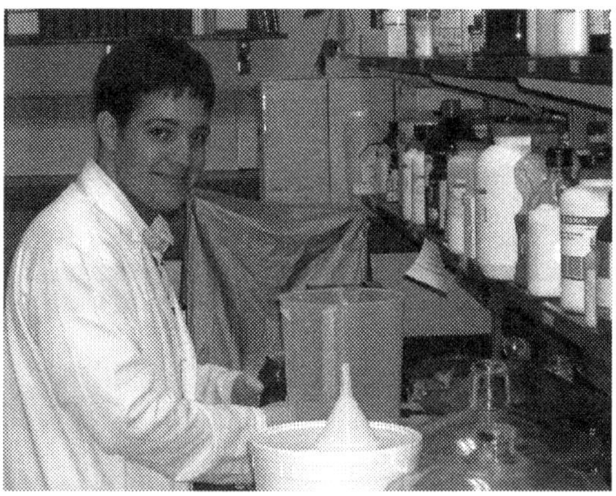

Adam Lauver

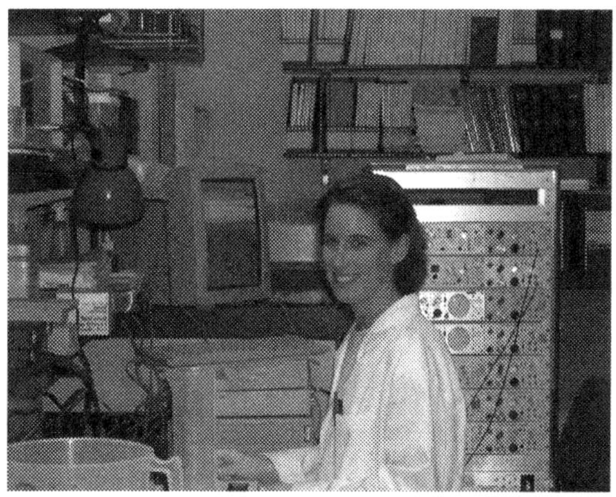

Erin Booth

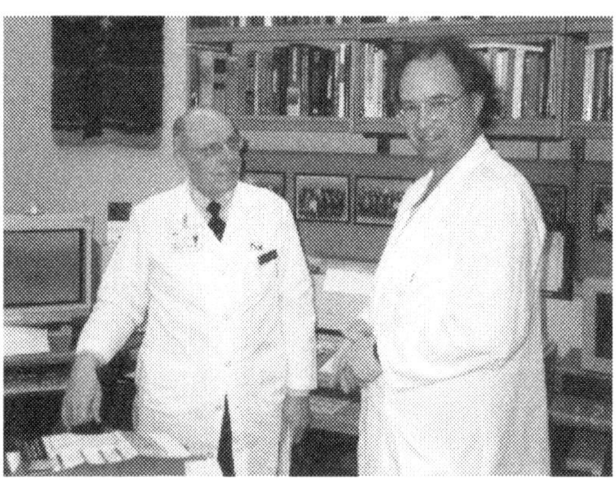

Dr. Lucchesi and Edward Driscoll

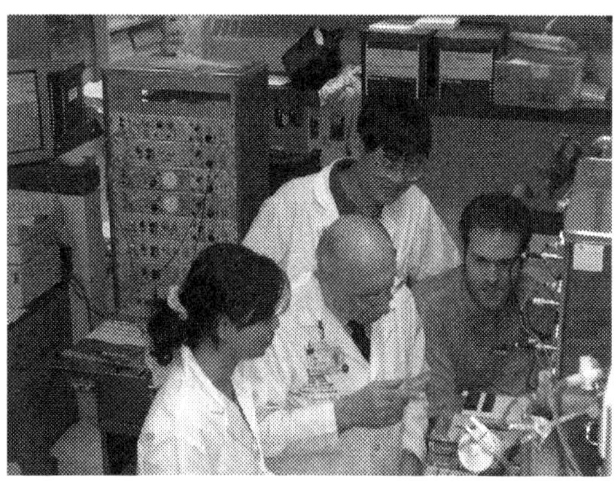

Ting-Ting Hong, Jinbao Huang, Andrew White and Dr. Lucchesi

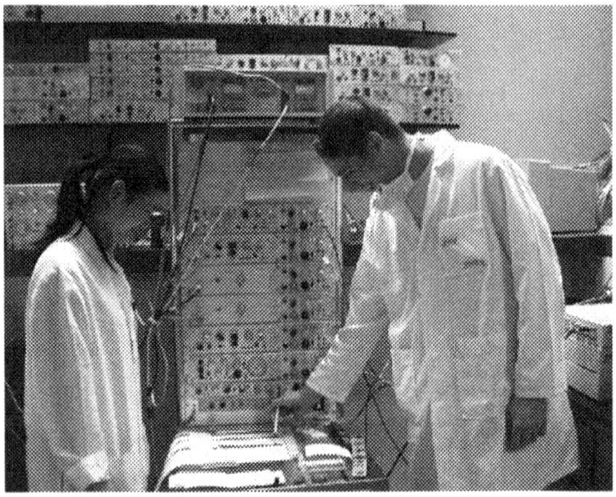

Ting-Ting Hong, Paul DiMusto

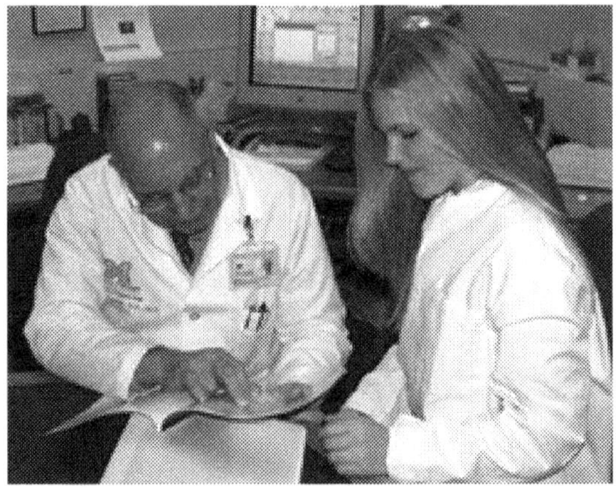

Dr. Lucchesi and Jessica Galaska

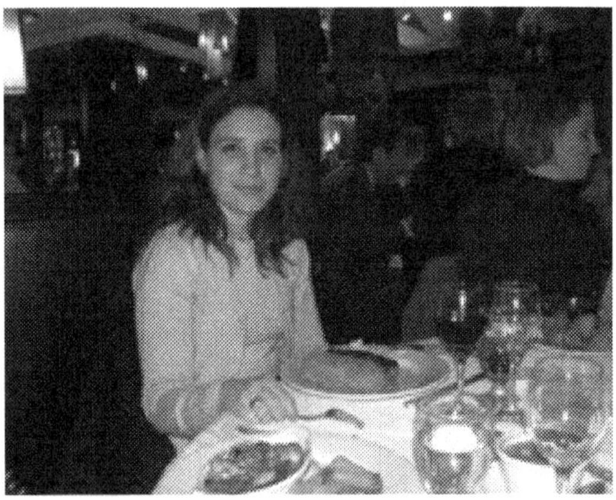

Marta Marchesi

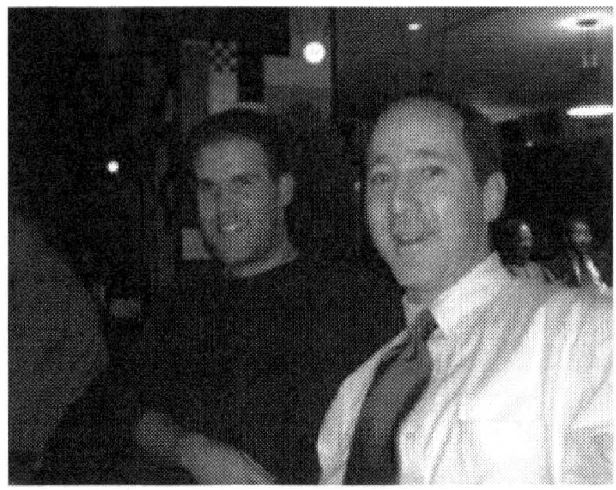

Andrew White and Peter Fischbach

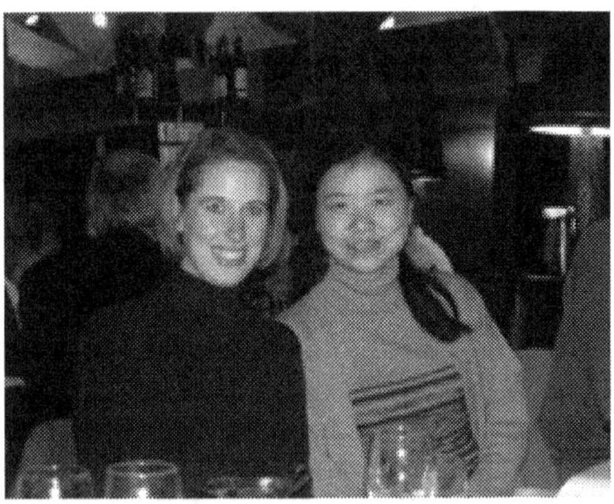

Erin Booth and Ting-Ting Hong

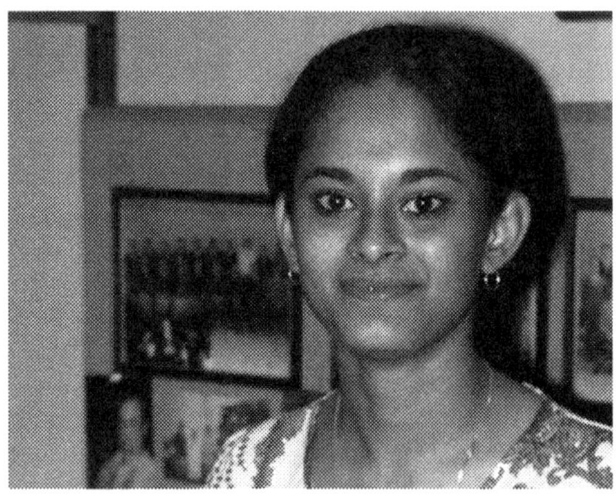

Treasa Davis

Dr. Jeffrey Martens' Research Interests

I am honored to be joining the Department of Pharmacology at the University of Michigan in the Spring of 2004. I received a B.S. degree in chemistry from the University of Florida in 1993 and remained at the University for doctoral training in Pharmacology. Following my post-doctoral training in the laboratory of Dr. Michael Tamkun, I joined the faculty as an Assistant Professor in the Physiology and Pharmacology Department at Oregon Health & Science University in 2001. The opportunity to join the faculty at the University of Michigan and be a member of such a respected and accomplished department is exciting to me. My wife, Lori, and I are native Michiganders and Lori was raised in Ann Arbor. So in a way, this is a homecoming for our family.

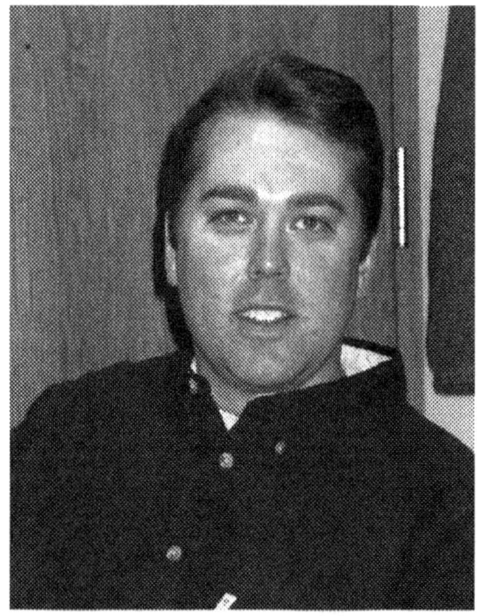

My research is currently focused on characterizing the role of protein-lipid interactions in ion channel targeting and function with an emphasis on understanding the details of K^+ channel/lipid interactions and how this is integrated into the broader context of normal cellular signaling and the pathogenesis of disease. Ion channel regulation within neuronal and muscle membranes is an important determinant of electrical excitability in the nervous and cardiovascular systems, skeletal muscle, GI tract, and uterus. Voltage-gated K^+ channels (Kv) play an important role in setting the resting membrane potential and determining repolarization in these functionally diverse systems and therefore represent significant therapeutic targets in the treatment of a growing list of diseases including cardiac arrhythmias, hypertension, diabetes, and cancer. Importantly, the subcellular localization of K^+ channels is necessary for proper electrical signaling. While progress has been made in identifying elements involved in channel targeting, clustering and anchoring, it is not yet clear how the number and location of channel complexes within the plane of the membrane are determined and how this compartmentalization affects channel function. Recently, we were the first to show that Kv channels differentially target to specialized microdomains, termed lipid rafts, within the plane of the plasma membrane. These domains are enriched in cholesterol and sphingolipids and concentrate a number of signal transduction enzymes. The differential targeting of Kv channels to lipid rafts represents a novel mechanism both for the subcellular sorting of K^+ channels to regions of the membrane rich in signaling complexes and for modulating channel properties via lipid based signaling mechanisms. Ion channel targeting to lipid rafts is likely to be clinically relevant in disease states such as atherosclerosis and neurolipidoses. Several ongoing projects in our lab combine techniques in molecular biology, protein chemistry, and electrophysiology to examine the mechanisms and functional significance of Kv channel targeting to lipid raft microdomains.

In addition to microdomain localization, a general research interest of my laboratory is the therapeutic modulation of lipids to control membrane excitability particularly within the cardiovascular system. Emerging evidence from our laboratory and others suggests that the regulation of cellular lipids such as cholesterol or sphingolipids can have dramatic effects on ion channel function. This is in turn can effect the excitability of cells expressing these channels. For example, the duration of the cardiac action potential can be altered or the contractile state of vascular smooth muscle cells may be changed with membrane lipid levels. Therefore, the alteration of cellular lipids, either by disease, dietary intake, or clinical use of lipid-lowering drugs may have profound effects on the electrical events within the body.

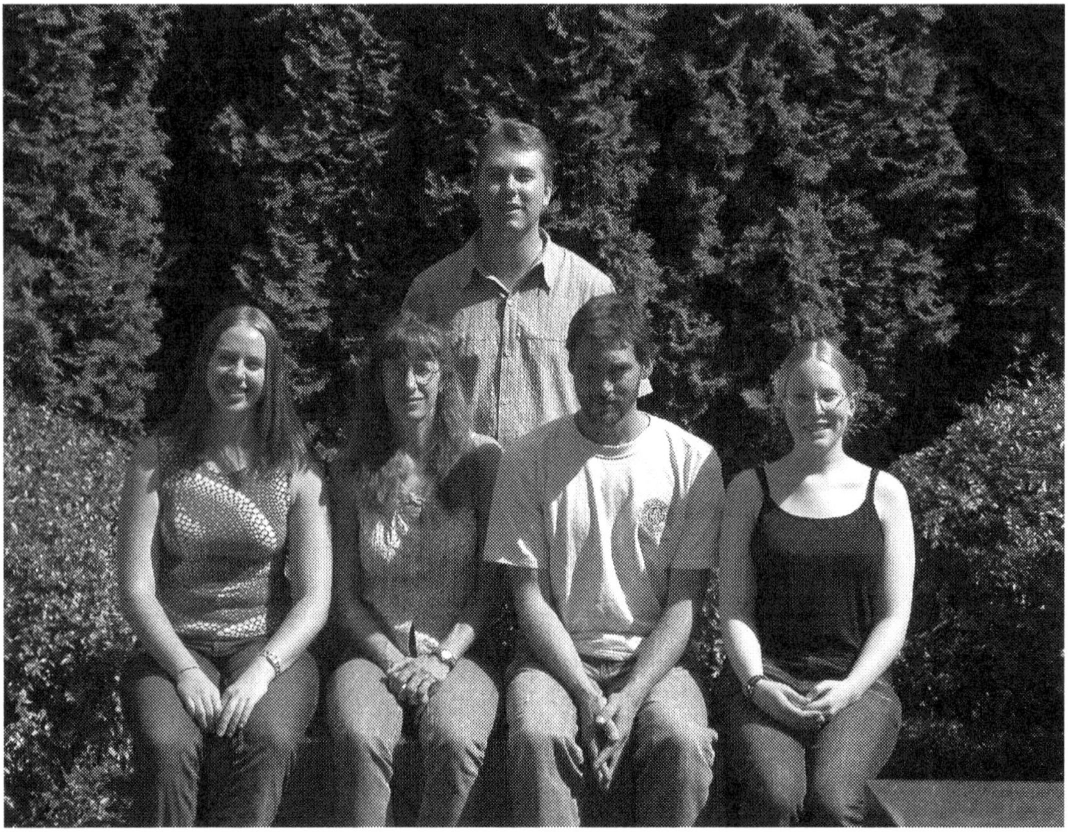

Fronmt Left: Karen Foster, Barbara Leighton, James Brady, Candice Erdman
Back: Jeff Martens

Dr. Jonathan Maybaum's Research Interests

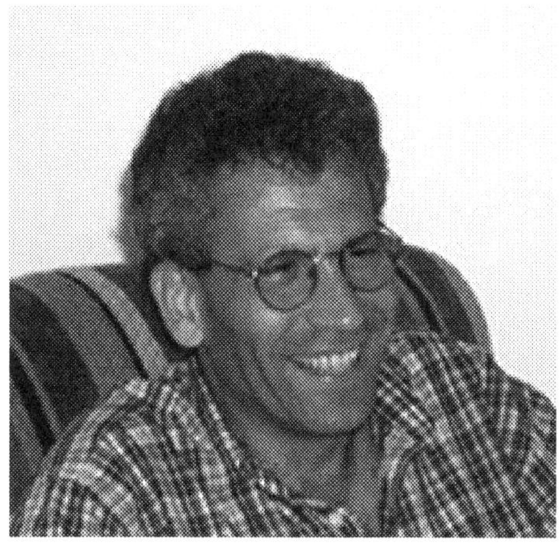

Dr. Maybaum's lab has long been interested in the mechanisms by which the initial biochemical lesions caused by anticancer drugs can eventually lead to cell death, cell cycle arrest and other fates. Much of this work has been directed towards understanding the mechanistic basis for therapeutic efficacy of agents that inhibit thymidylate synthase. Our current work is focussed on understanding how thymidylate synthase inhibition activates cell cycle checkpoint signaling pathways involving ATM, ATR, Chk1, Chk2 and related molecules, and how differences in response of these pathways among various types of neoplastic and normal cells can lead to divergent outcomes following drug treatment.

The lab also has made contributions toward understanding the mechanisms by which antimetabolites (such as fluoropyrimidines) can sensitize tumor cells to ionizing radiation, and we are investigating the role of checkpoint signaling in radiosensitization.

Finally, Dr. Maybaum has a long-standing interest in computing and information technology. He has served as Director of Academic IT Resources for the University of Michigan Medical School and is the principal architect of UM.SiteMaker (an institutional system for facilitating website creation and maintenance; see: UM.Sitemaker history). He is also working on a system to aid researchers in synthesizing and visually representing disparate pieces of information related to complex biological phenomena.

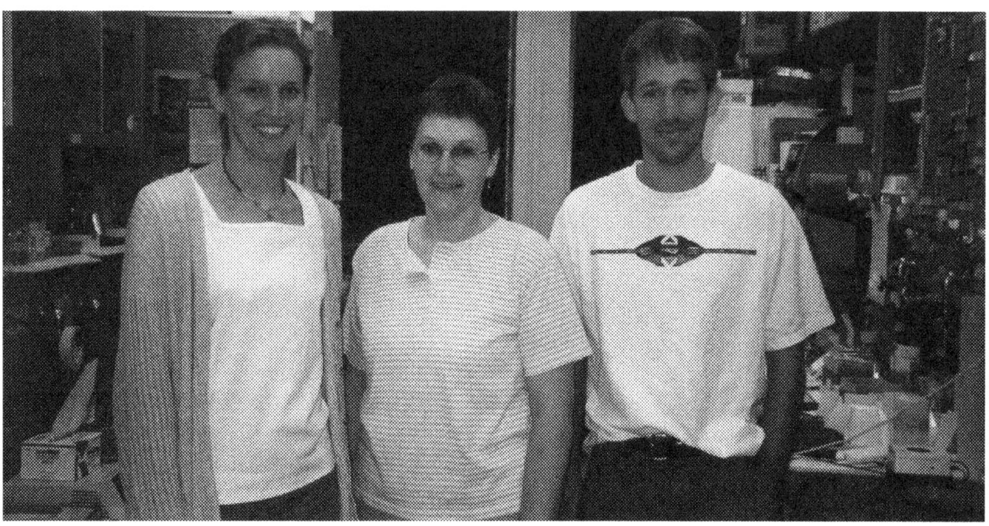

Leslie Parsels, Susan De Remer, Joshua Parsels

Dr. Richard M. Mortensen's Research Interests

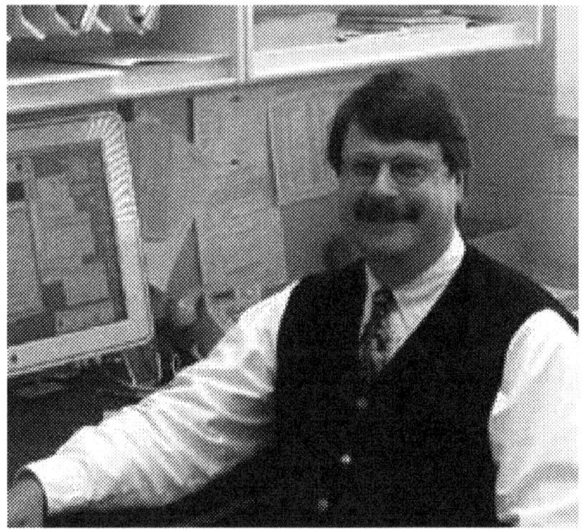

The focus of our laboratory is on understanding disease process in diabetes and cardiovascular disease and developing strategies in regenerative medicine to produce stem cells and differentiated cells for therapy and scientific study.

We are using both murine and human embryonic stem (ES) cells to study the formation and function of cell types in diabetes and cardiovascular disease.

We have also previously developed methodologies to genetically manipulate stem cells and have devised a "high antibiotic" selection method which allows the isolation of homozygous knockout cell lines using a single targeting construct. We have further developed this method using Cre-lox technology to allow for sequential targeting of multiple loci using a single selectable marker. We are now furthering these models by selection of differentiated cell type using cell type specific promoters driving selectable markers. Thus, we have utilized this strategy for cardiocytes and endothelial cells and are expanding it to beta islet cells, skeletal muscle, and adipocytes. These systems will allow the production of knockout cell lines and the analysis of the knockout in differentiated cells without producing a transgenic animal and we have used this system to study the phenotypes of a number of knockouts including ones which are lethal in animals. This methodology should be particularly appropriate for analysis of human gene function using in vitro differentiated human ES cells. Analysis of these cells will greatly contribute to our understanding these cells which have such great therapeutic potential.

We are defining gene targets in intracellular signaling cascades for treatment of cardiovascular disease. Cardiovascular disease remains a major cause of death and diseases such as hypertension, diabetes, and lipid abnormalities are large contributors to the risk of cardiovascular disease. My laboratory is determining the cellular signaling pathways that govern cardiac function (heart rate, contractility) and lead to cardiac and vascular disease and contribute to the many risk factors, particularly intracellular hormonal signaling and signaling in lipid and glucose metabolism. Our focus has been on G-protein mediated pathways and more recently regulation by the PPAR family of nuclear receptors. We use gene knockout and transgenic technologies to determine the importance of signaling molecules.

We have produced knockouts of the heterotrimeric G-proteins G%i2 G%i3 and G%o and have delineated specific signaling pathways through these family members. We have used these knockouts combined with electrophysiological, biochemical, physiologic, and immunologic analysis to determine the significance of these pathways in cardiac contractility, control of heart rate, cardiac apoptosis and growth in animals. In addition, we have developed and used methods of obtaining cell line knockouts to quickly determine phenotypes of knockouts.

We are developing expression panels using quantitative PCR to characterize transcriptional effects of various signaling pathways.

We have also begun to use PPAR-% and PPAR-y knockouts along with tissue specific knockouts to understand the roles of these receptors in cardiovascular disease. PPAR-% is important in controlling lipid metabolism in a variety of tissues including the heart. PPAR-y is critical for formation of adipocytes and is highly expressed in some cardiovascular tissues but its function is still poorly determined.

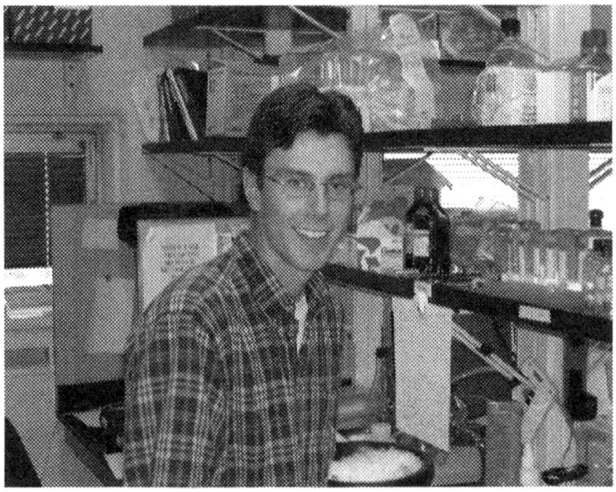

Matthew Merrins

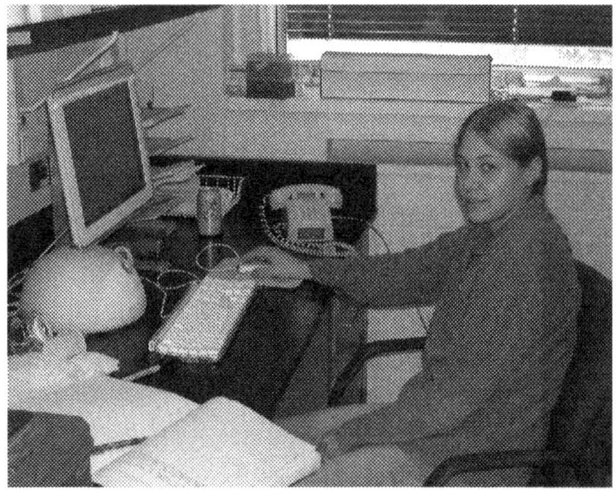

Kimberly Wearne

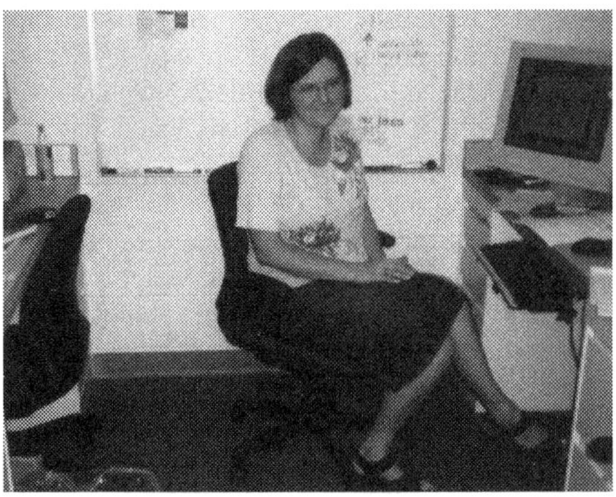

Christine Ivashchenko

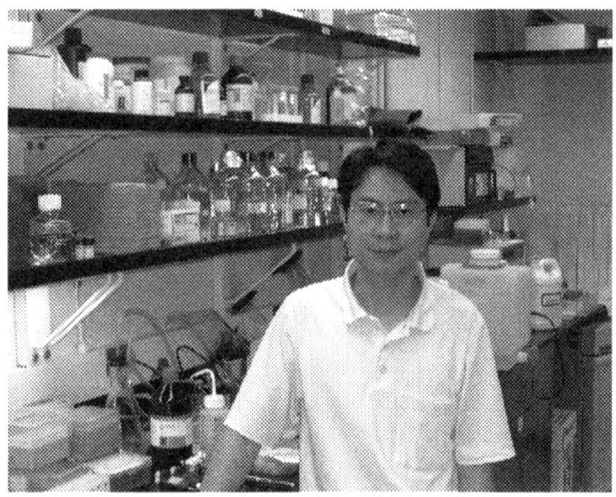

Shengzhong Duan

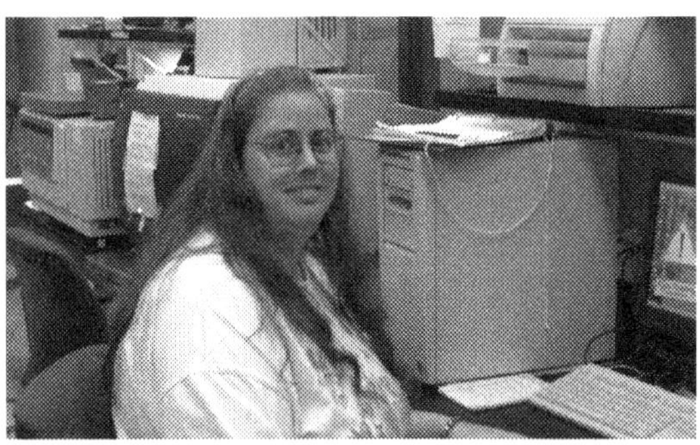

Debora Van Heyningen

Dr. Richard R. Neubig's Research Interests

Research in the Neubig Lab focuses on mechanisms of signal transduction through GTP binding proteins (G proteins) and the receptors that activate them. We are interested in structural and kinetic mechanisms of GPCR signals and the development of drugs that target novel sites in signal transduction processes. Three areas of recent interest are the novel family of RGS proteins, scaffolding proteins that contribute to specficity of receptor-G protein-effector signaling, and the structural basis of the receptor-G protein contact site.

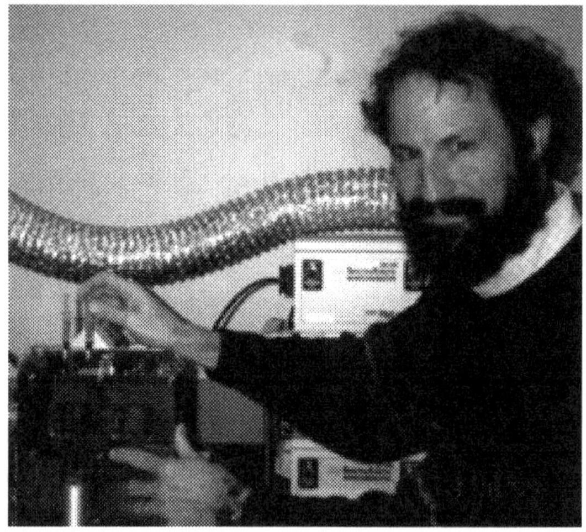

G Protein Mechanisms

The general theme of work in Dr. Neubig's laboratory is the cellular and molecular understanding of guanine nucleotide regulatory protein (G protein) mechanisms. G proteins are involved in the regulation of many critical cellular signaling systems. There are four projects/groups in the lab.

Recent areas of study in this project include the novel RGS proteins (Regulators of G protein signaling) and GFP-labeled receptors and G protein subunits.

RGS proteins play a critical role in controlling the timing and extent of G protein signals. We have developed three distinct approaches to study the function and specificity of RGS action in intact systems (genetic, ribozyme knockdown, and synthetic inhibitors). For the first, we are using mouse knock-out technology to better understand their role in physiology. We recently described the significance of RGS proteins as a novel drug target. Second, we are using RGS-selective ribozymes to reduce expression of distinct RGS proteins and have identified receptor-specific actions of RGS in vascular smooth muscle tissue. Finally, we are collaborating with the Mosberg lab in a structure-based design project on inhibitors of RGS4 function and are examining their specificity and activity in intact cell systems.

In examining G protein mechanisms, a major emphasis of the lab has been the use of real-time spectroscopic approaches to define the earliest steps in G protein signaling. This has included the use of fluorescence spectroscopic techniques to examine the structure and conformational states of G proteins. Fluorescence Resonance Energy Transfer (FRET) has permitted real-time measures of subunit-subunit and receptor-G protein interactions. Fluorescently-labeled GTP analogs have also been developed to probe the nucleotide binding site and conformational changes at the site. Drs. Wang and Zhong are involved in this project. Leighton Janes was a summer student as well.

Structural Basis of Receptor-G Protein Interactions

They are using a multi-faceted approach to understanding the structural basis of receptor-G protein coupling. A driving principle behind this work is the idea that the receptor-G protein interface may be a target of drug design. Several approaches have been applied to this question. First, synthetic peptides from the structure of the alpha2 adrenergic receptor have been studied in biochemical, structural, and functional experiments to identify the molecular basis of receptor-G protein coupling. In addition, classical site-directed mutagenesis and random mutagenesis and genetic selection in yeast have also been used to define the RG interface. A better understanding of the RG interface should permit its targeting in drug design to directly modulate G protein function bypassing the receptor. Duane Chung, Uma Gopalkrishnan, William Lim, and Sue Wade are primarily involved in this project.

Cell Biology of G Proteins

We are examining the hypothesis that receptors and G proteins move freely in cells and couple randomly based solely on the primary sequence of the partners in the interaction. Data from our lab and others shows that there is a more complex organization of these proteins in cells. The structural basis for and functional consequences of this organization is being explored. Drs. Neubig, Wang, Alec Schmaier, and Pete Clapp are primarily working on this project.

G proteins in cardiovascular function/disease

Dr. Wang is focusing on G protein and RGS function in the vascular smooth muscle. Min Liu works with her on this project. A collaborative human genomics project is also underway with UM cardiologists to define alterations in signaling molecules in cardiovascular function.

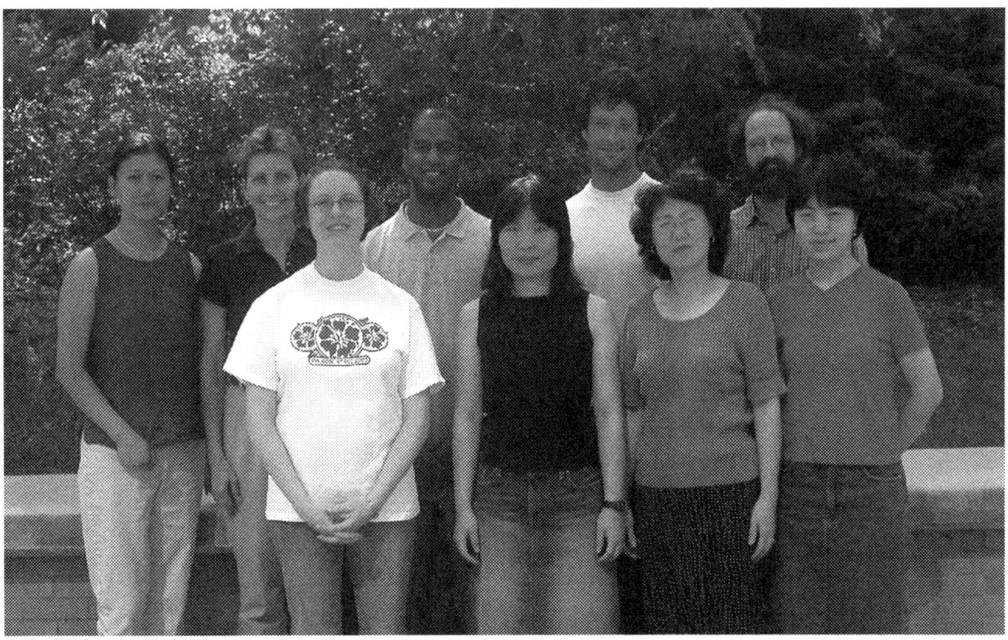

Neubig lab 2003
Front row: Becky Roof, Ying Fu, Qin Wang, Xinyan Huang
Back row: Min Liu, Sue Wade, Chris Evelyn, Pete Clapp, Rick Neubig

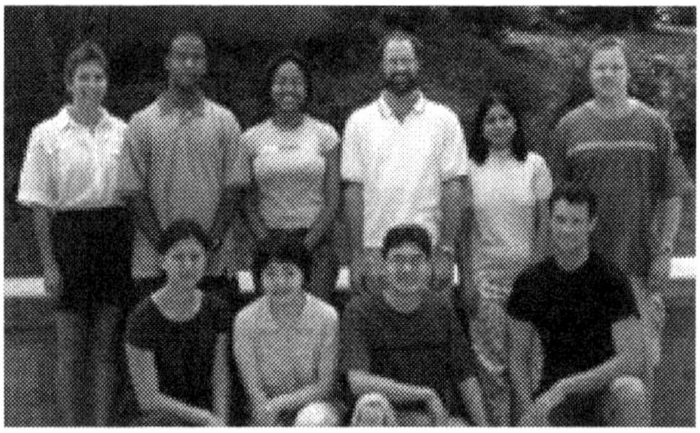

July 2002 Front - Min Liu, Xinyan Huang, Joe Lee, Pete Clapp. Back - Sue Wade, Chris Evelyn, Namandje Bumpus, Rick Neubig, Uma Gopalakrishan, Wayne Leifert (not pictured - Qin Wang)

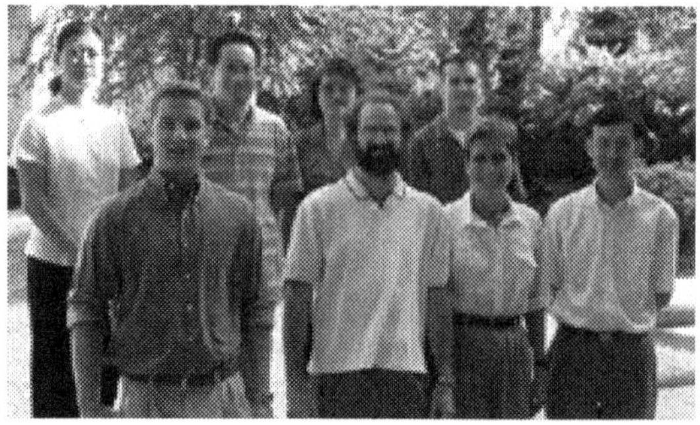

August 2001 Min Liu, Alec Schmaier, Huailing Zhong, Qin Wang, Rick Neubig, Brian Adams, Sue Wade, William Lim, not pictured Uma Gopalakrishan, Leighton Janes and Brandy Butcher

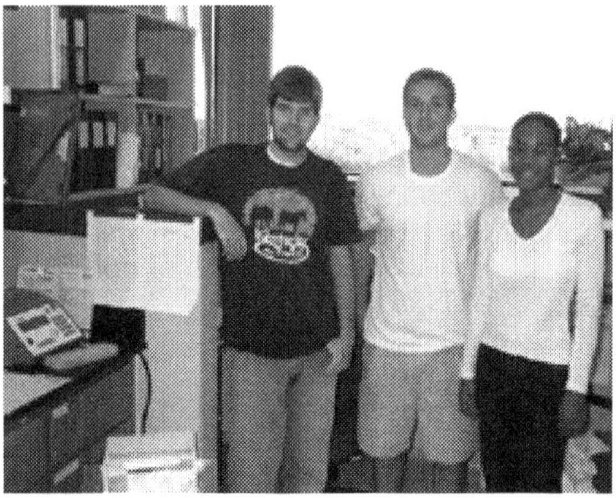

Summer Students 2001 Leighton Janes, Alec Schmaier, and Brandy Butcher

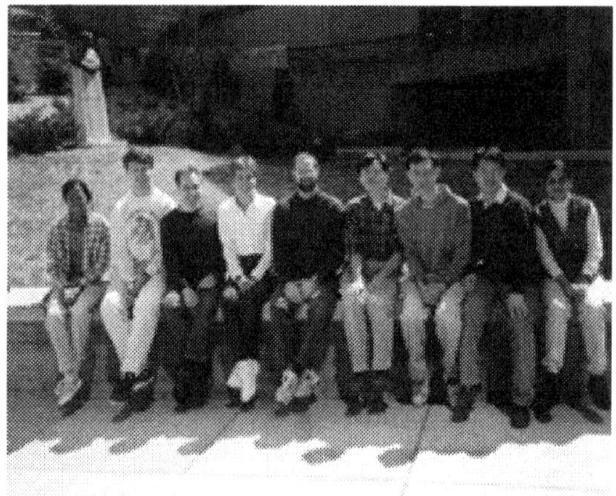

Neubig Lab Members 1999 - Erica Riddle, Dyke McEwen, Tiaan Brink, Sue Wade, Rick Neubig, Gary (Keng-Li) Lan, William Lim, Masa Nanamori, Uma Gopalakrishan

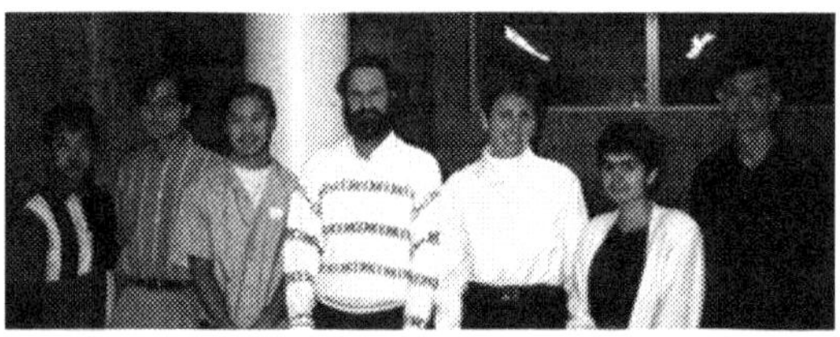

Neubig Lab Members 1998 - Masa Nanamori, Gary (Keng-Li) Lan, Duane Chung, Rick Neubig, Sue Wade, Noune Sarvazyan, William Lim

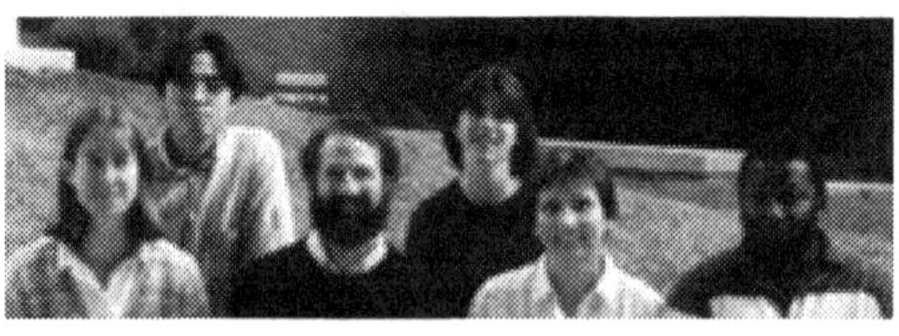

Neubig Lab Members 1997 - Ann Remmers, Gary (Keng-Li) Lan, Rick Neubig, Joan Taylor, Sue Wade, Joseph Thompson

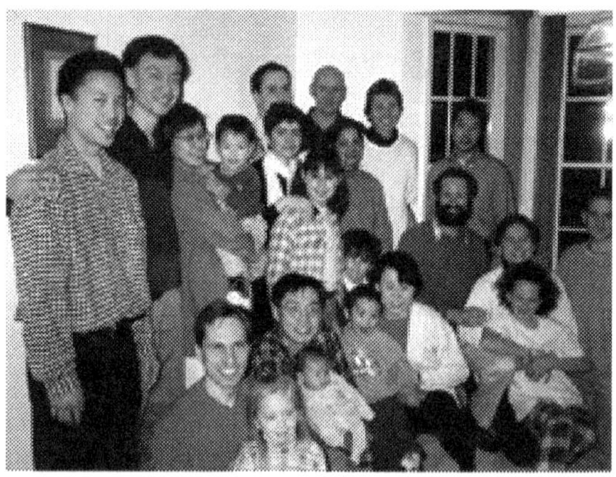

Lab Party for Keng-Li (Gary) Lan after his Ph.D. thesis defense, April, 1999

Dr. Roger S. Newton's Research Interests

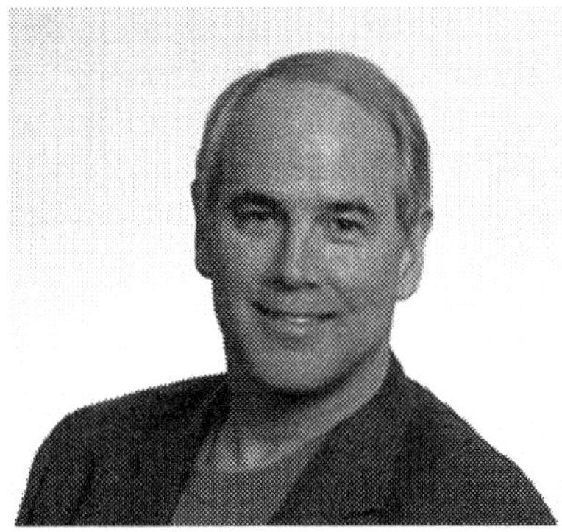

Roger S. Newton, Ph.D., FAHA, is a lipid biochemist whose research interests over the past thirty years have focused on the nutritional and pharmacological regulation of cholesterol and lipoprotein metabolism as they relate to vascular disease. He was initially employed as a Senior Research Scientist in Atherosclerosis Pharmacology at the Parke-Davis Pharmaceutical Research Division of Warner Lambert Company. During his tenure at Parke-Davis from 1981-1998, Dr. Newton became Chairman of the Atherosclerosis Drug Discovery Team during which time he researched the potential mechanisms to beneficially regulate cholesterol and lipoprotein metabolism by pharmacological intervention. His initial research focused on mechanism of action of fibrate drugs, which included gemfibrozil (Lopid®), the first lipid regulating agent.

Dr. Newton was given the responsibility at Parke-Davis to lead a program focusing on the discovery and development of new agents to inhibit the rate limiting enzyme in cholesterol biosynthesis, HMG-CoA reductase. The Atherosclerosis Drug Discovery Team worked over five years synthesizing and testing different chemical series before discovering a very potent and efficacious HMG-CoA reductase inhibitor atorvastatin (Lipitor®). Lipitor® is now the most widely prescribed cholesterol reducing drug and the largest selling pharmaceutical in the world.

In May 1998, Dr. Newton left Parke-Davis to co-found Esperion Therapeutics, Inc., and has been its President and CEO. Esperion is dedicated to the discovery and development of pharmaceutical products for the treatment of cardiovascular and metabolic diseases through the use of a new approach called "High Density Lipoprotein (HDL) therapy." Based on the company's understanding of HDL function and its role in reverse lipid transport, Esperion's biopharmaceutical product candidates are designed to be used as sub-acute infusion therapy to mobilize cholesterol from vulnerable, unstable atherosclerotic plaques, and as a result, reduce cardiovascular endpoints in acute coronary syndrome (ACS) and high risk patients. Recent results support a statistically significant regression of atherosclerosis after only six weeks by measuring a change in plaque volume using intravascular ultrasound (IVUS) in ACS patients who received standard of care and were also treated with ETC-216 (apo AI-Milano/phospholipid vesicles). Further studies will investigate the impact of mobilizing cholesterol from atherosclerotic plaques using HDL therapy and the effect on reducing cardiovascular-related endpoints including heart attacks and surgical interventions such as angioplasty.

Dr. Newton is also an Adjunct Associate Professor in the Department of Pharmacology at the University of Michigan Medical School and serves on the National Advisory Board for the University of Michigan Cardiovascular Center. In addition to being a Director on the Board of Rubicon Genomics, an Ann Arbor-based company, Dr. Newton has served on the Steering Committee of the Michigan Life Sciences Corridor. *Editor's note: Pfizer is now purchasing Esperion.*

Dr. Yoichi Osawa's Research Interests

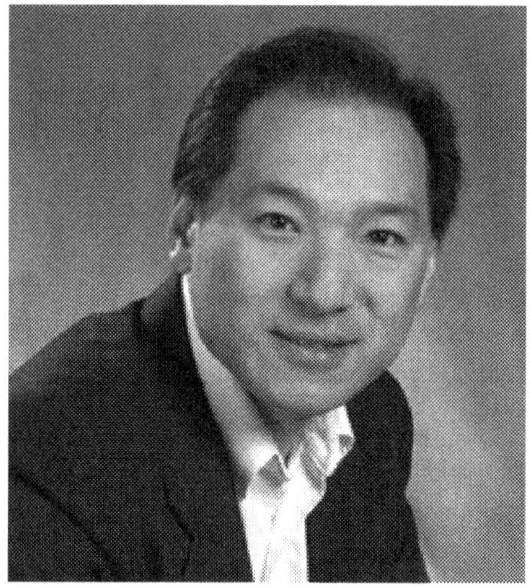

Yoichi Osawa is an Associate Professor of Pharmacology and Director of the Biomedical Mass Spectrometry Facility in the Medical School. Dr. Osawa is a recipient of the 2002 Henry Russel Award, which is one of the highest honors awarded to a faculty member by the University of Michigan for excellence in teaching and promise of distinction in scholarship. He has also received national recognition as the recipient of the prestigious Young Investigator Award in Toxicology from the Burroughs Wellcome Fund and the Established Investigator Award from the American Heart Association.

Dr. Osawa's research focuses on the fundamental question of how chemicals, such as drugs and environmental pollutants, cause toxicity. His discoveries have enhanced our understanding of a pivotal mechanism underlying the toxicity of a number of chemicals and explain how a toxic event becomes amplified and persists long after the body has been exposed to the chemical. This mechanism involves the metabolism of compounds by the body to highly reactive chemical intermediates, which subsequently interact with important cellular targets and lead to toxicity. Hemoproteins, such as hemoglobin, cytochrome P-450, nitric oxide synthase, and prostaglandin H synthase, have been of special interest to Dr. Osawa as they are important generators and targets of these reactive intermediates and have critical cellular functions, including synthesis of hormones and neurotransmitters. He is characterizing these interactions on the molecular level with the use of a variety of biological and chemical methods and evaluating the significance of these events in biological processes.

Dr. Osawa's long term aim is to use this knowledge to exert molecular control over these processes for therapeutic benefit in conditions, such as myocardial ischemia reperfusion injury, sexual dysfunction, or drug toxicity, where reactive intermediates play a role.

The Medical School has historically been a center of pioneering research in the field of metabolism and toxicology and Dr. Osawa aims to maintain and enhance this reputation of excellence in this discipline. To this end, he is currently building a state of the art analytical facility to study the metabolism of chemicals to toxic reactive intermediates. This facility will be a resource in a multi-disciplinary approach involving the basic and clinical sciences within the Medical School to explore ways to minimize chemically induced toxicity. Through these efforts, we aim to develop safer drugs through research as well as in the training of future scientists with expertise in toxic reactive intermediates.

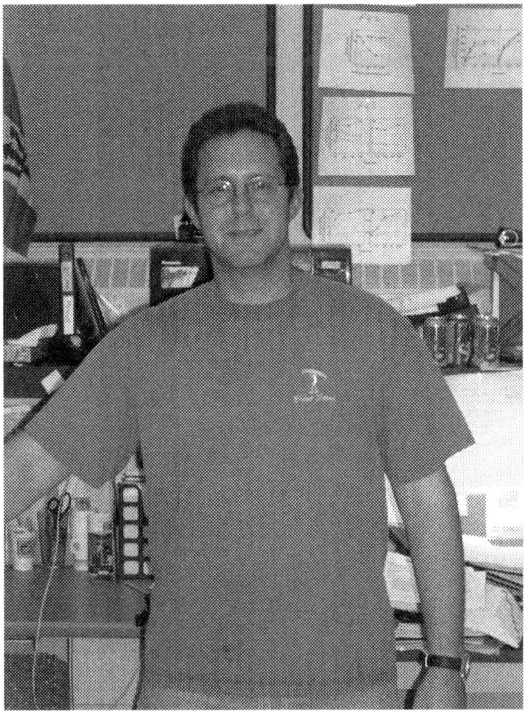

Scott Billecke

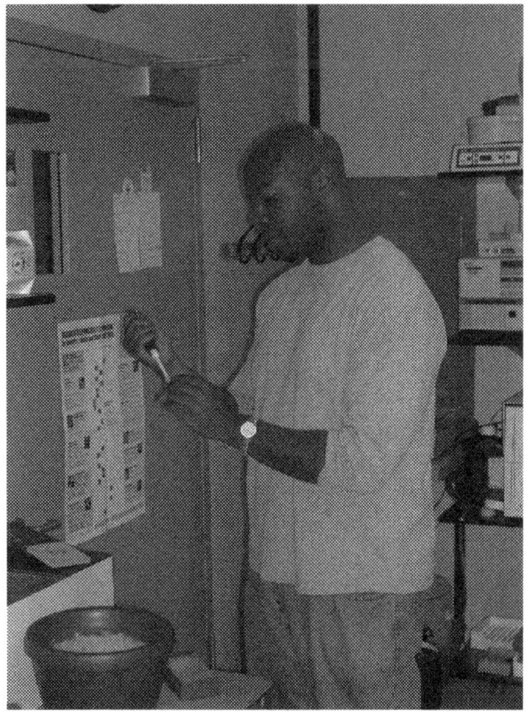

Anwar Y. Dunbar

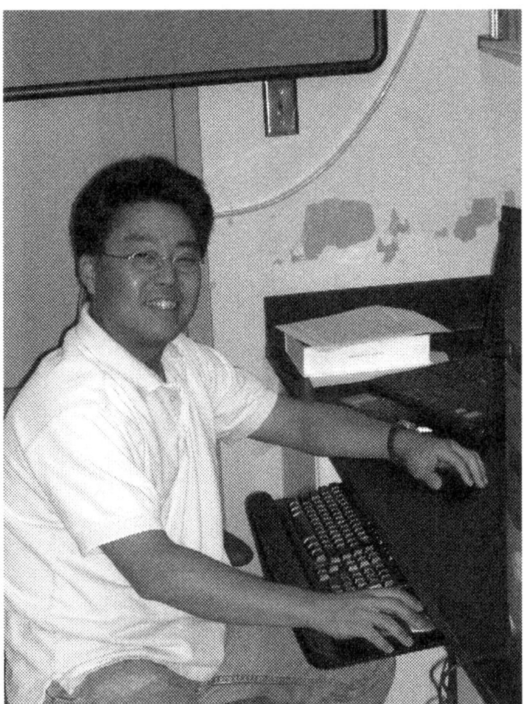

Anthony Lee

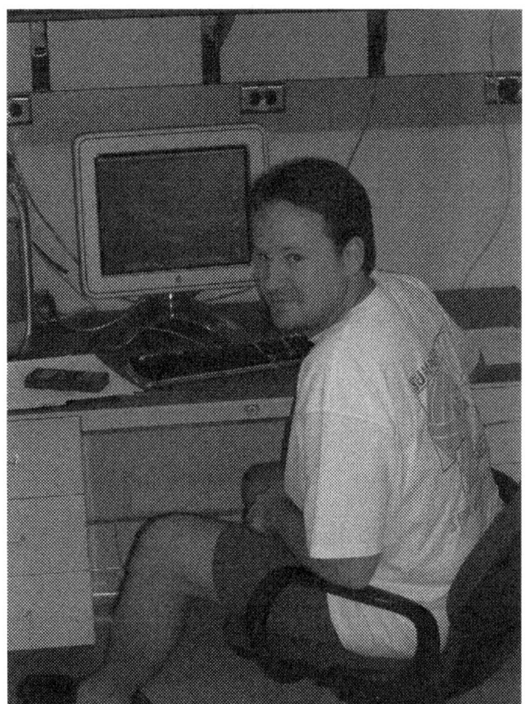

Gary Jenkins

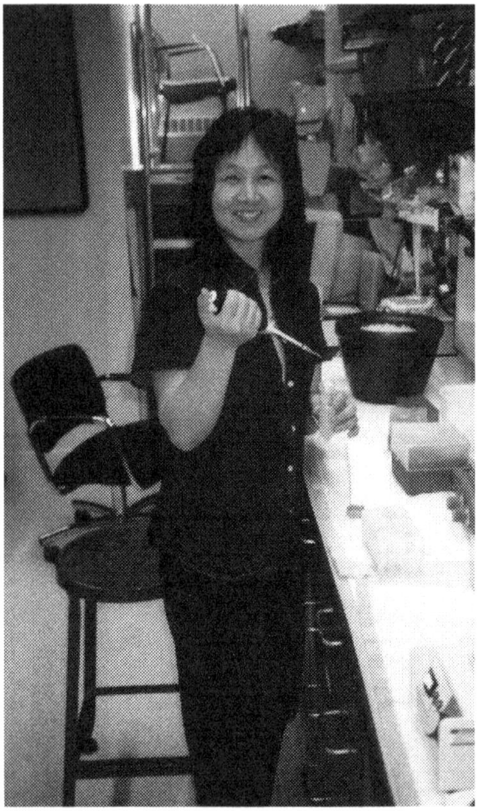

Hwei-Ming Peng

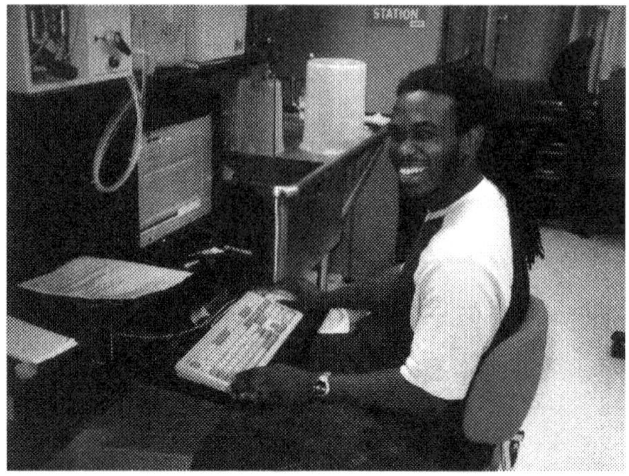

Ezra Lowe

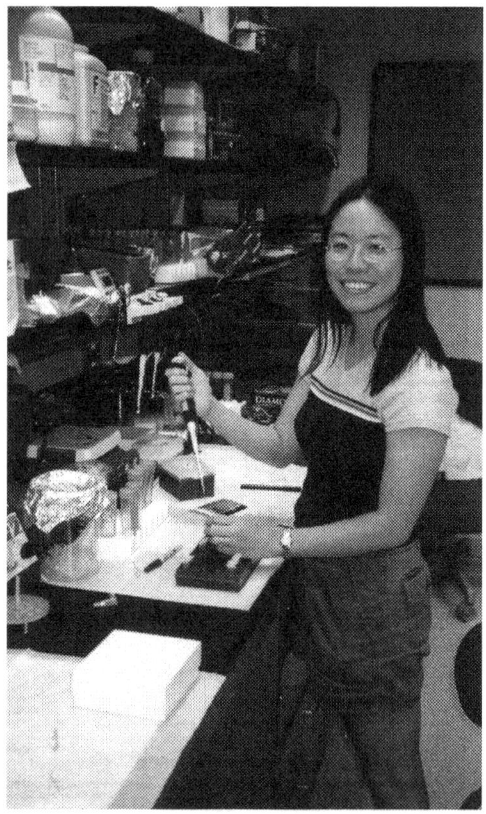

Maranda Lau

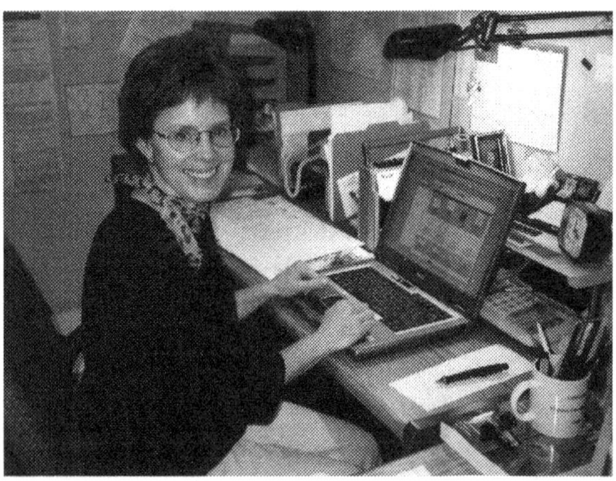

Dr. Kate Noon

Dr. Gabrielle Rudenko's Research Interests

Dr. Gabrielle (Gabby) Rudenko has recently joined the Department of Pharmacology as an Assistant professor and the Life Sciences Institute at the University of Michigan as an Assistant Research Scientist. Dr. Rudenko is a protein crystallographer by training. Dr. Rudenko earned a B.S. in Chemistry from the University of Amsterdam and her Ph.D. at the University of Groningen, Netherlands. She completed her graduate studies with Professor Wim G.J. Hol at the University of Washington and post-doctoral studies with Professor Johann Deisenhofer at UT Southwestern Medical Center.

While working in the lab of Professor Johann Deisenhofer at the University of Texas Southwestern Medical Center in Dallas, Rudenko was the lead author on a study that describes the LDL cholesterol receptor molecule. The LDL receptor stands on the outer membrane of a cell, and binds passing "bad cholesterol" and draws it inside a cell, where it may be broken up to make hormones, cell membranes, vitamin D and other essential molecular ingredients. One observer called her six-year effort to understand the receptor "a heroic effort."

Dr. Rudenko was born in San Francisco, and holds dual citizenship in the U.S. and The Netherlands.

Dr. Rudenko is a structural biologist, who is interested in determining the three dimensional structure of proteins that have important functions in the brain, by using x-ray crystallography. Her studies are augmented with biochemical and biophysical studies, as well as site directed mutagenesis. The brain is the most complex and least understood organ in our body. It is estimated that there are about 10^{10} neurons and about 10^{14} synapses.

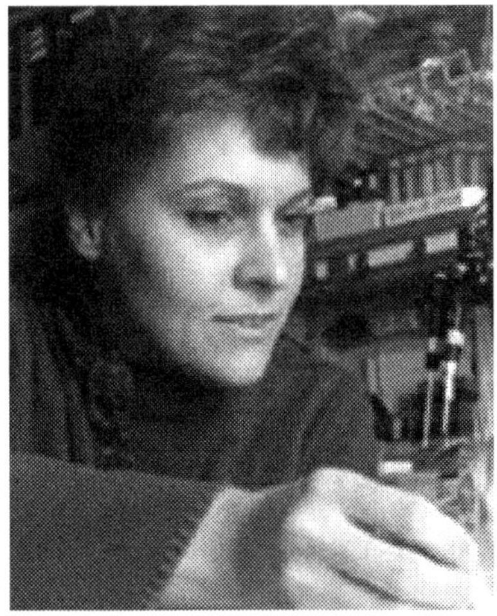

What makes us who we are, what we feel and how we act is somehow stored in the brain. At a molecular level, a tremendous wealth of proteins, including receptors, channels, cell adhesion molecules, transcription factors, different signaling cascades and a large number of enzymes all work together to carry out our mental processes. Understanding how these different proteins function at a molecular level requires intimate knowledge of their three-dimensional structure. Dr. Rudenko is currently studying a family of proteins implicated in the organization and adhesion of synapses.

Her latest work also focusses on a transcription factor that accumulates in the brain of rats upon chronic administration of certain drugs of abuse, anti psychotics, and antidepressants as well as after electro-convulsive seizures.

Dr. Rudenko plans to study other molecules that play a key role in the brain's ability to adapt to physical and chemical insults.

Dr. James A. Shayman's Research Interests

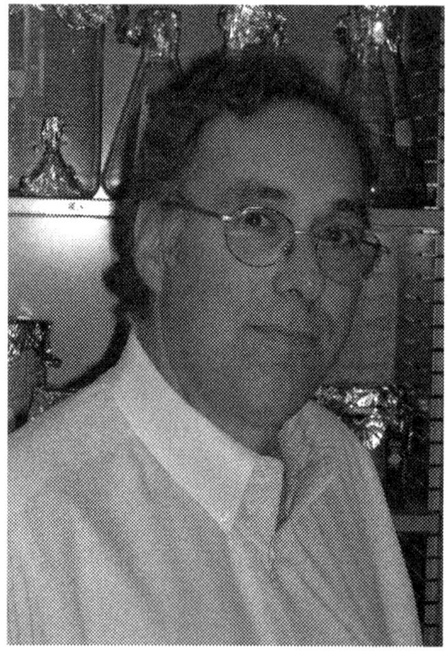

Sphingolipids are ubiquitous membrane components that were originally identified as the accumulated products associated with a variety of lysosomal storage disorders. Sphingolipids are very complex molecules consisting of a long chain base (sphingosine), a fatty acid in amide linkage, and a head group. Depending on the head group, the resultant products may be major membrane phospholipids (e.g., sphingomyelin), glycolipids (e.g., glucosylceramide), or the sphingolipid metabolites (e.g., sphingosine-1-phosphate). These lipids are not only the pathophysiological basis for the sphingolipidoses, but they serve various normal biological functions as signaling molecules, receptors, and scaffolding structures. Sphingolipid storage disorders are relative uncommon but are associated with significant morbidity and mortality for affected children and adults.

The Shayman group has studied the biochemistry, cell biology, and pharmacology of sphingolipids. Specifically, the group has focused on the first dedicated step in glycosphingolipid formation, the glycosylation of ceramide to form glucosylceramide. The group has explored three general areas of inquiry. The first area of inquiry is the role of glycosphingolipids in the regulation of cell signaling. Glycolipids are enriched in membrane domains termed lipid rafts. These rafts are hot spots for signal transduction events and contain receptors, G proteins, kinases and phospholipases. The group has discovered that sphingolipids play critical roles in the regulation of both non-receptor tyrosine kinases and phospholipase C.

A second line of inquiry involves the role of glycosphingolipids as the basis for the pathology associated with more common diseases such as diabetes and vascular thrombosis. The group has discovered, for example, that the glycosphingolipid that accumulates in Fabry disease, Gb3, is a significant mediator of arterial thrombosis.

A third line of inquiry has been the development of small molecule inhibitors of glycosphingolipid synthesis. The group has targeted the enzyme glucosylceramide synthase and has developed a series of compounds that are potent and specific inhibitors of glucosylceramide and of other glucosylceramide based glycosphingolipids. These compounds have been licensed for clinical development for the potential treatment of glycosphingolipidoses such as Gaucher disease, Fabry disease, and Tay-Sachs disease.

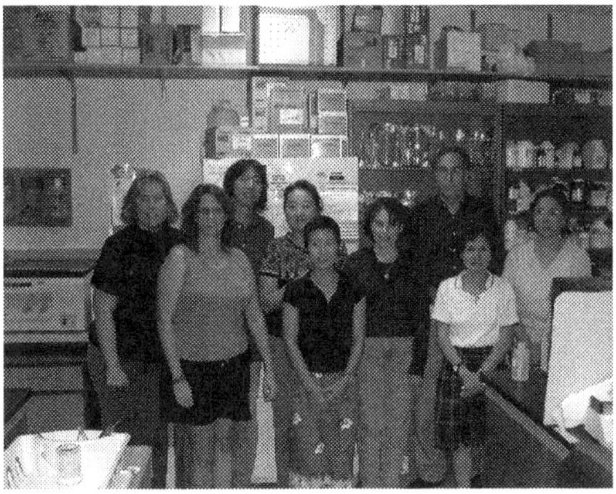

From left to right: Judy Hanson, Heather Poucher, Akira Abe, Miki Hiraoka, Yong Li, Sue Wild, Jim Shayman, Sherry Lee, Liming Shu

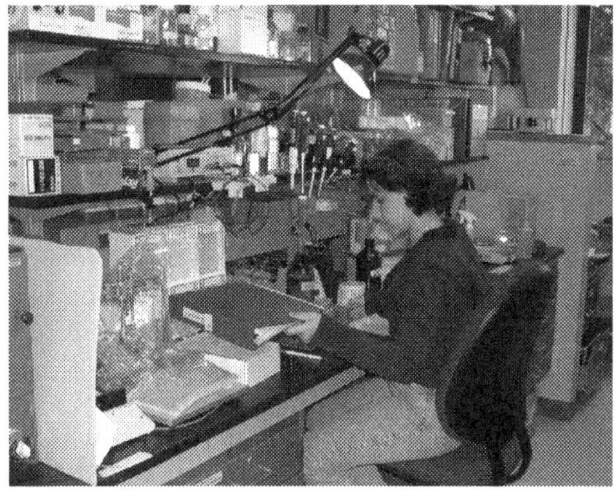

Sue Wild

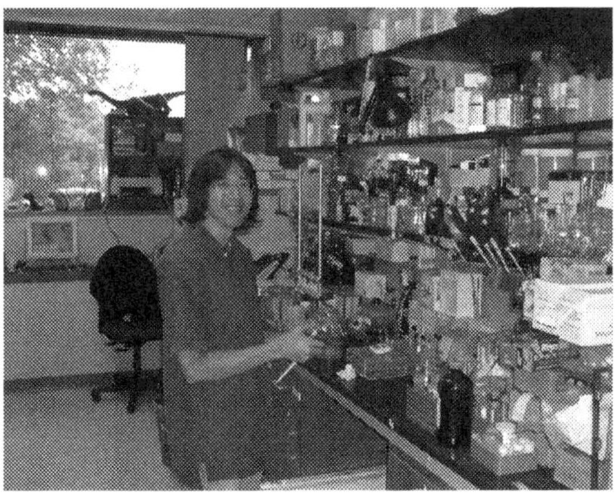

Akira Abe

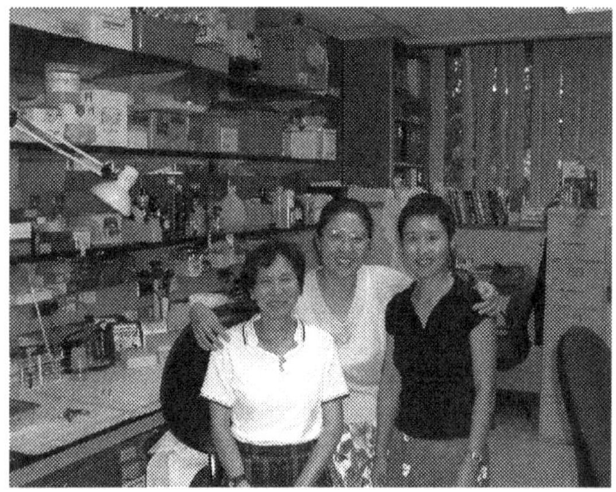

Sherry Lee, Liming Shu, Yong Li

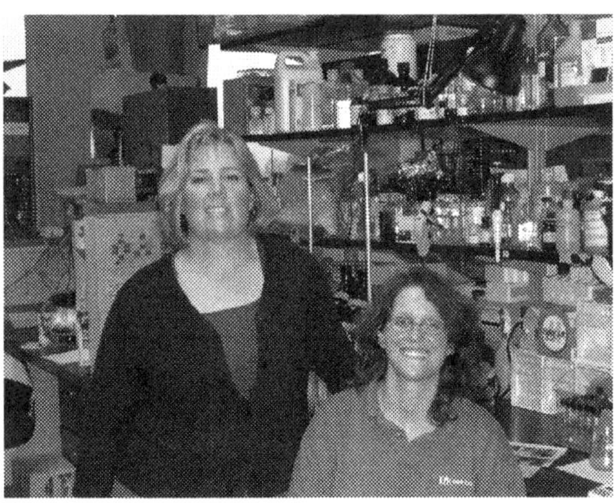

Judy Hanson and Heather Poucher

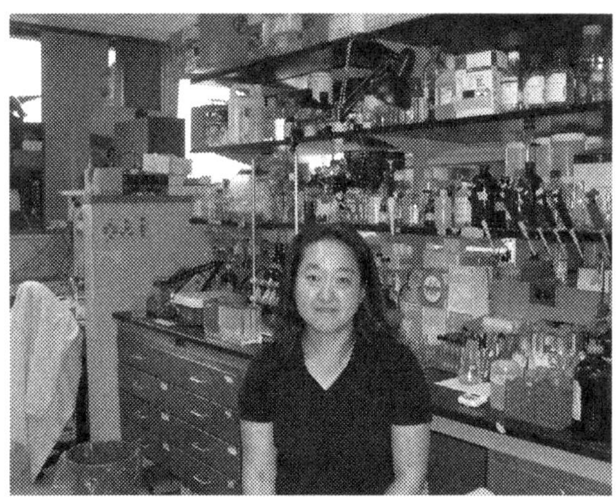

Miki Hiraoka

Dr. Donna S. Shewach's Research Interests

The Shewach laboratory studies the metabolism and mechanism of action for nucleoside analog chemotherapeutic agents, with the overall goal of developing approaches that will enhance the antitumor activity of these drugs. The two major projects currently being studied are: 1) gemcitabine, a deoxycytidine analog that is active clinically in the treatment of a variety of solid tumors, including pancreatic cancer and non-small cell lung cancer; 2) enzyme-prodrug therapy with herpes simplex virus thymidine kinase (HSV-TK) and ganciclovir.

The drug gemcitabine (2',2'-difluoro-2'-deoxycytidine) is phosphorylated readily in tumor cells, and both the di- and triphosphate derivatives contribute to the antitumor activity of the drug. The diphosphate is a mechanism-based inhibitor of ribonucleotide reductase, which results in a decrease primarily in dATP pools in solid tumor cells. The triphosphate can inhibit DNA polymerases and is incorporated into DNA. We hypothesized and then proved that gemcitabine is a potent radiosensitizer, and this property is conferred by the inhibition of ribonucleotide reductase by gemcitabine diphosphate. Our current hypothesis is that the gemcitabine-mediated decrease in dATP pools causes incorrect nucleotide incorporation into DNA, a lesion that can normally be corrected by the mismatch repair pathway. However, in combination with ionizing radiation, we propose that the DNA mismatches are either not repaired or repaired incorrectly, resulting in cell death. We are investigating this hypothesis in mismatch repair proficient and deficient cells, and using a plasmid-based shuttle vector assay to identify the exact mutations in DNA produced by gemcitabine. Other studies are identifying the role of cell cycle proteins in radiosensitization with gemcitabine.

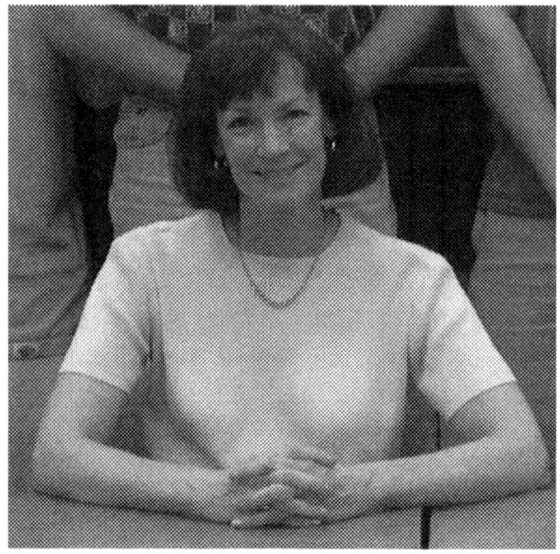

Gene Therapy Studies

The antiviral drug ganciclovir is normally non-toxic to cells, but in the presence of HSV-TK expression it phosphorylated to its triphosphate, which is a potent antitumor agent. Studies in my laboratory have demonstrated that ganciclovir is superior to other related antivirals due to its unique effects on DNA synthesis. Extension of our mechanistic studies led to the demonstration that inhibitors of ribonucleotide reductase enhanced the antitumor activity of ganciclovir. In addition, in cultures consisting of both HSV-TK-expressing and non-expressing bystander cells, these inhibitors synergistically enhance the cytotoxicity of ganciclovir to the bystander cells. We have demonstrated that toxicity in bystander cells occurs through transfer of phosphorylated ganciclovir from HSV-TK-expressing cells. Current studies are exploring the mechanism of synergy for ribonucleotide reductase inhibitors and ganciclovir, as well as elucidating the mechanism by which ganciclovir phosphates are transferred from HSV-TK-expressing to non-expressing bystander cells using in vitro and in vivo models.

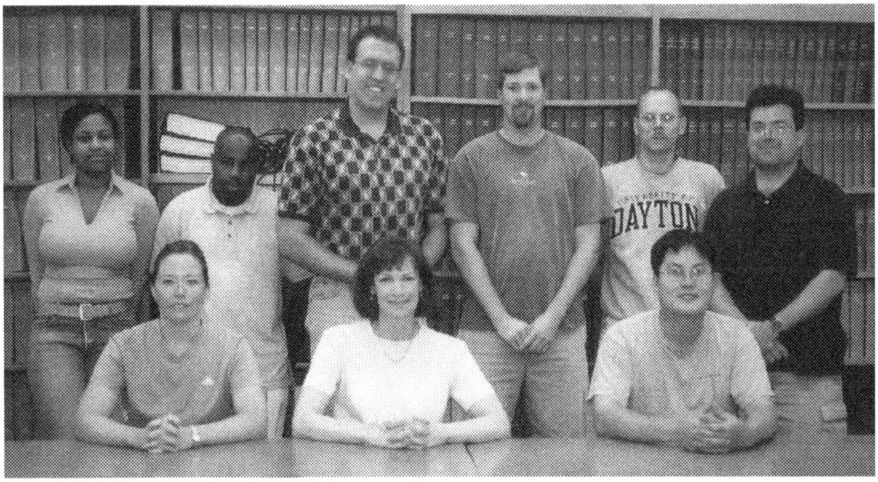

Front row: Sheryl Flanagan, Donna Shewach, Mike Im
Back row: Namandjè Bumpas, Joe Barber, Brian Gentry, Blaine Robinson, Leo Ostruszka, Paul Boucher

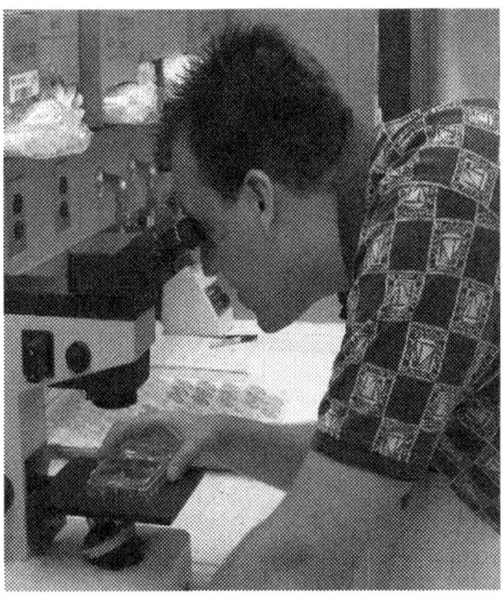

Brian Gentry

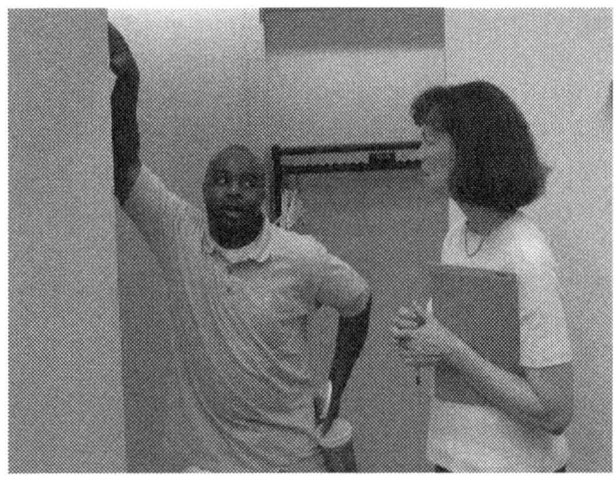

Joe Barber and Donna Shewach

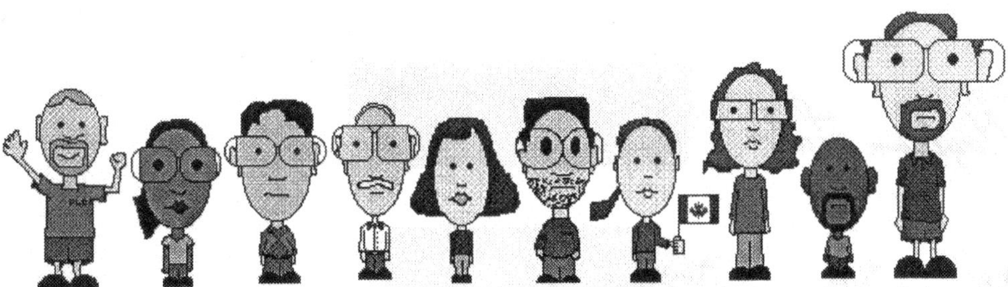

Dr. Marshal Shlafer's Research Interests

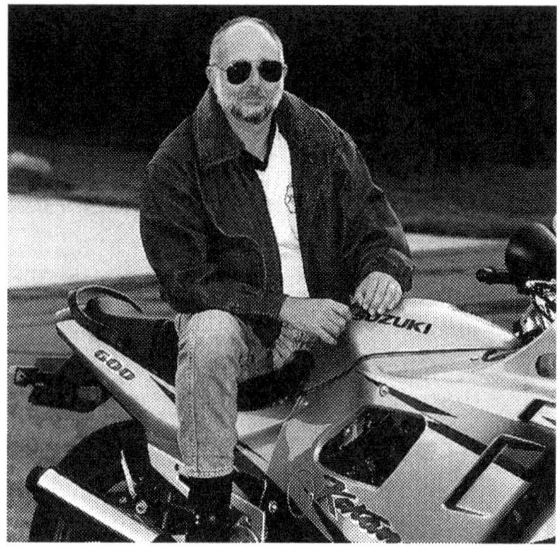

Dr. Shlafer's lab is closed. He still maintains an interest in his research area, the mechanisms by which oxygen deprivation due to ischemia damages the heart. His publications focused on the involvement of cytotoxic oxygen metabolites (oxygen radicals) that appear to be produced by the ischemic and reperfused heart. The research addressed the possible subcellular sources of oxygen radicals, the chemical nature of the radicals, changes in endogenous myocardial defensive mechanisms against free radical-induced damage, and pharmacologic approaches to preventing such damage. He is in his 23rd year directing the undergraduate nursing pharmacology course, Pharmacology 210. Recently he assumed directorship of the short introductory pharmacology course for the first year medical students, and codirectorship of the cardiovascular diseases sequence for the M2s.

Dr. Robert U. Simpson's Research Interests

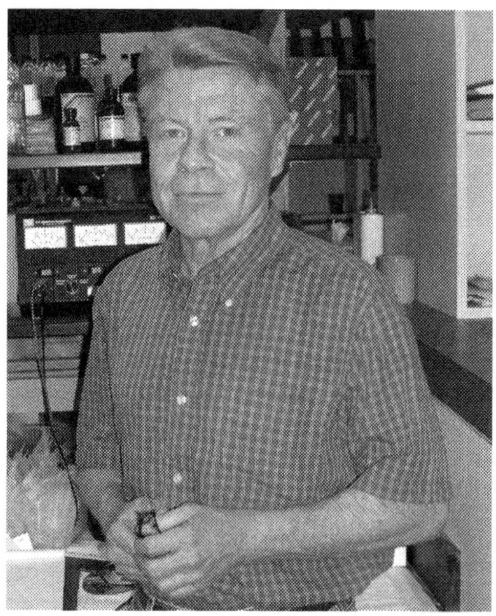

A goal of Dr. Simpson's research is to understand the mechanism of action of 1,25 dihydroxyvitamin D[1,25(OH)2D], the hormone derived from vitamin D. Studies examine the action of this hormone to regulate differentiation of cells as diverse as pre-osteoclast-like macrophages and heart myoblasts. Biochemical and molecular biology techniques are currently employed for the characterization of the actions of 1,25(OH)2D to regulate gene expression.

Dr. Simpson's group has recently shown that the expression of the genes for protein kinase C and c-myc protooncogene are controlled by 1,25(OH)2D. Research efforts are now focused on determining the cellular processes in which these gene products participate and how these genes alter cell function.

Dr. Jerry Stitzel's Research Interests

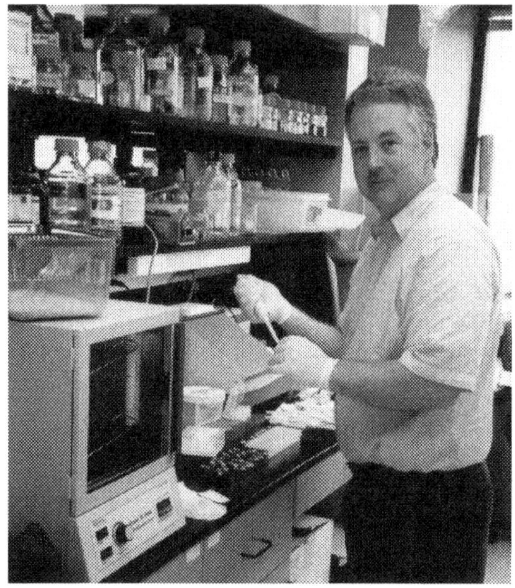

The Stitzel laboratory utilizes a genetic approach as a means to appreciate the role of the nicotinic cholinergic system in modulating behavior, physiology and development. The lab is also interested in understanding how naturally occurring genetic variability influences individual difference in the physiological and behavioral effects of nicotine and other abused substances. The lab currently has two major projects underway.

Project 1: Identification of naturally occurring polymorphisms in the mouse nicotinic receptor subunit genes. Neuronal nicotinic receptors are pentameric ligand-gated cationic channels. Many potential receptors subtypes exist in the CNS and PNS, each comprised of a specific combination of the subunits $\alpha2$-$\alpha10$ and $\beta2$-$\beta4$. The specific role of given receptor subtypes in normal, aberrant, and drug-related behavior and physiology is poorly understood. The objective of the project is to better understand the role of specific nicotinic receptor (nAChR) subtypes by evaluating the effect of genetic polymorphisms in individual nAChR subunit genes on behavior, physiology, and neuroanatomy. Single nucleotide polymorphisms (SNPs) in two of the nAChR subunit genes, Chrna4, and Chrna7, which encode the nAChR $\alpha4$ and $\alpha7$ subunits, respectively, are currently under investigation.

A missense SNP (threonine/alanine) in Chrna4 has been found to be associated with various behavioral and physiological responses to nicotine and alcohol (Stitzel et al., 2000; Tritto et al., 2001, Tritto et al., 2002; Butt et al., 2003). Biochemical studies have shown that the Chrna4 missense SNP affects basal receptor function as well as the ability of alcohol to potentiate the function of $\alpha4$ subunit-containing receptors (Dobelis et al., 2002; Butt et al., 2003). Electrophysiological analysis of the $\alpha4$ subunit variants suggest that the threonine/alanine polymorphism affects the ratio of high and low affinity $\alpha4\beta2$ receptors (Kim et al., 2003). The combination of these data suggest that individuals with different proportions of high and low affinity $\alpha4\beta2$ nAChRs are differentially sensitive to certain effects of nicotine and alcohol.

Polymorphisms in Chrna7 have been linked to the level of expression of $\alpha7$-containing receptors (Stitzel et al., 1996), sensitivity to nicotine-induced seizures (Stitzel et al., 1998), auditory gating (Stevens et al., 2001) and pre-pulse inhibition of the startle reflex (Yau et al., 2001). Chrna7 polymorphisms also are linked to mouse strain differences in hippocampal cholinergic and GABAergic neuroanatomy (Adams et al., 2001) suggesting that Chrna7 determined neuroanatomy of these systems might lead to individual differences in information processing and sensitivity to nicotine. Several of the SNPs in Chrna7 reside in a portion of the gene (intron9) that contains an alternative exon that is incorporated into a splice variant of $\alpha7$ (Saragoza et al., 2003). The potential role of the $\alpha7$ splice variant in neurodevelopment is currently under investigation. In addition, SNPs in the promoter of Chrna7 have been found to affect gene expression in a cell type-specific fashion. The mechanism through which these SNPs affect gene expression also is being explored.

Project 2: Identification of genetic loci that influence nicotine consumption in mice. Individual differences in smoking behavior in human and free choice nicotine consumption in rodents are significantly influenced by genetic factors. The objective of this project is to identify genetic loci that contribute to individual differences in nicotine consumption in mice in the hope that the genes identified will lead to a better understanding of the biological basis of nicotine consumption in humans. Currently, we are mapping quantitative trait loci (QTL) for nicotine consumption in an F2 intercross between C57BL/6J and C3H/HeJ mice. Although the QTL mapping is not yet complete, we have identified a major effect QTL on distal chromosome 1. This QTL accounts for approximately 23% of the total phenotypic variance in nicotine consumption. Interestingly, a QTL for alcohol withdrawal also maps to the same location on chromosome 1 suggesting a genetic link between nicotine consumption and alcohol withdrawal. Understanding the link between the alcohol withdrawal and nicotine consumption QTL on distal chromosome 1 may provide insight into the biological basis for the high co-morbidity between alcoholism and smoking in humans.

Editor's note: Dr. Stitzel has accepted a position as an Assistant Professor in the Institute for Behavioral Genetics at the University of Colorado in Boulder as of January 2004. Our loss is their gain.

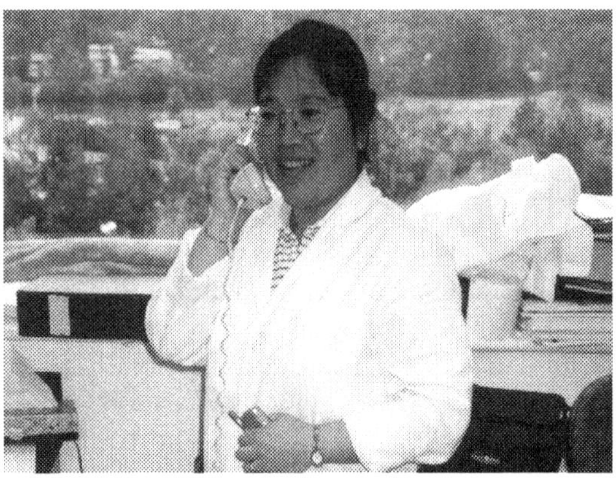

Xiao Chun Li

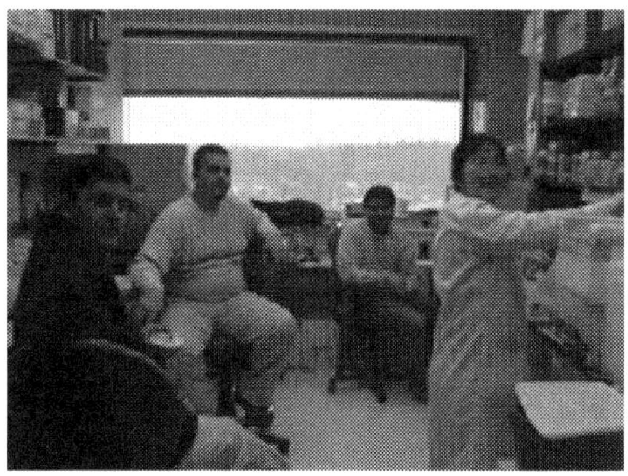

Mark Karadsheh, Paul Jenkins, Mohammad Shah and Xiao Chun Li

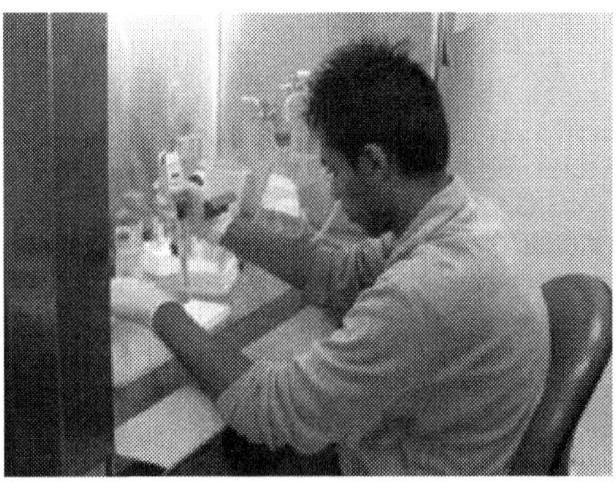

Meet Patel

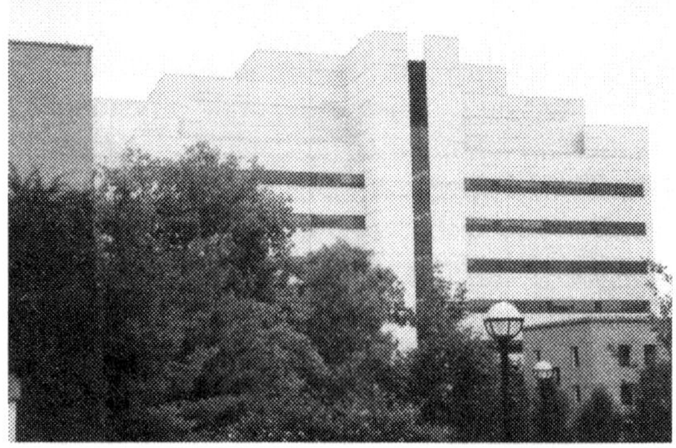

Cancer / Geriatric Center

Dr. Roger K. Sunahara's Research Interests

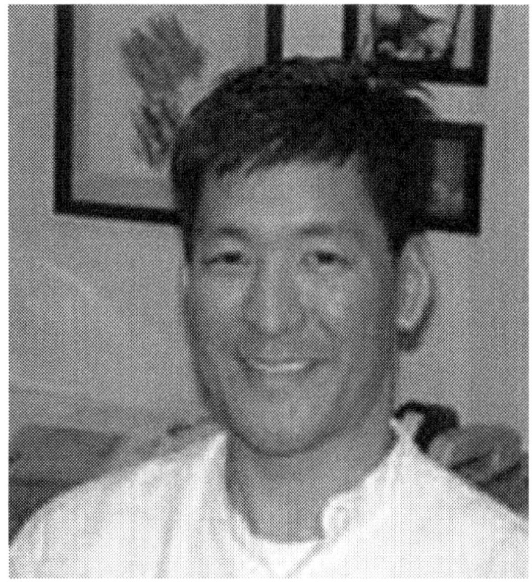

The Sunahara laboratory is primarily interested in the biochemical dissection the structural and functional consequences of signal activation and propagation. We address fundamental aspects of the G Protein-Coupled Receptor (GPCR) signaling cascades and have used the study of G proteins and the soluble portion of adenylyl cyclase as a model system. In previous studies we utilized several approaches to study the behavior of G proteins on regulation of adenylyl cyclase.

Advances in structural biology have resulted in the elucidation of the atomic structures of thousands of cytosolic proteins. Together with a plethora of functional data a firm understanding of how these proteins work has been appreciated. Unfortunately only a dozen or so membrane protein structures have been resolved. The structure of only one GPCR, bovine rhodopsin, has been elucidated thus far. Although it represents a monumental achievement, the X-ray structure revealed only slightly more than previously predicted by electron microscopy and other biophysical studies. The critical regions of the GPCR that are responsible for interacting with G proteins were unfortunately disordered and therefore not visible. Thus the question of how light-induced isomerization of the chromaphore results in G protein activation remains unanswered.

The necessity to understand the underlying mechanism of GPCR signaling is underscored by the fact that the majority of all therapeutics target GPCR signaling cascades (~ 60% of all pharmaceutics). Various genome projects have introduced even more potential therapeutic targets by uncovering hundreds of novel GPCRs, new G proteins and effectors. A firm understanding of the mechanism of signaling events will help the development of more potent and more selective therapeutics. High-resolution structural and functional characterization of GPCRs themselves will undoubtedly facilitate such goals. For example, knowledge of the three-dimensional structure of co-receptors for HIV, also GPCRs, could lead to the development of selective drugs that block HIV infection. A beta-adrenergic receptor structure will aid in the development of more selective and potent cardiovascular therapeutics. Most neuroleptics that target dopamine receptors, also GPCRs, have been successfully used for the treatment of schizophrenia, Huntington's chorea and Parkinson's syndrome. The development of more selective dopamine receptor ligands, with reduced side-effects, will improve drug efficacy, improve drug compliance and most of all improve the quality of life during treatment.

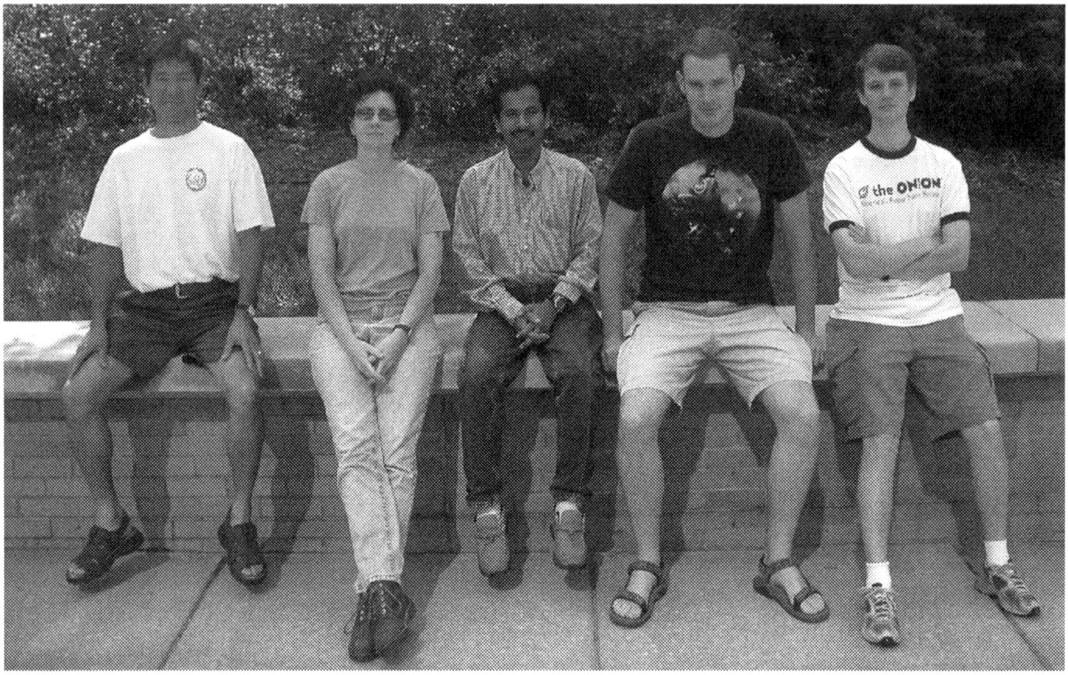

Roger Sunahara, Margaret M. Sadoff, Kannan Vadakkadathmeethal, Matt Whorton, Adam Kuszak

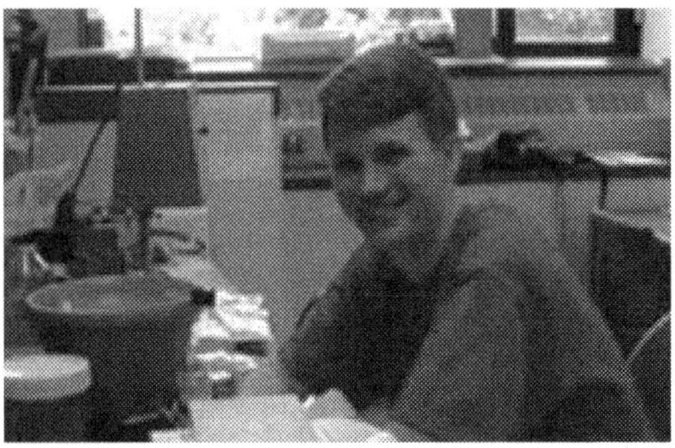

Adam Kuszak

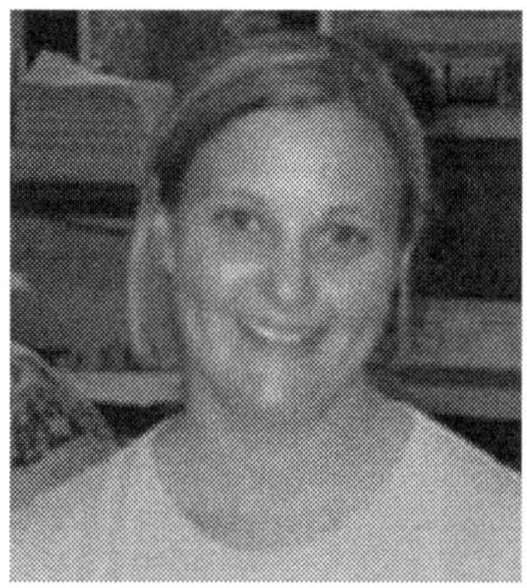

Aimee Felczak

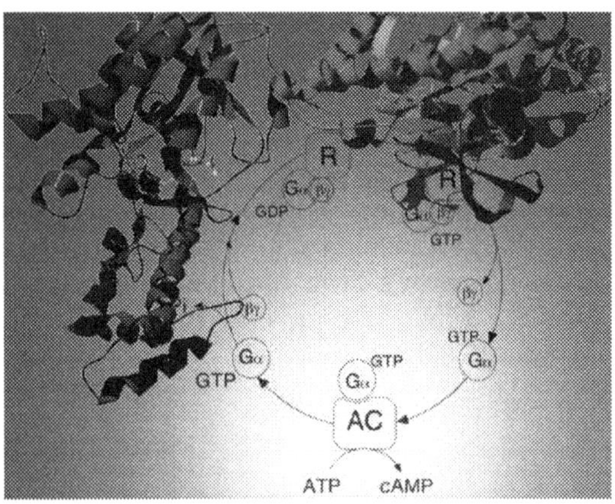

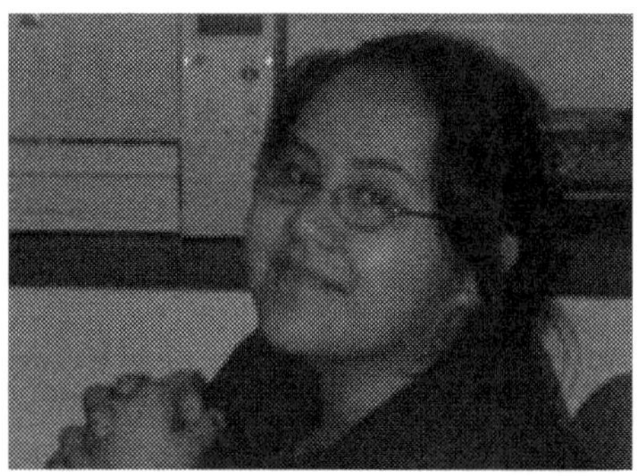

Jen Swift

Dr. John R. Traynor's Research Interests

The Traynor laboratory's research focuses on heroin and related drugs as part of the NIDA funded Narcotic Drug and Opioid Basic Research Center. According to the 1998 National Household Survey on Drug Abuse, an estimated 2.4 million people use heroin at some time in their lives, in addition, 2.6 million Americans use pain relieving drugs for non-medical purposes. We study the mechanism of action of opiate drugs (including heroin) and opioid peptides at a cellular/molecular level and in vivo in order to uncover mechanisms behind acute effects (e.g., analgesia and respiratory depression) and chronic effects leading to dependency. The goal is to provide better drugs for pain relief and medications for the treatment of opiate addiction. The lab is affiliated with the Drug Evaluation Committee of the College on Problems of Drug Dependence and the University of Michigan Substance Abuse Center (UMSARC).

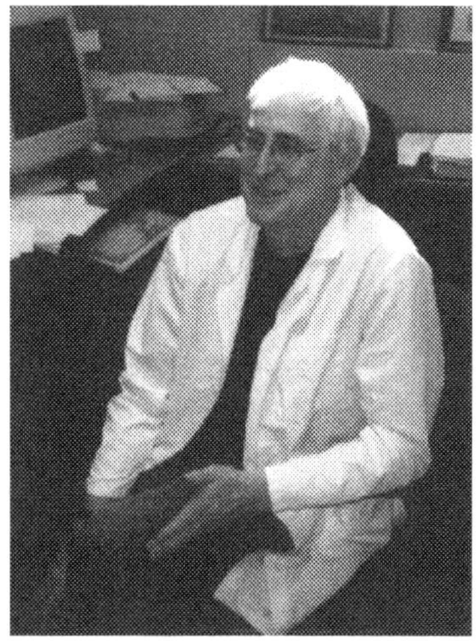

Current Projects

Heroin treatment medications. Methadone is widely used as replacement therapy in heroin abuse. Buprenorphine is an alternative recently approved by the FDA. Methoclocinnamox (MCCAM) has been proposed as a lead to a newer generation of medications. To develop improved treatment agents there is a need to understand the mechanisms of action of these agents. The work studies the cellular mechanisms of action of buprenorphine and MCCAM compared with methadone, using knowledge of opioid receptors, G protein coupling and cellular signaling pathways.

Identification of opioid properties in compounds submitted to the Drug Evaluation Committee (DEC) of the College on Problems of Drug Dependence (CPDD). The aim is to identify opioid activity in compounds for government agencies, industry and the academic community. This includes new compounds and compounds that have potential for abuse. Many different opioids are available but there is always a need for compounds with antinociceptive activity that have improved clinical profiles over available compounds, compounds that might be suitable as treatment agents and compounds with specific profiles for use as pharmacological tools.

Opioid signal transduction. Morphine and related opioid drugs act at a family of receptors that couple to heterotrimeric G proteins. There is only a limited understanding of the mechanisms of acute actions of opioids and especially of chronic actions that lead to the development of opioid tolerance and dependence; processes that contribute to abuse liability. We are investigating the functional significance of a class of proteins that regulate G protein signaling (RGS proteins) to these processes. RGS proteins are a family of proteins that regulate heterotrimeric G proteins by acceleration of the deactivation of G proteins. Thus over-expression of RGS protein should inhibit signaling and conversely expression of RGS-insensitive G proteins should promote signaling. We are studying the acute and chronic effects of opioids in cells expressing RGS-insensitive G-proteins and the effects of chronic morphine treatment on RGS protein expression.

Development of compounds as ligands for Positron Emission Tomography (PET) of opioid receptors. Presently only the mu agonist [11C]carfentanil and the non-selective antagonist [11C]diprenorphine are widely available for visualization of opioid receptors by PET; there are no available PET ligands with selectivity for other type of opioid receptors. In collaboration with Dr. Woods' group and Dr. Kilbourn (Radiology) we are designing imaging agents for the study of opioid receptor distribution and changes induced by pharmacological or physiological manipulation in rodents and monkeys and in different pathological states in man.

The therapeutic potential of delta opioids. Non-peptide delta opioid agonists reduce pain in allodynia and hyperalgesia in animal models. Such agonists are also active in a learned helplessness paradigm in rats. These findings suggest therapeutic potential for delta agonists in the alleviation of pain and in the treatment of depression. However, delta agonists also elicit convulsions. In conjunction with Dr. Woods' group, mechanisms behind these different behaviors are studied in order to realize the therapeutic potential of delta opioid agonists.

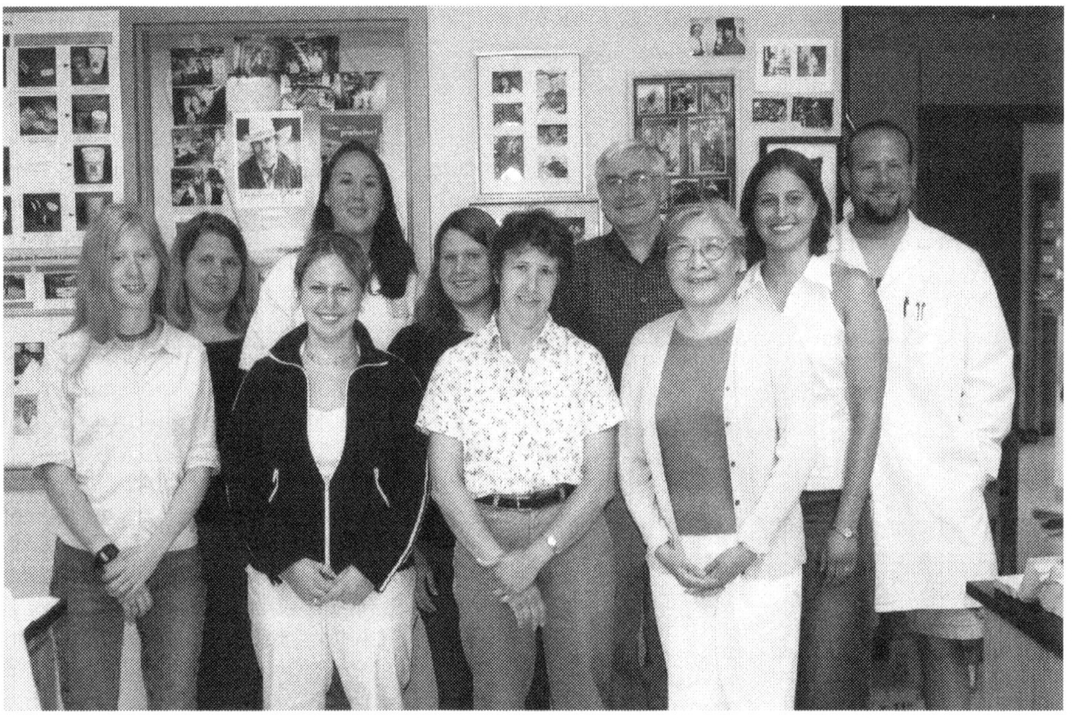

Front: Timra Gilson, Penny Rayner, Mary Clark, Hui-Fang Song
Back: Elizabeth Lapoczka, Mary Falgout, Shannon Andrews, Dr. John Traynor, Kelly Bosse, Tod Tharp

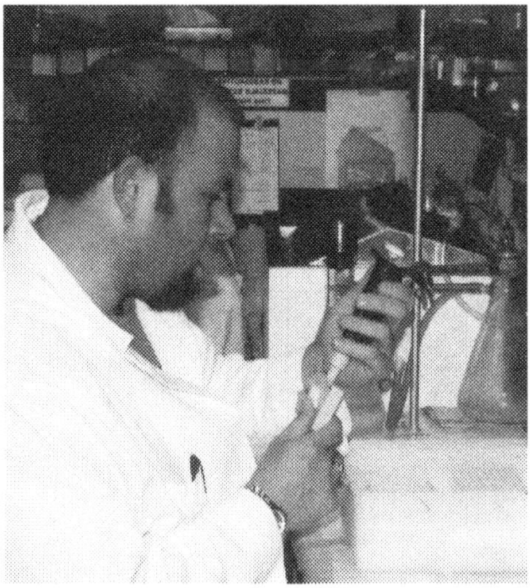

Tod Tharp

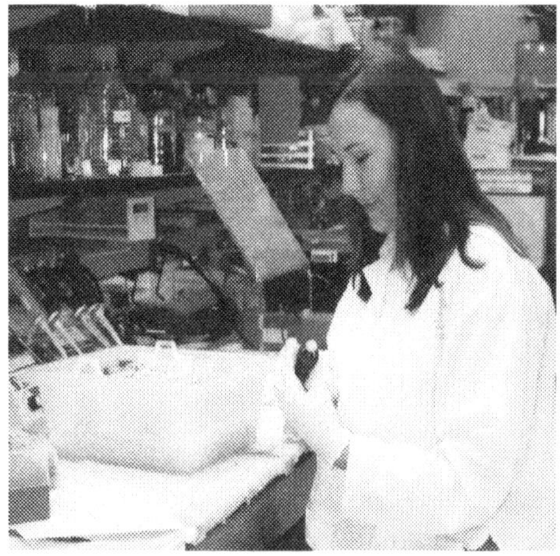

Mary Falgout

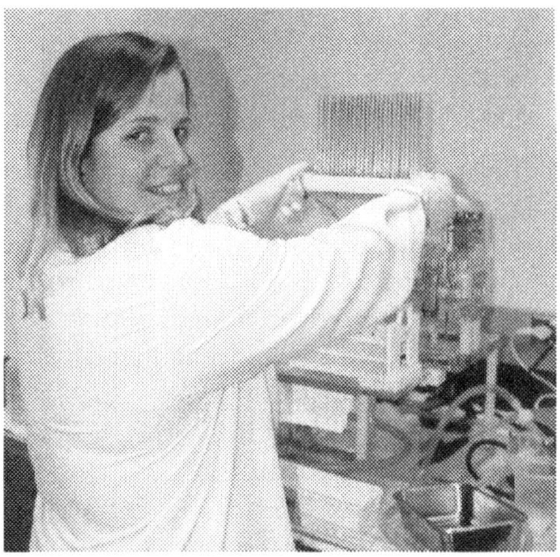

Elizabeth Lapoczka

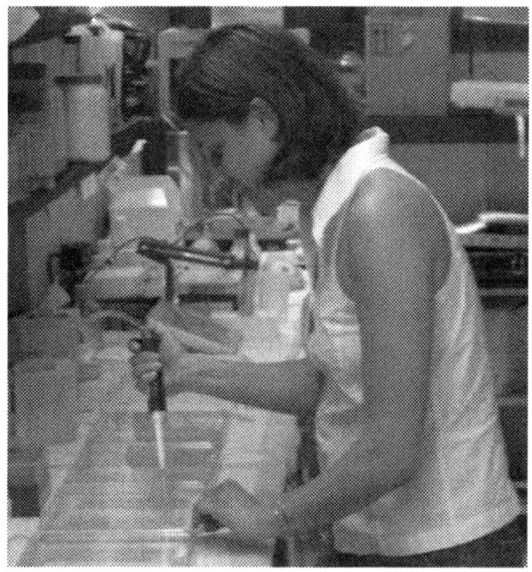

Kelly Bosse

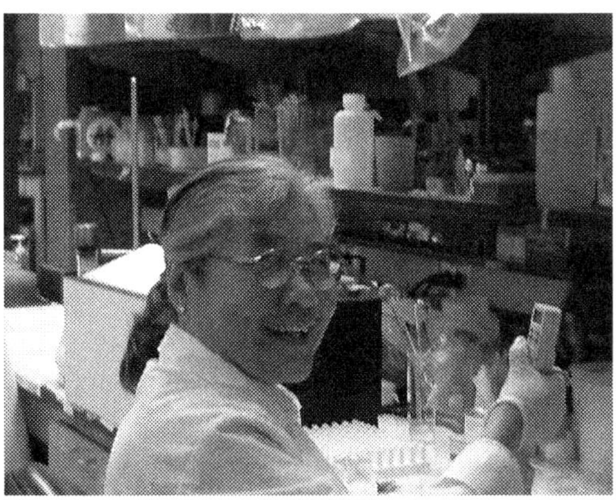

Hui-Fang Song

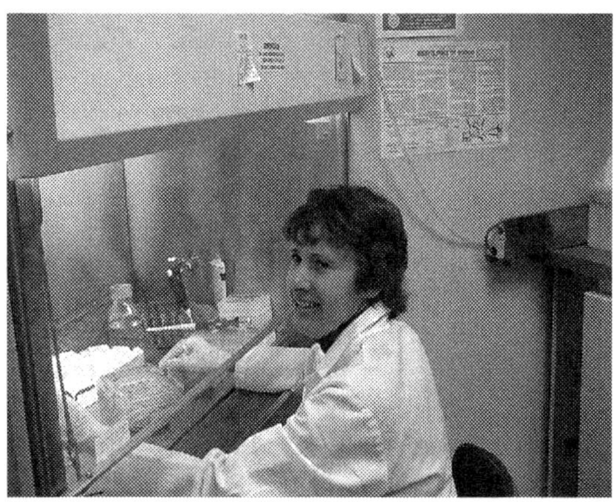

Mary Clark

Dr. Tetsufumi Ueda's Research Interests

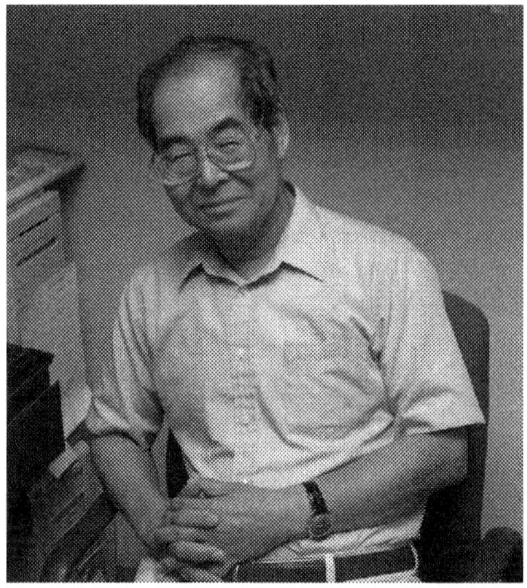

Our laboratory is concerned with the biochemistry, function and regulation of synaptic vesicles in the nerve terminal, and the role of glucose metabolism in synaptic transmission.

Glutamate is now recognized as the major excitatory neurotransmitter in the vertebrate central nervous system. As such, proper glutamate synaptic transmission is implicated in learning and memory as well as in basic neuronal communication. Abnormal glutamate transmission is involved in various types of brain diseases, including certain forms of seizures, stroke, Parkinson's disease, Huntington's disease, amyotrophic lateral sclerosis, and also potentially schizophrenia. Although glutamate is a common substrate involved in a number of metabolic pathways in all cells, it enters the neurotransmitter pathway via a specific glutamate transporter present in synaptic vesicles in the majority of nerve endings. Glutamate molecules accumulated in synaptic vesicles are eventually released into the synaptic cleft, the small gap between the nerve ending and the next neuron, when an electrical impulse propagated along the axon arrives at the nerve terminal. The synaptically released glutamate then excites the postsynaptic neuron through activation of a receptor/channel complex. Thus, the glutamate transporter in the synaptic vesicle membrane plays an important role in initially directing glutamate into the neurotransmitter pathway away from its metabolic pathways.

Since the vesicular glutamate uptake system functions as the gate for glutamate to enter the transmitter pathway, we postulated that this step might be subject to some regulation, and sought an endogenous substance inhibiting the accumulation of glutamate into synaptic vesicles. We found evidence for the existence of a proteinaceous factor inhibiting glutamate uptake into synaptic vesicles. We purified it to apparent homogeneity as a brain cytosol protein (M_r = 138,000) that inhibits glutamate transport. This "inhibitory protein factor" is referred to as IPF. The hydrodynamic properties of IPF suggest that this is an elongated protein. Partial sequence analysis shows that IPF is derived from the α subunit (M_r = 283,000) of fodrin, a protein implicated in several diverse cellular activities. IPF inhibits ATP-dependent glutamate uptake into purified synaptic vesicles, with an IC_{50} of ~26 nM, while showing no ability to inhibit ATP-independent uptake at concentrations up to 100 nM. Moreover, IPF inhibited neither norepinephrine uptake into chromaffin vesicles nor the Na^+ - dependent glutamate uptake into synaptosomes. However, IPF inhibited uptake of γ-aminobutyric acid into synaptic vesicles derived from the spinal cord, suggesting that inhibition may not be limited to glutamatergic systems. We propose that IPF could be a novel component of a presynaptic regulatory system. Such a system might modulate neurotransmitter accumulation into synaptic vesicles and thus regulate the overall efficacy of neurotransmission.

Despite the potent action of IPF and its striking sequence homology to α-fodrin, α-fodrin is devoid of the ability to inhibit vesicular glutamate uptake. How IPF is made from α-fodrin is an interesting question. Our sequence data indicate that the N-terminus amino acid of IPF is the 26th amino acid from the α-fodrin N-terminus. It is well known that α-fodrin is cleaved by the calcium-dependent proteolytic enzyme calpain into two fragments, one of which is known as the 155-kDa protein. However, we observed that the calpain digests of purified α-fodrin exhibit no inhibitory activity, even at high concentrations. This suggests the importance of a distinct, specific proteolytic enzyme which cleaves the bond between the 25th amino acid (Arg) and the 26th amino acid (Tyr), in generating IPF from α-fodrin.

When IPF, but not α-fodrin, is incorporated into isolated pinched-off nerve endings, it leads to a reduction in the amount of exocytotically released glutamate and GABA, presumably by reducing the amount of these transmitters stored in synaptic vesicles. This suggests that IPF is capable of a regulatory function in the nerve terminal *in vivo*.

We have also been engaged in the search for cell membrane-permeant, potent non-proteinaceous compounds which affect vesicular glutamate storage. We have found that the fluorescein derivative Rose Bengal is a potent inhibitor of vesicular glutamate uptake, with a K_d value of 19 nM, while fluorescein exhibits little, if any, effect. This raises the possibility that Rose Bengal could regulate exocytotic release via reduction of vesicular neurotransmitter storage. Thus, Rose Bengal might serve as a xenobiotic quantal size modulator for glutamate and represent a prototype for developing drugs targeting vesicular glutamate storage.

With respect to our study on the role of glucose metabolism in synaptic transmission, we have recently presented evidence that glycolytically produced ATP, in particular that produced by GAPDH and 3–PGK, but not mitochondria-derived ATP, is harnessed for accumulation of Glu into synaptic vesicles in synaptosomes; Glu transported into synaptic vesicles in this manner is released upon depolarization. Glucose is the major source of brain energy and essential for maintaining normal brain and neuronal function. Hypoglycemia causes impaired synaptic transmission. This occurs even before a significant reduction in global cellular ATP concentrations. The relationships among glycolysis, ATP supply, and synaptic transmission are not well understood. We demonstrated that the glycolytic enzymes glyceraldehyde phosphate dehydrogenase (GADPH) and 3-phosphoglycerate kinase (3-PGK) are enriched in synaptic vesicles, forming a functional complex. Synaptic vesicles are capable of accumulating the excitatory neurotransmitter glutamate by harnessing ATP produced by vesicle-bound GAPDH/3-PGK at the expense of their substrates. The GAPDH inhibitor iodoacetate suppressed GAPDH / 3-PGK-dependent, but not exogenous ATP-dependent, [^{3}H]glutamate uptake into isolated synaptic vesicles. It also decreased vesicular [^{3}H]glutamate content in nerve ending preparation synaptosomes. This decrease was reflected in reduction of depolarization-induced [^{3}H]glutamate release. In contrast, oligomycin, a mitochondrial ATP synthase inhibitor, had minimal effect on any of these parameters. ADP at concentrations above 0.1 mM inhibited vesicular glutamate uptake and dissipated the membrane potential. This suggests that the coupled GAPDH / 3-PGK system, which converts ADP to ATP, ensures maximal glutamate accumulation into presynaptic vesicles. Together, these findings provide an explanation for hypoglycemia-induced aberrant synaptic transmission and insight into the essential nature of glycolysis in sustaining normal synaptic transmission.

We are now extending work on the role of glycolysis in synaptic transmission. We are also in the process of expressing IPF-like proteins in bacteria as a step toward understanding the mechanism of action of IPF. Moreover, we are engaged in the search for a better membrane-permeant inhibitor of synaptic vesicular glutamate uptake.

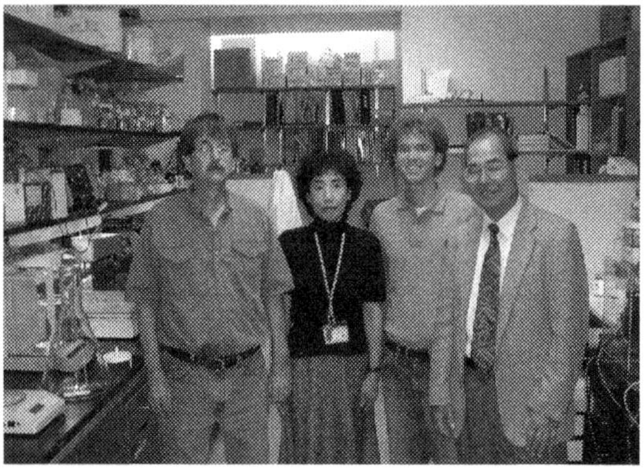

From left to right: David G. Bole, Yasuko Noda, Rafe Petty, Tetsufumi (Ted) Ueda

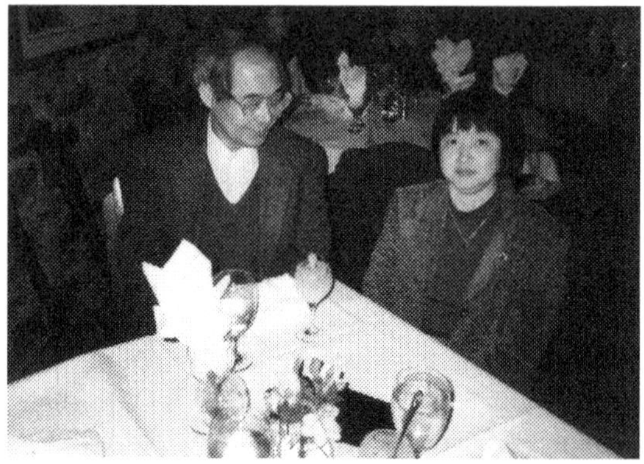

Ted and his wife Yasuko

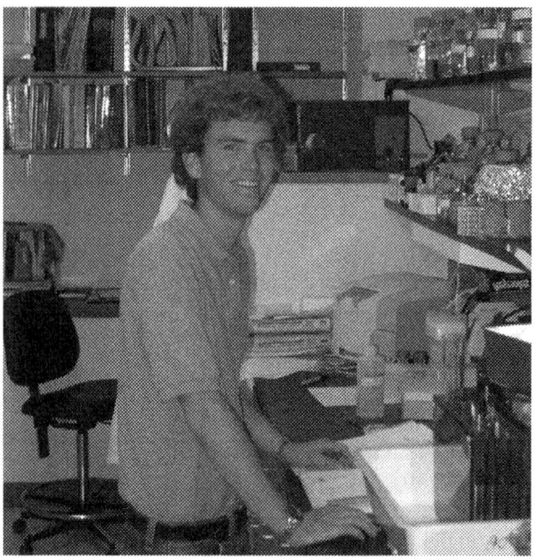

Rafe Petty

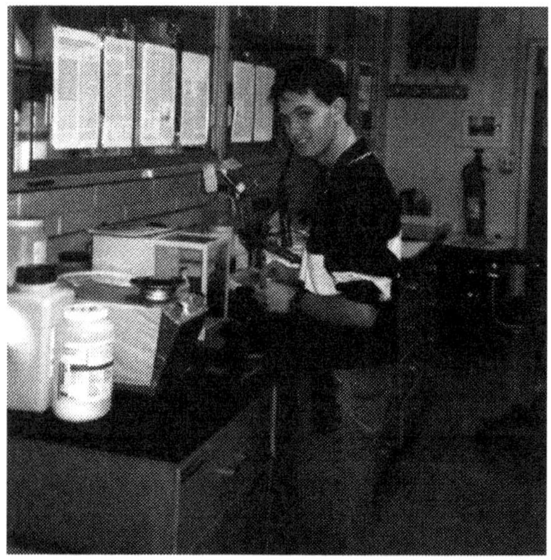

Eric Snyder

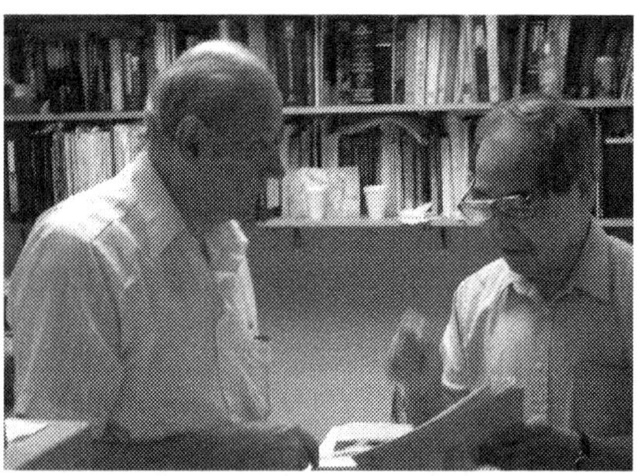

Ted Ueda emphasizing that glycolysis ensures maximal glutamate accumulation into presynaptic vesicles.

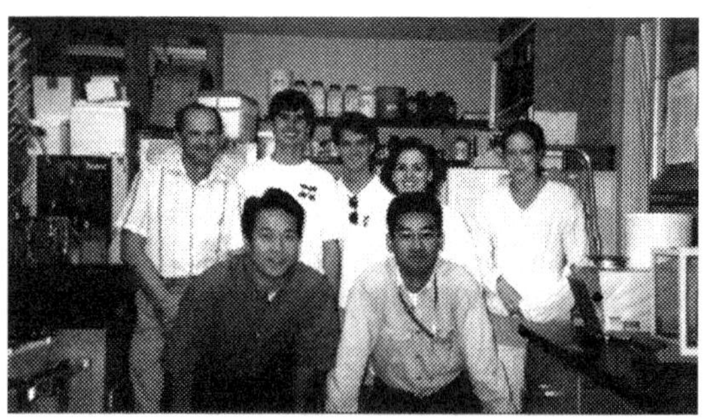

Front row: Kiyokazu Ogita, Koji Hirata
Back row: Alexander Margulis, Christopher Jones, Eric Snyder, Mary Kay Sisson, Chris Jones' friend

Dr. Wendell W. Weber's Research Interests

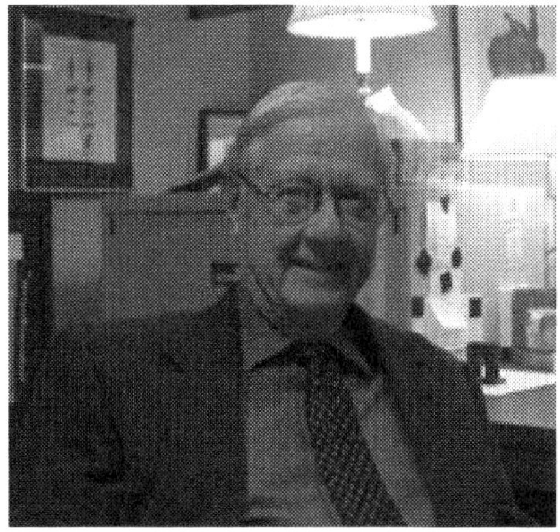

Dr. Weber's teaching and research has centered on the study of pharmacogenetic traits for nearly 4 decades. The main goal of his studies is to assess the variation of genetic susceptibility of human subjects to the dire effects of drugs, foods and other exogenous substances. Like other human genetic disorders, pharmacogenetic traits reveal themselves as molecular lesions in DNA that can be inferred from family inheritance patterns and detected by direct observation. With the maturation of the Human Genome Project, the analysis of genetic variation in human drug response on a grand scale, and the case for targeting and treating human disease through genomically-based, high-throughput research is rapidly gaining acceptance in today's world, and pharmacogenetics is moving from the basic laboratory to the clincal arena. By finding the genetic lesions that modify a person's response to drugs and other exogenous substances, risk profiles for individuals can be constructed to discriminate those who are susceptible to these traits from those who are not, and by linking these traits to their molecular basis, we expect to discover better therapies for human disease and improve prospects for individualized medicine. If medical treatment is guided by such profiles, physicians should be able to select the most appropriate drug treatment for particular patients, and greatly reduce, or avert therapeutic failure and drug toxicity.

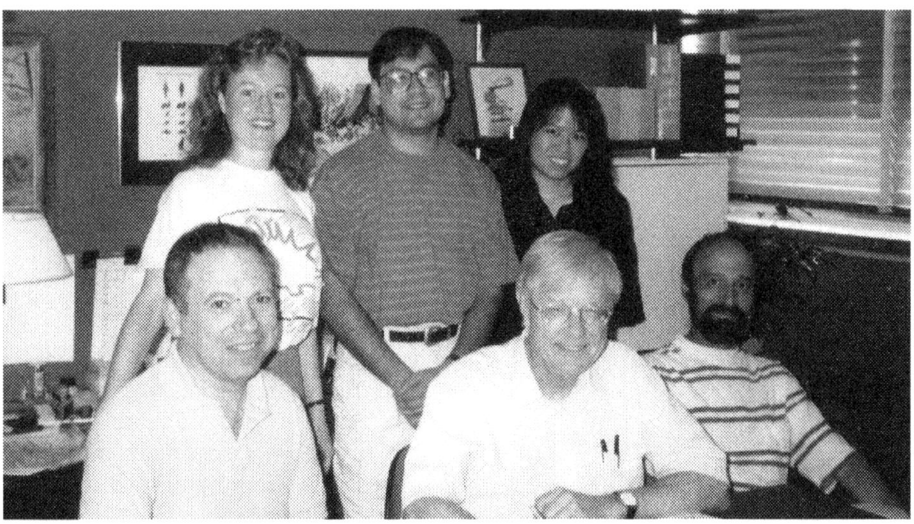

Front row: Jerry Levy, Wendell Weber, Gus Vatsis
Back row: Karen Martell, Jesse de Leon, Lily Hu

Dr. James H. Woods' Research Interests

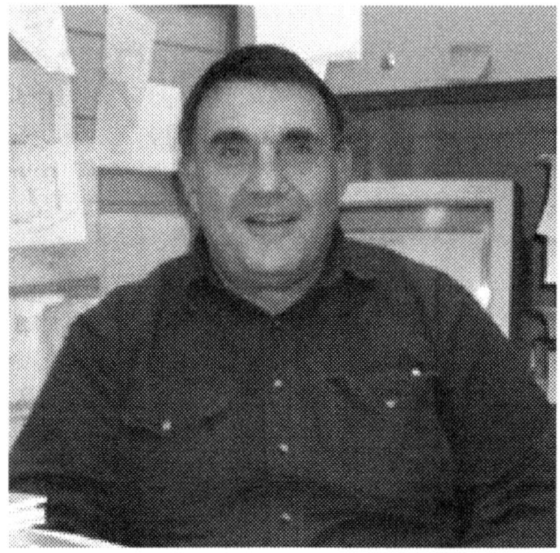

Jim Woods' fundamental research interest is in the interaction between drugs and their receptors, using in vivo procedures. He is particularly interested in the effects of drugs on behavior, and in the experimental study of drug abuse. He has a long history of research on the behavioral effects of opioid drugs and has characterized the effects of opioid agonists and antagonists on the three types of opioid receptors, mu, kappa, and delta, in behavioral studies in rats and rhesus monkeys.

A fourth opioid receptor, so called because of the homology that exists between this receptor and the other three opioid receptors, has recently been described. Although drugs that act as agonists at this receptor are not very promising when studied in rodents, Dr. Holden Mei-Chuan Ko, an assistant research scientist in Dr. Woods' laboratory, has found that these agonists may be very interesting analgesics in rhesus monkeys. An ORL1 agonist appears to produce analgesia in monkeys that is equal to that produced by morphine. This drug has not been shown to produce some of the side-effects that limit the use of morphine; it does not produce the itch sensation that most morphine-like drugs produce when they are given as spinal analgesics. With the help of Dr. William Fantegrossi, a postdoctoral student working with Dr. Winger, in the self-administration laboratory, Dr. Ko has found that an ORL1 agonist has limited reinforcing effects, suggesting that these drugs may not have the abuse potential that has been a major concern in the use of opioids as analgesics. Further work on the sedative, respiratory depressant, discriminative stimulus, and constipating effects of these agonists, plus evaluation of their analgesic effects in humans, are being planned.

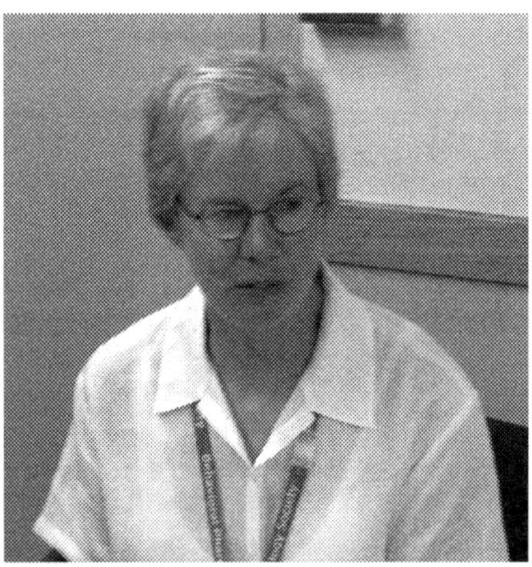

Dr. Gail Winger

Another example of the potential of novel opioid drugs for therapeutic use involves the study in the laboratory of the antidepressant effects of delta opioid agonists. Using a forced-swim assay in rats, Dan Broom, a former graduate student, and Emily Jutki, a current graduate student, determined that delta opioids are effective in this model of antidepressant drug action. Furthermore, these drugs may act much more quickly to relieve depression than do all of the currently available antidepressant drugs, a potentially important development. Mary Toregrossa, a graduate student in the neuroscience program, is finding positive effects in her study of the interaction of delta agonists on brain derived neurotropic factor (BDNF), a compound that has been shown to increase in the brain following administration of antidepressant drugs.

Opioid withdrawal is known to be stressful, and measuring withdrawal-induced increases in stress hormones initiated another research. There are a number of compounds that block the corticotrophin releasing hormone (CRH) receptors in the pituitary and/or in the brain. Work in that laboratory indicates that administration of these antagonists can modify levels of ACTH and corticosterone under a number of conditions of induced stress. The interaction between swim-induced stress and the parasympathetic nervous system is currently being evaluated by Susan Wood, a pharmacology graduate student.

Dr. Woods is a close collaborator with Dr. Winger in her research on the reinforcing effects of drugs in rhesus monkeys. They are developing behavioral economic procedures to help measure difference in the reinforcing effects of a variety of drugs of abuse, and determining whether combinations of drugs are better reinforcers than either drug alone. Dr. Chad Galuska, a new postdoctoral student, is heavily involved in this behavioral economic research. The self-administration laboratory has other questions of interest. Dr. William Fantegrossi, a former graduate student in psychology and a current postdoctoral student,

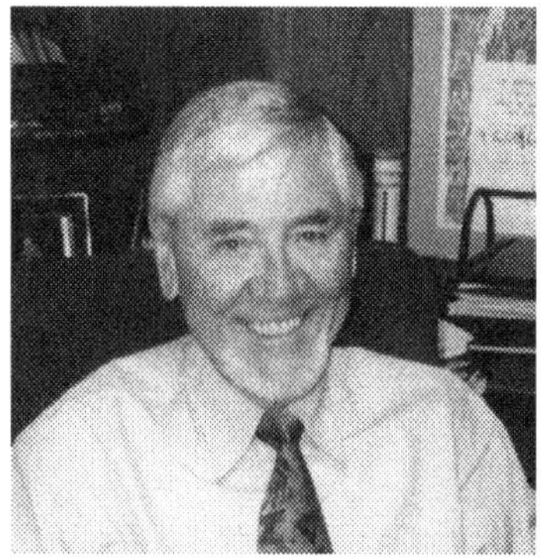

Dr. Bob Schuster

has evaluated the reinforcing effects of MDMA (Ecstasy) and its isomers in these monkeys and found that this drug looses its ability to maintain behavior over a period of several months of access. The possibility that this is a neurotoxin response to MDMA is currently under evaluation. Graham Flory, a psychology graduate student, is also involved in studies of the reinforcing effects of intravenous ethanol in rhesus monkeys that were raised under different conditions at the NIH. The possibility that these animals differ both in their reactivity

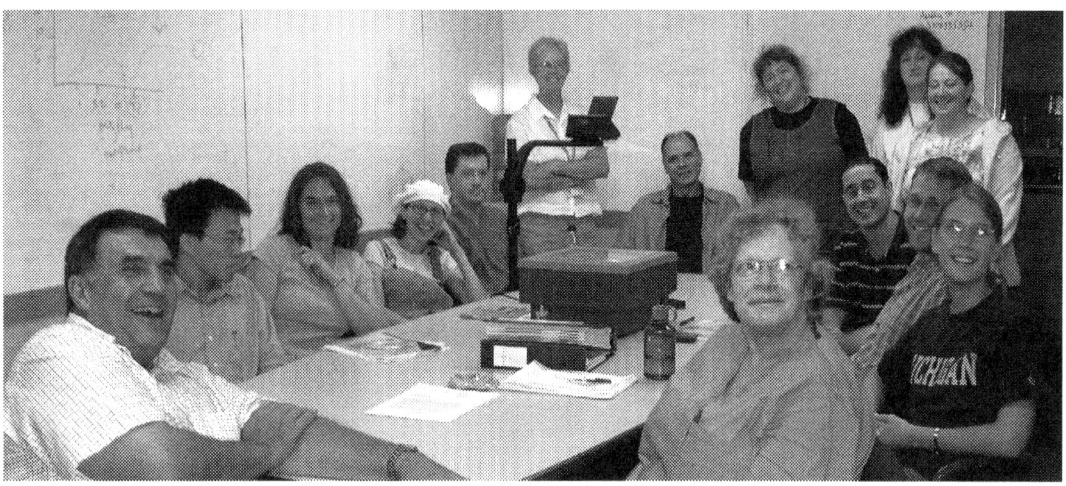

Around the table: J. Woods, M. C. Ko, Mary Torregrossa, Ziva Cooper, Graham Flory, Gail Winger, Al Bertalmio, Rebecca Mc Laughlin, Debbie Huntzinger, Kathy Chadman, Chad Galuska, Greg Collins, Susan Wood, Edie Frost

to stress and in their response to alcohol as a reinforcer is the primary question of Graham's Ph.D. thesis.

The NIDA X Center grant that has been funded for the previous 30 years is currently focusing on a new area of research, that of PET imaging of the various opioid receptors. This project requires a team of experts, and such a team had been assembled in the center grant. Dr. Steve Husbands at the University of Bath in England is a medicinal chemist who will be synthesizing potential PET ligands – agonists or antagonists at the mu, kappa, and delta opioid receptors. These will be evaluated initially in the laboratory of Dr. John Traynor in the Pharmacology Department here. Dr. Traynor will evaluate Dr. Husbands' chemicals and determine their specificity at the three receptors and whether they are primarily agonists or antagonists at these receptors. The most promising of the synthetic drugs will be given to Dr. Michael Kilbourn in the Department of Radiology at the University of Michigan and he will take on the task of radiolabeling these interesting compounds. Dr. Kilbourn has worked with Dr. Jon-Kar Zubieta in the Psychiatry Department using labeled carfentanil, a very potent mu opioid binding in humans.

Dr. C.R. Schuster and Dr Chris-Ellyn Johanson, in collaboration with Dr. Mark Greenwald, all from Wayne State University, have participated in Center Grant activities over the years. They have a human drug abuse research facility in Detroit and have studied the effects of buprenorphine and methadone in their heroin-abusing research subjects. Their contributions to the Center at the present time include evaluation of the binding potential of these treatment agents using labeled carfentanil and PET imaging. The general aim of the Center, that of understanding more of the behavioral and pharmacological mechanism of opioid drug action so that better treatment agents can be developed, and current treatment agents better understood is particularly well supported by these clinical investigators.

Dr. Charles (Bob) R. Schuster is currently Professor of Psychiatry and Behavioral Neurosciences at Wayne State University, and Adjunct Professor of Psychiatry at the University of Michigan. He is a former staff member of our Department from 1962-1968. As Director of the Addiction Research Institute at Wayne State University he provides the mechanism for the Clinical/Human transfer of basic animal research.

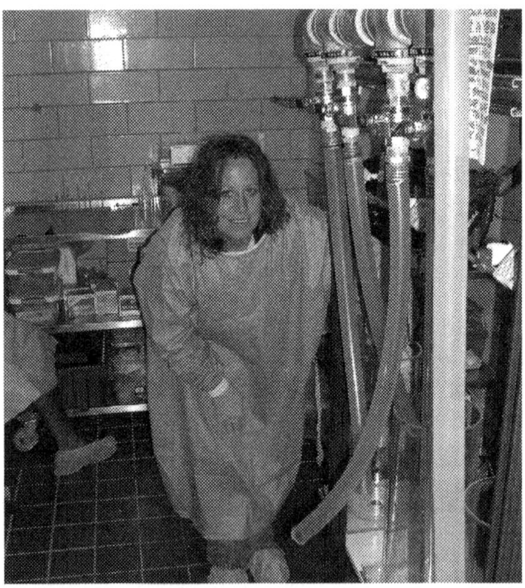

Penny Bruce working on the rat antidepressant assay

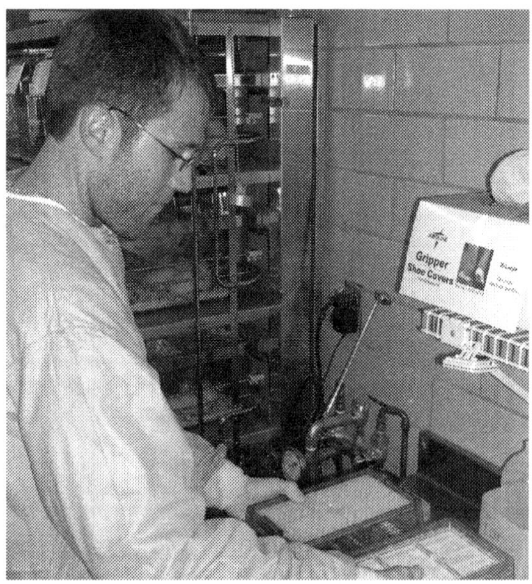

Greg Collins

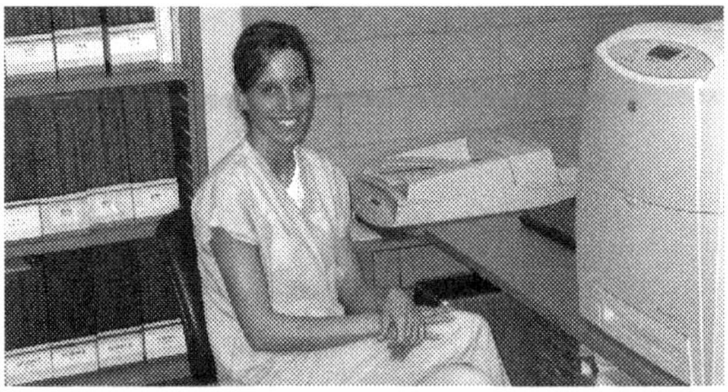

Julie Pirozzo

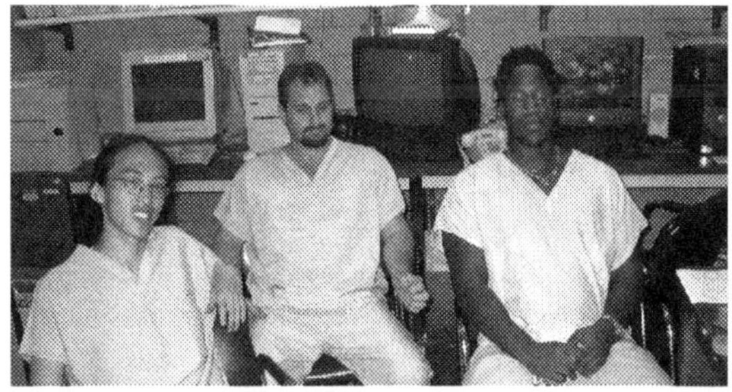

Wayne Yang, John Busenbark, Tristan Edwards

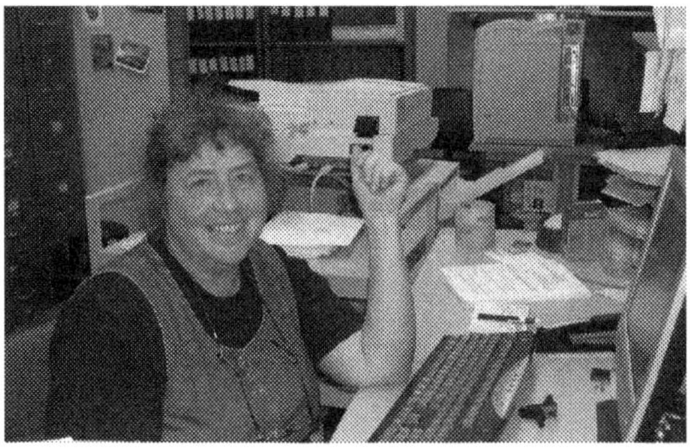

Beck— Smiling as usual

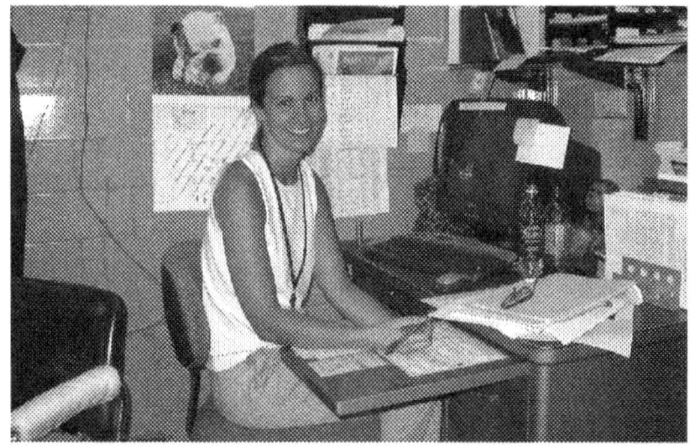

Tiffany Bass

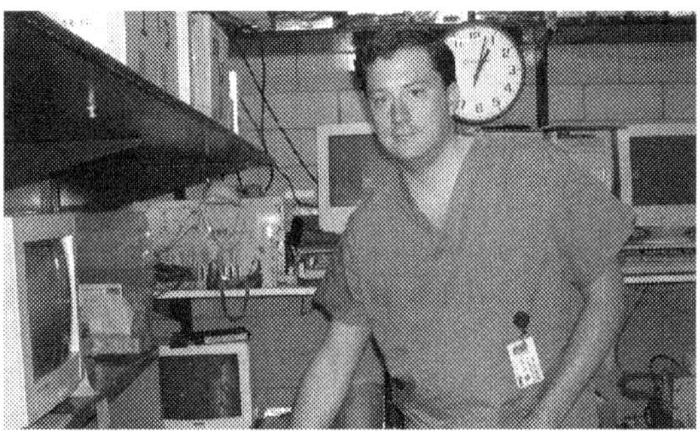

Graham Flory, a graduate student in Psychology

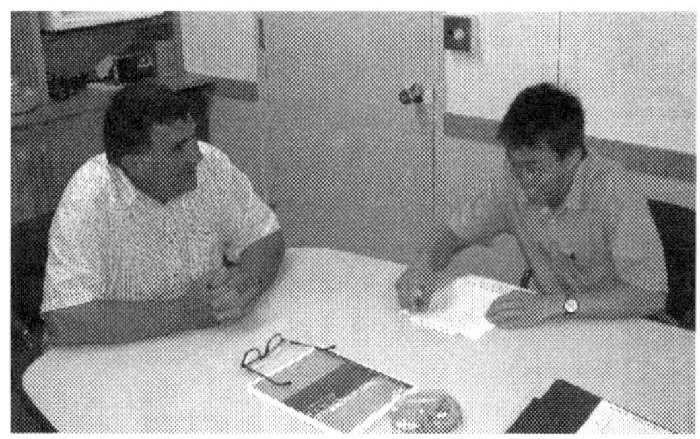

Dr. Woods in conversation with M.C. (Holden) Ko

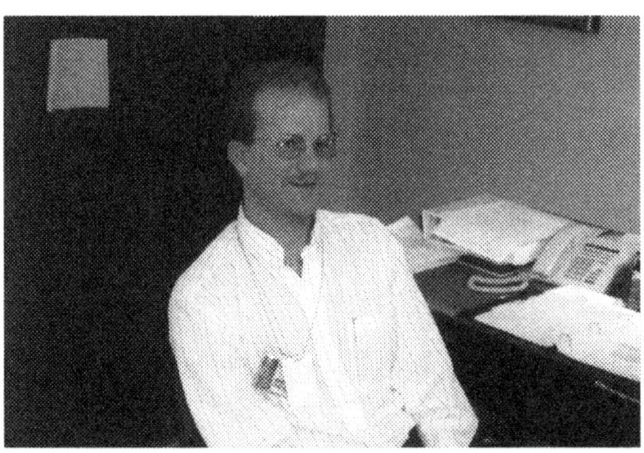

Dr. Mark Greenwald, WSU

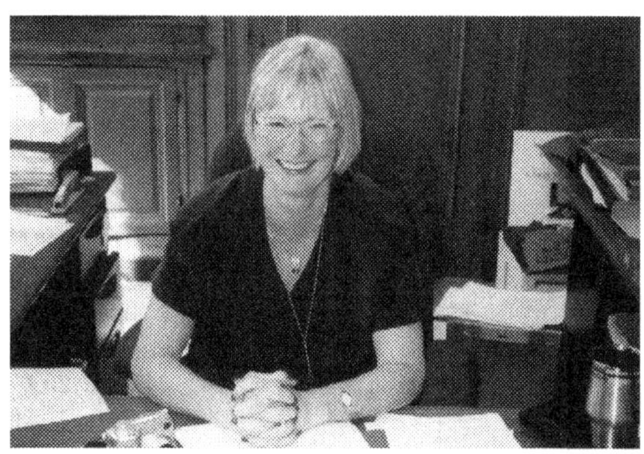

Dr. Chris - Ellyn Johansen, WSU

Dr. Vincent G. Zannoni's Research Interests

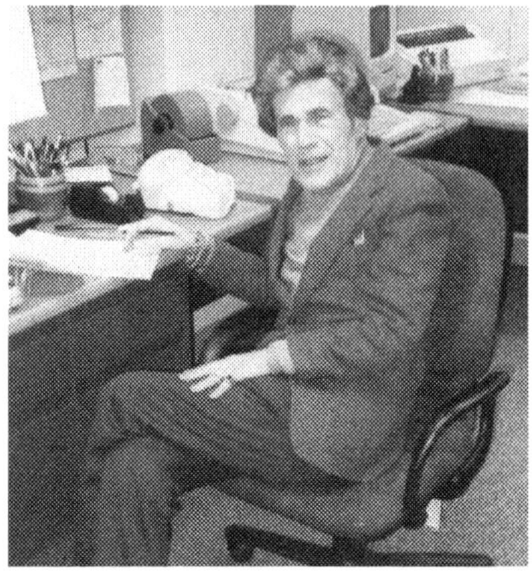

Dr. Zannoni's major research interests include the area of biochemical pharmacology; in particular, mechanisms involved in the mixed function oxygenase system responsible for the metabolism of a vast number of xenobiotics and environmental contaminants. In vitro and in vivo experiments include an integrated enzymological, pharmacodynamic and toxicological approach to investigate and evaluate the underlying environmental, genetic, nutritional and physiological factors responsible for the ultimate detoxification of pharmacological agents and environmental chemicals.

A native of New York City, Dr. Zannoni earned his B.S. degree in 1951 at the College of the City of New York, and his M.S. and Ph.D. degrees, in 1956 and 1959, respectively, at George Washington University. From 1954-63, he conducted research at the National Institutes of Health, and in 1963, he joined the faculty of New York University Medical School in the pharmacology department. He joined the faculty of the University of Michigan in 1974 as a professor of pharmacology.

While working at the NIH, Dr. Zannoni made several major contributions in the analysis of the hereditary enzymatic deficiencies underlying the metabolic disorders of phenylketonuria, alcaptonuria, and histidinemia. He also discovered a new polyphenol oxidase which seems to be involved in the formation and deposition of an abnormal pigment in the connective tissues of alcaptonuric patients. Dr. Zannoni's later research, which was internationally recognized, focused on the role of vitamin C in drug metabolism. He developed a chemical method which is still the best available to measure the content of vitamin C in biological tissues, and his group showed how this vitamin is involved in the metabolism of alcohol (ethanol) in man. He has conducted important investigations on the protective effects of vitamin C against the types of cancer produced by environmental chemicals and their relationship to mechanisms of drug metabolism.

In the Department of Pharmacology, Dr. Zannoni spent many years directing the graduate program in pharmacology. He was recognized as an excellent teacher, whose lectures were known for their clarity, superb organization, and humor. Dr. Zannoni has always taken great pride in the development and accomplishments of his students, many of whom are now conducting research in the pharmaceutical industry and in academia. Dr. Zannoni enjoys an international reputation as a productive scientist, a devoted and caring teacher, and a distinguished editor of Drug Metabolism & Disposition from 1983 to 1993, who has brought credit to the Department of Pharmacology and the University of Michigan.

The Regents saluted this distinguished educator and noted scientist by naming Vincent G. Zannoni professor emeritus of pharmacology in 1994.

Administrative Staff

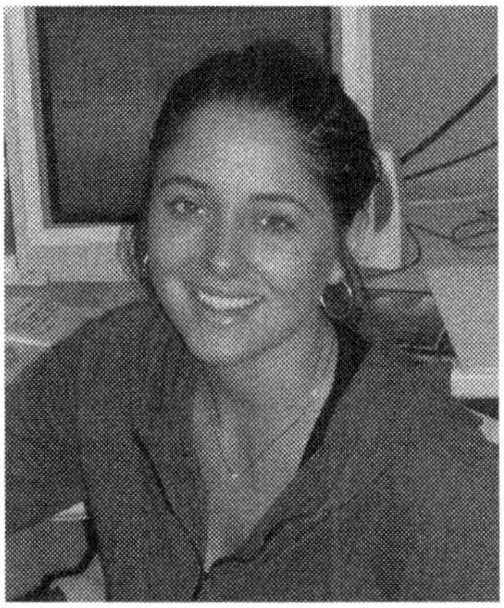
Rebecca Earwood

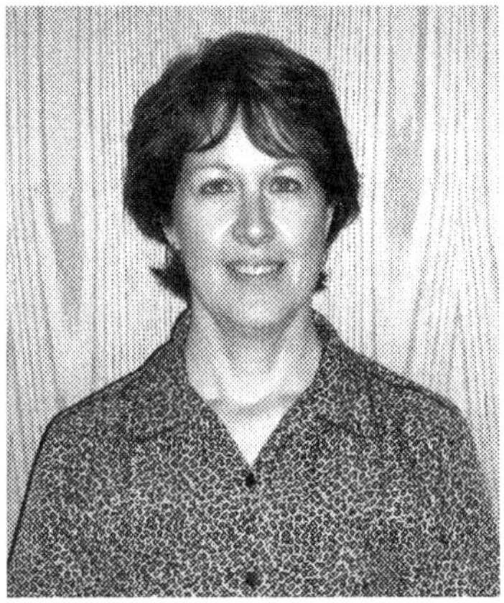
Eileen Ferguson

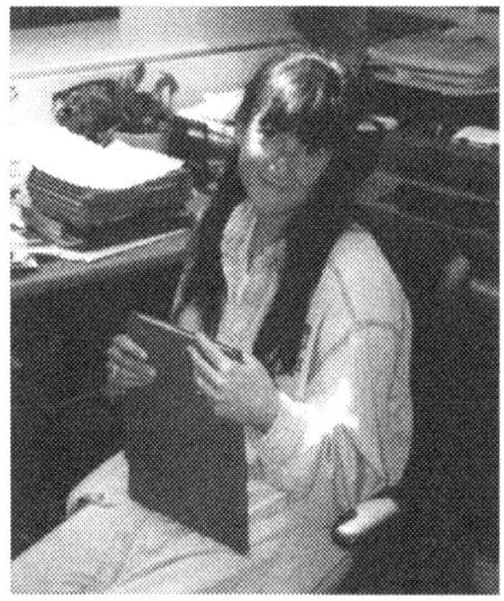
Denise

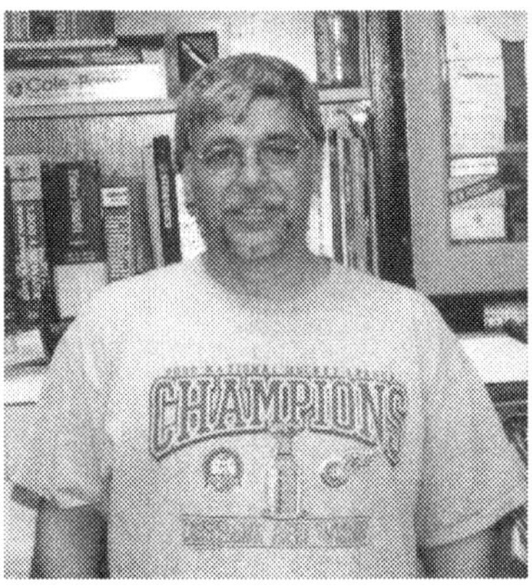

Tom Larmee

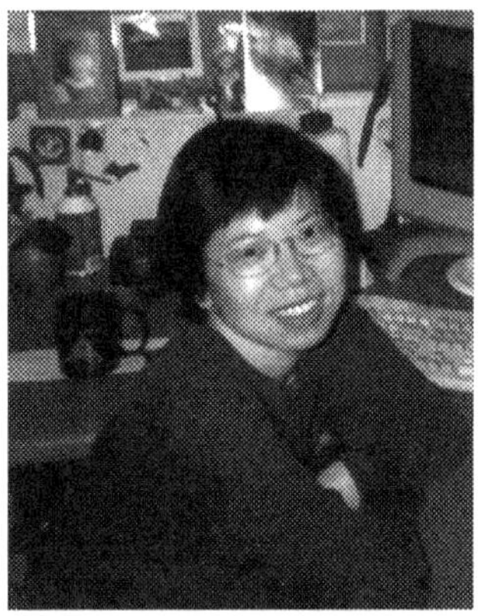
Dar-Wei Liao

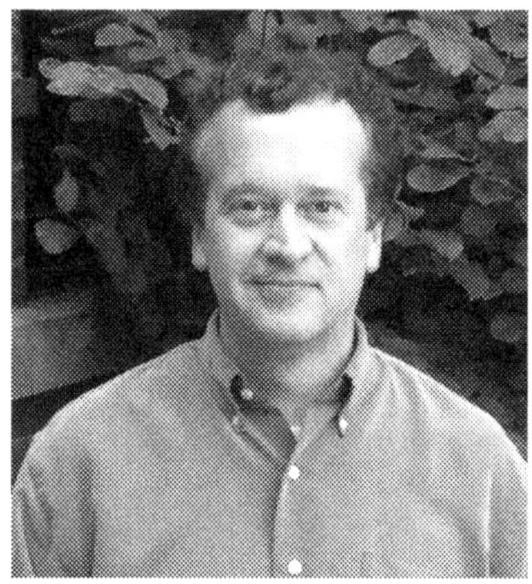
Dennis Ondreyka

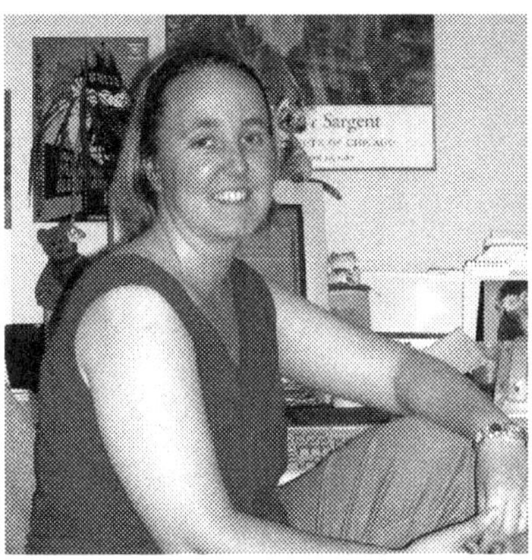

Anna Taylor

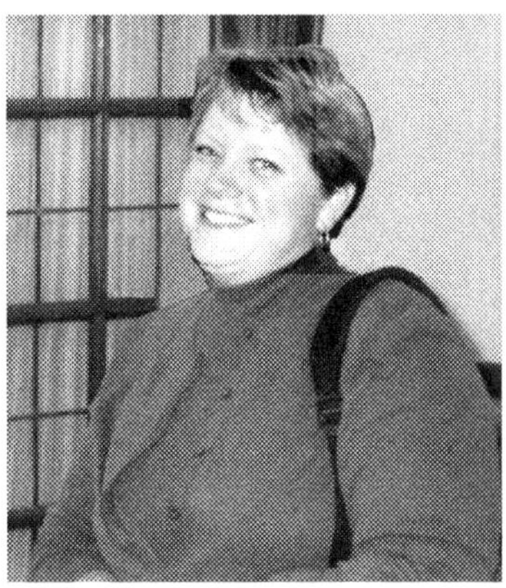
Ms. Ward

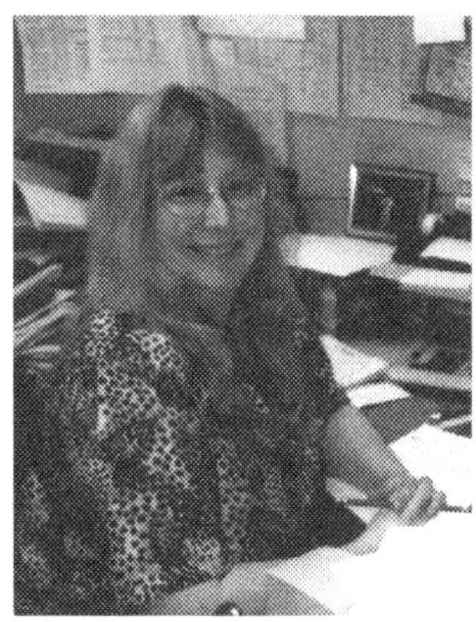
Paula Wilks

Shop Staff

Two important staff persons who have been in the Department for many years are Tom Larmee and Jim Ferguson. Tom is responsible to the Department chair Dr. Hollenberg and Jim to Dr. Woods on the Center Grant. Both Tom and Jim frequently work together on Center projects. If you need shop help call Tom first and get in line.

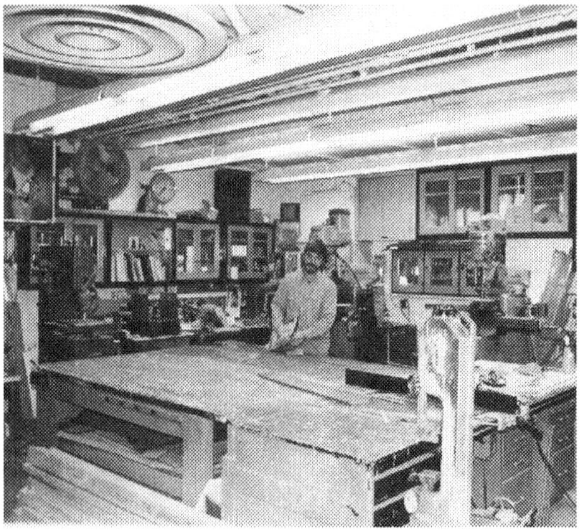

An organized shop, a long time ago

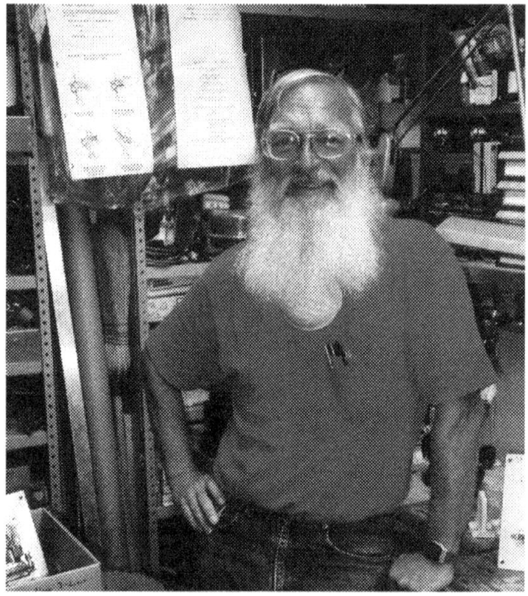

Jim Ferguson in his closet sized shop

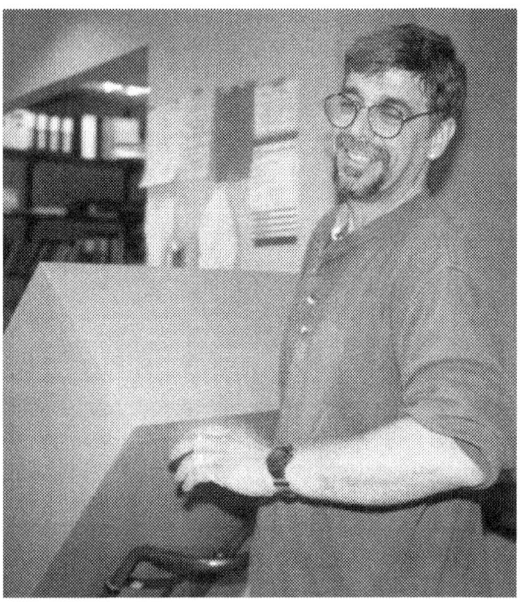

Tom Larmee hauling a repaired cabinet

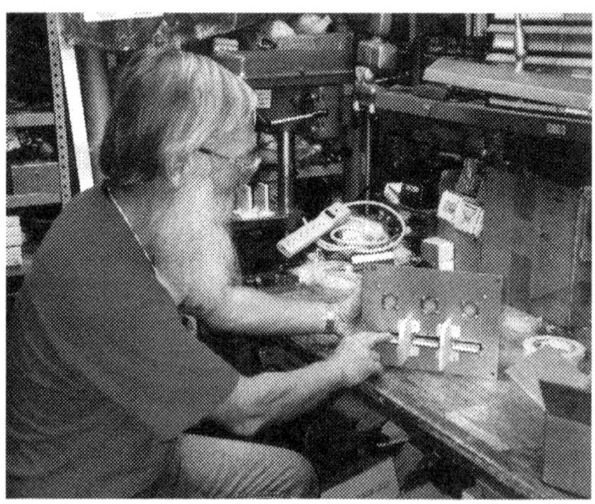

Jim's latest operant lever design

Recent Events

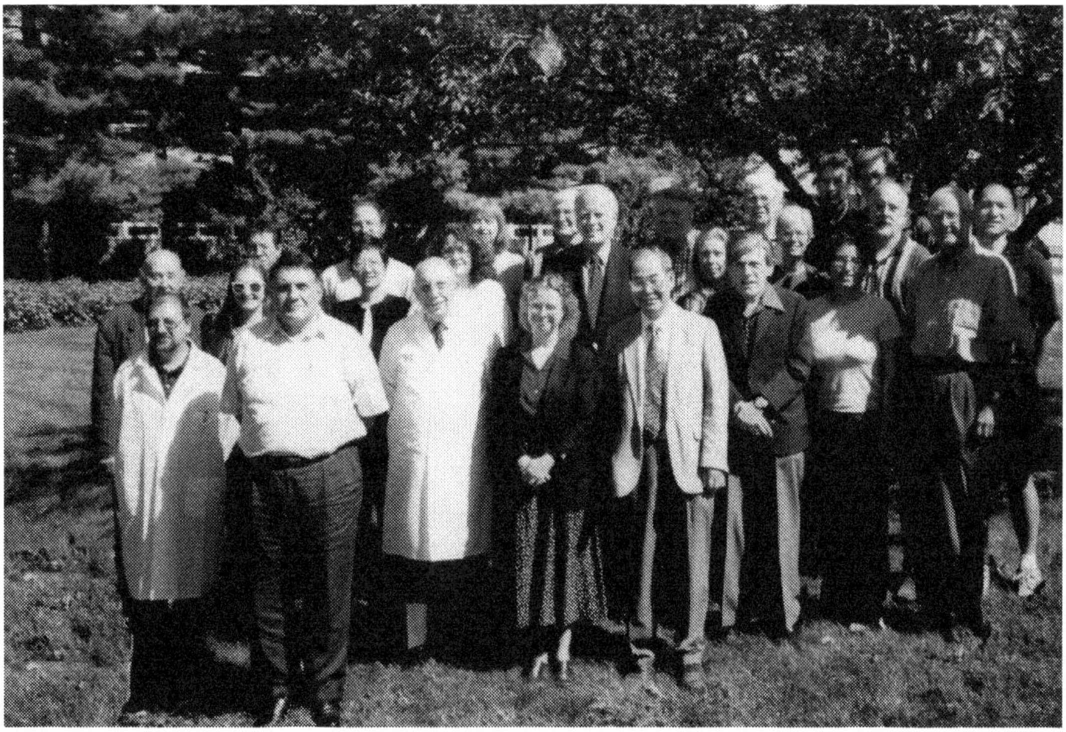

The Department faculty 2003

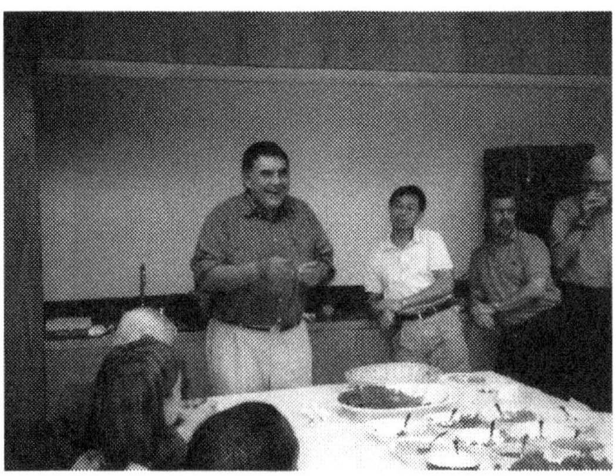

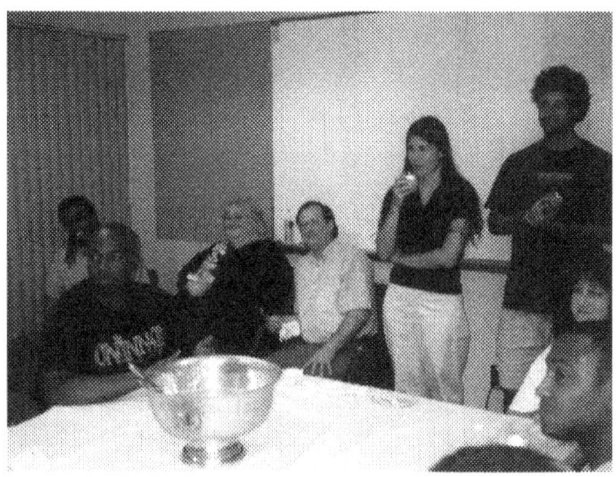

Celebrating Kathy Chadman's thesis defense

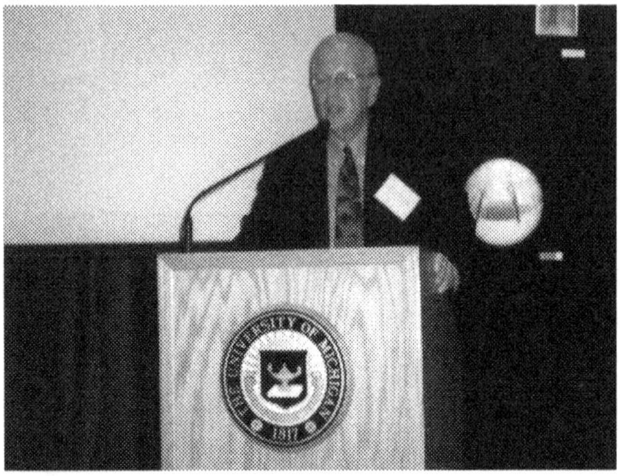

Dr. Hollenberg introducing

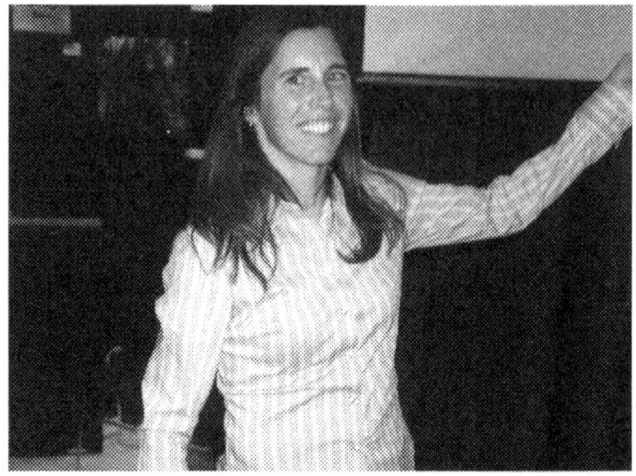

Dr. Joan Taylor speaking

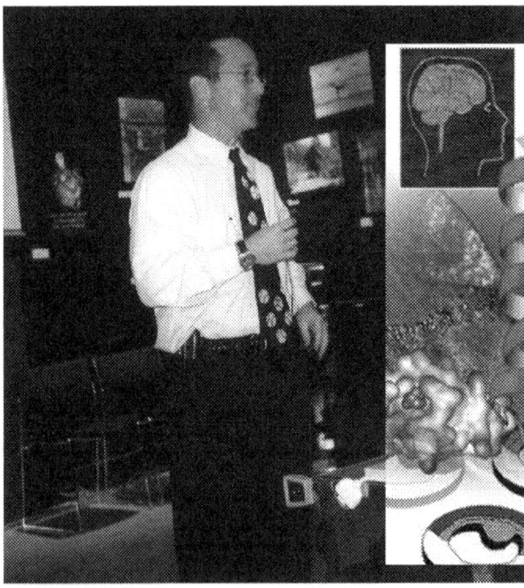

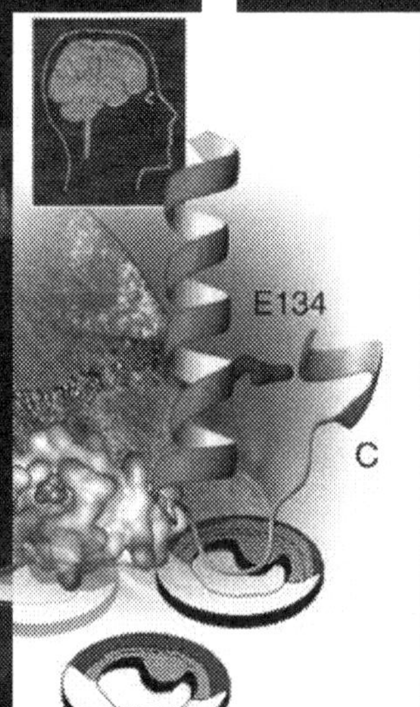

Dr. Peter Fischbach speaking

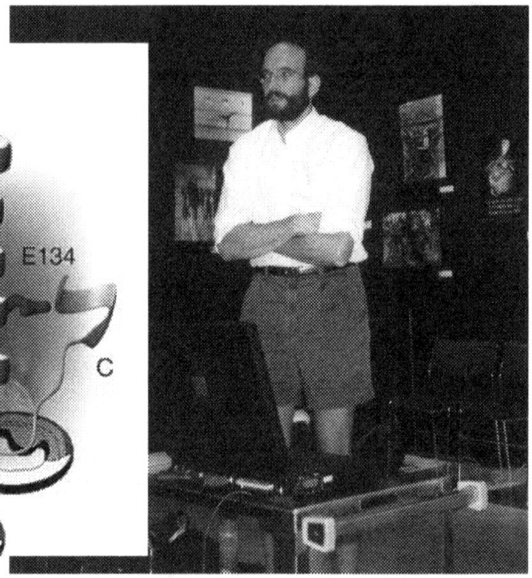

Dr. Jorge Iñiguez speaking

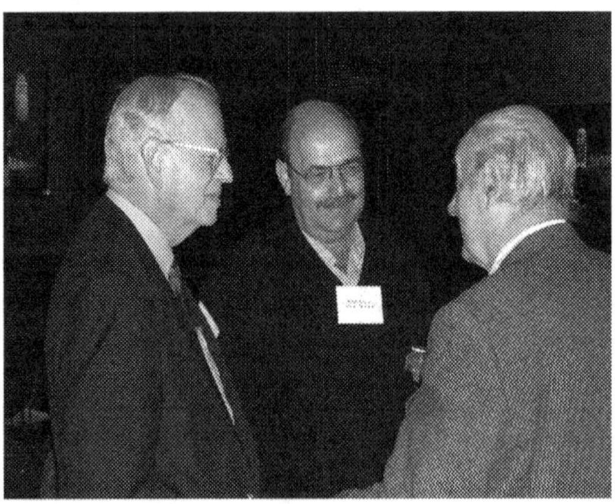

Paul, Harvey, and Ed talking

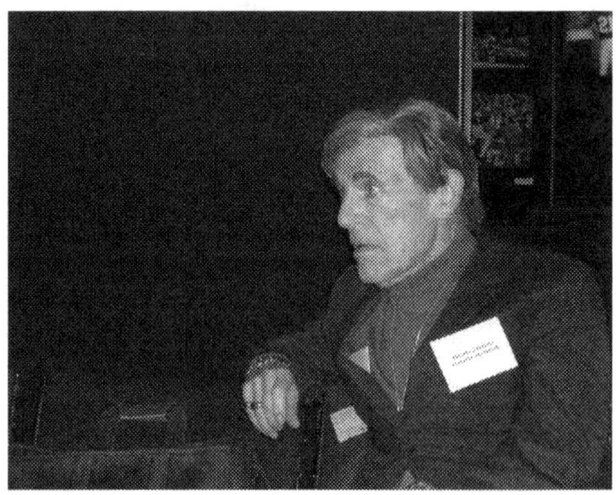

Dr. Vince Zannoni listening

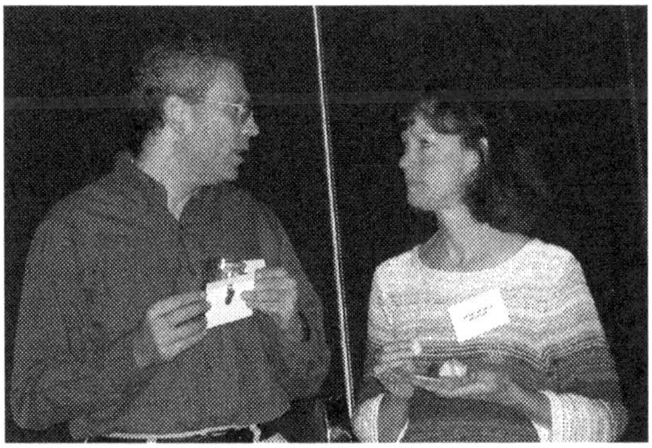

Jonathon and Donna

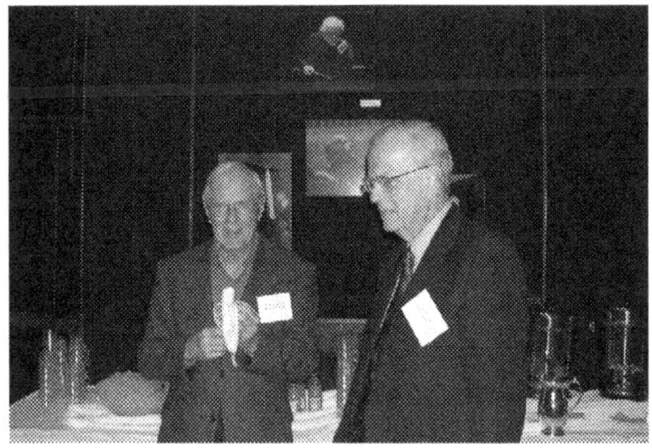

Wendell and Paul

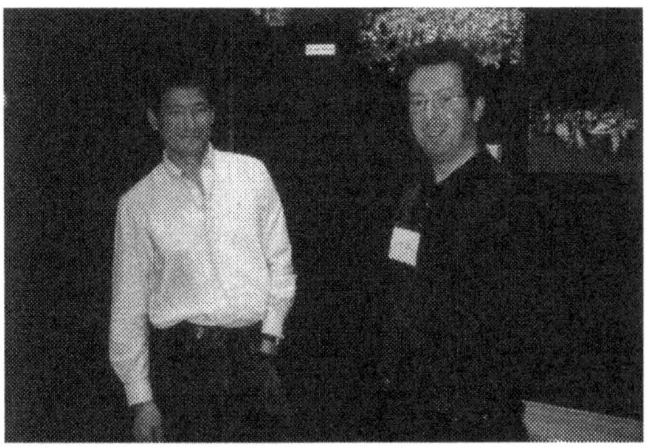

Roger and José

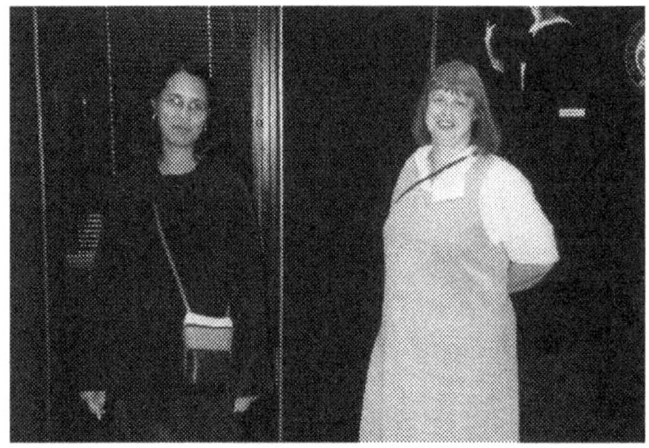

Helen and Mary

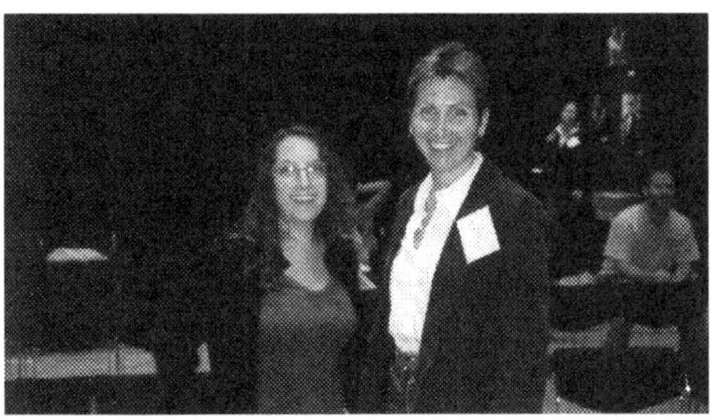

Emily and Sue

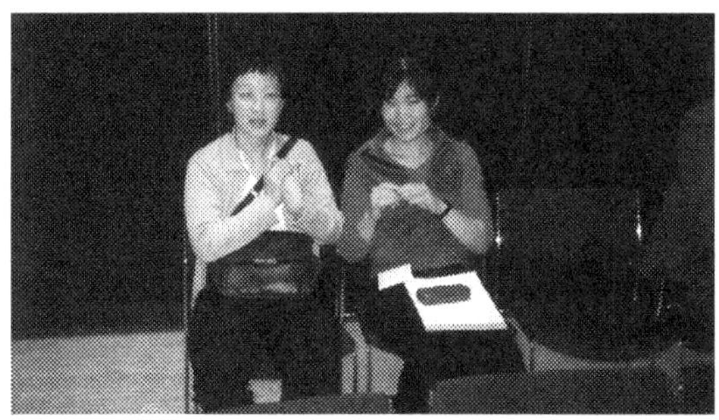

Lei and Ying

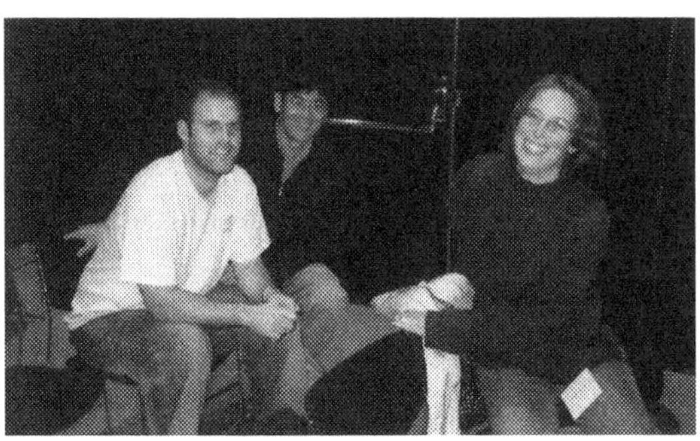

Andy, Jinbao and Erin

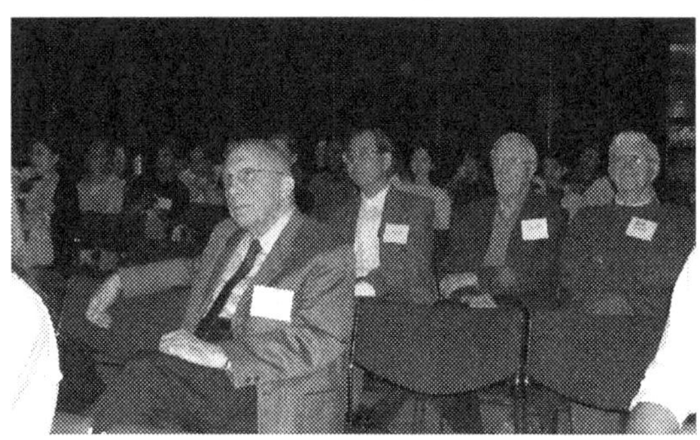

Ben, Ted, Wendell and Burt

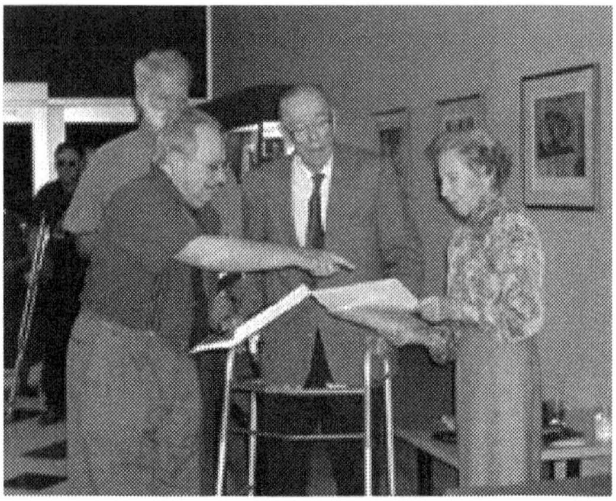

Billy Martin, Lou Harris, Lauren and Carol Woods

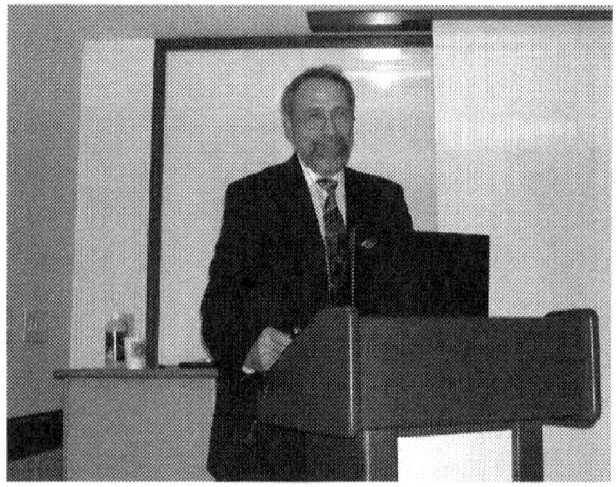

Lindsay Hough

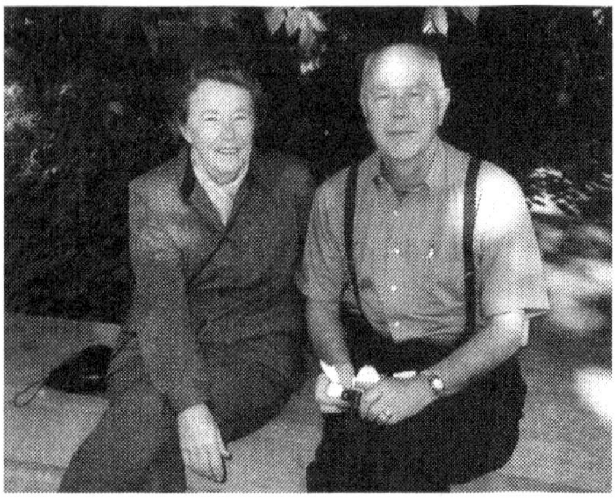

Margaret and Reese Jones

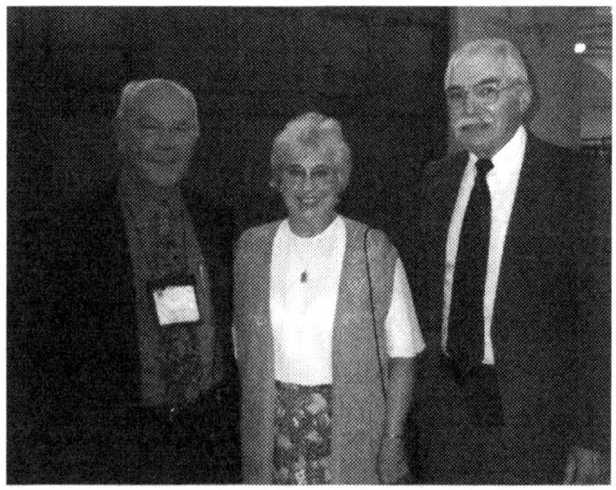

Reese with the Bairds

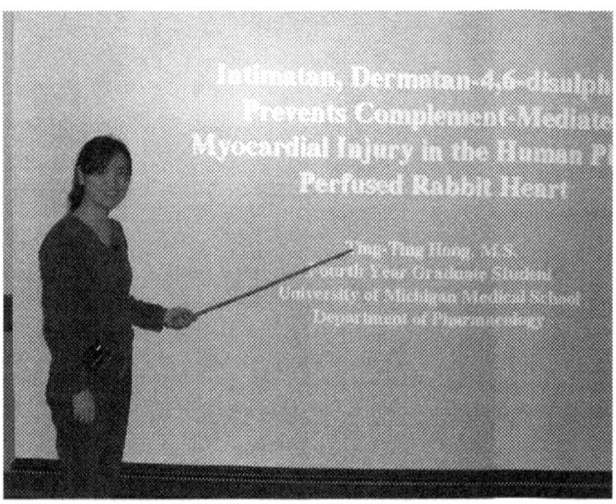

Ting Ting speaking

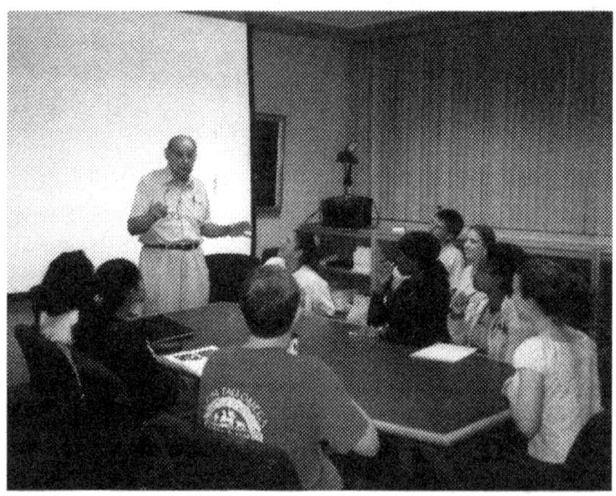

Ed lecturing

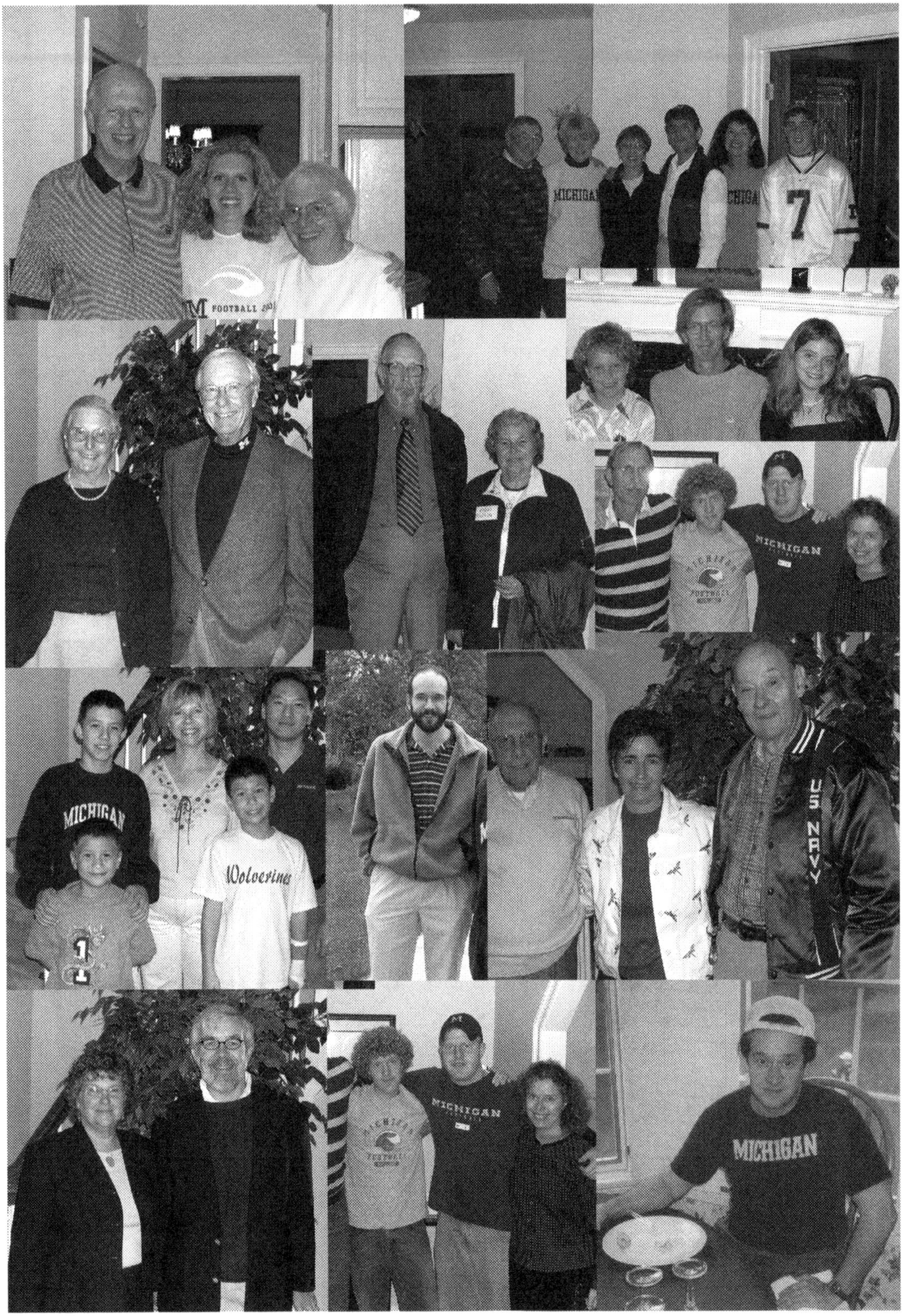
MICHIGAN
Wolverines
US NAVY
MICHIGAN

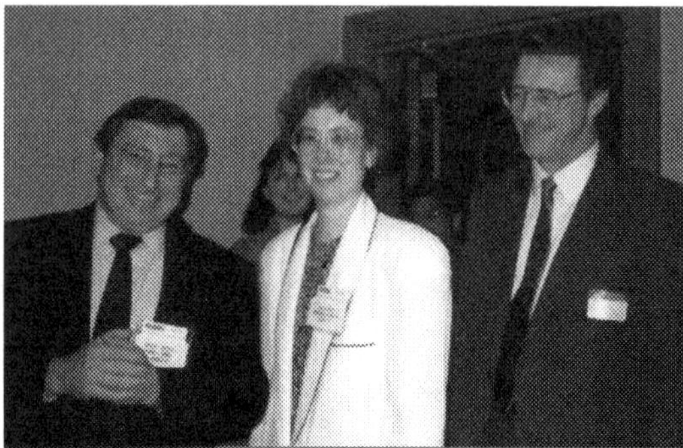

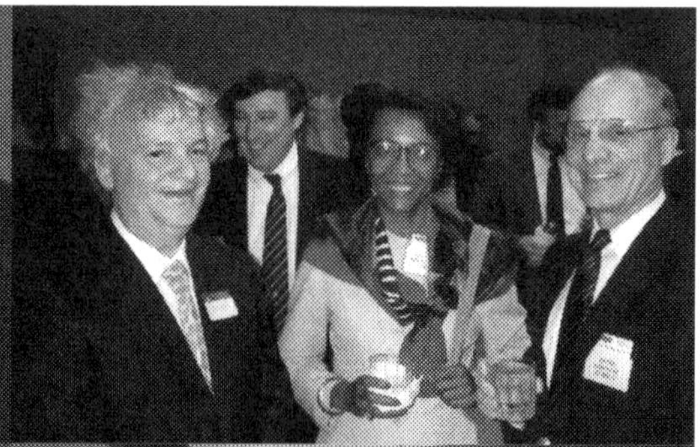

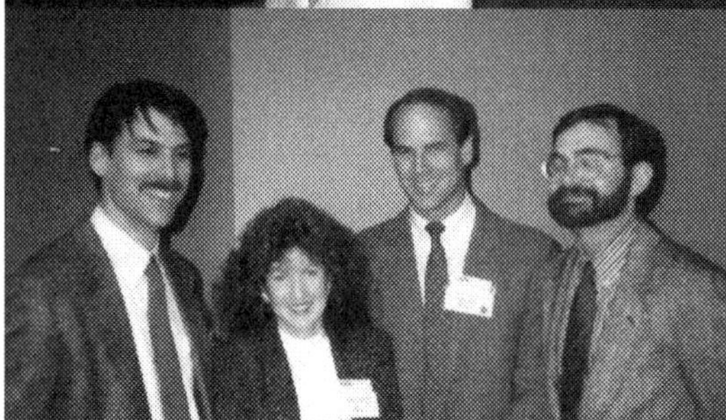

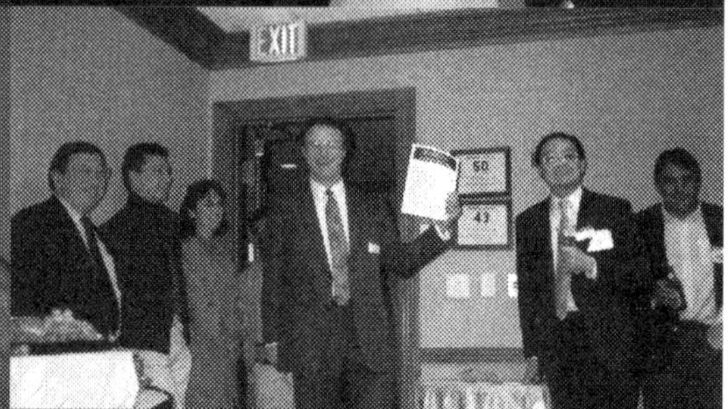
EXIT

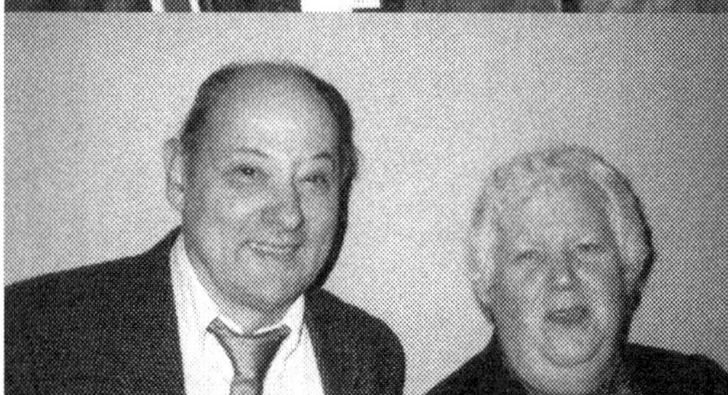

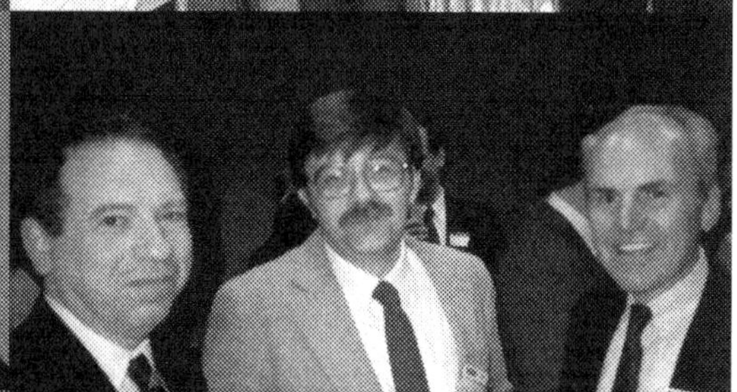

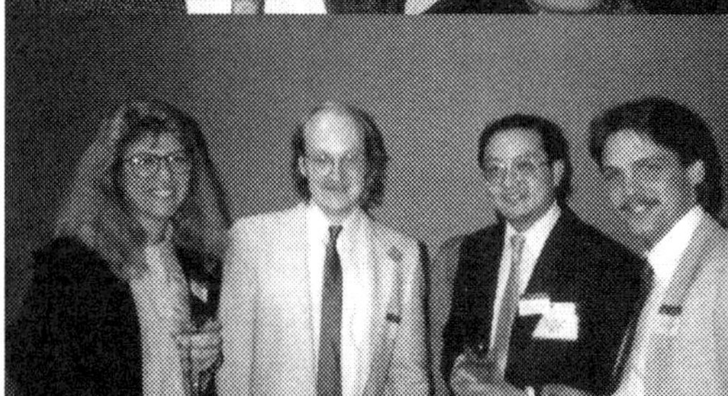

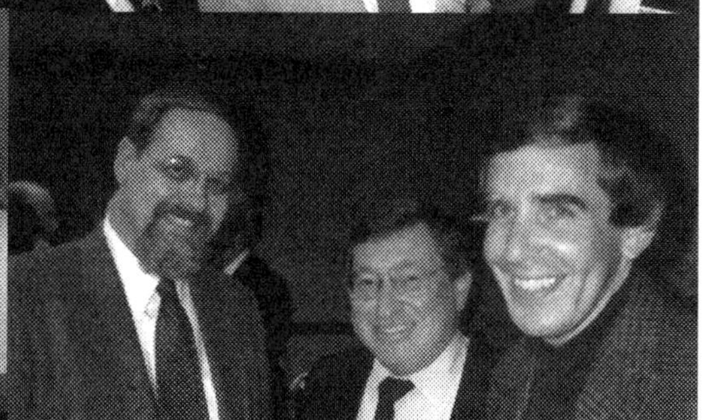

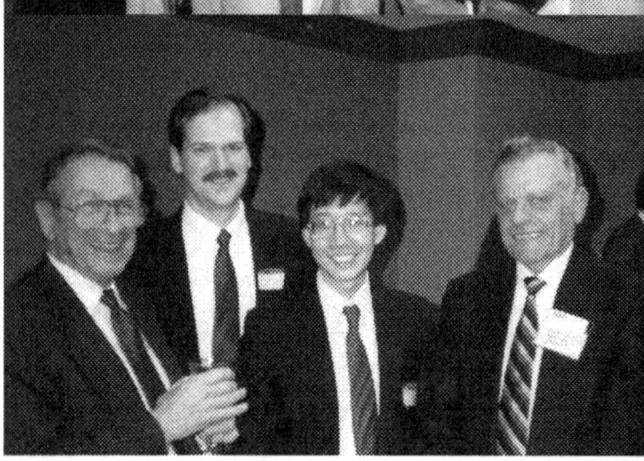

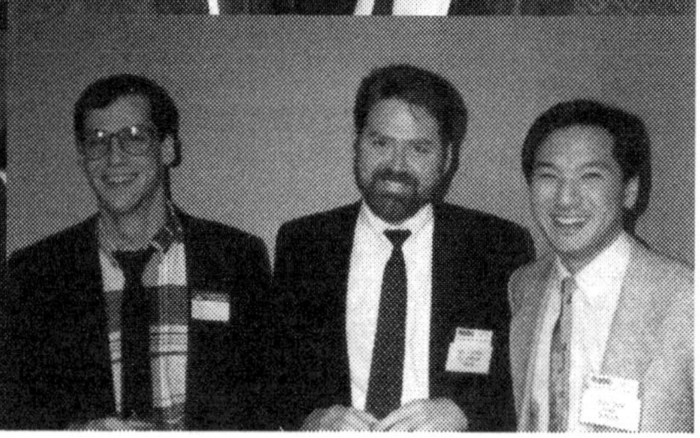

23

Outstanding Alumni Awards, 1989-2003

This award is presented annually to a former graduate of the Department to recognize those who have made outstanding contributions to pharmacology in research, teaching and service. The award consists of a small honorarium and a plaque, which is presented at a seminar given by the recipient.

1989
Dr. Harold F. Hardman

Dr. Harold F. Hardman was selected as the first recipient of the Department's Outstanding Alumnus Award. Dr. Hardman had an exemplary career as a teacher, researcher and administrator. He received his doctorate in 1954. During the next four years, he served as a part-time instructor in the department while he pursued his M.D. degree. In 1958, he was appointed assistant professor of Pharmacology in the department. Dr. Hardman then rose through the academic ranks at an accelerated pace. In 1960, he accepted the position of associate professor in Pharmacology at Marquette University School of Medicine and in 1962 he was appointed full professor and chairman of the department - a position he held until 1987.

1990
Dr. Paula Stern

Dr. Paula Stern was awarded the Outstanding Alumna Award in 1990. Under Dr. Ted Brody, Dr. Stern earned her Ph.D. in 1963. In 1966, she became an assistant professor at Northwestern University, and was promoted to professor in 1977. She is best known for her work with Vitamin D and the mechanisms used by drugs to affect bone and calcium metabolism. Dr. Stern was recognized for her contributions to both research and teaching, as well as for her outstanding leadership in several professional societies.

1992
Dr. Ken Moore

In recognition of his numerous contributions to pharmacology, Dr. Ken Moore was named the third recipient of the Department's Outstanding Alumnus Award for 1992. On October 2, 1992, Dr. Moore presented a seminar to the department, after which he was given a plaque to mark the occasion. The title of his seminar was "A Neuropharmacologist's Journey: The Road Less Traveled By." Dr. Moore received his Ph.D. in 1961 under the supervision of Professor Ted Brody. After several years in the Department of Pharmacology at Dartmouth College, he joined the faculty at Michigan State University in 1966. Since 1986, he has been professor and chair of the Michigan State University Department of Pharmacology and Toxicology.

1993
Dr. Raymond W. Ruddon

Raymond W. Ruddon was selected by the Alumni Steering Committee as the 1993 Outstanding Alumnus Award recipient. On October 1, 1993, he became the fourth recipient to be honored and was presented a plaque to commemorate the occasion. Dr. Ruddon received his Ph.D. in Pharmacology in 1964 under the mentorship of Lawrence B. Mellett. Three years later, in 1967, he received his M.D. again from The University of Michigan. After serving as chair of the Department of Pharmacology at The University of Michigan from

1981 to 1990, Dr. Ruddon was appointed the director of the Eppley Institute for Research in Cancer and Allied Diseases at the University of Nebraska Medical Center. The title of his seminar was "Protein Folding at Michigan and Nebraska."

1994
Dr. John S. Lazo

In recognition of his many achievements in the field of Pharmacology, John S. Lazo was selected as the 1994 Outstanding Alumnus Award recipient. In September 1994, he presented a seminar entitled, "Anticancer Drug Resistance and Apoptosis," or "Death and Differentiation After Michigan" to the department and received a plaque to commemorate this occasion. John received his Ph.D. in Pharmacology in 1976 and was a student of Ray Ruddon, the previous year's recipient. Dr. Lazo has served as the chair of Pharmacology in the School of Medicine at the University of Pittsburgh.

1995
Dr. Lora Rikans

The recipient of the Oustanding Alumna Award for 1995 was Dr. Lora Rikans (now deceased). Dr. Rikans earned her Ph.D. under the mentorship of Dr. Ray Ruddon in 1975, and in 1995 was Professor of Pharmacology at the University of Oklahoma Health Science Center. In October of 1995, she presented a seminar and was given a plaque in honor of the occasion. The seminar was entitled, "Aging and Hepatotoxicity, an Oral History."

1996
Dr. John McNeill

The recipient of the 1996 Outstanding Alumnus Award was John McNeill, Professor and Dean of the Faculty of Phamaceutical Sciences at the University of British Columbia. On September 27, 1996, John presented a seminar entitled "Phosphorylase, Receptors, Cardiomyopathy and Vanadium: Thirty Years of Pharmacology." John received his Ph.D. in 1967 under the mentorship of Ted Brody and was recognized for his many contributions to the field with a commemorative plaque for the occasion.

1997
Dr. Gerard Gebber

The recipient of the 1997 Outstanding Alumnus Award was Gerard Gebber, a professor in the Department of Pharmacology and Toxicology at Michigan State University. Dr. Gebber presented a lecture entitled "The Limits of Reductionism in Neuroscience: A Not So Random Walk Through Sympathetic Nerve Discharge" to the students and faculty. Gerry received his Ph.D. in 1964 under the mentorship of Lloyd Beck and was recognized for his many teaching and research contributions.

1998
Dr. Michael Vasko

The recipient of the 1998 Outstanding Alumnus Award was Michael Vasko, Professor in the Department of Pharmacology and Toxicology at Indiana University. Dr. Vasko presented a lecture entitled, "Eicosanoid-Mediated Sensitization of Sensory Neurons: How to Make it Hurt, Even More" to the students and faculty. Mike received his Ph.D. in 1977 under the mentorship of Ed Domino and was recognized for his many teaching and research contributions by the department.

1999
Dr. Stephen Holtzman

Dr. Stephen Holtzman was honored with the 1999 Outstanding Alumnus Award with his lecture "Acute Opioid Dependence." He entered our graduate program in July 1965 and received his Ph.D. in four years with Dr. Julian Villarreal as mentor. He devoted his studies to behavioral pharmacology. Dr. Holtzman was the recipient of Research Scientist Development, Research Scientist, and Senior Scientist Awards from National Institute on Drug Abuse (NIDA) from September 1, 1975 until August 31, 2005. From August 1, 1988 to June 30, 1998, he received the MERIT award for the NIDA Grant DA00541. In July 1997 Dr. Holtzman was also Honorary Professor from the Ningbo Drug Withdrawal Research Center in Ningbo, China. Now Dr. Holtzman is professor in Pharmacology at the Emory University School of Medicine.

2000
Dr. Jay I. Goodman

The Outstanding Alumnus Award for 2000 was presented to Dr. Jay I. Goodman on October 13, 2000. Dr. Goodman earned his Ph.D. under Dr. Thomas Tephly in 1969. Now a professor in the Department of Pharmacology and Toxicology at Michigan State University, Dr. Goodman gave a seminar entitled "Epigenetics, Altered DNA Methylation and Secondary Mechanisms Underlying Carcinogenesis." Dr. Goodman is active in the Society of Toxicology and was its president in 1999-2000.

2001
Dr. Fulton T. Crews

Dr. Fulton T. Crews received the Outstanding Alumnus Award on September 21, 2001. Dr. Crews is the Director of the Bowles Center for Alcohol Studies and a Professor of Pharmacology and Psychiatry at the University of North Carolina at Chapel Hill. He gave a lecture titled "Neuropharmacological Studies on the Progression from Experimentation to Addiction." Dr. Crews received his Ph.D. with Dr. C.B. Smith in 1978. He then was an N.I.H. Pharmacology Research Associate Award Fellow with Dr. Julius Axelrod at N.I.M.H. Dr. Crews and his colleagues are now major contributers to ethyl alcohol research.

2002
Dr. David W. Hein

The 2002 Outstanding Alumnus Award was given to Dr. David W. Hein. Dr. Hein's primary research themes were N-acetylation pharmacogenetics and discriminative stimulus properties of opioids. He obtained his Ph.D. with Dr. Wendell W. Weber as mentor from 1977-1982. After his years at Michigan, Dr. Hein was appointed Chairman of the Department of Pharmacology at the Morehouse School of Medicine in 1985, Chairman of the Department of Pharmacology and Toxicology at the University of North Dakota School of Medicine, and Chairman of Pharmacology at the University of Louisville School of Medicine in 1989 and 1997 respectively. Since 1999, Dr. Hein has been Acting Director of Center for Genetics and Molecular Medicine at University of Louisville. On October 11, 2002, Dr. Hein presented his seminar "N-acetylation Polymorphisms and Cancer Risk: Past, Present and Future."

2003
Dr. Lindsay B. Hough

Dr. Lindsay Hough was awarded the Outstanding Alumnus Award in 2003. He is a Professor of Pharmacology and Toxicology and Vice-Chairman of the Department of Pharmacology and Toxicology at Albany Medical College. He earned his Ph.D. with Dr. Ed Domino in 1978. He has been increasing our knowledge of the neuropharmacology and neurochemistry of histamine since his days as a graduate student. Dr. Hough presented a lecture entitled "Pain perception and the histaminergic system." He has several patents and over 80 refereed journal articles and numerous reviews and abstracts on his favorite subject.

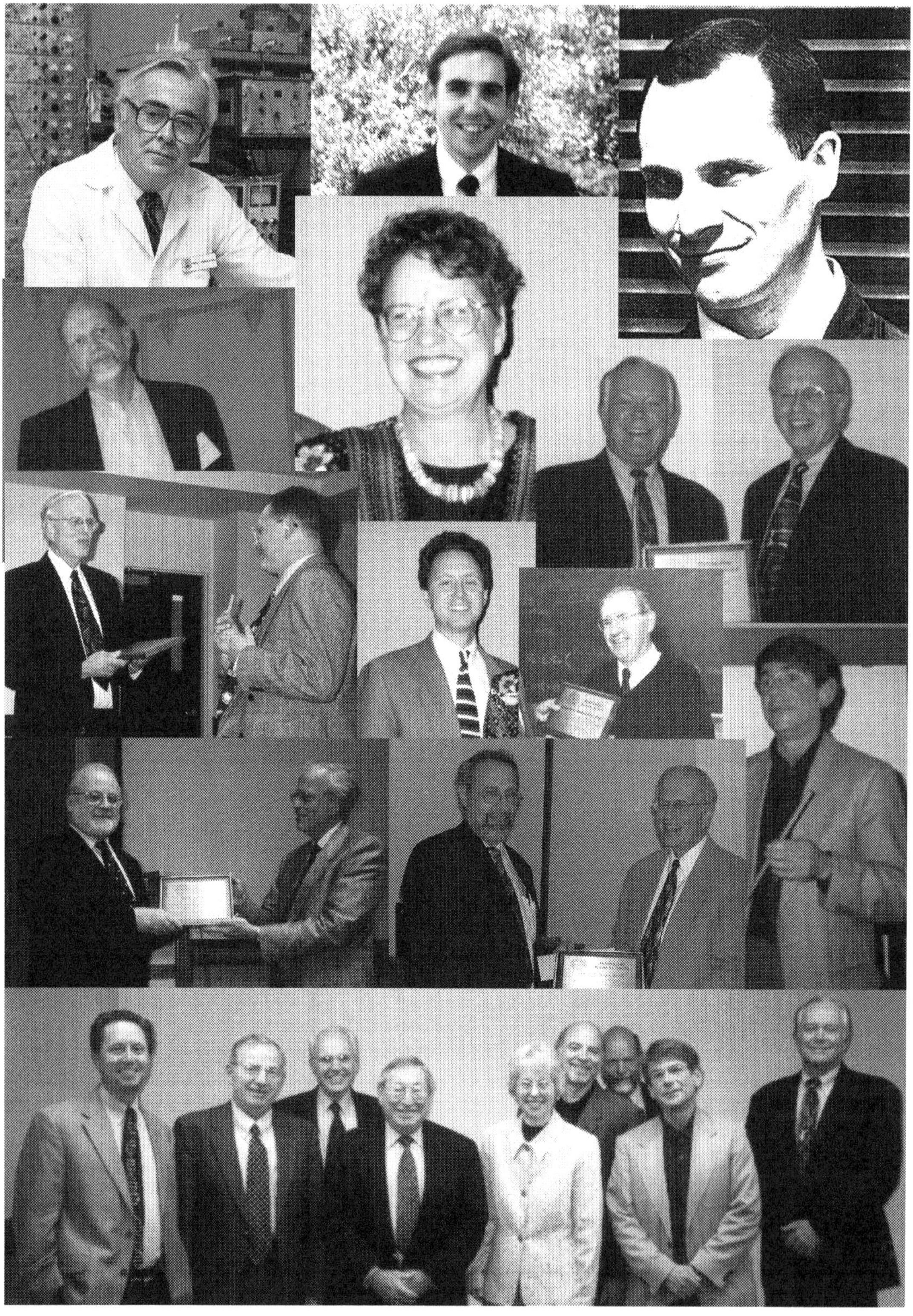

24

Reflections on the Past and Present, with a View of Pharmacology's Future at UM

Benedict R. Lucchesi, M.D., Ph.D.

Since the very first day as a member of the faculty in the Department of Pharmacology, I became intimately involved with the teaching of medical students, as well as students in the College of Pharmacy and the School of Nursing (Pharmacology 210). The latter was one of the most enjoyable assignments as I had an opportunity to restructure the course and expand the syllabus. Initially, Pharmacology 210 was required for all second year students in the nursing program. In later years the School of Nursing instituted a program for graduate nurses who returned to school to obtain a bachelor's degree in nursing. During the 14 years that I coordinated Pharmacology 210, I had the pleasure of coming in contact with undergraduate and graduate students in the School of Nursing. In order to provide instruction for graduate nurses I was required to travel to the Flint Campus of the University of Michigan during the winter term and to Traverse City during the spring and summer terms. Other faculty members delivered lectures in Kalamazoo and at the Dearborn Campus. The program proved to be successful in that it allowed graduate nurses to maintain their job-related activities while studying for their bachelor's degree in nursing.

As I reflect back on the early years of my career, I come to realize that many changes have occurred in our educational programs. For example, during spring and summer terms, the Department provided a course of instruction in Medical Pharmacology. The syllabus consisted of the same lecture topics offered to our second year medical students. The course was intended for registrants from other medical schools both from the United States and from foreign countries. The need for faculty to present lectures on a wide variety of topics in pharmacology was a means of expanding one's repertoire and to keep abreast with the advances in therapeutics. No faculty person, junior or senior, was exempt from teaching.

I also recall the many hours of instruction provided to second year medical students during the pharmacology course that consisted of ~125 hours of lecture during the year and six hours per week of laboratory instruction. The second year medical students were divided among eight laboratories located on the seventh level of Medical Science Building I. There were six groups of four students in each of the eight laboratories. In addition, one faculty member and two graduate students were assigned to each of the laboratories. It should be obvious that this undertaking involved the cooperation of the entire faculty, graduate student body and support staff. Each laboratory session required that the faculty and students begin setting up the experiments early in the morning so that the students could complete the laboratory assignments before the noon hour. Teamwork was the key to success and somehow we managed to do it.

Over the years the laboratory courses became "obsolete" as changes were made in the curriculum. Thus, the laboratory that once served as the primary venue in which graduate students had an opportunity to teach was no longer available, thereby leaving very few opportunities for predoctoral students in pharmacology to either develop their teaching skills or become familiar with many of the classic in vitro and in vivo approaches to the study of pharmacological agents. One outcome from the demise of the teaching laboratory was that the Department was among the first in the Medical School to make use of new approaches to teaching through the use of television. Both live TV demonstrations as well as carefully prepared taped videos provided valuable instruction to large groups of students. Among the most memorable demonstrations was that prepared by Dr. Edward Domino and the staff in the Department of Anesthesiology. Second year medical students were given the opportunity to view patients being administered every form of anesthesia in common use. Despite the passing of time and the advances in anesthesiology, the video prepared in the 1970s would continue to serve as a valuable means of instruction. Where today can students witness the induction of anesthesia by open drop ether, the administration of cyclopropane or the use of basal anesthesia? The ability to observe the various stages of anesthesia as they develop during the induction of anesthesia by diethyl ether is most likely never experienced today by students and clinicians. It is not meant to suggest that the administration of diethyl ether is a preferred anesthetic agent. However, the understanding, through observation, of how the central nervous system is progressively affected by general anesthetics was obtained best by visual observation during induction with ether. Each phase from the analgesia, the loss of consciousness, blunting and finally loss of reflexes, skeletal muscle relaxation and the suppression of respiration could be clearly defined as the emergence from anesthesia in which each of the phases occurred in the opposite order. This in itself was a "short course in neurophysiology."

The passing years were to involve other changes in the medical school curriculum. As a teacher who made every effort to perfect my understanding of pharmacology and therapeutics, I was witness to major changes brought about by student dissatisfaction with the overwhelming amount of information to be "memorized," rather than understood, during the first two years of the medical curriculum. The classical, time honored approach to classroom instruction gave way to the distribution of extensive handouts and examinations that required the student to memorize facts rather than demonstrate the ability to use deductive reasoning. In many instances students seldom attended class or laboratory sessions. Despite the lack of attendance, students continued to obtain passing grades simply by memorizing the faculty handouts and subscribing to notes transcribed from the class lectures. The classroom environment deteriorated to the point where faculty members were expected to "simply deliver the facts." The quiz and examination questions had to be structured so that the answers could be found in the faculty handouts. Any departure from this would engender student hostility and "challenges" to the test questions. A sufficient number of challenges usually resulted in the elimination of the question despite the fact that gifted students who are capable of reasoning do not have difficulty in responding correctly. Many of my faculty colleagues who teach third and fourth year students would often express disappointment when they encountered the students in the clinical setting and discover that most of the information presented in the second year of medical school has been forgotten. Pharmacology is not a subject to be memorized. An academic who only presents facts is not a teacher; a teacher is one who nurtures the learning process and thereby modifies behavior and patterns of thinking for a lifetime of self-instruction. A teacher is not one who strives only to obtain a favorable student evaluation.

The changes in the curriculum were not limited to the Medical School. Graduate education also has been changed dramatically. Some would suggest that the changes represent an improvement. Others, including myself, would refute that opinion. Those who accept the current state of affairs may not have a full appreciation for the scope of the discipline of pharmacology, or do not appreciate that learning and understanding of concepts and retention of important information requires a foundation upon which the information can be interrelated. This is the nature of pharmacology that by definition is an integration of molecular chemistry, anatomy, biochemistry, physiology, molecular biology and pathology. It is this broad based foundation that enables the student to understand why, when and how drugs can be used to treat disease.

This is the primary difference between pharmacology and the other basic sciences. The ultimate focus of the pharmacologist is human disease and its management through therapeutic intervention. In order to master the subject and to participate in the advancement of therapeutic interventions it is essential that the student be well versed in the normal physiology and then the pathophysiology and how the latter can be altered to treat a disease. It is somewhat incomprehensible that a graduate program leading to a doctoral degree in pharmacology can be considered complete when such core subjects as physiology and pathology, to mention a few that are no longer part of the curriculum. Furthermore, the near total elimination of comprehensive graduate level courses in the various subspecialty areas of pharmacology (e.g. cardiovascular, central nervous system, renal, immunology, etc.) only compounds the situation and ignores the fact that pharmacology is an "integration" of many disciplines. To paraphrase Dr. John Jacob Abel, let one person be more of a biochemist, another more of a physiologist, or another more of a clinician, but first they should be "pharmacologists."

The recent emphasis on molecular biology and the human genome project, while of tremendous importance, has captured the attention of funding agencies and program directors attracted to the sources of financial (NIH grants) security. It is becoming painfully evident that the distinction among the basic sciences and the training programs are blurred to the point were everything looks the same. This is not to say that the work being performed at the molecular level is not important. However, to put all of the funding and training resources at the level of molecular biology will result in a decline in areas of training so necessary for taking a new therapeutic candidate from the "bench to the bedside." In addition to contributing to an imbalance in the training of future investigators, the current approach to the training of basic and clinical pharmacologists will deprive academic institutions of experienced personnel capable of teaching in our medical schools and addressing subjects in a manner relevant to the needs of medical students and practicing physicians.

Unless there is a radical change in training pharmacologists, preparing graduates to address the needs of the pharmaceutical industry, and training physicians, the discipline will decline in its importance. In the future, pharmacology departments may be amalgamated with other basic science departments or have the teaching functions provided by faculty from various clinical disciplines. The latter possibility becomes ever more of a concern in times of financial uncertainty such as those confronting our medical schools and medical centers as they attempt to cope with the changing patterns in reimbursement for delivery of medical care.

All is not gloom and doom. As in the past, problems of a similar nature have occurred and the leaders have responded. One area in need of immediate attention is already undergoing intensive scrutiny, that being the "peer review" system. The system had been "broken" for too long and is in desperate need of repair. Despite the availability of research funds, there are too many productive and capable investigators being denied adequate support or having their programs interrupted due to lack of funding. All too often the negative comments are trivial and any perceived or real errors in a proposal could have been corrected by appropriate guidance from the reviewers rather than assigning a less than fundable score to the grant. The need to resubmit a proposal to correct minor points of disagreement does not seem to make much sense especially in our modern world in which communication can be carried out with the speed of light. What purpose does it serve to delay or prevent continuance of a project that has shown promise? How does the uncertainty about continued funding encourage the young scientist to remain in an academic setting? Would the situation be improved if an investigator were to be judged more on progress as opposed to having presented a well crafted, but untested hypothesis? How much more progress could be made if reviewers were more like mentors rather than judges?

Equally important is the need for leaders in academia to consider the stresses imposed upon non-tenured faculty who are at risk of losing salary support and/or laboratory space when grant funding is not obtained. How do such stresses impact upon the willingness of faculty to engage in other activities (teaching, scholarly works, administration, curriculum development, etc.) considered to be important to the functioning of a department and/or medical school?

Indeed there are problems to be addressed and eventually resolved. Overall I remain optimistic.

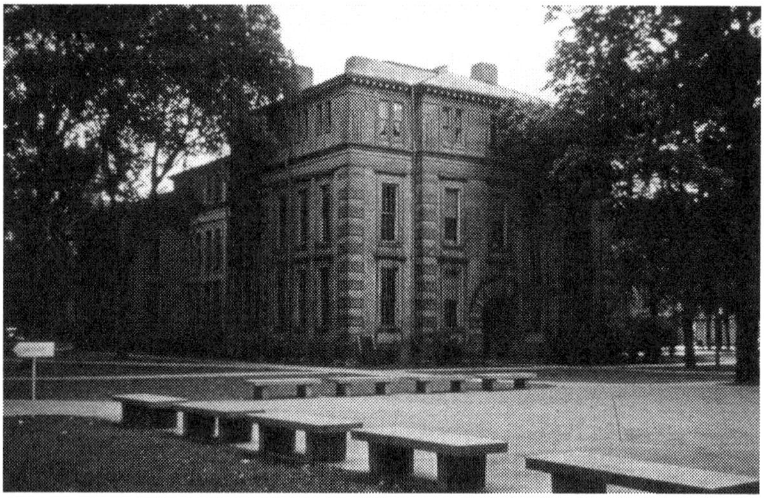

Past view of the old Pharmacology Building on the Diag

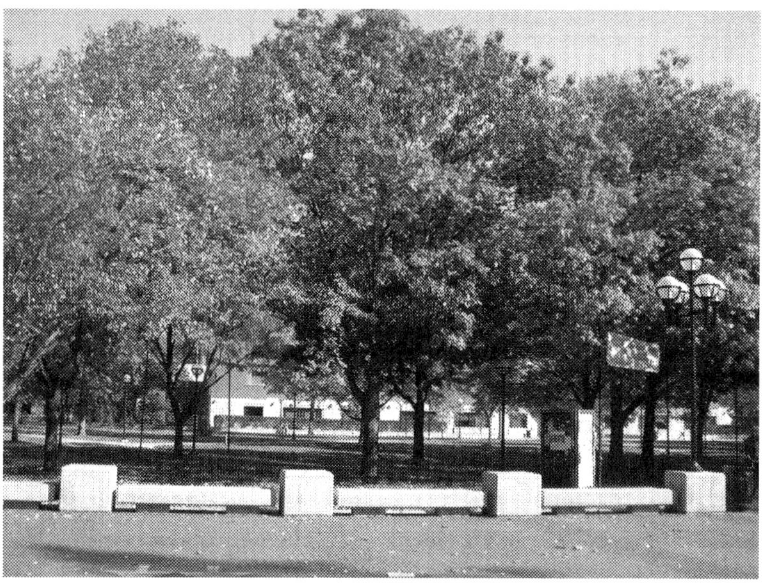

Present view of the Diag where the old building used to stand

25

Medical Student and Service Teaching by the Department of Pharmacology

Marshal Shlafer, Ph.D.

Synopsis of Our "Recent" Medical and Service Teaching

When we prepared a comprehensive review of our department's activities for Dean Joe Johnson in 1988-1989, we noted what could be called a modest load of medical student and service teaching (i.e., non-Ph.D. program courses). It appeared not to have changed significantly from what we had had for several years prior.

We presented 45 hours of "pharmy" (or just the monosyllabic pharm) to the M1 students, 60 hours to the M2s. We covered, we believe, the essential gamut of topics in a more than adequate, more than superficial, and well-received way. Animal labs had been a thing of the past for some time.

Ben Lucchesi, Hank Swain, and Ed Domino organized and delivered most of roughly 90 hours of presentations to about 25 M4 students in a Senior Pharmacology and Therapeutics elective. Many of our department's faculty (and many clinical faculty) helped out. It was a popular course in many ways, not the least of which was its timeliness (up to date, and happening not long before the students were to graduate and head into the world as interns and residents); its clinical bent with a distinct basic science reconnection; and the enthusiastic teaching faculty. Then, too, there were the Lucky Pierres, for which each student randomly selected some therapeutic topic, had overnight to work it up, and the next day had to present a lucid discussion to the group. Any faculty who attended these sessions were surprised and impressed with how good a job these "kids," — these almost-doctors — did and how we learned from them.

Dental students (in Pharm 602, a course that was for years led by Hank Swain and Ken Cochran) and nursing students (Pharm 210, headed by Ben Lucchesi for years) got 45 lecture hours each (in separate courses).

For several years before and after the 1989 report, there were some quasi-official off campus "assignments" for the Nursing School's off-site program to enable RNs to earn a bachelor's degree. These were truly complete pharmacology courses with 40-something hours of lecture. Tad Smith taught in Dearborn and Kalamazoo. Ben, and then his postdoc Ken Gibson and I, then Ken Kilgore and I, did Flint. (Ben's memory of Flint and mine coincide instantly on one major point: the drives to and from class in near-blizzard conditions, home in the pitch black of night.) Ben had another teaching activity that wasn't nearly as bad: nursing courses in the summers in Traverse City. Some years later several of our graduate students (Lori Mangels comes to mind) taught pharmacology to nursing students at Eastern Michigan University.

In the '70s and '80s we taught a separate two-term course (404 and 405) to the pharmacy (B.S.) students and our second year grad students. It was there that I got my first taste of course directing (with Ray Counsell) and teaching here. Eventually, partly because the College of Pharmacy did away with the B.S. degree program (in favor of a Pharm. D. program), and partly because of politics, 404 and 405 ended when the pharmacy students took their pharmacology course with the med students. That, too, would change and come full circle in a few years.

All this tallied up to over 300 hours of total lecture to medical and other health professions students a decade or so ago — off campus teaching excluded.

As we headed into 2000, our teaching responsibilities changed a bit overall, more significantly as it involved medical students. (Those of you who are interested in seeing more about what we teach now should visit our department's web page: http://www.sitemaker.umich.edu/pharmacology). Our faculty (counting just those with primary appointments in Pharmacology) now give about 25 hours of lectures to M1s (Pharm 525) and a mere 43 or so hours to M2s throughout the entire year, spread over various sequences. In short, our preclinical medical teaching was cut by a full one-third (and further cuts loom on the horizon for everyone, not just us). Ben Lucchesi and Ed Domino still run the M4 elective, but they and other Pharmacology faculty give only about 25 hours of formal lecture, total. Clinical faculty play a much greater role than before, largely because our faculty is pitching in less, at least in terms of actually presenting. Some of our faculty, however, have been more than generous with their time, serving as facilitators in the class while others present their material.

The dental course, now run by Jon Maybaum and Martha Somerman, still gave about 45 hours of lecture a year, in Winter term. The course has been revamped, in conjunction with folks at the Dental School, into a two-term course that apparently will keep the essentially the same lectures by our faculty, integrated with more clinical presentations by the Dental School faculty.

Tad Smith and Rob Simpson shepherd Pharmacology 659-660. In an earlier incarnation it was the 404-405 sequence that ended when pharmacy students were (for a while) assimilated into the M2 pharmacology course. Pharm 659 and 660 were born to provide a venue to teach the pharmacy students who had been moved into the medical course after they were moved out. The reasons were interesting, and political. On one hand, the Pharmacy School wanted a separate course tailored to just their students. When the medical school implemented its new curriculum, one administrative decision (decree is more appropriate; no votes were taken on this) was to ostracize all students who weren't medical students from medical student classes. No place for pharmacy students, nor for our graduate students. Thus, Pharm 659 and 660 were created out of a no other good options necessity, not by desire.

Tad and Rob have about 45 hours each term for two terms, with such colleagues as Bill Pratt and Peggy Gnegy organizing some of the courses' sections. Pharm 659 and 660 are our main course not only for the PharmD students and our second year graduate students; but for a new a cohort: students in the Acute Care Nurse Practitioner (ACNP) Program. They are working R.N.s going on for advanced training and certification to assume new and more participatory roles (including, they hope, if politics work in their favor, some prescribing) along with their M.D. colleagues. There was concern about how the ACNP students would do academically (many of them had been out of the study grind for years), and how they would contribute to or fit in with the class. From what I've heard from Tad and Rob, and others too, they appear to be motivated, bright, and enthusiastic learners. Their questions and other class participation (stemming from having much clinical experience already) add to discussions a valued spin that wasn't there before.

The undergraduate nursing pharmacology course on campus (210) grew, in 1999, from three credit hours to four, increasing lecture time to over 50 hours per term. This increase in contact time, OK'd by Paul Hollenberg and formally endorsed by the Nursing School Curriculum Committee, was unusual since it came at a time when teaching obligations were generally holding the line or shrinking, and the work loads for the nursing students were already heavy. Our Department is no longer involved in off-campus teaching, nursing or otherwise.

In summary, the most recent medical and service teaching tally, about 275 hours is only about 25 fewer annual hours less (on paper) overall than we were presenting on site 10 years ago — which does not look like a significant change.

Our current assignments are such that two or three different faculty may be teaching the same topic to different audiences. This sounds like duplication of effort, or inefficiency, and to a degree it is. Mainly, it's just perpetuation of the way things were. On a positive spin, this "duplication" of teaching efforts reflects a breadth of our collective repertoires, a matter I will come back to later.

What one needs to realize, however, is that a majority of those 275 hours is taught by a handful of faculty — older faculty who, in the next five to 10 years or so, are not likely to be here. We face a challenge. Moreover, just looking at the total doesn't adequately reflect how significantly our medical student teaching has been cut. Indeed, were it not for the forced rebirth of Pharmacology 404-405 in the guise of a new course (659-660), it might appear that our Department has taken a heavy cut in its formal teaching responsibilities — and our "visibility" to medical students and the others in the medical school who are "watching."

Teaching at Michigan: Evolution, Revolution, or Devolution?

The Medical School's reassessments of their philosophies about and approaches to basic science education have necessarily affected our department's involvement in it too. But it's gone beyond that. Financial and scientific factors have also affected service teaching for many of our colleagues. It's certainly affected me. If you read on perhaps you will see that our continuing educational evolution — or "revolution" or "devolution" or even "dissolution," which might be more appropriate terms — seems to herald more cuts in our medical student teaching. They could have an even greater and potentially highly negative impact on medical student teaching and education for those on both sides of the lectern. Changes wouldn't threaten the existence of the Medical School, or its accreditation by the national Liaison Committee on Medical Education (LCME), but what happens to the basic science departments may be another matter.

We face a Catch 22. If we reclaim more medical student teaching time or gain more service teaching (both unlikely), or even if our current teaching obligations stay as they are (likely, I hope personally), and if we don't recruit or prepare younger faculty to pick up a huge teaching load, the departure of just a few key faculty may impose an onerous burden on and challenge to those who remain or join new. If those who remain must suddenly take on new teaching roles, and spend abundant time preparing for them, other things such as research may be constrained. Conversely, no matter how many skilled teachers we might have, if our teaching obligations are cut significantly, a major raison d'etre for keeping alive a separate Department of Pharmacology may disappear in the eyes of the institution. Indeed, that concept of departmental dissolution is already being discussed and debated.

The Changing U of M Medical Center Campus

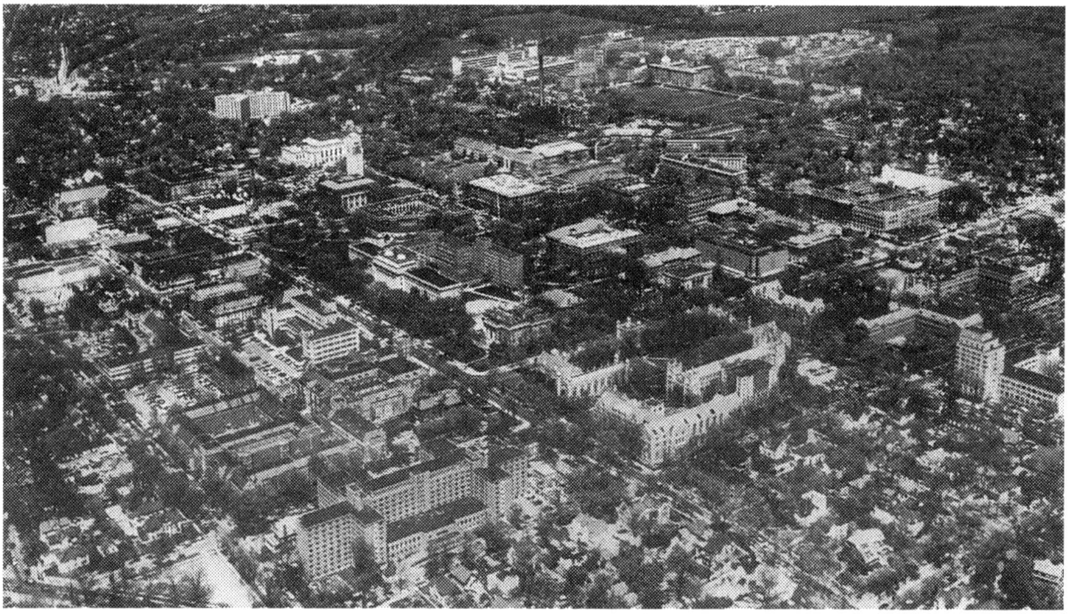

Can you find it? ca. 1960s

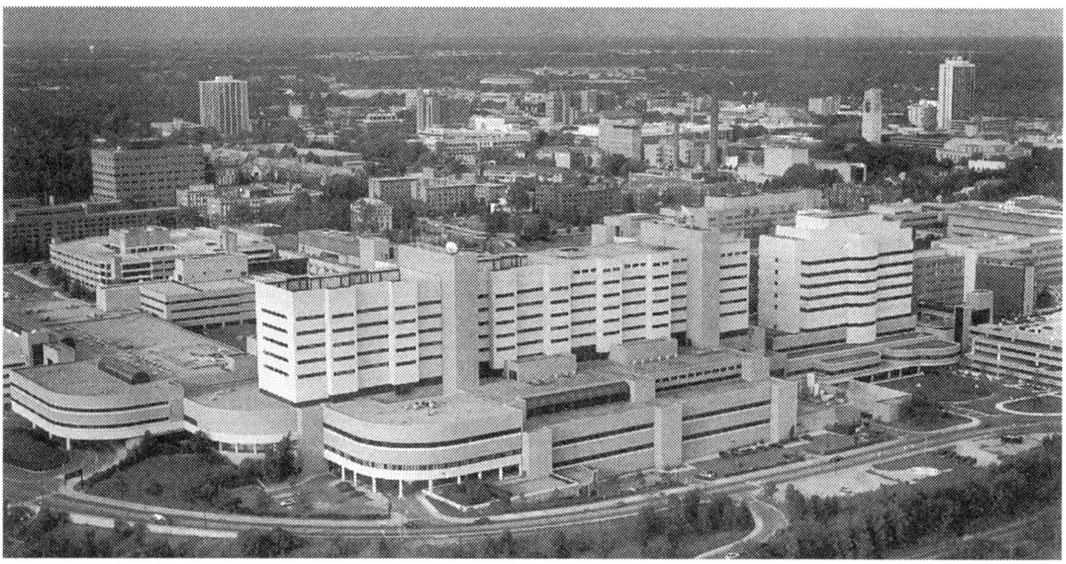

The Medical Center, ca. 1997

26

Excerpts from the Torald Sollmann Oration*

Theodore M. Brody, Ph.D.

We know that drug discovery and new observations in the field [of pharmacology] as well as in other disciplines, are largely based upon previous findings, which we ultimately attempt to build upon. In a similar fashion, what we attempt to accomplish during our careers is dependent to a large extent on individuals we encounter along the way, who ultimately shape our lives as teachers, scientists, and/or administrators.

Teaching pharmacology to medical students is now a critically important area for departments, and to some extent the viability of the discipline may depend on our ability to deliver the appropriate information to medical students in a palatable format that will be helpful in their future roles as physicians. Currently, it is difficult to distinguish one basic science department from another, relying solely on ongoing research in the unit. As pharmacologists we should demonstrate that we provide something special. Basic pharmacological concepts and the information base of the discipline should be presented in a format that is clinically relevant. Generally this is not difficult in problem-based learning sessions, which have a clinical flavor. Formal stand-up lectures, however, sometimes present a problem, depending on the lecturer.

In 1952, 50% of the 277 pharmacology faculty members in US medical schools were medically trained. Today, of the 1500 faculty members in medical school departments, only 75 faculty, or 5%, have M.D. degrees. We now have 125 medical schools compared to 76. Thus there are now 12 faculty members per department, compared to four or less in 1952. While we may have many fewer medically-trained pharmacologists now than 40 years ago, we cannot turn back the clock. Nor, in my view, will training more clinical pharmacologists be especially helpful. Even non-medically trained faculty should be familiar enough with the clinical aspects of their teaching area to keep abreast of the medical students' clinical knowledge. If relevant teaching, or the "right stuff" continues to be a problem with faculty, then perhaps our graduate programs need restructuring, or perhaps that individual faculty member has little interest or is unwilling to spend the necessary time to become an effective teacher.

The unthinkable alternative may be a mandate by the medical school dean that clinical faculty play a significant role in the teaching of pharmacology. While many would view this as a disaster, contrary to popular opinion, many clinicians are willing and able to assume that role. It is not unreasonable, however, to invite clinical faculty to provide some of the lectures, as long as control of the overall course still resides with the pharmacology department. On the other hand, curriculum committees and deans are extremely short-sighted in attempting to reduce the hours devoted to pharmacology. Deans are surely aware that today, as has been the situation for many years, "drugs" are the most frequently used modality in the treatment of disease. This reflects a need for greater emphasis on the teaching of pharmacology in medical schools, in terms of both adequate hours and the "right stuff." Pharmacology will never be in jeopardy as an independent discipline, or in trouble with "bot-

* Reprinted with permission from *The Pharmacologist* Volume 37- No 4, Fall 1995.

tom-line devotees" in deans' offices, as long as we provide the appropriate information to our medical students in whatever teaching mode the dean thinks is important!

Just a brief thought about the status of our graduate programs and research in pharmacology departments. Many have decried the role of "molecular pharmacology," which is now a principal research emphasis in many departments. This is really no different than in 1952, when I began my career as a "biochemical pharmacologist."

I quote here a paragraph written by Maurice H. Seevers in 1965 that well reflects my views on what some consider to be a significant problem:

"The ultimate goal of pharmacologic research is an understanding of the mechanism of action at the molecular level. While fascinating, worthy of extensive pursuit, and probably in the long run a most important approach, it is a very specialized area. Success requires an unusual training, a creative mind not hampered by convention, an interest in theory rather than practice, and other talents not possessed by all who would enter pharmacology. All need not, and should not, undertake it. In terms of the prime functions of pharmacology as a basis for rational therapeutics, and in the protection of the public health, the role of molecular pharmacology is no more and no less exalted than any other subdivision of pharmacology. "

While the goal in most departments is to determine the mechanism of action of a drug at the molecular or cellular level, it is also critical that students understand the relation of the molecular mechanism of a drug to its action in the intact human with its full component of biochemical, physiological, and pathological influences. Sadly, this latter relationship is missing in Ph.D. training programs in many departments. It has always been my philosophy that any in vitro observations must be consistent with findings in the functioning intact animal or organ.

It is equally discordant and distressful that some grant-funding agencies have placed undo emphasis on molecular biology and view any studies in the intact animal as being less relevant in the current competition for funds. Therefore, proposals that include studies in the intact organism or in functioning tissues, which may actually have greater relevance to the public health, have less likelihood of support. It is also imperative to find a mechanism to distribute more research dollars to young new investigators, so that we are not in danger of losing an entire generation of biomedical scientists. These are important problems that cry out for resolution.

In my view, equally discouraging is the falling attendance at Pharmacology Society meetings. This will only change when students and faculty are firmly convinced that attendance is in their own best self-interest.

Also disappointing is the action of some departments to rename their units, "Department of Molecular Pharmacology" or "Department of Molecular Biology and Pharmacology," etc. Such changes are premature and defensive. Does this mean that the department knows little about other subdivisions of pharmacology or does not teach them? Is Pharmacology now a subdivision of Molecular Pharmacology? Certainly this approach does little to reinforce the distinction between pharmacology and the other basic science disciplines, which is important if we are to flourish as independent units. For my part I have always been a pharmacologist and an "ASPETer." Although I have published extensively in JBC and AJP, I have never found it necessary to belong to either of the parent societies.

Although I have described several negatives, there are also positives. In most medical schools, pharmacology departments continue to do well, and play major roles in institutional teaching and research programs. Cooperation and collaboration is still the name of the game.

27

Whither Pharmacology at the University of Michigan

Edward F. Domino, M.D.

Many of us in departments of pharmacology are necessarily excessively occupied with competing for funds and resources to survive and, if possible, to pursue individual research interests. We tend not to be concerned with the place of pharmacology as a scientific discipline. It is now a fact that most basic science departments in any health science professional school are far more similar than different except for their teaching responsibilities. University administrators give much lip service to the importance of teaching, but woe betide the department that is annually financially in the red. Fortunately at present our Department is not. We all assume that as long as an academic department collectively brings in adequate research funds its survival is assured. Funded areas of research are constantly changing, the number of basic scientists continues to grow, and the now obvious limited funding opportunities exist. Those less willing or unable to change research directions will suffer. After all, change is inevitable. Many major decisions are made only by administrators. Frequently, individuals on the academic or research track have little input other than to cope with those decisions, good or bad, as best one can.

We all must realize that the primary mission of pharmacology is defined in its name, "pharmakon" meaning medicine or drug and "ology" meaning science – thus the science of medicine or drugs is what pharmacology is all about. As the number of useful medicines continues to grow, there is an increasing need for drug experts. Furthermore, as we learn more about cell biology, and the wondrous complex mechanisms within as well as between cells and organ systems, new drug targets will continue to emerge. Many scientists from diverse disciplines will always make important contributions to pharmacology. The science of pharmacology does not belong exclusively to pharmacologists. Our field will always be dependent on inputs from many different scientific disciplines. However, pharmacologists, if they choose, have a unique role in studying and teaching the mechanisms of drug action, and in integrating that information from a chemical structural, molecular, intracellular, and extracellular (to organs, intact animals, and humans) point of view. Our field will surely rapidly incorporate the new knowledge of molecular genetics and apply it in a practical as well as theoretical context.

Pharmacology as a science seems to be growing exponentially, but what kind of a home or homes will it have in future academic settings? The Department of Pharmacology at the University of Michigan now has its base in the Medical School. Historically it has interacted with all schools and branches of the University. That has been its strength! At the present time, its place in the Medical School curriculum has markedly shrunk and is being compromised. Our Department needs a real presence, not only in the first two years but also in the senior clinical year of medical school. We need to interact with clinicians far more than is the case at the present time. The existence of our Department needs to depend on more than just getting grants with their associated overhead. Some day soon a dean in our Medical School may well conclude that he or she could save enormous resources by combining basic science departments. Why pay for two or more chairpersons, their associated administrators and office staff when one administrative unit would do?

I fear that our young people, who prefer to publish only in journals of biochemistry and molecular biology, and who feel that the teaching of pharmacology to medical students is a minor or even irrelevant activity, will some day find themselves without a department of pharmacology in a medical school. That may well be their desire! Today, a medical school dean can easily take the position that pharmacology is better taught to medical students by internists and a few faculty from the Pharmacy School. As the number of staff members in pharmacology become increasingly involved in fundamental biochemical mechanisms in which drugs are merely tools, one can make a stronger case that they are less capable than internists or Pharm.D.s to teach pharmacology to medical students. This is already true at several medical schools in the United States. The current trend to train Ph.D. medical scientists with a common curriculum of basic sciences and specialization with a major and a minor will create Ph.D.s in pharmacology who may or may not be committed to the field of pharmacology. The organ system approach to teaching medical students provides less time for pharmacology and frequently is better taught by clinicians interested in therapeutics than by members of many current pharmacology departments, including our own here at Michigan.

Inasmuch as no one person can master a field as diverse as pharmacology, it is necessary that a variety of experts at the chemical, molecular, biochemical, genetic, physiological, pathological and clinical levels constitute a broad based department of pharmacology. Experts from other scientific fields will always be welcome as pharmacologists, so that their contributions can advance the discipline. Currently, too many of us are more concerned with what we can do to enhance our own research status rather than what we can give to the discipline. We must ask ourselves how can we contribute to the discipline of pharmacology as well as help in the mission of the school of which we are part, i.e., medical, pharmacy, dental, nursing, etc. Similarly, pharmacologists in research institutes or in pharmaceutical industry must contribute positively to the mission of those organizations.

It is a curious fact that the more we learn of the genetics of cellular biology, the greater the need to knock in or knock out specific genes in intact animals such as the mouse. It appears that there will still be a very important place for intact animal pharmacologists to take advantage of these new developments. Why does a mouse whose acetylcholinesterase has been knocked out live? Why does a mouse without the beta subunit of sodium channels have seizures?

Basic and clinical pharmacologists need each other. Basic pharmacologists must, of necessity, work at the molecular level in order to determine the chemical mechanisms of drug action. However, we need clinical pharmacologists to study the effects of drugs in humans. As pharmacologists, we must have a broader point of view than molecular biologists. We must think at the molecular, macrocellular and intact animal and human organism levels. If we do not, I believe we will become a dying breed. Whether our discipline survives at the University of Michigan for another century plus, as it has since the days of Abel, will depend on our administrators and our younger staff members. The number of retired professors in our Department has increased, leaving potentially serious gaps, particularly in pharmacogenetics, cardiovascular pharmacology, and clinical pharmacology. It will be interesting to see at the end of the first decade of the 21st century where our Department ranks as an entity in the priorities of our Medical School and University. It is a curious fact that our University currently has a John Jacob Abel Professor of Life Sciences instead of Pharmacology. Pharmacologists especially, but also biochemists, revere Abel as crucial to the history of their discipline. It appears some feel he is a suitable model for a life scientist as well. Whither pharmacology at the University of Michigan!

28

A Curriculum for the 21st Century : A Diminished Role For Pharmacology in Medical Education

Marshal Shlafer, Ph.D.

The Road to A New Curriculum

While Giles Bole was Dean there was renewed discussion about the need for a new curriculum for the medical students. Giles described the current one — then nearly 20 years old — as a train that had gone down the same track too long, and it was time for a change. Many faculty were skeptical, if not adamantly opposed to, any significant change, and they had been soured by prior and rather botched attempts to redo the plan of study largely by fiat. But this time Giles wisely knew that the motivation for change, and the nature of any change, had to come up from the faculty, rather than being crammed down our throats.

As the '80s waned, Bole charged Wayne Davis, his new Associate Dean for Medical Education, with the task of enlisting widespread faculty support and participation to put a new curriculum together. Arguably, the Dean couldn't have found a better person to lead the way for curricular reform than Wayne — whether locally or nationally — the only alternative being someone who had experience as a classroom teacher for medical students.

Wayne got the faculty involved from the get-go in a new curricular plan, eventually to be called MD2000. He set finite timetables to accomplish specific tasks, and by God expected them to be met. He kept the faculty at-large frequently informed of goals, objectives, and progress, and listened to concerns. He masterfully picked his allies in the drive for a new curriculum, and did what was necessary to neutralize nay-sayers or actual adversaries. Wayne was, in essence, an administrator *par excellence.*

The process to get us a new curriculum took several years, thousands of faculty and student rep hours, many hundreds of committee meetings. (Davis' staff kept meticulous minutes and agendas, putting the meeting number for each committee at the top of the packet. The number of meetings for some committees that continued long after the curriculum was launched reached well into the hundreds.)

I started serving on several planning committees, initially as one of our departmental representatives who wanted to ensure that the "basics" of pharmacology didn't get short-shrifted (for us or for the students), and that we were the ones responsible for teaching at least the bulk of pharm material. Several colleagues in our Department added significant input.

One overriding goal of MD2000 was to encourage students to become more "independent learners." Another was to help students acquire the fundamentals of clinical skills, including interviewing and risk assessment, earlier than before. Fostering students' "self-directed life-long learning skills" would be accomplished in a simple way: limit formal lectures to no more than 15 hours a week, total. That was at least a 20% cut in formal lecture time from what the preclinical students had had for a long time.

Sweating the Details

The new M1 year (now dubbed "Component I"— who knows why we needed such a highfalutin term for what everyone else recognized simply as the M1 year) was to be a "basic sciences fundamentals" year. A new multidisciplinary (multi-departmental) cell and molecular biology course, plus another one dealing with clinical skills (called Introduction to the Patient; ITTP) would be the flagships, spanning both semesters. Still other new courses, including one entitled Host Defenses, were assembled. A few more or less traditional department-based courses (anatomy, histology, pathology, genetics) were kept. Pharmacology initially wasn't one of them.

Component II would be more basic sciences, at a more advanced and integrated level of course, with considerably more clinical connections to ITTP. Eleven multidisciplinary M2 sequences (courses) were identified. Each would focus on some body system or process and cover things from pathologic, physiologic, pharmacologic, and other basic perspectives in an integrated way. They would replace all department- or discipline-based courses, which had been around for years. Bye-bye pharmacology in the M2 year.

We soon discovered that only one small portion of what our Department had taught to medical students for years would come out of the extensive revision process unscathed. That was the Senior (M4) Clinical Pharmacology and Therapeutics elective. That course, organized by Ben Lucchesi, Hank Swain, and Ed Domino (with contributions varying over the years) was held out as the exemplar of an activity that would become a mandatory "Science in Clinics Experience" for the M4s. While Senior Therapeutics itself wasn't required, the concept was that M4s must "revisit" basic science issues with a more clinical and more advanced thrust and connection before they could graduate.

Most of you will remember that in the long-time "old" curriculum pharmacology had a very identifiable presence. As Ernie Harwell would have said, that course, which covered general principles of pharmacology plus the major groups of drugs individually and as they interrelate, now was long gone. We didn't know precisely how or where core pharmacology material would be presented, but we knew for sure that a portion of what there was would be spattered throughout both years.

How the New Curriculum *Really* Came About

The new M1 year would be launched a year before the other components, giving the folks working on the M2 through M4 years a break. Detailed plans were worked out well before the students arrived, and all eyes were on it and the folks who put it together and ran it.

Organizing the new M1 year would be a managerial and political nightmare. The political issues derived from the fact that most departments lost their courses, and so, their control over what was presented. That loss of ownership was not received too positively at first. Limiting formal lecture time to 15 hours per week (whether in the new M1 or M2 years) meant that departments would be, in essence, competing with one another for precious teaching slots. The matter was complicated by the fact that Bole repeatedly enunciated more reward (translation, dollars) for teaching. But even the dullest of minds realized that less teaching would mean less compensation from medical school funds. "We'll reward the faculty more for more teaching, but the faculty will teach less" was the message we inferred.

Every basic science chair (and most rank-and-file faculty) became extraordinarily and almost instantly protective and territorial about medical student teaching. Researchers who disdained teaching (at best) morphed into medical education advocates. Like it or not, they knew that if their teaching assignments disappeared or got cut radically, compensation for them and their departments might too. I remember distinctly how so many teaching faculty who before would "just as soon not teach" (and some who, for various reasons, shouldn't be allowed within a hundred yards of a medical student classroom) suddenly became possessive of their teaching time and worried that their lectures would be cut.

Early on, as I saw how things would pan out, I pitied the poor slob who'd be charged with not only coming up with the overall curricular plan, but also having to decide ultimately which departments had their teaching cut, and by how much. As fate would have it, that job landed in my lap. I had been appointed as the first director of the new Component I; I had to sweat the details. Fortunately I got Joe Fantone, from pathology, to come aboard as assistant director.

Putting the M1 year together was difficult, help or not, time commitments aside. Joe and I had to get away from a long history of temporal mismatches in the sequence of presenting content. No longer would, say, physiology be doing cardiovascular while anatomy or histology did the reproductive system and biochemistry focused on something completely different.

Everything had to be "in synch" as much as possible so students could learn and see, from different perspectives, similar or connected things at the same time. Doing this with nearly a dozen courses, scores of faculty from different departments, each with some measure of self-interest in mind, and a whole year of medical student education, was more than a challenge. One new course, that flagship element of Component I — was to be multidisciplinary, and it was obviously to be controlled largely by one department.

Since there were faculty in many other departments who had previously given content that would go into the new course, there were spats over who would do what… which department would get the credit for the teaching. So one the main roles Fantone and I faced was mediating occasional turf battles waged by departments or individuals who had had lots of teaching time before. Naturally, at many times we had to make an administrative decision that didn't leave some folks too happy.

I faced a personal conflict because it was clear that pharmacology teaching as we knew it and believed it should be would be relegated to a small spur on Bole's new railroad. In fact, initially there was no planned time *anywhere* in the M1 or M2 year for pharmacology to teach even general principles of the discipline: pharmacokinetics, drug metabolism and other aspects of pharmacodynamics; or any autonomic pharmacology (which, we know, is critical to understanding many areas of pharmacology and therapeutics). It certainly couldn't go well into the new M2 year, since that was systems-based and there was no good place for general fundamentals.

Pharmacology found a spot in the new M1 year, but it was not ideal. I insisted on and got a short basic principles and introduction to autonomics course. It would be presented in about 20 hours at the very end of a long, tiring M1 year — just in time for students to start thinking ahead to their last free summer for years; just in time to forget content over that summer so that, when they needed to recall that knowledge as M2s, they could say "gee, we never got that stuff." One of my departmental colleagues headed up the new course, cognizant of the challenges. By accident — literally — I assumed directorship of that M1 course several years after its inception and managed to "sneak in" two more lecture hours a year here, another two or three next year, and so on, till we eventually had about 30 hours of contact time. I added topics that I thought were important: general concepts of adverse drug effects and drug-drug interactions; alternative medicines; OTC drugs; implications of age on drug therapy; and medication errors.

Perceived Pitfalls

And what about the rest of our old but successful two-term M2 pharmacology course? For sure it would be fragmented, but no one knew which pieces would ever fall in place, or where or when. Our chance (or anyone's) to teach some content could be overlooked or eliminated altogether, or trimmed and pigeon-holed in sequences where content didn't fit best in our opinions. And we wouldn't know precisely what would happen for a long time, because the M2 year wouldn't start for a full year after the new M1 year came on line. Most people outside our Department seemed not to understand our concerns over providing reasonable pharmacology content, or even care. We didn't have impartial sympathetic ears to listen to us, even though pleas were coming from a few of us who had, for various reasons, a vested interest in (if not many years of commitment to) teaching.

Regardless, M2 pharmacology teaching was largely out of our Department's control. We could lobby, remind, and prod, but in essence there was little we could do to force things to come out our way. That's because in most cases clinical faculty became co-directors for the M2 sequences (and generally had much more clout than their basic science counterparts). They assigned lectures to their clinical colleagues (often junior faculty), who presented things from their perspective, overlooking or being plain ignorant (in many ways) of the basic pharmacology or the wide net that a particular area of pharmacology casts over other areas.

From our Department, only two people became sequence co-directors from the get-go: Ben Lucchesi (cardiovascular) and Donna Shewach (Infectious Diseases). Yet with the clinical dominance in directorships, to this day, to me, a look at many of the M2 sequences reveals a definite clinical superspecialty bias in content and contact time, at the expense of solid basic science material. Alas, there was plenty of basic science superspecialist material too. It's Michigan, after all.

As many students (and I) would lament after the new curriculum got rolling in 1992, the demise of our cohesive and comprehensive pharmacology course took away something with which students developed a love-hate relationship: the comprehensive, integrated final exam on all of pharmacology at year's end. To be sure, it was an onerous exam for some (many?) students, but coming right before Part 1 of the NBME (now Step I of the USMLE), it was a dandy way to kill two birds at once: preparing for the pharmacology course and the pharmy part of boards, just a couple of months away, at the same time.

Validation

The success of the new curriculum was "validated" using a host of subjective and objective measurement tools developed internally. Based on feedback the curriculum was perpetually and inexorably being tweaked, which was good. On the other hand, radical revisions were coming to the table again, served up administratively in a somewhat "eat this" fashion. Student (and faculty) "satisfaction" with the curriculum and other aspects of med school life went up. Our site visitors from the Liaison Committee on Medical Education — that austere group that holds monopolistic control on medical school accreditation — found things to complain about (their *raison d'etre*), but all went well.

While all of our internal assessments of the new curriculum were comforting, they masked one secret angst. We were waiting for, if not secretly fearing, what some felt would be a more pragmatic measure of success: performance on Step 1 of the USMLE. Well, that didn't change a bit, any more than it changed from year to year, or phase of the moon, as in years past because our students are, generally, exceedingly bright.

But What About Pharmacology?

Our internal evaluations were frequent, if not incessant. By most measures there was great student satisfaction with the medical school overall, and with the curriculum and the many elements of it. Indeed, our little M1 course gained growing respect and admiration from the students, such that in about 5 years it had gone from being rated "about average" by students, in terms of overall quality, to the second best. (We were ranked right behind Gerry Abrams's pathology course, and without a doubt Gerry was deservedly acknowledged as the best and most-liked teacher in the preclinical years.) But then I became aware of an exhaustive survey of students in all four classes, conducted at the end of 2003. The findings were shocking to me, and warrant a summary here. Nearly 120 students in the M2 class that year (roughly 70% of the class) completed the survey. Among the things they were asked to comment on was their perceptions of the adequacy of curricular time devoted to studying the various basic science disciplines. For pharmacology, 21% of the respondents marked "not nearly enough" pharmacology — compared with 2% of students saying the same, on average, for each of the other basic science disciplines. (That's a 10-fold difference, folks!) Thirty-nine percent of respondents said they got "somewhat too little" pharmacology education. That compared with 10% giving the same response for the other basic science disciplines, and only 4% saying that their education in basic biomedical sciences overall was a tad on the low side. (It's worth noting that 66% of the same student evaluators said they got "somewhat or much too much" exposure to another basic science discipline, and 44% of them indicated that the quality of instruction in that discipline was either poor or fair.)

The data were disturbing, at best. I was initially restrained in my concern about pharmacology education, figuring that perhaps once students completed the clinical phase of their education they'd be able to see or appreciate better what they had learned in terms of pharmacologic knowledge. That wasn't the case. Forty-four percent of the class that graduated in 2003 stated that their education in basic pharmacology was inadequate or too little. Such high numbers were far bigger than those given to any other basic science course or discipline.

One would expect, if not at least hope, that with a huge number of students feeling that they needed more formal or better education in pharmacology, that issue would be addressed appropriately.

That was not the case. In the Fall of 2003 (before data on student perceptions about the adequacy of pharmacology content were analyzed) we launched yet another new curriculum. This one, again mandated from the Dean's Office, did not receive the widespread faculty support given the prior revision. Indeed, nearly every faculty member with whom I spoke (and there were many dozens) was opposed to it. Moreover, the question "what's going on with the new curriculum?" was uttered often, and with concern, since planning for main parts of this new go-round went right down to the wire. Students planning to matriculate in 2003 had no idea of what kind of "new curriculum" they'd experience. They were being sold the proverbial pig in a poke. The reason they didn't know anything about the new curriculum, of course, was that we didn't know. (It is no stretch of truth to say that some new M1 courses weren't put together, aside from a crude framework of start and end dates, until a couple of weeks before the activity was to start.)

And pharmacology? You know… the discipline that many students found lacking in attention.... Our well-running, highly-regarded short course was disbanded altogether. The same happened with our sister discipline, physiology. The new M1 year now evolved around systems-based sequences, in parallel with the M2 year. Topics we taught were now to be scattered throughout the sequences with little opportunity to provide cohesiveness. (As I write this, there's little information on what will happen with some key elements of our little course, because they will go into the Winter semester, and that simply hasn't been mapped out in any satisfactory detail.)

However, there's a plan (from the administration) to have our successful senior therapeutics elective become mandatory for the upcoming M4s. Great idea, mandating a revisit of pharmacology. Unfortunately, if our faculty are to be running that course we have several problems: those who have been in charge of the elective are very close to retirement; I sense no groundswell of willingness from the rest of our Department's faculty to take on that responsibility (some of the likely candidates for that course are teaching 50 or more hours in other courses); and the plan is to give that course three times each year so we can rotate the entire class through it. We simply don't have the resources to do that (well), and so no one should be surprised if that excellent course falls into the hands of the clinical faculty, out of ours.

So, one morning in April of 2003, I gave the last lecture in a series of pharmacology courses started over a hundred years ago by John Jacob Abel.

We Don't Need Be Disinvited From Teaching: We'll Make Ourselves Extinct

How and *why* did we get to a point where, I think, we're becoming irrelevant to teaching such students as those in medical school, or at least not needed?

Is this apparent demise of a separate, identifiable, and cohesive pharmacology curriculum at Michigan solely the administration's fault? Is it a national trend? Do we as a Department, or individual members of it, share some responsibility? What about the future of medical school pharmacology education by pharmacologists? Have we responsibilities there, too? Do we have the ability to keep on teaching pharmacology as we did for many years?

One can argue that because our Department has an active and well-funded research base, with many productive faculty (young and older alike), our research efforts can prepare us to teach undergraduate medical students, and do it properly. I'm not so sure. An interesting but not surprising concept that bears on the subject was articulated by some external reviewer who was invited here, I believe I recall correctly, for one of our periodic departmental evaluations. To paraphrase, "Look at the lab notebooks and publications coming from most pharmacology research labs nowadays, and if someone didn't tell you in which department the work was gone you'd be hard-pressed to figure it out on your own." In essence, similar work could be (and was being) done just as easily with the PI residing in a department of physiology, biophysics, cell biology, biochemistry, genetics.... well, you catch on.

A clear implication is that you don't need to be in a pharmacology department to do research that has pharmacologic impact. A corollary of this is that, perhaps, you don't have to be in a pharmacology department, or have formal training in pharmacology, to teach pharmacology to students other than graduate students. Are we on our way to making ourselves extinct and irrelevant by becoming or at least appearing homogeneous with all the other basic science disciplines?

It's particularly troubling to me when teaching is concerned. We hire top-notch faculty, at least in terms of their research credentials and promise. But are we instilling in them an expectation to get on the teaching wagon soon? Are we expecting of our junior faculty a desire (nor just a responsibility or burden) to teach health professions students, to become fully immersed in all that's required for optimal teaching, and to view teaching just as important as research? Do we hold their heels to the teaching fire, just as we do in terms of getting funded, expecting not only quantity but quality? Do we expect that our faculty have any formal training in basic pharmacology? After all, as our consultant noted, having that training certainly isn't necessary to do great, fundable research.

I concur with many colleagues who argue that having a Ph.D. in pharmacology isn't necessary to be a "good" teacher of pharmacology. But I think it helps, or at least makes it easier, more efficient, and ultimately more on target, content-wise, for both the instructor and the students. Both teachers and learners need what I feel is a perspective that goes (or at least can go) beyond the confines of the precise topic area as defined by the lecture or textbook title. It certainly must extend past the title or theme of one's latest grant or research publication.

Then there's the notion that if one can do an outstanding job of presenting a research seminar, one will automatically be a good teacher of such individuals as medical students. I don't agree; I've seen too many cases where the excellent seminar presenter has laid a leaden egg in the classroom.

Another notion is that regardless of

one's background (but assuming one has a doctorate in some science or bioscience), just picking up Goodman and Gilman, reading the material that relates to their assigned lecture topic, and getting onto the stage in front of 170 bright medical students, is just about all that's needed to teach optimally.

Goodman and Gilman, the bible of our discipline, is, of course, encyclopedic. But learning a discipline from an encyclopedia isn't the best or most efficient way to go, especially if you then have to teach. We used to tell our students to "read the big print" in G & G, and that's gone. But it still takes time and other forms of prior and newly acquired knowledge to figure out what's "important" to teach when you're limited to an hour to present a subject that could stand many more hours. To do that, the teacher must know what's important, and that can be derived only from being totally immersed in the specific area, and related ones, over years of exposure and learning.

To do what I think is an adequate preparatory and teaching job, you need to look at and understand other topics or concepts that may be more or less related — those other groups of drugs, or disorders for which they're used — and that in one way or another impact on the drugs you're teaching about, or the disorders for which those drugs are given. The good pharmacology teacher also needs (I maintain) a basic understanding of the underlying physiology and pathophysiology, and perhaps some anatomy too, whether to provide the more complete and lucid explanations or simply to prepare for that "good question" from a student. Not easy to do if you haven't had training in physiology or pathology, or any of the sister disciplines.

And when the audience is health professions students I think you need a reasonable grasp of clinical medicine, which is changing just as rapidly as most of the basic science disciplines. You need to pull out a copy of Cecil's or Harrison's, for example (and have the where-with-all to understand it). You need to read NEJM, Annals of Internal Medicine, and other general or specialty journals or texts for even just a little current clinical perspective. If you're teaching about local anesthetics, for example, you have to go beyond a discussion of the ins and outs of sodium channels; an overview of drug therapy of diabetes mellitus has little wiggle room for discussions of insulin synthesis of the hormone's x-ray crystallographic attributes. One's latest and rather focused research findings must not intrude on precious lecture time when you have an abundance of older but still important and widely validated information. But when the latest research is hot, and it's the most familiar stuff to you, there's a natural tendency to give it too much play in a lecture in front of students who probably don't need to hear about it at all.

I'll add another potential problem: as stellar as our faculty are with research and mentoring future scientists (those who will graduate with a PhD in pharmacology, for example), the "younger generation" is largely devoid of pharmacologic and therapeutic cultural literacy, and so it's difficult for faculty to serve as optimum role models for future teachers of health professions students. This is partly an experiential matter: fewer and fewer young faculty receive broad-based graduate educations, whether it's in pharmacology or other basic biomedical disciplines, and so it's difficult at best to pass such an appreciation on to one's students if you yourself don't have it. It is also, perhaps more so, a matter of conscious or unconscious choice and necessity: research productivity and funding helps most with professional stature, promotion, and salary.

Regardless of the root causes of a failure to instill a broad appreciation of the discipline, the emphasis is on research. Teaching is a dreaded nuisance that takes time from the "important stuff" — teaching large classes of undergrad health professions students is to be avoided except for what will count towards promotion.

Our students (even I) rightly see the many necessities for and benefits of research; likewise, I think many of them see faculty disdain for teaching (at least to students other than graduate students) and assimilate it in their attitudes, behaviors, goals and objectives, and even fears. And they may have heard the message "If you lose your grant you have to teach more." That, to me, instantly lessens the institutional value of teaching, and puts it more in the light of punishment than a worthwhile activity for which, I believe, we're here in the first place. No wonder students (and faculty too) would rather do research than teach. While I haven't had any grad students since 1996, when I went into medical administration and then focused exclusively on teaching and writing, I've gotten to know many of our grad students reasonably well. And, over the 20 or so years I've been running my nursing pharmacology course I've had about 40 grad student teaching assistants from our Department. I'd be generous if I said I've encountered more than three or four of them who expressed any deep desire to teach as part of their long-term career plans, beyond what their future employers might consider to be the bare minimum requirements for an academic position.

Whither Pharmacology

Whatever the causes of what I perceive as problems, I wonder what we're doing in a substantive way to remedy them. Some say there is no problem to fix anyway. Some say we can just let the clinicians do all the teaching. (I've often encountered "real docs" who would gladly teach more, and believe they could do a better job than we basic scientists. But when push comes to shove they're too busy in the clinics, or on the wards, and teaching becomes oh such an annoyance that also hurts the revenue stream. Clinicians, especially the superdocs we find here in abundance, aren't the ideal solution either.)

Where pharmacology (as a discipline) goes, what it will become or how it will look, depends to a great degree on how we "define" pharmacology — not simply as the title on a building directory or journal, but as a discipline that is unique in both the scientific and educational sense. I think most of us will agree that one of the beauties of our discipline is that it encompasses and even enriches the other basic science disciplines. There are interrelations with biochemistry, physiology, and cell biology (as examples); there is room for (and we rightly embrace) all sorts of methodologic approaches or "orientations," whether they are the more traditional systems-oriented approaches (transitional research) or those of an immunologic, molecular, or genetic nature; they can be oriented towards neural, cardiovascular, behavioral; and so on.

Where we go, what we look like — indeed, even if we survive — is up to us. If we just look at academic institutions like ours, a necessary blend of both educational and investigative missions, and ignore the future needs of drug companies, you may see that there aren't many people besides ourselves who are advocating and rooting for our future. Some don't even know what it is we do — at least do differently, when it comes to research. Others may have a better sense of our missions, but feel that we don't "own" the roles and responsibilities, and we're not the only or best ones to take on those tasks. The support needs to come from on top: the deans. However, I believe most medical school deans would just as soon do with one less department, one less administrative layer (although they will, no doubt, add more administrative layers of their own), and "ad hoc" the educational mission.

29

*Projection to the Future**

*Maurice H. Seevers, M.D., Ph.D.***

It was easy in 1939 to portray to the Council of the American Society for Pharmacology and Experimental Therapeutics why, as a relatively young man, I contemplated deserting pharmacology for a more promising field. Survival of the subject as an independent discipline was at stake.

In 1947, the course of events had furnished the background for survival, but strong action was needed. It was not difficult, as President of the Society, to join with the survivors and the newer generation in the Rockefeller Foundation-sponsored Conference on Graduate Education in Pharmacology to chart a course that could assure pharmacology a respected place among the medical sciences.

In 1969, need for unusual action is not apparent. The corpus of pharmacology is strong and expanding rapidly. Few doubt its importance or despair for its survival. Excellent young men are entering the field. What more is there to say? Why, then, should one who will not participate in future developments in pharmacology attempt to project its future?

With misgivings for having accepted this task, I hoped, with plagiary in mind, to find a precedent for "futures" in other historical accounts, but without success. However, a paragraph in the foreword to the History of The American Physiological Society, Semicentennial, 1987-1937 by Walter J. Meek, one of my beloved preceptors, gave a possible clue to what was consciously or subconsciously in the minds of those oldsters, like myself, who have had this assignment. Today, many of Meek's statements about physiology apply equally well to pharmacology:

> The American Physiological Society, from its foundation, has been an important factor in the scientific life of our country. It has become a notable American institution. It is a forum in which are presented the current researches in the physiological sciences. It is the owner and manager of two great journals. It is the mother of other societies. It is a vital, growing organization. Not only has its past been honorable and productive, but at the present moment it is more prosperous in point of number and scientific activity than any period of its history. There is every indication that its value and influence will continue to increase as the years go by.

This Committee has limited my task further by defining clearly and specifically the knowledge gaps in modern therapeutics that may constitute the areas of future research in general pharmacology. I have assumed, therefore, that the choice of one who has survived the rigors implies some qualifications for discussing the future in light of the past – a tacit admission that somehow the fears that

---

* Written in 1969, reprinted with permission from *The American Society for Pharmacology and Experimental Therapeutics: The First Sixty Years*, 1908-1969, Edited by K.K. Chen. 1969. Pp. 207-220.

** Deceased

plagued earlier generations of pharmacologists have not been entirely dispelled – or have others emerged to take their place?

I have attempted in what follows to evaluate and discuss certain fundamentals that have always confronted pharmacology and are important to its future, its scope as a science and its independence as a discipline, its relation to the other biomedical sciences and to clinical medicine, its importance as an interpreter of drug and chemical effects in the interests of the public health, and its evaluation of the effects of drugs on society as a whole. If this discourse appears to lack organization, it is because of the interlocking nature of these problems.

From the beginning, pharmacologists, even Buchheim and Schmiedeberg, found it difficult to circumscribe a specific body of scientific knowledge and say, this is the substance of, and therefore belongs exclusively to, the science of pharmacology. Its very nature requires that pharmacology be dependent on the physical and biomedical sciences for concepts of normal cell and organ function and for methodology. In the early days, a majority of the leaders in the biomedical sciences viewed pharmacology as an applied branch of physiology or biochemistry, not worthy of recognition as an independent discipline. Some still do.

In 1924, when I began the study of pharmacology, my preceptor A.L. Tatum was the only pharmacologist in a joint department with physiological chemistry. In those days, the subject was commonly subordinated to physiology or physiological chemistry, scientifically and politically, or left alone to deal with materia medica and therapeutics, an ill-defined and lackluster castoff, below the dignity of most clinicians. In short, pharmacology was held in low esteem by scientists and clinicians alike and with more than a little justification. The few who arose in its defense had great difficulty in citing specific contributions of pharmacology on which to base their case. But in that same year, 1924, Abel made a gallant and worthy try in a letter to Abraham Flexner:

> ....all of these substance are drugs and constitute a great part of the proper field of the study of the pharmacologist. I am fully aware that they also constitute the field of study for the physiologist, the pathologist, and other medical scientists. The scope of this domain is so large that there is ample opportunity for all the above-named individuals to work without ousting the pharmacologist or subordinating him to some other field....I care little for labels and names – you can extend the use of physiology to clinical medicine; you can call pathology abnormal physiology; you can call pharmacology applied physiology; and make otherwise use of this term. All of this, however, does not alter the fact that the increasing and steadily growing contents of pharmacological science which is applying physics and chemistry in the most advanced and minute way to the problems of cell action, which is almost daily making new additions to our armamentarium of drugs, cannot be subordinated to physiology which has its own problems which may or may not interlock with pharmacology....The science has its own problems and quite aside from achievements that are of immediately assistance to the physician, which are of fundamental character and allied to physiology but, in reality, belong to the vast realm of experimental biology and medicine. To these problems, the pharmacologist brings his own viewpoints and methods, just as the biochemist or the physiologist may do....I have always maintained that the more varying types in the way of

> pharmacologists, physiologists, pathologists, and anatomists the better. Let one pharmacologist be more of a chemist, another more of a physiologist, another more of a clinician. The main thing, I think, is taking ability for granted, as this is the main requisite – that all of these men should be more than mere pharmacologist or physiologist or what-not, but that their interests should be broad, that they could be classed as students, or investigators in the broad field of experimental medicine and biology....I hope that pharmacology will keep on accumulating, along with its practical discoveries, an increasingly great amount of such apparently, for the moment, useless knowledge.

Although this demonstrated Abel's breadth as a man, scientist, and physician, his effort did not alter the trend.

In the darkest days (the 1930s), pharmacologists, in dwindling numbers, found principal preoccupation with the question: What is the matter with pharmacology? Attempts were made to redefine the subject, give it a different name, shift it from a biological to a physical science (pharmacy), and the like. Many deserted for fields that offered a better future.

The development of the sulfonamides and the antibiotics, the coming of the atomic age, the great achievements in organic and physical chemistry and biophysics associated with World War II, and the phenomenal advances in the knowledge of cell and organ function in all of the biomedical sciences furnished the substance from which a new pharmacology was built. The passage of the Food and Drug Amendments of 1938 created a new demand for pharmacologists in industry and government; politicians, impressed by the effectiveness of large-scale wartime research efforts, furnished the funds, not only for research, but also for training – a most important need.

Today, pharmacology no longer needs to be sharply circumscribed to find its place in the scheme of things. In this era of molecular biology, defining pharmacology to encompass the action of all chemicals on all living matter is accepted with little debate. Even a few decades ago, such a definition would have elicited snorts of derision.

In spite of having some of the earlier fears— engulfment by clinical medicine or physiology, or dominance by industrial scientists if they were permitted membership in the Society— alleviated, some disquiet still exists among pharmacologists. For example, there are those who, viewing the current administrative trends in some medical schools, especially the appointment to important chairs of scientists who cannot qualify as pharmacologists, would again raise the specter of survival, not only for scientific, but for political reasons. They point out that molecular biology finds no need for traditional lines of separation of the biological sciences, and they argue that the threat to pharmacology lies in the fact that the other biomedical sciences can also be defined in terms of the action of chemicals on living things. Ergo, merge them all into one unit, possibly under what is called today "biochemistry."

This specter, I think, should be laid to rest. If such a threat does indeed exist, it does not apply specifically or solely to pharmacology, and, for practical reasons alone, it seems improbable in the foreseeable future. However, defining pharmacology in terms of the universe creates some problems with which pharmacology must deal.

Any individual scientist in the physiological or biological sciences, or even in the social sciences, can identify as a pharmacologist by examining, or even contemplating, drug-cell interactions. Very often, such an individual has little, if any, knowledge of the principles that govern such interactions or the complexity of the biological systems with which he is dealing. The height of absurdity is reached when such persons extrapolate their data to human therapeutics. This makes a large contribution to the vast rubbish literature of pseudopharmacology, of which I shall speak later.

A second and very significant problem for pharmacology is created by those who leave the impression that molecular pharmacology is the only thing that really counts. Without discounting the great importance of this facet of pharmacology, there is clearly a vast knowledge gap between the many theories and the few facts relating to conformation analysis of receptors, and the many facts concerning drug-enzyme interactions, for example, and the demonstrable action of drugs on the intact organism as a basis for the intelligent and safe use of drugs in man. Indeed, one can logically raise the question, if molecular pharmacology represents the basis of pharmacology, what is pharmacology?

Clearly, a dichotomy in thinking existed among the current leaders of American pharmacology who prepared the report of the Pharmacology and Toxicology Training Committee. In the section on "General Pharmacology at Present" we find:

> Pharmacology as we know it today is little more than 50 years old. In this time, as any informed layman knows, its record of accomplishment is truly phenomenal. The advances in pharmacology in this century have constituted many of the familiar medical miracles. The medical practitioner today enters the sickroom backed by a therapeutic armamentarium that has been developed largely by the scientific methods of pharmacologic discipline.

Contrast the optimisim expressed in this paragraph with the pessimism of the section on "Molecular Pharmacology:"

> Biochemical pharmacology has suddenly gained importance, in fact is bound to replace "classical biochemistry" after decades of latency.... The development of modern biochemical pharmacology demands great expertness in physical sciences, enzymology, and biophysics, requirements that are hardly met within "classical training" in pharmacology as visualized by empirically oriented proponents. Yet this trend is inevitable, and the other one (termed "classical training") will merely furnish raw material, incapable of dealing with its true problems. Society has the choice to support costly, future (empirical) hit-or-miss games, providing only temporary successes followed by greater confusions (new drugs vs. old drugs games), or to invest in the difficult but predictably successful approach, which is bound to produce as hard realities as did the relativity theory in form of present-day nuclear chemistry.
>
> At the present, arguments in favor of abandoning "the old trend" are numerous (e.g., inability to solve cancer, old age as a disease, etc.), and true successes in molecular pharmacology are yet few (e.g., mode of action of antibiotics, contribution to genetic chemistry). But "lack of success" in the case of empirical pharmacology is, in fact, an overriding argument for turning to the novel enterprise.

It would appear to an old fossil that society also has the choice of whether to maintain the "status quo" as far as new drugs are concerned for an untold number of years, or to pursue the "old trend" with reliance on the most modern pharmacologic technology until the "natural laws which permit 'coordination' of enzymes into biological function processes" are discovered – clearly not an easy task with over 100,000 known organic substances and 700-800 enzymes.

Apparently, I am not the only one who is confused about the use of the terms "molecular" and "biochemical" pharmacology. It would seem from the Statement of Purpose of our new Society journal, Molecular Pharmacology, that this term embraces about everything chemical, physicochemical, biochemical, biophysical, theoretical, or practical. This is somewhat difficult to harmonize with the statement quoted above "true successes in molecular pharmacology are yet few (e.g., mode of action of antibiotics, contributions to genetic chemistry)." If molecular pharmacology encompasses everything chemical and is synonymous with biochemical pharmacology, it has been with us a long time and would not appear to need the hard sell.

In the summary of the Pharmacology and Toxicology Training Committee report, we find a somewhat less forceful and more mature and meaningful appraisal of molecular pharmacology: "When one considers the number of drugs, it is clear that this important field is in its infancy, if not still in a gestation period." Evidently, a majority hold that some growth must occur before this infant can fill adult apparel and that "molecular" is not synonymous with "biochemical" pharmacology.

Be that as it may, pharmacology might appear to be free of the paranoias of the past if the present generation is willing to challenge "classical" biochemistry and assume responsibility for the solution of cancer and old age.

I would not chew this bone unless I believed strongly that even the suggestion that "classical" pharmacology be abandoned represents a predictable risk in loss of perspective, not only for pharmacology as a scientific and political entity, but for the individual investigator as well. It would be a great disservice to pharmacology as a discipline if the scientists who followed the "classical" approach were relegated, even inferentially, to a category of second-class citizens solely because their interests and skills did not utilize a biochemical approach.

In the area of central nervous system pharmacology, for example, most of the clinically proven drugs were discovered by scientists or clinicians who were trained in observing and interpreting behavioral responses. In the few instances where their actions are clearly identified with enzymes as inhibitors or competitors, these attributes were determined secondarily and still serve largely as a means of screening new drugs for potential behavioral studies.

Who will acquire the facts needed to fill the knowledge gap between molecular pharmacology and the application of pharmacologic knowledge to human therapeutics or in the public health? This is a research area involving what was once called the physiological approach— information obtained by conventional physiological methods and/or direct observation and analysis of drug-induced behavior in the intact animal. This type of research may be less spectacular, but it is equally important and, in some ways, more difficult than molecular pharmacology.

Is this area to be relegated to those who do not qualify as pharmacologists either on the basis of their training or knowledge? It would seem unwise. To create such a vacuum would assure the usurpation of this vast area by the poorly trained and incompetent, a first step in the scientific and possibly in the political demise of pharmacology.

In a field of such scope as pharmacology, any individual investigator may expect to make a significant contribution in only a very limited area of research. Wisdom would counsel that, other things being equal and having made his choice, the investigator persists in a limited area of research until he becomes a master. The history of biomedical research reveals that the advent of each new major advance in knowledge creates a "gold rush" of many investigators to apply these new findings to their own problems. A certain few, with the proper background and good fortune, may strike a rich vein; many with an inadequate academic stake, finding the work tedious, the competition tough, and the nuggets few, may become disenchanted and desert the entire field.

What, then, is pharmacology and what makes a pharmacologist? I cannot improve on the substance or perspective of paragraphs from the summary of the same Committee Report:

> Pharmacologists, guided by a set of principles which allowed them to organize their observations of the effects of chemical substances on living structures in a meaningful way, have brought many drugs of great usefulness for man's benefit to positions where they can be employed with maximum safety and effectiveness, despite the fact that the intimate mechanisms of action of these drugs are not well understood.
>
> Many of these principles are so important to the proper examination of the effects of chemical substances on living systems or their components – whether these are being studied in the whole and exceedingly complex human in a clinical situation or at any point along the continuum of organizational levels down to submolecular events now being probed by a few molecular pharmacologists – that the principles themselves merit brief review in this summary. These principles concern: 1) the relationship between the concentration of a chemical compound (drug or poison) and the response of the living reactor or its components, 2) the time-action curve, 3) the factors of absorption, distribution, binding, biotransformation, and elimination, 4) chemical structure-biological action relationships, 5) bioassay in some instances, 6) factors of repeated drug use, such as tolerance, cumulative effects, chronic intoxication, habituation, addiction, and adverse reactions, 7) antagonism or enhancement of one chemical's effect by another, 8) the localization of the site of drug action within the living system or its components, and 9) most difficult of all, the mechanism by which the action is brought about.
>
> All pharmacologists and toxicologists must have a thorough understanding of these principles. This group of scientists is bound together by these common concerns, even though they may be widely separated along the spectrum of specialties required for working with the effects of chemicals on systems as complex in one direction as the submolecular events involved in the intimate action of a drug molecular on a single sensitive type of macromolecular component of a cell and as complex in the other direction as the subtle behavioral changes observable in a person who has ingested a relatively few molecules of, for example, a powerful hallucinatory drug.
>
> The extreme diversity of conceptual and technical capabilities required for an effective attack on the unsolved questions in these fields of pharmacology and toxicology makes it, in one sense, practically the most interdisciplinary of the medical sciences. The development of increasingly specialized research in these fields is, therefore, not at all surprising.

Like other biomedical disciplines, the subject matter of pharmacology has become so great that division into subspecialties with their own journals was inevitable. Some hold that pharmacology as an organized society is poorer today for failing to have circumscribed chemotherapy, toxicology, and psychopharmacology, and worry about further splintering of the subject.

Pharmacology as a broad discipline will suffer only if the organizations representing the subfields fail to support training in general pharmacology as a basis for their specialty programs or go their own way, failing to recognize the importance of the common functions and goals that unite pharmacology as a discipline.

I hope we would not become so interested in the anatomy of pharmacology that we lose sight of its function. Pharmacology, as a political entity, is more likely to survive because of its function than because of its substance. Without doubt, the founders of the Society visualized its prime function in terms of establishing a scientific basis for therapeutics. Modern developments have broadened the scope to include all chemicals that affect the public health.

Seventeen of the 18 founders of the Society were physicians; many were full-time practitioners. The early identification of pharmacology with medicine and medical schools has colored its subsequent existence. In contrast with some other biomedical sciences, it has never flourished apart from a clinical association. Although it is no longer necessary, nor desirable, that all pharmacologists be physicians, many should be— even some who may not follow clinical pharmacology as a specialty. It is important to pharmacology as a discipline that it be interpreted to the clinician by one who knows from experience how the problems of the clinic differ from those of the laboratory.

It may be of great importance for the future of pharmacology that physician-pharmacologists heed the precept of A.L. Tatum: remember you are a physician first, a pharmacologist second. It was his strong belief that the strength of pharmacology in medical schools comes in convincing the clinician that pharmacology has something unique to offer the medical student and the practitioner, something that is not forthcoming from other basic sciences or from the clinician himself. It was his equally strong belief, amply supported by historical events, that if pharmacology depended for its strength on biochemistry and physiology, it would remain an anemic weakling in the medical school hierarchy, if it survived at all.

Today, medical educators seem to have finally solved the chicken-egg game with the basic sciences versus clinical medicine by concluding that both come first. The resulting curricular shifts, without altering subject content, have significantly left pharmacology, like all basic sciences, at loose ends. Some of this restructuring will upgrade the educational process if it breaks down the long-existing artificial barriers between the basic sciences and the clinic. Some changes are wheel-spinning, others academic spelunking. Where such changes distort the relative importance of the essential elements that a physician needs to practice modern medicine— for example, submerging therapeutics to diagnosis— then pharmacology has reason to be concerned.

After 60 years, we hear echoes of the cries from some of the charter members of this Society who objected to the use of "Experimental Therapeutics" in the Society name. Will pharmacology in medical schools be disenfranchised by clinical medicine?

Since preparing this discussion, an article has appeared: "Pharmacology: Its Nature in Medicine" (Science 161: 443, 1968). Thomas H. Maren, the pharmacologist-author, discusses in detail and with good perspective the problems confronting pharmacology as an administrative and teaching unit in medical schools, emphasizing the chronic shortage of leaders in the field capable of filling the critical positions in universities, government, and industry.

Let me say this. If pharmacology is submerged it will be in institutions where the pharmacologist, even though medically trained, identifies pharmacology only in laboratory terms. It is not likely to happen where pharmacology occupies an important position in the basic and clinical teaching of medical students throughout their educational program; where clinical pharmacology conducts training programs at the postdoctoral level and is recognized as a bridge between general pharmacology and clinical medicine; where the clinical pharmacologist is trained in both; where he is formally and physically associated with both; where he interprets laboratory findings in clinical terms and serves as a coordinator in all things of a clinical-pharmacological nature. In the long run, it may be that this type of cooperative activity will be a principal reason why general pharmacology, as an independent discipline, will survive in medical schools.

Unless pharmacology continues to assume the role of principal interpreter of the effects of chemicals and drugs in man, it will have abandoned its heritage, since this is its only function that is unique.

The biochemical pharmacologist fragments the organism in order to study its component parts; the organ-oriented subdivisions of pharmacology are engrossed with specific technics and interests; the clinical pharmacologist, while dealing with drug effects on man, is also a specialist: toxicology is too often identified only with small animal pharmacology. In order to bring perspective to medical and public health problems concerning drugs, information from all sources, subcellular to the whole organism, must be evaluated with a minimum of bias. Often, the pertinent information is found only in indigenous medicine. Often, the picture must be constructed primarily from witnesses from the past. Competence for such reconstruction requires a broad background in the laboratory, with more than a passing knowledge of the clinic, a "composite" pharmacologist, if you please.

This is pharmacology.

The broad nature of the subject matter of pharmacology lends itself with particular ease to encroachment by many kinds of pseudoscience and pseudoscientists. Unfortunately, there is a substantial group of individuals, some scientists, even in "high places," practicing what, for a lack of a better term, I will designate "pseudopharmacology." This includes those who lack the background or desire to bring perspective to the problem of drug action. It includes the hypercritical as well as the uncritical and those who purposely distort facts to support what they consider a worthy end.

Many of the most difficult public health problems (alcoholism, drug dependence, tobacco smoking, air and stream pollution, pesticides, food additives, over-the-counter drugs), involving as they do the total population, become the special province of a whole array of "experts"— well-meaning but scientifically ignorant reformers; commentators and writers in communications media who misinterpret facts to fit their own bias or create spectaculars; politicians who find this a rich potential for popular appeal; scientists who do not limit their pronouncements to their own area of competence, including even some pharmacologists.

I can best illustrate what I mean by pseudopharmacology as practiced by scientists by citing a few examples: inflation of inconsequential data by elaborate statistical treatment, masking poor design and inadequate data by disguising them as hypotheses, acceptance of data obtained with gadgetry even if they conflict with observations of behavior, extrapolation of data obtained by chronic administration of unrealistic doses in small animals to prediction of drug or chemical toxicity in man, ignoring long-time human experience in favor of arbitrary margins of safety in animals as a measure of safety in man, and many more. Pseudopharmacology of scientist or lay origin weakens the integrity, devalues the importance, and dilutes the effectiveness of pharmacology as a biomedical discipline. It not only confuses the public, but may glamorize the hazard it purports to expose. If pharmacology is to achieve its greatest stature in the future, pharmacologists in responsible positions must be willing, as individuals, to sacrifice their own private and research time to combat these hazards to pharmacology and the public health.

We are in an extraordinary time in history when change takes over on a wholesale basis. The research and development revolution is transforming nearly all aspects of our daily life. The explosion of knowledge, coupled with the obsolescence of knowledge, makes it impossible to predict future developments. Continuous automation and the computer have changed the machines and skills required to operate them. Biologists are expected to keep pace.

It is extremely difficult to explain to the public, or even for biomedical scientists to bear in mind, that one machine remains the same – the most complex of all, the animal and human body. It operates with remarkable efficiency and fidelity, yet we know comparatively little about how and why. The pharmacologist can speed it up, slow it down, in whole or in part, but he cannot make it create any new function. He can take it apart and study the pieces, but he cannot reassemble it.

Pharmacology must be prepared to adapt itself to new and future developments in science and medicine. Clearly, the scientific and medical facts that presently constitute the substance of pharmacology will expand greatly in the future; the need to acquire new facts about drug-cell interactions at all levels of biological organization will continue to accelerate; and although interpretations of drug actions may change remarkably, the need for the rational application of these facts and interpretations to the art and practice of medicine and to the public health will become even more important. Whether this body of knowledge and its interpretations remain in the hands of those who today call themselves pharmacologists depends on how well they take cognizance of the strengths and weaknesses of pharmacology as related to other scientific and medical disciplines.

The young man, intrigued with the glamour of medical science, who contemplates for the future, or has already begun, a life work in pharmacology might do well to consider the following.

Wisdom dictates an early decision to enter the field since proper qualification requires many years of dedicated effort. The scope of pharmacology is great. A broad as well as an intimate understanding of drug action requires a substantial knowledge of mathematics and the physical and biological sciences. Hopefully, he would superimpose this special training on a general education in the humanities and social sciences. With this background, he should seek the highest quality training in general pharmacology, regardless of his ultimate goal as a research specialist. He must be a pharmacologist first. Abel, who was one of the founders of the Biochemical Society as well as the Pharmacological Society and more of a biochemist, said, "Let one pharmacologist be more of a chemist, another more of a physiologist, and another more of a clinician." He did not say, let one be a chemist, one a physiologist, and another a clinician.

Society expects returns on its training investment in terms of individual research achievements. Pharmacology pulls in may directions, but unidirectional research effort is usually more rewarding. It is to the advantage of the investigator to utilize the most advanced equipment and technology, keeping in mind, however, that none has been devised that compares with "a seeing eye to a thinking brain."

The ultimate goal of pharmacologic research is an understanding of the mechanism of action at the molecular level. While fascinating, worthy of extensive pursuit, and probably in the long run a most important approach, it is a very specialized area. Success requires an unusual training, a creative mind not hampered by convention, an interest in theory rather than practice, and other talents not possessed by all who would enter pharmacology. All need not, and should not, undertake it. In terms of the prime functions of pharmacology as a basis for rational therapeutics, and in the protection of the public health, the role of molecular pharmacology is no more and no less exalted than any other subdivision of pharmacology. It is not likely to yield many new drugs or contribute much to the public health in the foreseeable future.

With a solid foundation in general pharmacology, postdoctoral training in a specialized field is highly desirable. Serendipity favors the prepared mind.

Pharmacology is an interdisciplinary science. The advantages of division of labor in reaching major research objectives should be recognized early in the career of a pharmacologist. But he should know that cooperative projects are difficult and often require submerging individualism to a common goal.

Pharmacology attracts persons from all walks of science. Each may make an important contribution, whether in academic, industrial, or government employ. The horizon of a pharmacologist will be expanded greatly if he works with individuals in these several areas, who may follow other routes to the same objective. Like the art of medicine, there is also an art of pharmacology; the ability to make choices, decisions, and even projection from pieces of the whole.

Constantly aware of the prime function of pharmacology as a basis for therapeutics and in protecting the public health, one should always be cognizant of the weakness inherent in the extrapolation of data from lower forms to man; training in medicine, although not essential, may give him a better perspective.

The proper interpretation of pharmacological data in the interests of the public health requires that the pharmacologist recognize his own scientific limitations, respect the opinions of other knowledgeable persons in other fields, even while disagreeing, and have disrespect for, and a willingness to stand out against, pseudopharmacology in all its forms. The ability of a pharmacologist to bring perspective to public health problems involving drugs or chemicals is one of his unique functions.

My search for an American whose career as a pharmacologist had not only a profound impact on pharmacology but also on medicine because he possessed many of these attributes was not difficult. Of all the pharmacologists of my acquaintance, none had human qualities more worthy of emulation, or more common sense, than Torald Sollmann. Joseph Seifter, his last student, said of him, "He did not base the future of pharmacology on spectacular discoveries, but on steady growth. He considered those engaged in his field as ordinary humans with a capacity for hard work, imagination, and self-development rather than possessors of unusual genius." In addition to his contributions to pharmacology and toxicology, his administrative duties as a medical school dean, and his scholarly pursuits as an artist and poet, he gave of his energies to matters of medicine and of the public health. He was a charter member of the Council of Pharmacy and Chemistry (now the Council on Drugs) of the AMA, serving continuously for over 50 years, more than 20 years as its chairman. Those of us who were fortunate enough to serve under him in this capacity never found him devoid of knowledge about drugs or men, or out of perspective, or failing in his concern for the future of pharmacology and its relation to medicine and the public health. Although past 90, always looking to the future, he was still revising his famous textbook, which was the "bible" of my student days. His advice to pharmacologists, present or future, is timeless:

> You younger men and women: keep your eyes on the mountains, but do not stop cultivating the plains. "All this is very fine, but let us cultivate our cabbages" – "C'la est bien diet, repondit Candide, mais il faut cultiver notre jardin"— Do not expect to be always dining on pheasant and artichokes; do not make the mistake of despising corned beef and cabbage: they give you strength to scale those mountains, and the mountains cannot be scaled without them– ONLY– never rest content with humble results. Be not as he who digs for treasure and is happy when he turns up a fishworm.
>
> "Mit gier'ger Hand nach Schatzen grabt
> Und froh ist wenn er Regenwurmer findet."

30

Epilogue

"One area of concern is whether the basic science departments, as [their] research programs and faculty expertise focus on cellular and molecular processes, will possess the necessary faculty with expertise to support the [undergraduate] medical student educational program in traditional areas of organ physiology, histology, and pharmacology. This might require realignment of teaching from the basic science departments to the clinical departments and other units possessing necessary expertise. The Associate Dean for Medical Education... is working with the Department Chairs [sic] to assure that faculty expertise is present to support the [undergraduate] medical education program."

Quoted from the *University of Michigan Medical School Institutional Self-Study Task Force Report on Medical Education*, submitted to the Liaison Committee on Medical Education. December 2003.

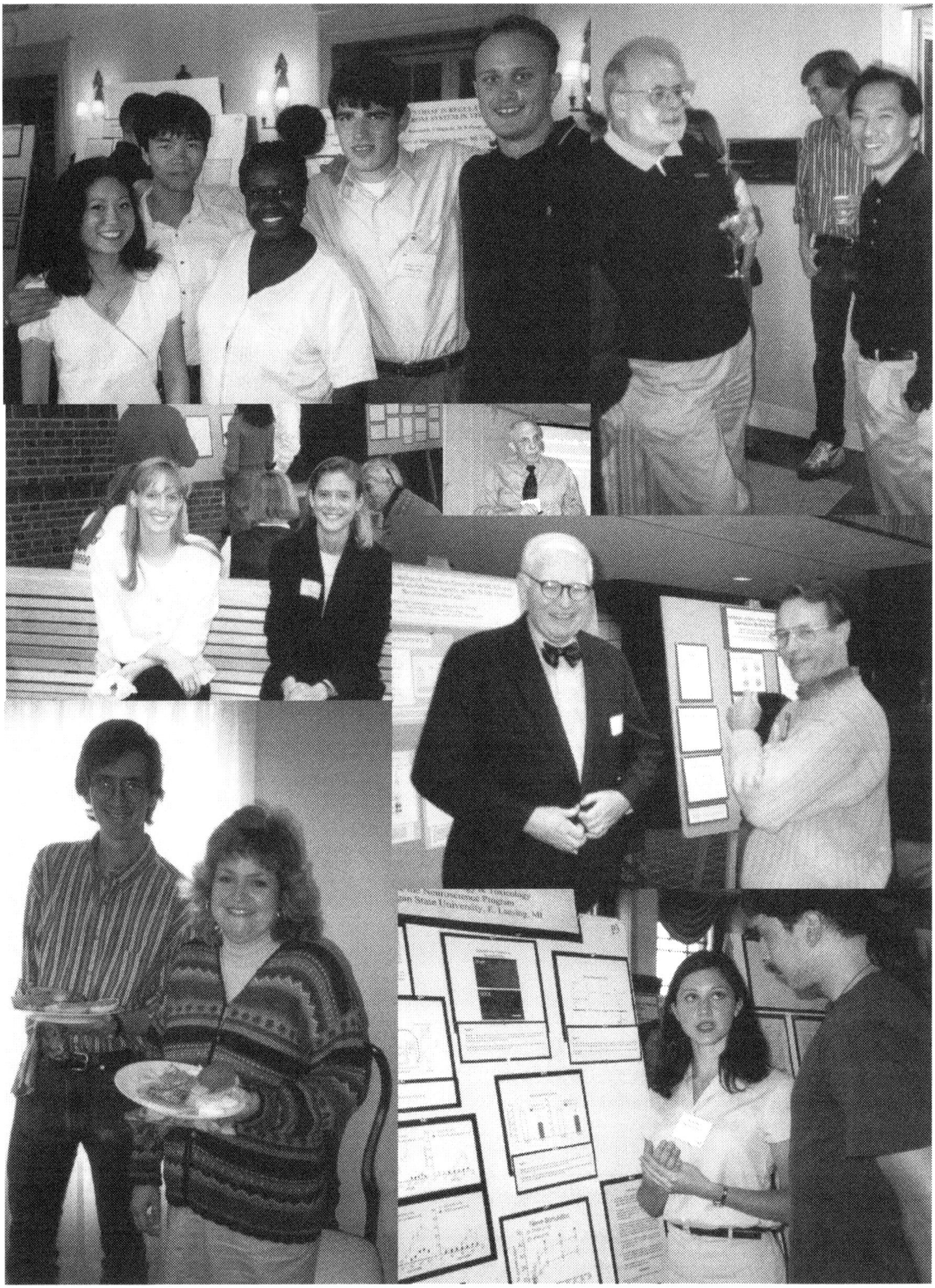

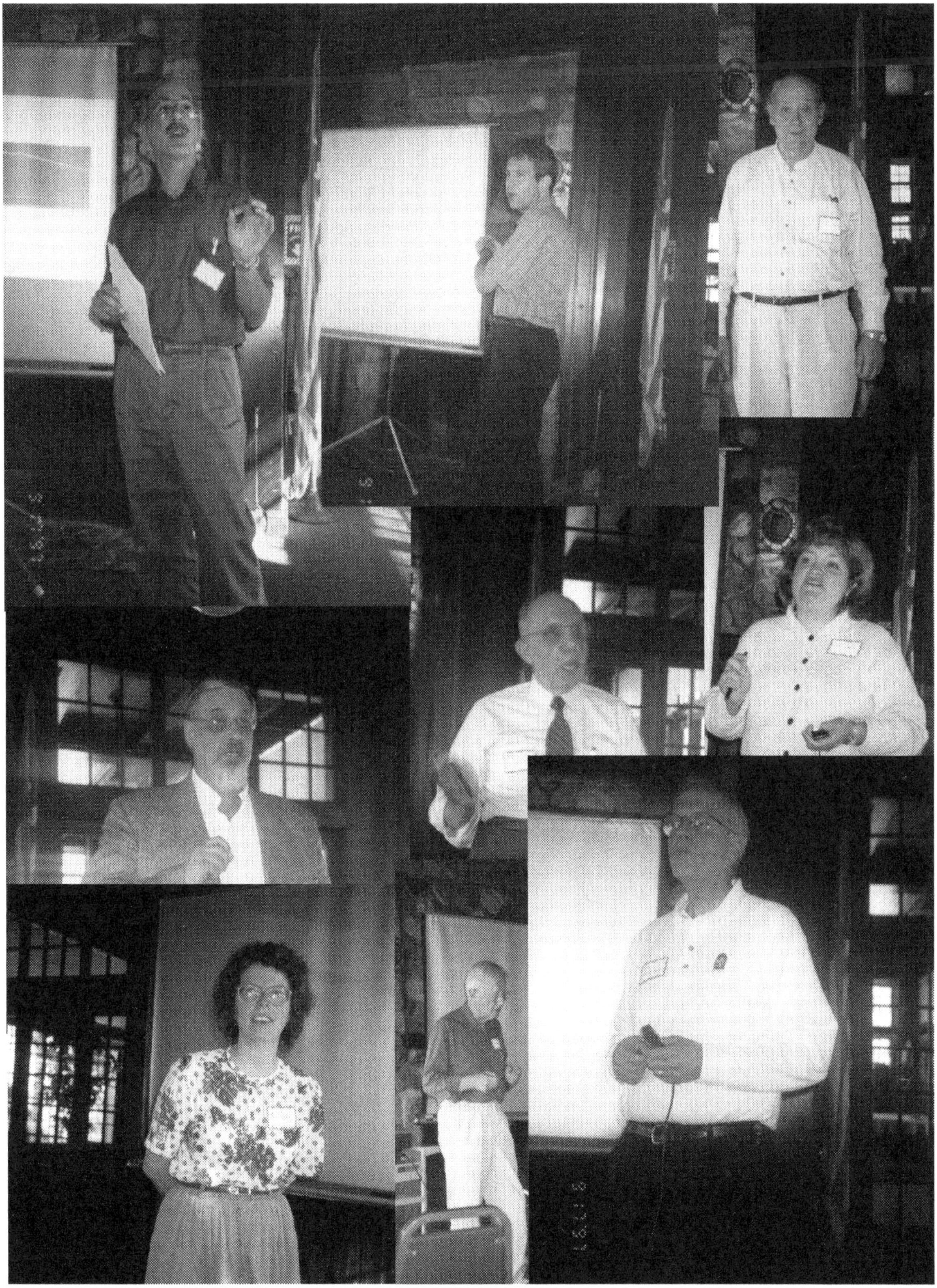

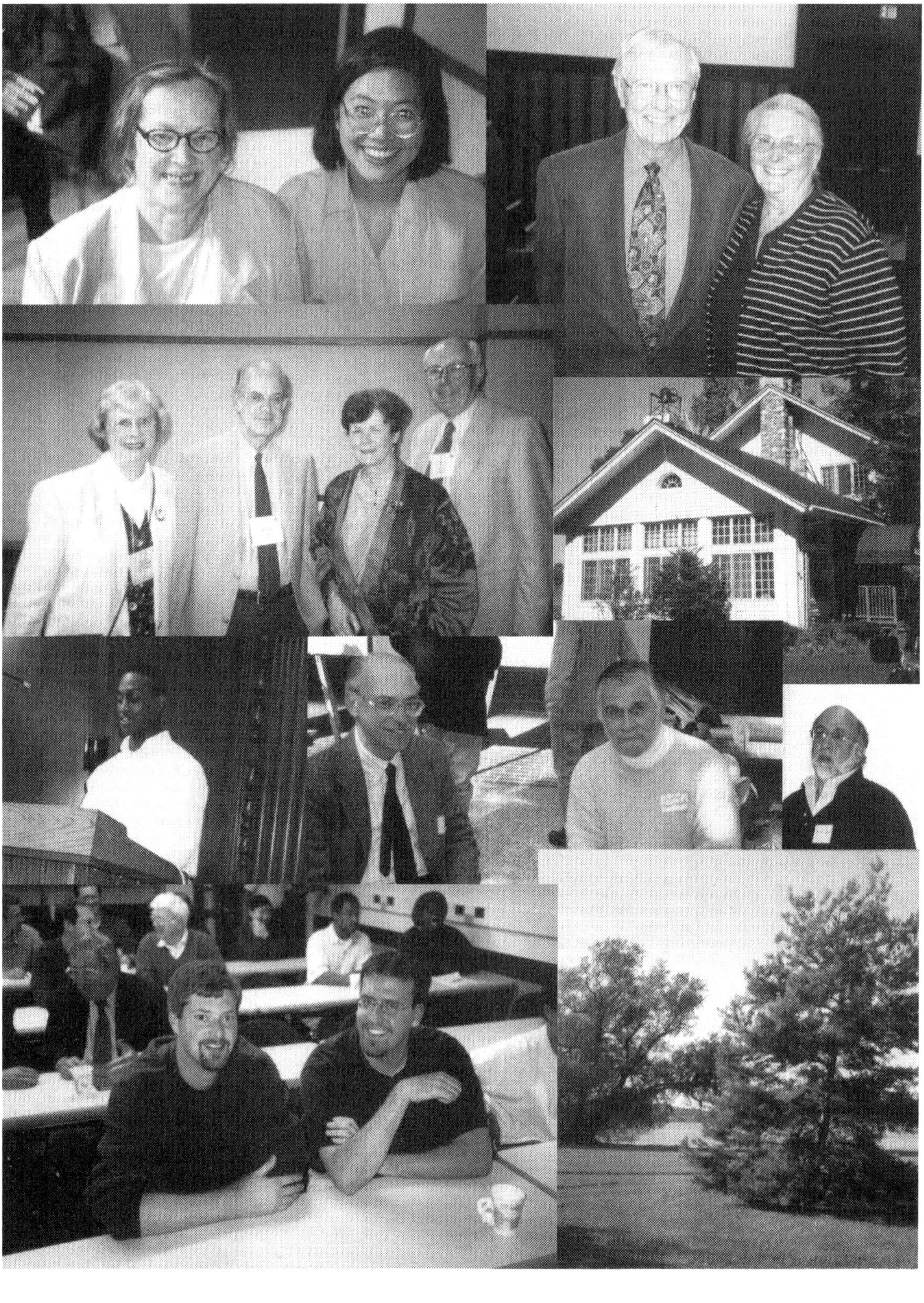

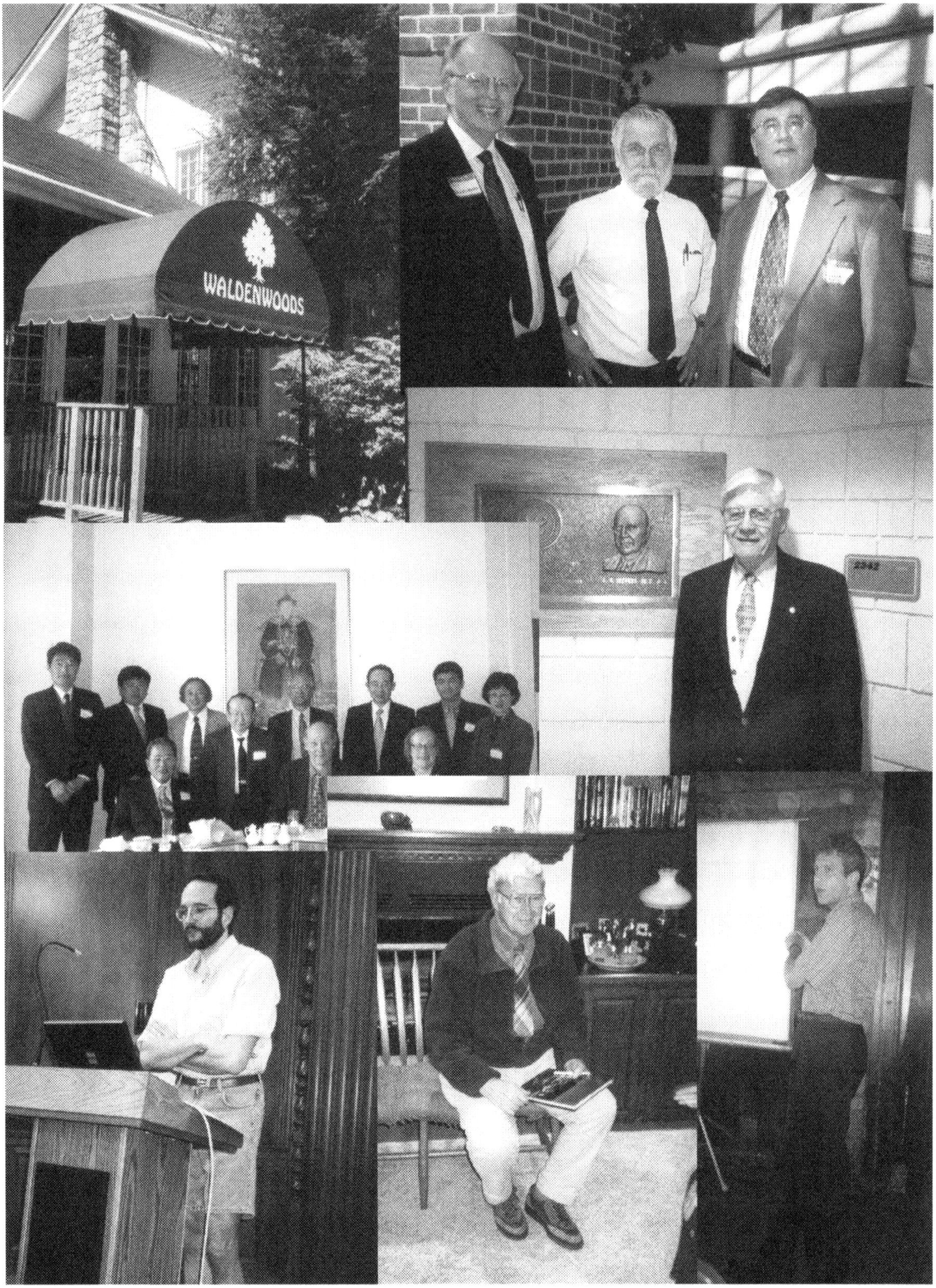
WALDENWOODS

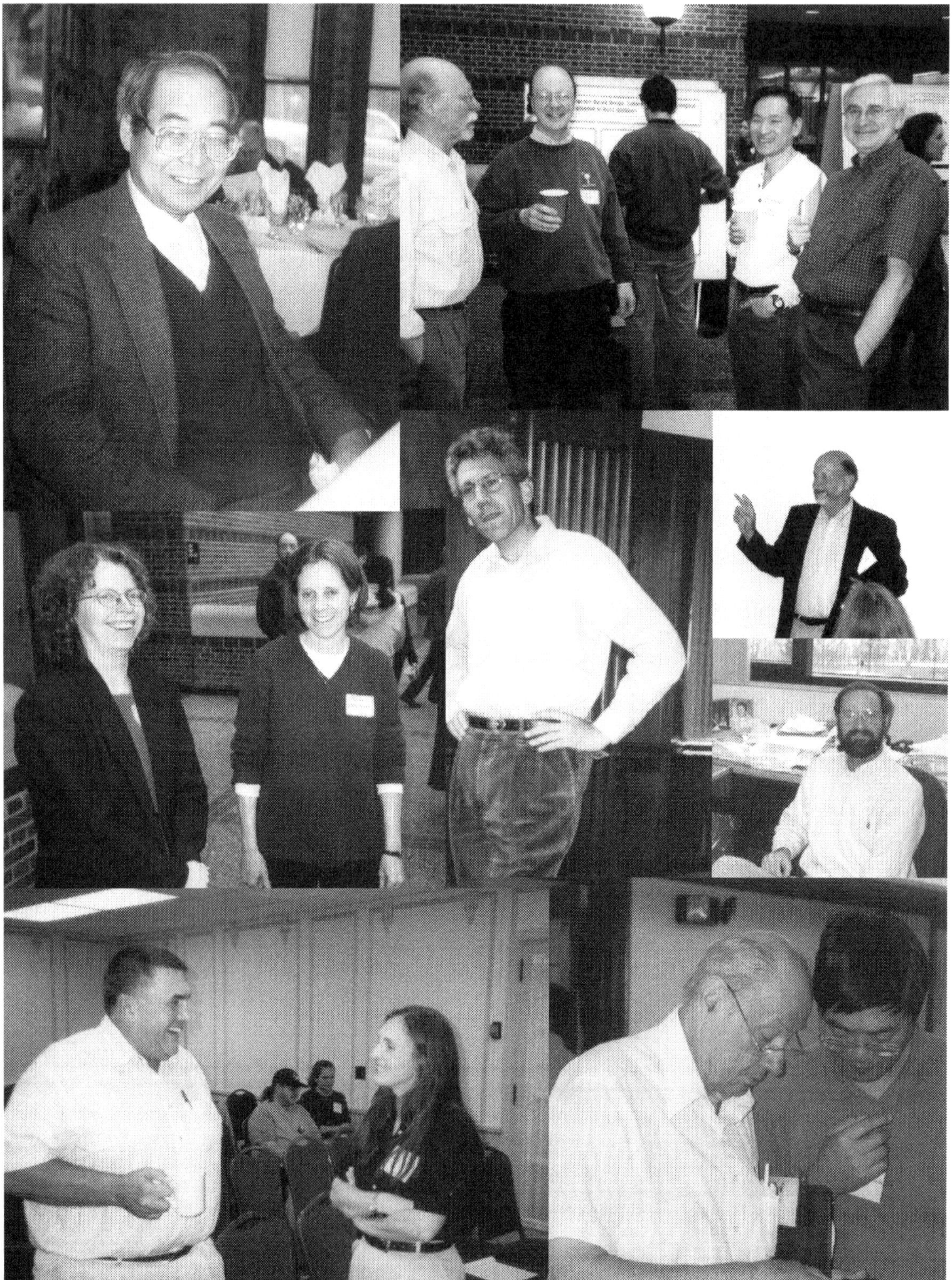

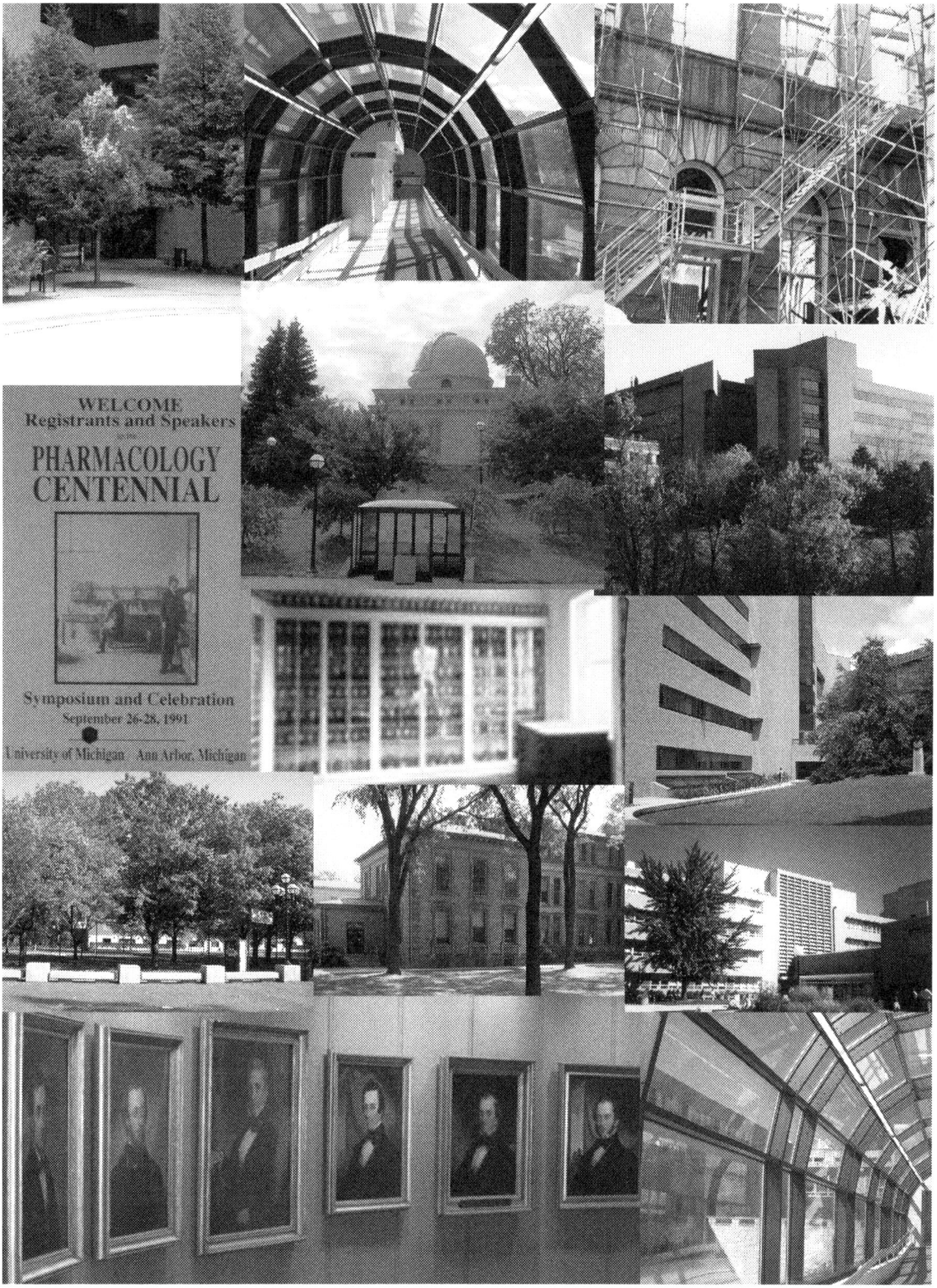
WELCOME
Registrants and Speakers
PHARMACOLOGY
CENTENNIAL
Symposium and Celebration
September 26-28, 1991
University of Michigan Ann Arbor, Michigan

www.ingramcontent.com/pod-product-compliance
Lightning Source LLC
LaVergne TN
LVHW082028200926
848481LV00010B/2941
9780916182137